WHAT IT TOOK TO RAISE MY SON WITH AUTISM

TO BE HIS OWN PERSON, LOOSE IN THE UNIVERSE

Reach for the stars and always keep dreaming!
Mary Jane White and Dr. Ruffin White thank Dr. Doreen Granpeesheh and Senior Therapist Evelyn Kung of CARD with this memoir.

Download it to a phone, computer, or Kindle for $0.00 from Amazon's Kindle Unlimited.

Click "Read Aloud" in the play menu to hear it read to you!

PRAISE FOR MARY JANE WHITE'S EARLIER BOOK
DRAGONFLY. TOAD. MOON. POEMS. (Press 53, Winston-Salem, N.C. 2021)

    How to be a poet and a mother both? Hard question, asked by many, and not to be answered, or worthily asked, except in the living of it. How to be a poet and the mother of a child with autism? Harder question, and harder in the living as well. In this extraordinary collection of poems, Mary Jane White allows us into the pain-ridden, privileged space of world-constituting devotion. How do the disciplines of lyric form rhyme with the luminous sense-making of "A waist-high web of string," for example, woven by a child who has walked in the night "from doorknob to doorknob . . . cabinet door to doorknob to cabinet door" after dismantling the crib that was meant to keep him safe? How does the mother who sees the sense of it and, yes, the beauty too, as well as the difficult entrapment, help the child make his way to larger freedom? Clear-eyed, exquisitely crafted, stripped of easy sentiment, the poems in *Dragonfly. Toad. Moon.* unfold for us the foundational strangeness and wonder of what Heidegger called our "thrown-ness" in the given world.

    – Linda Gregerson, author of *Prodigal: New and Selected Poems, 1976-2014*

    What a delightful book of poems that will resonate deeply within the heart of any parent of a child on the autism spectrum. It is a perfect mix of delectable words and images that massage old bruises and sing to any soul that has ever wondered if anyone else "gets it." Mary Jane White "gets it" beautifully.

    – Shannon Penrod, host of *Autism Live,* the #1-rated Autism podcast

    Mary Jane White's *Dragonfly. Toad. Moon.* is a book highly attuned to perception. The poet's intuition and gift for language runs parallel to her neurodiverse son's artistry, the clay he throws becoming "A vase that flows out and, breathing, closes in / Upon what is now a nearly perfect lip." As a mother learns her son's modes of expression, she cares for him with a fierce intelligence and desire to understand his vocalizations that might otherwise go unheard. *Dragonfly. Toad. Moon.* is a beautifully complex collection. A wonderfully human, humane, and empathetic achievement.

    – Denise Duhamel, author of *Second Story*

Mary Jane White describes raising her son with autism the way he and all of us experience our lives — in blinks — sometimes in the moment, sometimes not. She talks straight but underneath the straight is poetry that is all her own. And no matter how difficult things get, you have the sense that in the end, Ms. White's patience and the depth of her love for her boy will prevail. And in three clicks — dragonfly, toad, moon — they do. This is a tender and fearless book.

– Lola Haskins, author of *Asylum: Improvisations on John Clare*

Mary Jane White's *Dragonfly. Toad. Moon.* speaks to the mute heroism endemic to caregiving and to how patience is less a virtue than a survival skill. Deploying an ear honed on the music of Modernist masters, her lyrics oscillate between the sweetly, and sadly, personal and the divinely cryptic, and the current they produce powers a humane, thoroughly adult vision.

– Richard Katrovas, author of *Poets and the Fools Who Love Them: A Memoir in Essays*

A child with autism is a mysterious blessing. In *Dragonfly. Toad. Moon.*, Ms. White perfectly captures this. For parents and teachers of these children, this book will be a strong comfort after exhausting and challenging days. I remember my wife and I meeting Ruffin; she, who had never met a person with autism before, remarked, "He seems like a regular child!" Indeed, he did — at five or six, after years of ABA therapy. All the more so that sweet Ruffin changed many lives because Ms. White battled for critically necessary ABA services (woodenly, and like teaching a parrot to talk), and sent out dozens of copies of her efforts to other parents whose sleep-deprived days were filled with experiences similar to those she recounts herein. An inspiring read for all of us and should be required reading for the decisionmakers who impact all the Ruffins in the world. I wept and smiled as I read it.

– Sonja D. Kerr, Connell Michael Kerr, LLP

Writing both as the young daughter of parents and as the ferociously dedicated single mother of a son with autism, Mary Jane White's vivid snapshots, her poems, burn into the mind. A web of knotted string fills a room. A struggling naked boy hurls a curtain rod, makes four empty swings swing together precisely, is swaddled, raging, in a towel. With his mother, we endure horrifying images of children with autism who could not be taught. But then, finally, as tensions relax, the blessed beginnings of learning. The language of this poetry is as hard-edged and compressive as the images it shapes. The poems are unlike any I have ever seen, as unforgettable in method and content as the story they depict. Had White named her remarkable book with adjectives instead of nouns, she might have called it *Hard. Bright. Fierce.*

– Judith Moffett, author of *Tarzan in Kentucky*

I have spent over forty-five years working with and observing children with autism, their families, seeing how they overcame the difficulties and experienced the emotional significance of this life course. It takes an artist, a poet, to capture the experience, the upside-down communications, the anxious expectations. Certainly, there can be, after all, the most hoped-for successes, but there is always love.

– Dr. James A. Mulick, Ph.D., Professor Emeritus in Pediatrics,
The Ohio State University

WHAT IT TOOK TO RAISE MY SON WITH AUTISM

TO BE HIS OWN PERSON, LOOSE IN THE UNIVERSE

By Mary Jane White

GRATITUDE PRESS, LLC
P. O. Box 345,
Decorah, Iowa 52101

ISBN 979-8-9899527-0-0

WHAT IT TOOK TO RAISE MY SON WITH AUTISM
To Be His Own Person, Loose In The Universe

First Edition

Copyright @ 2024 by Mary Jane White

All rights reserved under International and Pan-American Copyright Conventions, including the right of reproduction in whole or in part in any form except in the case of brief quotations embodied in critical articles or reviews. For permission, contact publisher at maryjanewhite@gmail.com or at the address above.

Cover photo by Mary Jane White
Author Photo and Back Cover Photo by Chip Peterson

Library of Congress Control Number 2024903753

FOR MY MOTHER,
JANE ODIL WHITE,
ALWAYS MY TEACHER

Acknowledgments

The author thanks the editors of *Adelaide Magazine* where an early chapter of this book first appeared in a different form.

Contents

INTRODUCTION 15
CHAPTER 1: JULY 12, 1994: ALONE AND IN A HURRY..............17
CHAPTER 2: GETTING BUSY, COMING TO TERMS....................31
CHAPTER 3: EVALUATIONS 44
CHAPTER 4: FIRST IEP 57
CHAPTER 5: SCHOOL BEGINS...68
CHAPTER 6: ASKING FOR LOVAAS AND AIT 83
CHAPTER 7: WHAT DID YOU EXPECT? 99
CHAPTER 8: WHAT DO YOU THINK? 111
CHAPTER 9: A NEW PRESCRIPTION....................................127
CHAPTER 10: EVELYN 137
CHAPTER 11: I LOVE YOU. I LOVE YOU...............................148
CHAPTER 12: A MID-WINTER IEP 160
CHAPTER 13: CURT..168
CHAPTER 14: CHRISTMAS BREAK 176
CHAPTER 15: TIME IS OF THE ESSENCE 185
CHAPTER 16: THE UNIVERSITY OF IOWA 191
CHAPTER 17: DOWN TO IOWA CITY...................................195
CHAPTER 18: LETTING SEAMUS LISTEN.............................206
CHAPTER 19: CARRYING COALS TO NEWCASTLE 214
CHAPTER 20: LOS ANGELES 220
CHAPTER 21: SEARCHING FOR THE MAINSTREAM 230
CHAPTER 22: SPRING, AN UNSETTLED SEASON 238
CHAPTER 23: PREPARING. FOR WHAT? 249
CHAPTER 24: WET COW-PIES 256
CHAPTER 25: PUTTING MY FOOT IN IT 264
CHAPTER 26: DO YOU HAVE A FAX?...................................272
CHAPTER 27: AUDITORY INTEGRATION TRAINING...............283
CHAPTER 28: DEMANDING TO BE HEARD 287
CHAPTER 29: MIDSUMMER HEAT 297

CHAPTER 30: FIRST ANNIVERSARY 304
CHAPTER 31: THE PAPER CHASE 310
CHAPTER 32: DOWN TO THE WIRE 317
CHAPTER 33: MEDIATION 324
CHAPTER 34: BLOWBACK 329
CHAPTER 35: PROOF OF OUR SUMMER'S PUDDING 338
CHAPTER 36: TERROR AND JOY IN EQUAL MEASURE 344
CHAPTER 37: WHO TO TRUST? 356
CHAPTER 38: BACK TO GUNDERSEN 365
CHAPTER 39: PACING LIKE A TIGER 376
CHAPTER 40: THE INCLUSION KERFUFFLE 384
CHAPTER 41: MY OWN WORST ENEMY 393
CHAPTER 42: THE LESSONS OF EAVESDROPPING 406
CHAPTER 43: WHY CAN'T WE? 417
CHAPTER 44: PLEASE BRING YOUR PARENTS 429
CHAPTER 45: ARE WE IN DISAGREEMENT YET? 439
CHAPTER 46: PLAYING HOOKY! 450
CHAPTER 47: A BUCKET OF BLOOD 462
CHAPTER 48: GONE. ON VACATION. 475
CHAPTER 49: CURT FILES FOR DUE PROCESS 482
CHAPTER 50: ANOTHER SUMMER ON THE HORIZON 491
CHAPTER 51: PONY UP, OR I WILL 497
CHAPTER 52: BEFORE DUE PROCESS 505
CHAPTER 53: LEAVING NOBODY OUT, OR IN THE DARK 512
CHAPTER 54: I TESTIFY 516
CHAPTER 55: OTHERS TESTIFY 525
CHAPTER 56: MID-HEARING... 530
CHAPTER 57: END OF HEARING 538
CHAPTER 58: AWAITING SOME DECISION 544
CHAPTER 59: SORRY, TO EVEN BE HERE 551
CHAPTER 60: DECISION.. 558
CHAPTER 61: A NECESSARY LITTLE MOTION 563
CHAPTER 62: TWO WASPS IN A BOTTLE 568
CHAPTER 63: SHE WHO SETS THE AGENDA 573

CHAPTER 64: DID YOU KNOW, MOM? 579
CHAPTER 65: READY FOR SUPPORTED INCLUSION? 586
CHAPTER 66: FINDING THE LRE 591
CHAPTER 67: A ROSE BY ANY OTHER NAME 598
CHAPTER 68: THAT'S THE PLEP 601
CHAPTER 69: KIM AND EVELYN 603
CHAPTER 70: THE DEVIL IS IN THE DETAILS 609
CHAPTER 71: AIMING FOR FULL INCLUSION 613
CHAPTER 72: AFTER LUNCH, WHOSE OX? 615
CHAPTER 73: CARD: HOW TO FINISH? 617
CHAPTER 74: WHO? "MOE" AND ME 623
CHAPTER 75: MONEY IS CRUCIAL AND SO IS PEACE 628
CHAPTER 76: HERE, ABOVE THE WORLD 636
CHAPTER 77: A HEART MAKES CHAIRS SWIM 646
CHAPTER 78: PLOWED UNDER LIKE A SEED 651
CHAPTER 79: THE DIGNITY OF BRAVERY AND AUDACITY 657
CHAPTER 80: RUFFIN CUT LOOSE IN THE UNIVERSE 662
APPENDIX OF ADDITIONAL DETAILED TESTING RESULTS 671
APPENDIX OF THEORY OF MIND DRILL LIST 681
ACKNOWLEDGMENTS 683

Introduction

With every dark cloud is a silver lining.

One cannot fathom the fear and despair a parent must feel when told their son or daughter has been diagnosed with autism. *What is autism, how will it affect my child, what can I do to help, do I have the strength . . .*

After despair comes hope; treatments grounded in applied behavior analysis (ABA) have over 50 years of empirical science to back them up. Research outcomes suggest children who receive early intensive behavior intervention (EIBI) starting at four years or younger can achieve the following outcomes as adults: 47% achieve normal functioning; 43% make considerable gains with deficits in the use and/or understanding of spoken language; and 10% make no measurable gains.

It takes a unique parent to decide on the path of EIBI. It is a complex intervention that requires significant parent participation. Parents report it's like having another job. The usual course of treatment is three-to-five years — a marathon with life-changing consequences for parents and children.

Some children like Ruffin may be born with savant-like skills, but many skills are developed over the course of treatment. Children's IQ can increase 30-40 points. Language and social understanding has the potential to explode. At times, there is understanding of complex subjects such as robotics, molecular science, aeronautical engineering or chemistry (Einstein) that goes far beyond the ability demonstrated by typical learners. For most, however, the results are not as glamorous. The majority of children with autism who receive EIBI will make gains but will not "catch up" to their typical peers. Most children in the "non-best outcome" group will need lifelong custodial care, and the parents of these children will live their lives worrying about their children, particularly about when they pass, and the children are left to survive without them.

I would like to offer a special thank you for Mary Jane White, though not for her dedication to helping her son Ruffin, which is remarkable, to say the least. I would like to thank her for continuing to advocate for the field of applied behavior analysis long after her son recovered and lives as a fully functioning adult. Parents who continue advocating for autism treatments after their children are finished with ABA hold a special place.

Erik Lovaas
Founder and CEO
The Lovaas Center US
The Lovaas Center Spain
Fundación Erik Lovaas para El Autismo Spain

Chapter One

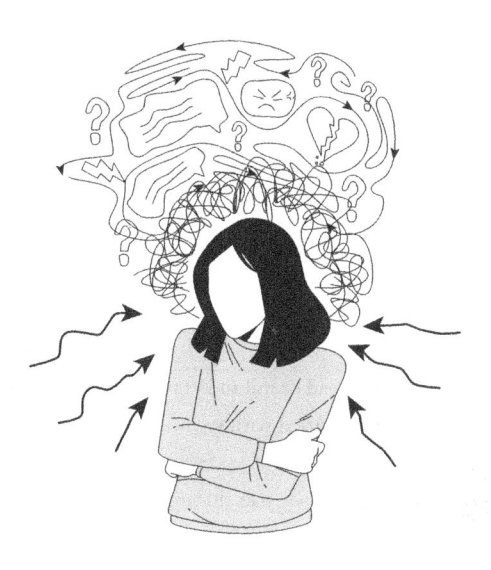

July 12, 1994

ALONE AND IN A HURRY

I sped down the eastern bank of the Mississippi from the big Gundersen Clinic in LaCrosse. We would come soon to the rattling grid of a narrow open-decked bridge, slow there enough for me to glance back at Ruffin — still fretting inconsolably in his car seat — and then take the sharp left into Lansing, that small, shadowy river town. We were back in Iowa under the river's high limestone bluffs. For a moment I felt safer. A familiar two-lane ridge road climbed toward the prairie through several switchbacks. I could pick up speed again as we topped those, drive directly into the blinding sun to our hometown library's gold-lit glass doors. I needed to look up the word that had produced my alarm: *autism*. "Autism" was Dr. Caldwell's word. And *Rain Man* the first resource he offered me, as a movie I might rent.

Myself, I hadn't sat through a movie since *Dr. Zhivago*. I confessed that readily. Both this new word and the movie were unfamiliar. The pediatric neurologist lifted his eyes as if to consult heaven, then threw me a brief, odd, knowing look. To help me understand, or maybe just to give me something to carry away, he bent his head over a half sheet of paper. His eyebrows shadowed the glasses sliding down his nose toward a tight smile. Then he handed me a hand-drawn diagram:

AUTISTIC SPECTRUM DISORDER

Mild	Ruffin	Severe
Asperger's Syndrome	Pervasive Developmental Disorder	Autism

I was focused on what was ahead of me and crammed that into my briefcase. I needed to navigate Ruffin — his hair curled with sweat, his kicking feet, his hand reaching out or seeming to flick small insects out of his eyes — with all his gear, his stroller, his sticky plastic toys and the soggy diaper bag through Gundersen's clean hallways, into and out of its elevators, quickly, to make our next appointment with a developmental occupational therapist. Familiar and cheerful, Lexi had followed Ruffin at regular intervals as a part of the neonatal follow-up clinic, ever since his premature birth.

After Lexi had struggled to finish her developmental testing, I mentioned that Dr. Caldwell had just drawn me a little diagram showing Ruffin's place on the autism spectrum. I pulled it out to show her. Her face fell, went white. Her involuntary, uncensored reaction was confirmation. Her unveiled expression of alarm, more than his sketchy diagram, sent me to the Comprehensive Child Care Clinic desk. This was where Dr. Caldwell planned to refer Ruffin for a full autism screening.

I tried to schedule an immediate appointment. But the receptionist who peered into her glowing green screen reported the next available date would be well into next year. I must have appeared frantic. This was my first encounter with a wall I would run into, again and again. Nowhere, it seemed, was a new diagnosis of autism treated as a form of emergency for which time might be of any essence.

In her effort to calm me, to help me calm myself, the receptionist looked up to catch my eye, "Don't you worry," she clucked. "When we can schedule an appointment, we'll be able to get an IQ for him."

"An IQ? He's three!"

"But you can expect him to do so much better, you know, if we find he has an IQ above 50."

I didn't know. But, with that remark, doubtless meant to be reassuring, I finally entered some form of shock. I gathered Ruffin up, and backtracked down to neurology, insisting on speaking to Dr. Caldwell again. He emerged briefly to scribble the name of a book I might find in the library, and Ruffin and I hurried off into the stifling summer afternoon to get home before the one I knew in our small town would close for the evening.

In the chill of the public library, in the first long, wooden drawer of the card catalog, with Ruffin still at my feet, kicking and straining against the belts of his stroller, I found the title: *Children with Autism, A Parent's Guide,* by Michael D. Powers, Psy.D. By scanning it quickly, I gathered that this autism was worse than I had imagined. The mother of all learning disabilities, apparently. *Incurable.* At that moment I felt unsteady on my feet, as if I were barefoot on sand that had just been washed by a receding wave. My heart beat with the force of primitive reflex: I could have made a huge mistake, having this child as I did, with Seamus.

It was enough to send me into the library's small bathroom, backwards through the heavy door, pulling Ruffin in his stroller in with me, and letting the door fall shut. Here was a small welcome privacy. Could this autism be our punishment, Seamus's, and mine, inflicted on our innocent son? A long no-life? And would my own life from now on be no more than that of his lifelong caretaker? Another long no-life? I knew myself well enough. I did not have the courage to face this. I was not constituted with the patience to do this.

And, I knew Ruffin's father, Seamus, well enough, years into our settled, arm's length relationship. I would probably be doing this alone. More or less, by myself.

One quick look in the mirror before facing the world. I still seemed to be here, as myself, as my startled self. A woman who still looked like a schoolgirl, far younger than the nearly forty years I had lived. Wire-framed glasses hid my green eyes, distorted to be smaller than they really were, behind my thick Coke-bottle lenses. For some, they might have marked me as a woman from an earlier century. My lips were taut, careful as an Appalachian basket weaver not to reveal an irreparable gap between my front teeth. Who would ever take me to heart now? Myself, with this newest baggage, this unwelcome diagnosis?

I count it as a small blessing now that I did not hear Dr. Caldwell's fuller prognosis until the next day, when I called him with my follow-up questions. Over the phone, he opined more freely. He told me Ruffin might never speak, might never work productively, was likely never to marry, nor ever understand that I loved him. He warned that the cost of Ruffin's lifetime care would be high, and that if I had as much as five million dollars to set aside and invest, I should do that. Now. As the experienced trial lawyer I was, who had hung my own share of crepe to lower client expectations about unpredictable outcomes, this struck me as truly dark, as bleak.

Even without hearing all that, that first night, I remembered a brief clip from National Public Radio: Japanese mothers who found themselves disgraced by some unaccountable failure or abandonment walked with their children into the sea. *Oyako shinju*. To hold them close as they drowned. But we — Ruffin, Seamus, and I — lived in the American Midwest, in Iowa, in fly-over country, too far from any ocean for my resolve not to falter before I got there. And, although I had also trained as a poet, I was not ordinarily given to operatic gestures. Those of us raised Presbyterian were not like that. Nor had I evolved to be a Buddhist, or to ever be deeply religious. Checking myself again, I couldn't feel any real disapproval raining down from the eyes of the gods, if there were any.

But, for the first time ever in my life I gave active thought to suicide. I had been raised to be hopelessly practical. At least about this — death — as any final solution. It would mean killing Ruffin first, and then killing myself. My tinny red hatchback was parked in the garage, with the dark eye of its sooty tailpipe. Carbon monoxide. I needed to think. Technology had never been my strong suit. My garage was ancient, wooden, and hopelessly leaky. It would never hold a dense cloud of exhaust long enough; it would ravel away. I couldn't be certain. At worst, Ruffin would die, and I would not. I would be found out in the dark: groggy, bereaved, incoherent, disgraced, prosecuted, and guilty. How could I? I was already hopelessly in love with him. Just as hopelessly as I thought I was in love with his father.

How could I ever lay hands on Ruffin, who was so beautiful, sleeping now, after our long day at the hospital? His face seemed utterly relaxed and perfect, his mouth slightly open, breathing. He was breathing. As I bent over him, small particles of dust swirled off his warm scalp, out of his curls. The sweet smell of milk and of clean sharp urine struck my nose and watered my eyes. I couldn't possibly ever lay hands on him. Never just pick him up and carry him out into the night.

For the moment, I couldn't think what I was going to tell Seamus or imagine how I was going to tell him. Certainly, I wouldn't be able to tell him anything right away, not until I could figure out what to do about this. He would want an explanation and need an answer. He would call sooner or later. Likely, he would have his own answer, like as not at odds with my own.

I let all the trapped breath out of my body and turned back to the beginning of my new library book. I could read this mindlessly all night. I did read, but attentively.

All night, as if it were some holy text — from cover to cover. I came to a long chapter outlining the *Individuals with Disabilities Education Act* — the *IDEA* — Senator Edward Kennedy's signature legislation, setting out how to wield its powerful legal swords and shields.

By morning, I was able to call my mother in Carolina with the word: *autism*. And a plan.

My mother and I might seem to be very different women to most people, but that would be a superficial misunderstanding. My mother, Jane Eve Odil, married my father, Thomas Boyett White, in her early twenties to start a family. That fall of 1952, she taught math in the prestigious Myers Park high school in south Charlotte all morning through the late afternoon, then took a slow, wandering bus across the city to teach night school on the community college campus. When would she have eaten? Or rested? When she nearly collapsed, pregnant with me, on the warm, damp concrete steps to their apartment, a kindly neighbor sat her down and suggested that if she happened to be bleeding, she might want to see a doctor.

To avoid miscarriage, the doctor offered her the latest remedy for so many medical conditions at the time, a synthetic estrogen, diethylstilbestrol (DES). A magic pill. Out of love, and in fear, to be certain of avoiding catastrophe, to be certain of a good outcome, my mother swallowed two courses of this prescribed medication during our first trimester together. Sometimes, this is how love and fear, and good intentions have their way with us. I was born the next June, on a Sunday, midmorning, to the ringing of church bells, on Flag Day, within two weeks of her first wedding anniversary. No injury to me was apparent.

First memory. Outside our small red brick apartment in Southern Pines, wearing a little plaid shirt, I leaned into the camera among the white violets on a gentle slope, on the thick grass, prickly with long pine-needles. This was where I lived with my mother, my father, and my year-younger little brother, whom I could not remember ever not having. Next door lived my friend Wanda Blue, whose name I heard as *Wander Blue*. My father brought home a stereo. From its two boxes, metallic sound entered each ear differently. It was country music, Nashville music, Hank Williams, Chet Akins, Flatt and Scruggs. Then he brought home a television. On its screen of four rounded corners our bald and grave President Eisenhower flickered.

I was still little, three maybe. Ruffin's age. Winter and summer, my own skin, the inner side of my arm, was as white as the underbelly of a fish. In the sun, my hair bleached. I played outside alone without a shirt. No one thought anything of it.

When I was old enough to enter kindergarten, our mother took my brother, Michael, our infant sister, Cathy, and me in for our annual physicals. I would go first. I had been tasked to be brave and take my shots without crying. Our mother had asked me to do this in front of Michael, to set him a good example. Of course, the sacrifice of my example was worthless. All it afforded was a chance for Michael to escape the examination room and the doctor's office, so our mother had to run to catch him out in the gravel parking lot. Then the doctor measured and weighed me and pronounced me average. I was proud to have been found average. I was privileged to believe I was destined to be completely normal.

The morning after Dr. Caldwell's diagnosis of Ruffin, I rang the regional office of the Bridgewater area special education agency and talked my way past a single, amiable receptionist, Joy. I might have babbled too much. Later, when I gathered the voluminous educational records of calls and meetings about Ruffin, I could see that Joy had written out a pink telephone message slip she had marked, URGENT: "Three-year-old son with autism. What type of programs do we have? (Think she is an attorney.)" Joy had passed it along, up to her boss.

I suppose because it was summer, I succeeded in getting The Man, Bridgewater's regional director of special education, on the phone later that morning. Either he called me back, or I had anxiously called in again. It wasn't as if I let on to having been on the brink of suicide the evening before, but I was more than a bit punchy from reading all night.

"Hello, this is Mary Jane White. I have a three-year-old with autism. Diagnosed yesterday, up in LaCrosse, at the Gundersen. I need . . . I mean, I understand what *we* need is an evaluation for a planning meeting, so my son, Ruffin, will be able to start special education in August. When I think it is that school starts here?"

The Man interrupted, speaking in a deep register to slow me down, "Well, I can tell you, Ms. White, is it? Right now, everybody here, except myself and Joy who took your message, is on summer vacation."

"Okay, so August, then?" I suggested. I tried to offer him some slack, some accommodation, although six weeks of waiting seemed endless to me.

"Let's say better after things settle down in the fall. We can pull together a multi-disciplinary diagnostic preschool team once we get back to school, probably in September or October."

"I know," I told him, a bit sharply, "that summer school is a part of special education services." Hadn't I just read that last night? I wondered that he didn't seem familiar with the concept, as he continued to offer forms of comfort that struck me as determinedly evasive.

"It will be easier for us after things settle down in the fall. The beginning of school is always a hard time for these meetings. For new students starting in the fall, we ordinarily hold meetings ahead of time. In the spring. We like to hold these meetings in the spring."

Now, I interrupted him, "Do we have to wait that long — until spring? Don't we need to get an evaluation done before school starts? I mean, he has autism, according to the neurologist up at Gundersen. So, Ruffin should begin school right away with everyone else when it opens? Shouldn't he?"

I had ended with a question, reckoning it was always good to ask a question to back off a bit. He responded, "I would need to make some calls first, find enough of my people who might be around, back from vacation, and see who might be willing to come in on single-day contracts . . ."

"Yes, that would be good! Lovely. Thank you."

At least I had shifted him from his royal we into the singularity of a moveable person. I deluded myself that I had made a friend. Director August Albert Montague. The Man! Why not? By my insisting on going right to the top. I congratulated myself. Well, no, I might well have made an impression as a memorable annoyance.

In the days and years to come, I learned that all too many families in the early 1990s were given a wait-and-see, comfortable clinical evasion that hardened irreversibly into "suggestive of infantile autism," or "pervasive developmental disorder, not otherwise specified (PDD-NOS), probably autistic disorder" by the time their worrisome child reached the age of seven or eight. Since any form of autism's downstream cascade of developing disability would have been dangerous to ignore, whatever Dr. Caldwell called it, however he connected Ruffin to autism, it came as something of a relief to have a name for everything that seemed to be wrong. Certainly, it was a gift — to learn Ruffin's diagnosis early.

It helped to have offered Dr. Caldwell audio and video recordings of Ruffin's more unusual behaviors that spring at home: his aimless activity, his forever twirling things and then breaking them, his toe-walking, his nightlong babbling, and explosive breathing which usually began around sundown, and which by mid-May had begun to invade the day.

As for Seamus and me, ours would be a common enough difficulty. Two parents always seem to grieve the autism diagnosis of their child differently, and at different paces, so each parent's journey of grieving grows to be separate and lonely, as the grief and disappointment intrude on the original joy of first crossing paths.

Well before July's diagnosis — wasn't it just before Christmas? — Seamus had let drop, quietly enough, a few remarks that I imagined made it clear he didn't think I was fit to handle Ruffin. I began to think sourly that he must think, "Why did you have him, if you don't know how to raise children?" Then, over my kitchen table, all that spring came long accounts of his three older sisters who had raised so many out on their farms.

"You think you're so smart, but you should listen to me."

I let Seamus talk. He talked softly enough, but I didn't seem to hear anything that sounded useful. Nor was I able to learn anything even remotely helpful.

That spring my mother had urged me not to put off Ruffin's next developmental check-up.

"I know you had to be in court, but you need to reschedule it. It could be important."

She was the one who made the first audio recordings during Ruffin's sleepless nights at my parents' home and thought someone needed to review them.

Yes, however tenderly I felt about Ruffin, however much I loved him, I had to admit to myself that I was having increasing trouble managing his behavior. I found him both difficult and mystifying. Grunting was how he spoke to me. A thing he wanted was somewhere. I needed to find it by looking everywhere. At all costs, I wanted to avoid a tantrum. It would not do to move so much as the salt or pepper. He did not want me to move anything. Did this avoid his asking me, "Where?" Would this avoid a tantrum? I seemed to be a thing in his world he might love, but would avoid by looking elsewhere — to avoid his tantrum?

This was not the plan. What had been the plan? My plan had been to have a perfectly wonderful baby.

My early marriage in my twenties had seemed odd to my poet-friends and legal colleagues alike. How could such an accomplished young woman fall for an old, bearded geezer with custody of two children from his second marriage? I had always kept my medical history, my repeated bouts of cervical cancer, a close secret. It was nothing I thought of confiding to my friends. This marriage to a man twice my age, which I had made the mistake of proposing, was an opportunity to have children, when I couldn't myself.

It had come to a predictable enough end. I had been walking down the road with a client with whom I had been spending too much time helping round up his sheep.

That, and helping repair his fencing seemed more effective and more amusing than trying to fend off the lawsuits threatened by his neighbors, when — on the fact of his unkept fences — he was clearly in the wrong. As they say, nothing had happened — yet.

My client disappeared from my side at the first shot, slipping nimbly into the nearest concrete culvert.

I ran for my life to escape, being less familiar with the lay of his land, stumbling in my farmyard boots, diving into the other road ditch for cover. I buried myself face-down, hoping not to be shot there. Not in my face, please. I hoped as I breathed and waited — such a long time it seemed — for the shooting to stop, counting seven shots as the ammunition ran out, counting on it to run out.

Alert then for any telltale sounds suggesting a reload.

When there were none, I got up out of the ditch and walked up to the shooter, my husband, who invited me to get in the open trunk.

"No," I reached up and shut it.

Just then, a man and his family in a pickup passed us — a man with a gun and a woman arguing — without stopping. Before cell phones, they had to go somewhere to call 911. I was already saying by then, very calmly, "You need to go. Go turn yourself in."

"Get in the front seat then, with me."

"No."

Wheels spun past my feet as his car roared out of the gravel.

My rescue, after the convergence of two counties' worth of sheriff's deputies in bulletproof vests would be a front-page scandal. It blew up my run for political office — my modest ambition to serve as a local prosecutor.

After a few weeks, after the lost election, this mess resolved itself in a public hearing I would sooner forget. Despite a full front courtroom-pew of women from the local shelters and agencies, my witness failed to result in much of any consequence. After all, it was just a .22, no more than a rabbit gun. No more intention than to scare me. To chase me back home.

No need to brand this lovely older gentleman, my husband, the custodian of two half-grown boys, as a felon. The case would be dropped after a brief period of supervision — to cover the uneasy time needed to complete a divorce.

There was going to be a divorce, wasn't there, the judge asked, his suggestion — offered to my husband.

In my mind, it would never be over. It was the sort of thing that no one later dared breathe about in direct conversation but would not likely be forgotten about me.

Immediately, it became my colorful past. Rumor had it I had wanted to have a baby of my own. I worked to live it down. I persisted in showing up weekly in the same courtroom where I'd been a witness, not really anyone's victim, in my blue or grey wool skirt-suits, in my expensive silk blouse, rising for the same judge when called upon, standing by counsel table in my low, black or brown heels.

"No, your Honor, I wasn't thinking of going anywhere."

Rumor was right. I had been to Minneapolis for exploratory surgery early on when I was twenty-three, a married stepparent, but still hoping to have a baby of my own. How much damage had my DES-exposure done? I seemed to have survived the early cervical cancer it brought on first at seventeen. But had it rendered me hopelessly infertile? "If you wake up with just a band-aid here," the famed Minnesota teaching-surgeon had said kindly, as he patted me above my bellybutton, "we won't have been able to help you." It turned out it was hopeless. We could cancel the appointment for the reversal of my husband's vasectomy.

Seamus was a new man offering to hold my small purchase if I wanted to make some further bid on something else maybe? A man I had visited with on the phone, didn't I recall, about buying a table? Yes, hadn't I laughed, as I was telling him I had lost a beautiful cherrywood table in the great divide?

Yes, in my divorce. I smiled. I remembered that soft, low voice over the phone, asking more questions than offering answers about the oak table he had advertised for sale — the one I was interested in buying as a replacement.

That voice, here it was again.

Whether Seamus considered me delicious, as he claimed, maybe strawberry, one of his favorites, as a flavor, I felt that I was vanilla, a sort of default or flat flavor, and worse, it seemed I was getting far enough on to being overlooked from here on out, not just because I was a woman — I was accustomed to that — but on account of my age.

That summer Seamus was a reasonable seven years older, a comfortable several inches taller, broad-shouldered, slim-hipped, and brawny from hard work outdoors, the back of his neck and arms brown from the sun. He had those narrow Irish eyes set high up in his face. I adored his crisp, black hair, whether it was curled with sweat, or fresh from the shower. Seamus would arrive, and we would dress to go out. He would grin, flashing his white teeth with pointed canines, and announce it was a fine time to head into town, to go drive around to find some place new.

Usually, it was the first time of the day I even stepped out to notice the weather, the smell of the earth, or the rolling Mississippi. I worked all week and every weekend that summer in concentrated seclusion on my final preparations to try a single, complex case of business fraud, *Ezzone*, named for its victim, my client.

I didn't need to have Seamus with me all the time to be happy. I didn't need to be married to him to be happy. I was absorbed in my work on this difficult case. I worked with discipline, careful to avoid all excesses — even of happiness. I was happy to have Seamus, amused to see him flirt with every hostess, singing waitress, and slender cashier, even as I was usually the one to pick up the check. For me, that early summer was all the proof I needed that I was never going to have a baby, not without considerable medical help.

My focus sharpened. In my late-thirties, I was still fierce, smart, and skilled in the legal profession I had wandered into and could still hole up and write or translate poems whenever I found myself flush. So far, I had yet to encounter a problem I couldn't solve or manage. Of course, Seamus presented an entertaining and insoluble mystery I could toy with interminably, at a safe distance that suited me. I didn't want to propose another disastrous public marriage. I didn't want to entertain anyone's proposal either. I didn't need to pick up or wash socks, or cook on schedule, or attend church to please some in-laws, negotiate this or that holiday between families, or bring hot dishes to backyard gatherings. I was free to work at night, all night if I liked, or write.

But the most important thing to me was the arms-length distance. That represented a necessary freedom. And emotional safety, after the mistake of my terrifying early marriage. I would find a way to become pregnant on my own. Women did. Seamus and I talked about it. His name, of course, would never be in question. Nor would be any financial contribution, ever. Seamus had no real money, no great land. Money and land were never what I thought Seamus had to offer me and were not what I needed. Could we try, you know, if I wanted to? But I could see Seamus considered it the remotest of possibilities, no threat to the calm horizon we had settled on.

I wrote to our three nearest medical centers: Iowa City, Minneapolis, and LaCrosse. On ethical grounds, Iowa City did not serve unmarried women with fertility issues. Nor would Minneapolis see me again. The records they pulled up to send me showed that I would be a hopeless case.

In the 1990s, only Dr. Hector Manuel and his new infertility group at the smaller, private Gundersen Clinic in LaCrosse seemed willing to take my money to try to help me. No insurance coverage for this. But he seemed young, eager, dark-eyed, and handsome with a warm smile. He was just starting out. He and his wife, Lucia, also an infertility specialist, had joined Gundersen in 1987, after training at the University of

California San Diego. Already, a small corkboard outside their joint office was crowded with celebratory photographs of new babies with their new parents, new families.

Dr. Manuel and I started with a medical record review of my earlier band-aid surgery. Then, he ordered new tests. The tenaculum's hooks gripped what remained of my DES-damaged cervix, so the contrast medium, an opaque dye, could be injected. Dr. Manuel's tests showed that nothing whatsoever would flow through my Fallopian tubes. At this point, it became a struggle against humiliation to maintain a cheerful fascination.

In June of 1990, Dr. Manuel operated several hours to reconstruct and open a single stunted Fallopian tube he thought might still function. It lacked fimbria, the waving fingers to beckon, "Come here, little one," and was too fragile to risk further medical testing. Even so, Dr. Manuel thought it seemed to be what he called patent, capable of doing its job. And it was, because by late September, I knew — by my little plastic stick with its magical, chemical window where the wished-for sign had appeared — I was pregnant and expecting.

I called Seamus, who sounded stunned. What did he expect? But he had always been an obliging man, and remained so, very calmly obliging, as he took in my latest news. I called my mother, too, who was in Houston visiting her older sister. As the mothers of so many children between them, they were thrilled. My whole family had been resigned in their disappointment that I would never be a mother.

Then I drove north, up the Mississippi to LaCrosse, to be certain. The ultrasound technician pointed to beating tissue, eighteen days into a heart's making. Then, smiling with delight, she drew my attention to the ovary opposite my reconstructed tube, to the site where she judged an egg had erupted. "We suspect this sort of traveling happens, but here you are, our proof!" Then she printed me a picture I could carry off to my next appointment.

My gynecologist, one of Dr. Manuel's young associates, did something surprising when I showed it to him. A handstand! In the examining room, all his loose change, glittering pennies, nickels, and dimes, cascaded out of his pockets, hit the hard floor, bounced, and rolled here and there, under the papered table, the sink, coming to rest along the baseboards. When he gathered himself on his rolling stool, he confided that he and Dr. Manuel had calculated my chances of ever becoming pregnant at something under 2%. He couldn't have been more pleased with himself. Nor could I.

Gently then, he began to raise my awareness. Mine would be a high-risk pregnancy because I was of advanced maternal age. How strange this made me seem to myself, a veritable crone. Was I really that old? He proposed a cerclage at sixteen weeks, should I still be pregnant. This inpatient procedure, under general anesthesia, was not usually offered until after an initial pregnancy loss, so the rules would need to be bent in my case. To make up for my cervix's obvious incompetence, the surgery would introduce a double purse-string suture to cinch me shut for the duration of my pregnancy, for as long as possible. Amniocentesis would be called for, of course. Finally, he sent me off with this exclamation, "And we'll need to find an obstetrician with brass balls to deliver you!"

He and Dr. Manuel referred me to Dr. Cody T. Wyatt, a tall blond, slow-talking Texan, who, it seemed, had been well-briefed by both of them on just how to manage me, this odd woman who always arrived with a long list of written questions to slip out of her briefcase. Too many to address in Dr. Wyatt's allotted time. With no eye contact, no small talk, and no bedside manner, Dr. Wyatt evinced zero interest in offering me long explanations. He suggested I visit the clinic's medical library. He would arrange borrowing privileges for me to check out the most recent OB-GYN textbook, a title he scribbled for me like a prescription. "Just get it and read it." He told me to come back every two weeks or so. His nurses would see me, weigh me, and counsel me.

"Now, off you go," he said, ushering me out. "Our medical library is that way."

The textbook was as thick as the usual open dictionary displayed on a library pedestal. A large item to prop on my delicate round belly, but exactly the intellectual red meat to have thrown a voracious, over-educated pregnant woman to keep her distracted.

As with many mothers whose children develop early childhood autism, my amniocentesis was normal. In 1990, there were no known genetic markers to look for or to find for autism. Even today, there are only a few newer prenatal genetic tests for autism-related conditions such as fragile X, Rett syndrome, and tuberous sclerosis.

By Christmas, I had my cerclage and another ultrasound that showed my child would be a boy. I would name him Ruffin, after a grandfather whom I had never met, my father's father, a civil engineer with the Army Corps, who had managed the Mississippi levees in Arkansas. The cerclage was holding well enough that I was able to drive from Iowa to Cleveland to gather with my family at my sister Cathy's home, with her children and my parents. Her home was the only place I ever suffered any morning sickness, likely from my failure to eat well on the road.

When I returned home after the New Year, my doctors and nurses sat me down for a serious visit. I couldn't continue to drive cross-country, or even visit my usual circuit of seven northeast Iowa counties to attend court. "It's time you go on bed rest," the nurse said. "Better to lie on your side. And remember, always — your left side."

I made a note. "Got it."

The nurse handed me a box, "This is the band to go around your belly, so let's open it and I'll show you how you'll download your data. And here's the modem to transmit the data to your monitoring nurse in Minneapolis, who will work with us. We will want to know if you're experiencing any contractions, and to monitor your baby's movements. Understand?"

I nodded again, although I didn't.

"Your nurse will call you every day to advise you, based on your latest data, whether you may stand, whether you may sit up a bit, whether you may bathe, or even wash your hair."

That got my attention.

I went back to practicing law out of my home, a log house, an old stagecoach and Pony Express stop situated on rough, low, soft bottom ground, cut by a stream, and closed in between two runs of steep, forested hills. The place was over a dozen miles from the nearest hospital in Decorah, Iowa. At first, I found it awkward to type while lying on my left side, a little difficult to manage to continue to practice law while on bed rest. But my clients continued to drive out to consult me even if I welcomed them in my pajamas, with my hair unwashed. I held court on an old hospital bed set up against a patch of limestone wall on the first floor, in the corner nearest the bathroom.

All my kindly back-to-the-land Iowa neighbors organized themselves to bring in my breakfast, lunch, and dinner. Coming and going in shifts, they brought in the mail and carried the outgoing mail up to the box at the end of my driveway. My law practice and I lived and died by the mail. No one ever missed a visit. No one was ever late. Regular as clockwork, Seamus called every night.

One warm night, in the earliest false spring of April, I was visited by a little green snake who crawled out of a crack in the limestone. Unafraid and right at home, he looked me in the eye. I have come to think of that little snake as the harbinger of the rampant bacterial infection and viral fever that rose and spiked in Ruffin and me — when my double cerclage finally broke up.

Chapter Two

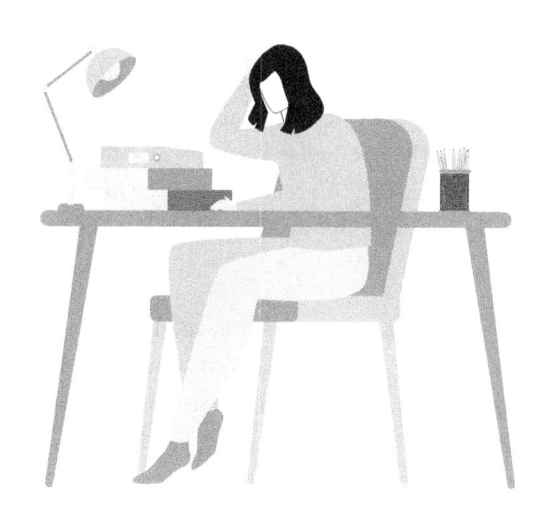

GETTING BUSY, COMING TO TERMS

A nine-page, single-spaced form had arrived from Gundersen for me to fill out to help their medical team prepare for Ruffin's autism clinic evaluation. It began, "What questions would you like answered as a result of your child's evaluation?" My reply was, "What is the best result I can reasonably expect of Ruffin as a functioning person? How can I best pursue that best result?"

Then I entered as much clinical and historical data as I could muster, working my way through all the supporting pages of the form. This make-work arrived as a comfort, did help me think, helped settle me with some measure of grace into addressing Ruffin's issues. It was clinical. It was work, like my own careful trial preparation, the gathering of every available detail. I summarized Ruffin's medical history, and his and mine throughout my pregnancy. Significantly, or not, I was on *terbutaline* for the last two months. I felt a distinct twinge of remorse. Just like my mother, I had taken what the doctor prescribed to be able to start a family. And I had been given antibiotics for the wicked intrauterine infection as my double-cerclage broke up, triggering Ruffin's premature birth by C-section at a bit more than 30 weeks.

I entered Ruffin's birth weight: 5 pounds, 4 ounces; his length: 17 inches. I recalled, "I was with Ruffin, actively caring for him all 18 days he was in the pediatric intensive care unit (PICU). Since he was not developed enough to nurse or swallow, I was taught to gavage feed him, threading a tube down his throat to reach his stomach, being careful to avoid threading it off-course into his lungs, and was allowed to take him home. Thankfully, I was very well trained at PICU. I fed him breastmilk by gavage until he was able to nurse."

Then Ruffin was on an apnea monitor at home. Those had been a terrifying first five months, with the monitor's alarms ruling my sleep and my attention. No one would agree to babysit him. Seamus wasn't trained on the equipment. It seemed excessive to him. After all, Ruffin was going to live. My parents had driven back to North Carolina, having never unpacked the funeral clothes they had been advised to bring. My father was still working.

So was I. In my heels, up three flights of stairs of dangerous, fraying courthouse carpet, I dragged Ruffin to court with me, or sat through lengthy depositions with him in a bassinet at my feet with all his wires and beeping boxes. But he had improved, and gained weight steadily, had stood and walked free of all that, I thought.

But, for his doctors now who were curious about his play with other children, I recalled a summer trip to the park. Ruffin had toddled over to a group of four swings. He pushed them until he brought them into an alignment that pleased him, without noticing or seeming to care about the three other children nearby — unless their play disrupted his careful pattern of empty swing and empty swing, of the crossing arcs of thing and thing, two pairs of swings doubling.

Ruffin began attending day care at fifteen months and was, as his sitter Julie described him, the "angel" of his playgroup. "Never a disciplinary problem." But he didn't talk there, where he was with a group of several boys and a girl his age. He played outside the group. He did participate in some of their dancing. I was grateful that Julie would take my toddling Ruffin as I returned to work more regularly to support us. Julie came recommended to me by Seamus. Her towering husband, Erik, was Seamus's own childhood friend. Among us it lay as an open secret that Ruffin was Seamus's son from the other side of the blanket, not that it was spoken of often.

On Gundersen's long checklist of problems I might be aware of now, I checked off these:
- Expressing himself
- Playing appropriately
- Behavior

I filled in the given blanks:
- Favorite activities: Walking, dancing without any music, mechanical experiments
- Least liked activities: Bathing, changing clothes, changing direction
- Favorite toys: Mechanical — sticks, strings, balloons, trucks, cars
- Favorite foods: Chocolate milk, yogurt, cereal, strawberries, any vegetable, and bananas

On the next checklist, I noted and detailed his difficulties:
- Frequent earaches, colds
- Appears not to listen in groups
- Doesn't speak as well as others his age
- Can be understood only by family members
- Difficulty following simple directions, seems unwilling to dress himself, pull up pants, etc.
- Difficulty understanding concepts, open/closed
- Seems "mincing" in his steps and gestures
- Tantrums, cries, or whines often — when asked to change his mind — new shirt, new direction in walk
- Seems uninterested in other children
- Doesn't play with toys appropriately

I felt stumped by this last item. What did that really mean? Appropriately? Ruffin's world was rich with toys, stuffed animals, little trucks, blocks, and colored rings in graduated sizes for stacking on a plastic stick. We had books like *Goodnight, Moon*, which somehow, we never managed to get to the end of when I tried to read to him. His attention wandered. *He* wandered. He paced the floor in patterns, up on his toes, singing, *Ninga, ninga, ninga,* meaningless syllables. He lined his toys up in neat rows along the back of our couch. His tiny chin pressed down into his chest as he bent to spin the wheels of trucks turned upside down, fascinated, and enthralled. Just as he was fascinated by the turning of locks and the flipping of light switches. I thought back over all I knew of him, checked this item, and offered, "He plays with the mechanical aspects of a train, but not the enactment of a 'journey' or any 'story.'"

In mid-July, The Man, Mr. Montague, sought written permission to consider Ruffin for special education and asked me to sign medical releases. He sent me a parents' rights brochure and some basic information on autism. All this seemed familiar enough from my first night's reading, and so, somehow, it arrived as an odd comfort in this changed world of my upended expectations. A pre-school early intervention screening clinic was scheduled in our town for early August. Mr. Montague encouraged me to take Ruffin. But really, all of this felt overwhelming. Somehow, Ruffin, my little love, my child, seemed to have become another troubling case — with a file.

Ruffin played at my feet. Would he look up for a smile? He would not. He was focused on his own business of breaking the plastic blades off the spinning flower of a lawn ornament, an object we had been unable to leave the drug store without buying. I needed to pick him up, to interrupt him before he broke them all off. As I did, he squirmed in my arms like a feral cat. I hugged him tightly, turned his face up so I could tickle his nose with mine. No, he didn't like that. It reminded me of whenever I tried to sing Ruffin a lullaby — he put his hand over my mouth in a clear enough gesture: *Stop!*

I couldn't stop. Through all the remaining days of July, I continued to gather and circulate as much medical information as I could about Ruffin's early development, including all the materials from Ruffin's follow-up visits after his premature birth.

As part of a standard protocol for following premature infants, Ruffin had been seen regularly by a developmental therapist, first within a few days of his birth, again at 4 1/2 months, again at 14 months, and finally on the day of Dr. Caldwell's diagnosis, July 12th, when he was 3 years, 3 months old.

Those reports had documented, even as Ruffin was diagnosed, that when offered tools and demonstrations, Ruffin was able to copy a circle and a vertical line but failed to copy a cross. Maybe he failed to notice it. He seemed to learn to hold scissors easily enough, and held a pencil correctly, stacked blocks as requested, and removed or dumped peas from a container.

But looking back over all those records, I could see that as early as 14 months, there appeared to have been a 4- to 6-month lag in the development of Ruffin's adaptive behaviors and language — his abilities to function as a person appropriate to his age, and to speak with others — well behind the obviously unimpeded development of his motor skills. Ruffin's robust physical development was no accurate proxy of his cognitive development. So, the now noticeable, growing lag between the two presented an obvious danger: Ruffin was nimble, agile, and mobile, without being able to appreciate either the social world around him or any verbal warnings or directions offered him. He had his own agenda, determined to explore his own world in his own way, annoyed by any interruption to redirect his attention, whether to a bug in the grass or the moon overhead.

I recalled then that when Ruffin was 2 years, 8 months old, I had felt a small, gnawing concern that his development seemed to have slowed to a crawl. I pulled out the pamphlets that had been sent home and tried to score Ruffin's progress against the 2-year and 2 1/2-year developmental benchmarks.

Now I pulled out all those pamphlets again. At 3 years, 3 months, Ruffin exhibited all the skills of a typically developing 18-month-old. I jotted down my assessment to circulate to his educators. "Ruffin can and does regularly exercise all the skills of the typically developing 2-year-old, except the use of plurals. I have never counted his speaking vocabulary, but 300 words seems large. Certainly, he understands that many words, and a great many more."

In this, my first naïve assessment of Ruffin's *receptive* language — his understanding of words spoken to him — I learned later that I had been sadly mistaken, a common-enough mistake of new parents, and many teachers, too. Put it down to wishful thinking. But I realized even then that by pulling out those pamphlets, I had been acting upon my own gnawing doubt about Ruffin's development. With growing sadness, I was beginning to revisit those feelings, and beginning to sense I couldn't spend too much more of Ruffin's time caught up in wishful thinking.

We might be out on the porch or the street where Ruffin was fearless, all too ready to approach perfect strangers who might be carrying something intriguing, or the neighborhood children who might be playing with their toys. He waved to passing walkers, other porch sitters, or wandered off into crowds lugging one of his cats — with no concern for where I was — held up in conversation and unable to follow him. But he was easily upset when any stranger approached him with a purpose — whether it was a friendly older child wanting to direct his play. "You be the cowboy, okay?" Or a lady at church, kindly asking his name and age. He wouldn't even hold up his fingers to answer. Certainly, he would be upset if a doctor needed to examine his ears or have him open his mouth for a wooden stick.

Only once or twice, coming in from spending time out on the farm with Seamus, did Ruffin try telling me about anything that *had* happened. "Broke." They had felled a tree, Seamus explained. "Big truck." That would be Seamus's wrecked truck, up on blocks. No need to visit that touchy subject. Nothing about people. Ruffin had no understanding of simple time concepts: "last night," "tomorrow," or "wait." For Seamus, too, he didn't seem to grasp the concept of "wait."

"He's impatient. He takes after you," Seamus chuckled softly.

As to his impatience, Ruffin did. But otherwise, strikingly, he did not, and had not.

If Ruffin were going to attend school without being able to talk, his teacher needed to know Ruffin didn't know his name or his colors, or his letters, or his numbers. He seemed not to understand when he might be tired, or that a nap might help.

All that past spring and summer, Ruffin and I seemed to have been living a life slowed to the flow of cold molasses. My mother had succeeded in toilet training him over the five long weeks of my *Ezzone* trial by using M&Ms but hadn't managed to get him to give up his bottle or his single favorite food after weaning — chocolate milk. As a trained teacher, she was frightened by his night-long babbling. With me, he struggled against changing into new clothes, and protested leaving the house, so he and I were always the last to arrive at Julie's daycare. By midmorning, her home would be busy, loud, and hot, and Ruffin wouldn't really want to stay there, but if I kept him with me, I couldn't get any work done unless he happened to be sleeping. Not housework, not the legal work that I needed to do to support us, and certainly not the scheduled, focused meetings my clients expected, when Ruffin demanded my constant attention. Usually, he and I struggled through a good part of the morning, just to get out the door.

With Ruffin in daycare for a long afternoon, I gathered up all his previous medical records, eye exams, hearing exams, too, to bring to the early August Bridgewater appointment. Obsessively, I photocopied all Ruffin's baby books in which I had recorded his early developmental milestones, visits to doctors, physical growth, little accidents, and falls, back to the development of his suck reflex, his early sleep and crying patterns.

The first time Ruffin had called me by name as "Mama," as opposed to copying the word as a sound, had been May 10th, when he was 3 years, 1 month old. He surprised me. He wanted up, lifting his arms. "Up," I said, as I lifted him up onto my heaving chest, through my tears. He *did* recognize me as his mother. Wasn't that what this "Mama" meant? This was the first occasion I felt he had used language to call me "Mama." He continued to do so and did so regularly now — except when he was excited and called for attention by saying, "Julie," the name of his sitter. Looking back over

Ruffin's baby books, it was curious to see that I never really noted when he recognized any other family member. I must not have been sure that he ever did.

Following up on other contacts provided by Mr. Montague, I placed calls to the Autism Society of Iowa, and to the mother of an older child with autism who lived several counties south. From her, I learned there was an autism resource team network in Iowa, led by a state autism specialist Sue Baker, at the University of Iowa's Hospital School. Sue was identified as the person in Iowa who knew the most about autism, and who enjoyed a reputation for being the most helpful. So, I called her, too.

My first question was whether health insurance would cover treatment for a child like Ruffin. Sue was clear: private insurance was not a promising avenue for funding either care or treatment. Most children and adults with autism eventually qualified for and depended upon Social Security Disability and Medicaid for a modest income, health care, respite care services to give their parents a break in caretaking, and eventual group home placement when life at home was no longer possible.

Sue also alerted me that Bridgewater's special education evaluation team was likely not very well versed in screening for autism. This marked my introduction into the world of competing autism experts, who seemed not to think much of each other, or of each other's skills and methods. As an alternative, she outlined the procedure for Ruffin to enter the state's autism evaluation network of Iowa professionals who were using the then relatively new *Psychoeducational Profile-Revised* (*PEP-R*), as an assessment instrument to administer to young children with autism. Ruffin's individual educational plan (IEP) could then be written based upon the *PEP-R* assessment findings, to avoid having his educators try out less useful general special education methods.

Basically, Sue offered me sound advice. Expert assessment by experienced professionals was fundamental, so that Ruffin's IEP team, including me as his parent, could choose appropriate, effective educational methods to reach reasonably high goals, step by step, using measurable objectives. An early assessment would be key to the identification of Ruffin's true, primary deficits — before any secondary limitations began to pile up on top of any early, un-remediated problems.

Sue also suggested getting a separate speech evaluation of Ruffin's *echolalia* — his tendency to parrot back the speech of others. She explained echolalia as having several functional types, both immediate and delayed, and suggested *The Sequenced Inventory of Communication Development* as a good assessment tool to gauge Ruffin's communication skills. As I did my own further reading, I found a helpful list of six communicative functions of echolalia: turn-taking, assertions, affirmative answers, requests, self-regulation, and rehearsals to aid processing.

Most important, I learned from Sue that echolalia was a good thing, because it meant there was no need to engage Ruffin in a long course of learning the more fundamental skill of verbal imitation — *ah, mmm, ma, mama* — before beginning to teach him the attachment of specific meaning to a given sound, or *receptive* language — that *mama* means Mama — so that *expressive* language might develop to replace echolalia.

Echolalia had been so often the occasion for musing about Ruffin. Whenever Seamus would drop in, daily, usually in the late afternoon, I would drop everything. Then he and I would go round and round with each other, over my kitchen counter, before I would need to go pick up Ruffin.

"But Ruffin does speak," Seamus would protest, as he left.

"Ruffin speaks in a mysterious and special way of his own," I would say, as calmly as I could manage, on my way out.

Ruffin's echolalia would hardly function well as social communication except within a confined world of those who understood him. For example, Seamus and I knew that Ruffin's echo of a Disney movie snippet from *Hello Dolly* meant he wanted a certain toy train because he associated it with the train running behind the opening credits. But I began to wonder whether echolalia couldn't be shaped into meaningful, ordinary speech, more useful to opening a wider world for Ruffin, socially, at school, and eventually, at work and beyond — into a life independent of us both.

For the moment, though, Ruffin, Seamus, and I continued to struggle. I hardly dared bathe Ruffin alone. To wash his hair was some danger. He might thrash the tub wall with his head. It took the two of us, Seamus, and me, both, manhandling him together. Seamus could not seem to take in why this was. Or, with his calm and obliging nature, could not seem to *bear* having to do this. To struggle so much over a simple bath. Ruffin hated any wetness. Even to change his shirt led me to drip water down his back, on purpose, more than once. Getting him wet like that made him undress.

Seamus and I had been talking outdoors, with Ruffin at our feet, when he cut himself on bottle-glass. It seemed he no more felt the pain than if his blood were water. He didn't look up for comfort, or cry. His blood was nothing until its wetness somehow bothered him. Only wet made him complain, look up. Not the cut.

"Mary Jane, look, he's cut himself."

"On *your* broken bottle, you didn't pick up."

Ruffin and his troubles were beginning to come between us.

Social skills were a core deficit — perhaps *the* core deficit — in autism, according to Sue, so it was puzzling to me that the only assessment she could suggest for Ruffin's social skill development was informal observation — close, careful, and thoughtful watching. She thought Ruffin should be placed in a center-based classroom at a schoolhouse with a group of variously disabled students, rather than be kept at home and taught directly by a devoted teacher, as Anne Sullivan had taught Helen Keller. Ruffin should be with other children to develop social skills, since he was being raised by me, as a single parent, and as an only child.

But Ruffin had been with other children since he was a toddler, well over half his life — with other friendly, outgoing, typically developing children — with his longtime day care provider, Julie. Julie and Erik's home had long been given over to childcare, with Erik having built a separate basement entry for children and their parents to walk into the house's large playroom. Their entire backyard was an organized playground fit for a public park. Erik was proud of his wife's work, supportive and tolerant of a changing cast of little visitors. I wondered how a classroom at school could be any better socially.

Julie and I sat down at her kitchen table after her long day. There were bags of animal crackers, popcorn, and cheese doodles Erik had brought in from Walmart. Her strong square face was the setting for two dark bright eyes, and her short square body sat heavily on her chair as her legs stretched out, and then tucked under her, while she leaned forward with interest in what I struggled to disclose.

"Ruffin has been diagnosed with autism," I finally said, flatly.

Erik came back to lean in the doorway and listen as Julie continued telling me what she had been holding back.

"He isolates himself. Curls up and rocks in his corner, while all the others go out to play."

I had come to know Julie as a close, careful, and thoughtful observer, herself a mother of four. A thoroughly good-hearted soul, she had been reluctant to offer me these and other classic observations of a child with autism.

Sue had let me know she kept an autism library at the university in Iowa City, but that would entail a six-hour round trip. With Ruffin still often unwilling to dress or go out, it was simply easier to order in any resources she recommended. I subscribed to *The Journal of Autism and Developmental Disorders*. I ordered the complete series of *Current Issues in Autism*, Series Editors, Eric Schopler, Ph.D., and Gary B. Mesibov, Ph.D., and I read all their volumes, covering topics from diagnosis to adult placement, and every educational and behavioral issue in between.

Dr. Schopler was the developer of the *PEP-R* assessment instrument Sue favored and was a founder with Dr. Mesibov of the then highly regarded model TEACCH program for the education of children with autism in North Carolina, and in many other partial copy-on states like Iowa. The essence of the TEACCH model seemed to depend upon a commitment by society and government to structure a life-long supportive environment around children with autism using visual cues, so they could grow into adults with autism trained for sheltered workshop piecework or make-work laid out for them in visual jigs. This was a worthy social goal, but I thought it would be highly vulnerable to social service funding fluctuations.

I briefly considered moving back to North Carolina where my parents lived to enter Ruffin into TEACCH's cradle-to-grave autism support system there. But I couldn't bear to think of leaving Seamus behind. Over our time together, I had quietly accepted that he would never leave his large extended childhood family, his parents, brothers, and sisters and all his aunts and uncles and cousins, or his family farm home in northeast Iowa. It would have been impossible to uproot them all.

Really, at the moment, I couldn't bear to think of leaving northeast Iowa myself, or of leaving my new, carefully restored Victorian home on Main Street, my clients, my established law practice, to undertake the ordeal of a new bar exam. Those were my excuses, the nonsense I offered myself. Truthfully, I couldn't bear the thought of moving back as a failure, to become dependent upon my parents again. There must be a less embarrassing way out of the mess I seemed to have made of our lives. What I said to everyone was that whatever North Carolina had to offer was not enough for Ruffin, or for me. Somehow, there had to be a better answer to what would be best for Ruffin, one that would be closer to my own heart, my ambitions, and the home I had made in Iowa.

In my earliest reading about autism, a few reports of rare instances of "recovery" intrigued me in Schopler and Mesibov's most relevant volume in their series, *Preschool Issues in Autism*. Neither Schopler nor Mesibov were able to ignore a 1987 research study published by O. Ivar Lovaas, Ph.D. of UCLA who claimed to have "recovered" nine children from early childhood autism. Schopler and Mesibov gave Lovaas, seemingly their chief academic rival, their sharpest critique. Nor could they ignore similar, earlier clinical results — recoveries reported by a private autism school in Princeton, New Jersey. I was curious to learn more about these UCLA and Princeton methods, both described as "intensive" and "behavioral," because those results seemed nearer to what I wanted for Ruffin and needed for myself — something more effective and ambitious.

No one else I was communicating with about Ruffin — none of the medical people, none of the school people, none of the special educators, not even Sue in Iowa City — seemed to know about these ways to "recover" children from autism by a scientific and proven method. Whenever I brought up the possibility of "recovery," no one else seemed even mildly curious, and that truly puzzled me.

So what if I knew very little about autism? I lived with it and with Ruffin. So what if all these people were paid to know more about autism, as professionals, than I did as his mother? I wasn't certain they had all the answers. Or the right answers for Ruffin, Seamus, and me. Maybe nobody did. But I was more strongly motivated than anyone else — more than Seamus, I had to admit — to find the best answers for Ruffin. And I wanted to keep asking questions widely, and to listen — receptively, but critically.

During our several long-distance conversations, Sue offered me two leads that proved immediately helpful, and powerfully helpful in the long run.

First, she told me about Bernard Rimland, Ph.D., an early autism parent, Navy psychologist, award-winning book author, and independent autism researcher based in San Diego, California, who published a regular newsletter *Autism Research Review International*. My first issue arrived in late July, recommending megavitamin therapy, principally B-6 plus magnesium, and dimethylglycine (DMG), a substance similar to a B vitamin, first used by Russian doctors in treating autism.

In late July, Ruffin began taking B-6 plus magnesium, formulated to Dr. Rimland's specifications by Kirkman Labs as Super-NuThera, together with DMG. His behavior and attention improved markedly, and he began speaking in 1- and 2-word utterances to people other than me. Also, I quickly discovered that withdrawing any DMG after midday helped Ruffin crash at day's end and sleep some nights, which came as a welcome relief to us both.

Second, Sue let me know about Lois Fergus of Compuplay. She was based at the YMCA in Cedar Rapids, a hundred miles south of where we lived. There she kept a lending library of new computer programs for students with autism, especially for younger children with few language skills. I gave her a call. No, the programs she offered wouldn't run on IBM DOS, my law office machine. I would need to buy a Macintosh personal computer for Ruffin to use at home. Since that would be a hefty purchase at $7,500, I decided it was worth the inevitable tantrum to drive Ruffin down to Cedar Rapids, where Lois could work with him in person and see what programs might be appropriate, whether he could manage to use a mouse, or whether he might need some more expensive equipment like a direct touch screen or a large button switch.

The next day, after a big tantrum and the long drive, I walked Ruffin into the cool green hallways of the Y. Lois greeted Ruffin simply and took him directly to several machines she had set up in advance. Ruffin's only distraction while exploring these came when a train rumbled through town. Its whistle drew Ruffin to the nearest window, where he looked out, turning his head like a cat, listening with first one ear, then the other, *Where is it? Where is it coming from?* Once the train passed, Ruffin took to the cursor like a fish to water.

Lois encouraged me to buy Ruffin a Macintosh and borrow three software programs published by *Edmark*: *Bailey's Book House, Millie's Math House,* and *Sammy's Science House*. As soon as their packages arrived on our front porch in late July, I sat Ruffin down in front of his new personal computer, and he began using his mouse to explore *Bailey's Book House*. These were his first sustained acts of joint attention. I sat with him. It was important that I sat with him, to move him along when he perseverated or persisted in clicking over and over to stay with a single presentation by the program. It was important that I sat with him, to nudge him along, because this was also the teaching of joy, the joy of accomplishment, the joy of him smiling with his eyes, the joy of pride, the joy of showing off.

Later on, Ruffin graduated to *Living Book Broderbund* programs, *Grandma and Me*, and *The Tortoise and the Hare*, and began working through several *Laureate* and *Micro-LADS* programs designed by speech pathologists to teach language — especially the meaning of verbs, by means of clear, uncluttered animation — to children with language delays, whether as a result of Down syndrome, autism, or aphasia.

As I read more deeply into autism research, I wondered if these computer programs weren't the best way for Ruffin to encounter language — as the written word persistent across time and space — rather than become lost in a classroom teacher's real-time noise that seemed to be far more demanding for him to process.

These computer programs flashed up individual, discrete tasks and responded instantly to Ruffin's mouse clicks with brief, highly rewarding visual and auditory special effects — or not, if he clicked on a wrong choice.

By late July, I had a list of questions to pass on to Ruffin's PICU team leader RN Fay Hill at LaCrosse Lutheran Hospital for her to send along with all Ruffin's earliest medical and developmental records to Dr. Carol Reed at Gundersen's autism clinic. And would Fay please urge Dr. Reed that Ruffin be fully evaluated quickly, much earlier than January? I hoped I could count on Fay to appreciate my desperation.

I told Fay I wanted to know Ruffin's IQ or "mental age," whether he was mentally retarded, how early his autism might have been evident in his developmental records, or in our home videos, and exactly what type of autism he might have. Could the autism clinic group rule out disintegrative psychosis, rare genetic disorders, childhood schizophrenia, tuberous sclerosis, and epilepsy? Could Ruffin have just a speech disorder or some simpler learning disability? I was eager to know the group's opinions and experience with various treatments, including mega doses of vitamin B-6, magnesium, fenfluramine, and other drug therapies. And I wanted to know exactly who would be examining Ruffin and advising me. Would someone from the autism clinic group call me?

After the hand-over meeting, Fay called with the good news that Dr. Reed had screened Ruffin's early May audio and video recordings, the ones I had sent Dr. Caldwell earlier, and had agreed to assemble a full multi-disciplinary team, quickly, including a very experienced clinical speech and language pathologist, Mila Sokolov, whom Dr. Reed could call out of retirement. Then Dr. Reed herself called to assure me Ruffin would be seen in early October rather than January. I was grateful and relieved.

Given all she had seen and heard of him on the recordings, Dr. Reed made a pointed request that I bring a second adult to watch Ruffin during the afternoon-long final meeting after the many autism clinic appointments so the various professionals would be able to confer with me without distraction — a very sensible suggestion, I agreed, given Ruffin's difficult behaviors.

CHAPTER THREE

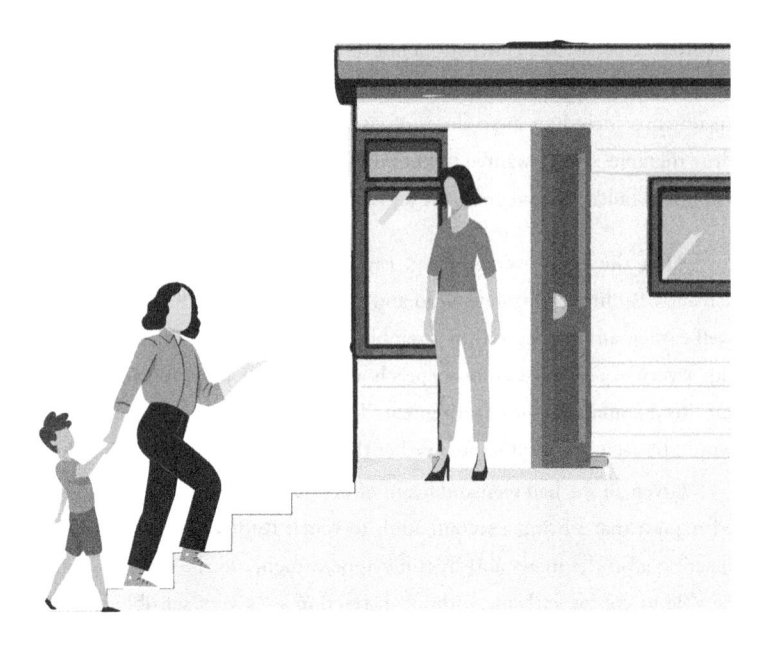

EVALUATIONS

I held Ruffin's hand late in the afternoon of August 1st as we walked together toward a couple of Bridgewater double-wide office trailers parked across from the blacktopped playground of the junior high. There had been a trace of rain. I could smell asphalt rising in the steaming heat, as Ruffin mounted the first step with his right foot, stood on it a moment to gather both feet, mounted the next step, paused again to gather both feet, mounted another slowly, up four or five shaky metal steps to the entrance, where a slender woman named Inge Nilsen, introduced herself. She waited, holding the steel door open for us as a cool waterfall of air-conditioning poured out.

By that time, I imagined I felt prepared — meaning I no longer expected anyone to confide this autism was all a mistake, a nightmare from which I was destined to wake, yawning, and stretching.

With a handshake, Jack Wallace stepped forward to introduce himself as Bridgewater's sector coordinator, putting a face to his voice which I already knew well over the phone. He was here to supervise Ruffin's screening and evaluation team. A large, shambling, warm-hearted heavy-footed man, before long, he was down on the floor with Ruffin, prompting him to roll a ball, delightfully, back-and-forth.

Inge was Ruffin's front-line team leader, an early childhood special education (ECSE) consultant, and the coordinating author of the screening and evaluation report that would be issued after our meeting. As I got to know her better, Inge impressed me as a person who worried about people, and had devoted her life to special education.

Ruffin's school psychologist, Emily Knight, was a scholarly-looking, bespectacled, dark-haired, rather reserved figure. It would be up to Emily to review Dr. Caldwell's medical disability diagnosis and to assess Ruffin's mental development by choosing and administering an appropriate educational test. She chose *The Bayley Scales of Infant Development-Second Edition*.

The answers Ruffin offered Emily were nearly inaudible, with one exception, when he loudly and proudly named a giraffe without being asked. By moving objects in relation to each other, he seemed to be able to show he understood a single preposition — "in." Working in concentrated silence, he matched 4 basic colors for her, and then identified 8 out of 10 basic pictures in whispered bits of echolalia: shoe, dog, house, clock, book, fish, star, and car. I was pleased Ruffin had somehow learned how to echo these words and colors and was able to draw on his knowledge here in this new place, among all these strangers.

Ruffin even seemed to have surprised Emily once. She had demonstrated a 3-block tower which Ruffin copied readily enough. When she asked him to add more blocks on top of his tower, he seemed to ignore her, or not to understand what it was she wanted of him. He seemed ready to wander away. But, as she demonstrated a 10-block tower, he understood immediately and showed her that he did, by building one of his own. Ruffin could not understand the language of even simple directions. However, he could understand and copy physical demonstrations. I found this encouraging to know. As Emily concluded, Ruffin was a "visual learner."

Later that afternoon, after we gathered around a conference table, Emily reported back to us that Ruffin had earned a mental development index of 50. I knew from my first night of reading that this amounted to the rough equivalent of IQ 50, or moderate mental retardation, when IQ 100 was the norm. IQ 50: I could let that sink in, very nearly thankfully, because of the Gundersen autism clinic receptionist's earlier remark the day of Ruffin's diagnosis. Somehow, I was able to take this result Emily offered us as better news than I might otherwise have, had I been taken completely by surprise.

Nevertheless, Emily explained how this fell within "the significantly delayed performance range," with Ruffin "functioning at the level of a 26- to 27-month-old." It was a dreary prospect. Anyone at our table could do the math. This amounted to an overall developmental delay of 13 months that Ruffin would need to make up. At the time, I imagined that was the purpose of special education — to do whatever might be necessary for Ruffin to catch up. Surprisingly, at this meeting, I began to learn this was not true.

In her report, Emily offered no quarrel with Dr. Caldwell's diagnosis. "Behaviors observed and those reported by the parent reinforced the physician's provisional diagnosis of pervasive developmental disorder. Further medical testing will be done to rule out other diagnoses (i.e., fragile X, organic brain syndrome, PKU). Ruffin does qualify for placement in the preschool handicapped classroom." Although this was exactly what I had wanted and had been my whole aim in bringing Ruffin in for this evaluation, it was still hard to read those words — "placement in the preschool handicapped classroom" — through anything but a trembling film of tears.

Seamus arrived that night for supper, hungry. We were eating in the kitchen, at the breakfast counter, perched on hard wooden stools. Ruffin had snagged his bottle and squirmed up into my green leather chair to get to his computer — in the formal dining room I had converted into a home-office. He was out of earshot. I told Seamus Ruffin's IQ, matter-of-factly without tears. He didn't care for tears.

Seamus looked over in the direction of the wide passageway where we could both see Ruffin.

"Mary Jane, look at him. What three-year-old has his own computer?"

"It was recommended," I reminded him.

"Wasn't it expensive?"

"It was. He likes it. It keeps him busy, so we can talk, so it was worth it."

"You need to be careful with your money. Don't you think he's too big to still be on a bottle? Do you have him drinking chocolate milk again?"

I responded by teasing him. "Yes, like father, like son. Or are you just mad there wasn't enough left for you?"

"Maybe," he admitted. I'd gotten a grin out of him.

Then he said, with a side-long glance, "Won't Julie be disappointed if you send him to school?"

"Maybe," I admitted. "I'll need to tell her, too. Ruffin will still need somewhere to go after school. You know, on those days I have afternoons in court out of town. It's hard getting back in less than an hour, especially if there's weather. I think there might be a bus."

"Well," Seamus said, sliding off the seat of his stool and pushing himself up from the counter, "You'll need to talk to Julie. Erik says she always has a waiting list. She might be able to keep Ruffin and take someone else in for the morning. When you visit with her" — and here he looked at me to be sure he had my attention — "you might mention that." Then, he was off to work, across the river for a late shift at the factory.

A summer stand-in speech and language pathologist (SLP) had also tested Ruffin, after carefully watching him work with Emily, and after visiting with me about Ruffin's long history of ear infections. To establish a baseline, she chose *The Preschool Language Scale-3* "to determine Ruffin's abilities to comprehend and use language productively," and the *Iowa Severity Rating Scale for Communicative Disabilities Revised*. Ruffin would come to be rated by these same measures repeatedly over the next 28 months.

Like Emily, she found that Ruffin could make whispered use of a good basic vocabulary and follow simple directions when a visual cue was offered to him. But Ruffin seemed unable to use verbs or adjectives, numbers, or prepositions. I had to wonder then; how could he manage to communicate without them? Could they be taught to him? With an IQ of 50, could he be expected to learn them? She had rated Ruffin a 3 on Iowa's severity scale. At the conference, she explained how this scale ran from 0 to 4, with 0 indicating an adequate performance, and every number above expressing a greater degree of disability. Well, I comforted myself, Ruffin could have been a 4, but thankfully, he wasn't.

She went on to explain that she judged Ruffin to be speaking at a 2- to 3-word stage, at a language age she pegged at 25 months, although she had overheard longer phrases while he was playing alone. I had heard them, too — too many times. They were always the same phrases, over and over again. "Big truck," and "*Ninga, ninga, ninga*" were already driving both Seamus and me batty, very nearly crazy. Before I could put that out on the table, she continued, offering everyone there what she had found to be the most encouraging: she thought Ruffin had a strong ability to imitate with his gestures, and by echoing her words. This seemed to mean Ruffin *could* learn, since imitation was one way all of us who develop more typically also learn.

As I came to appreciate the various forms of special education testing, what emerged as significant was that Ruffin gave a misleadingly hopeful impression of speaking like a 28-month-old child, when he could understand no more than a 21-month-old. At first, I found this measured discrepancy more than a bit odd. But this was an example of why it was nearly always more important to consider the sub-scale scores in testing young children with autism, because differing sub-scale scores were more richly informative than the averaged score — 25 months in Ruffin's case — which tended to erase these differences and obscure the effect of Ruffin's meaningless echolalia.

As I learned more about autism, I grew to appreciate, as Sue had suggested to me earlier, that the acquisition of *receptive* language skills — listening with understanding — logically and necessarily preceded the acquisition of *expressive* language skills — speaking with meaning. In her written summary and recommendations, this first speech and language pathologist seemed to have gotten the cart before the horse, by recommending speech and language therapy to help Ruffin "improve his *expressive* language skills so he could increase his knowledge of basic concepts."

While Ruffin was being tested, I kept track of him out of the corner of my eye. I had been ambushed to report to a special education nurse, who recorded the answers she could pull out of my distraction. "Tell me about Ruffin."

"He can be very demanding, very insistent when he wants something, or doesn't care to do something. No amount of reasoning seems to help. Once he wants something, or wants me to find something for him, I can't seem to distract him."

"And, when you have to, how do you discipline him?"

"If he has a tantrum, I try to take him to his bedroom, until he winds down. Once he's quiet, I go in, and say, 'Better.' Occasionally, I've had to swaddle him in his blanket. That's something I learned to do when he was a preemie in intensive care to help him calm down or bring about self-regulation. That's how his nurses explained it to me there. It still works well."

"And when does he seem to have these sorts of tantrums?"

"Anytime we need to hurry or give up what he's doing. You know, leave to go anywhere. But since I've learned he has autism, I find if I can tell him simply what we are going to be doing ahead of time, that works better. Sometimes . . ."

"Does he get good sleep?"

Even as I was certain it continued to work for Ruffin, I wasn't sure whether Dr. Rimland's Super Nu-Thera formula wouldn't sound a little California New Age — a little too "out there" as a form of alternative medicine to this starch-faced nurse — so I simply reported that Ruffin's sleep had been erratic but was improving.

"He might go to bed around 9:30 and wake up at 8:00 the next morning."

"Does he still nap?"

"Yes." And, whenever he slept, he liked to pack himself tightly in his crib, with bed pillows, sofa pillows, rolled up blankets like bolsters, all the pillows and blankets in the house. "Yes," I recalled, "he has to nestle himself to his own satisfaction . . ." but since

I had never done anything like that myself as a child or seen my brother or two sisters or any child I had ever babysat do that, I broke off describing this because it seemed an odd thing to come out with, and probably inappropriate to offer at the moment. I might have already ventured too far.

As she watched Ruffin continue to work intensely with the other members of his evaluation team, the nurse made an observation of her own about Ruffin's unusual breathing patterns. "He appeared to inhale, hold his breath momentarily, then blow it out."

She made another note I thought might be significant. Ruffin's head circumference of 53 centimeters fell into the 95th percentile. This was a measurement Ruffin had not permitted Dr. Caldwell to attempt earlier at Gundersen. Ruffin turned out to have an exceptionally large head. In 1994, this was thought to be a sign associated with autism.

Then the special education audiologist took Ruffin in hand and tried to test his hearing, without much success, since Ruffin objected to wearing earphones. He was having none of it, pushing them off his head and flinging them. The audiologist persisted in trying more informal testing by speaking to him in a whisper and playing taped sounds to prompt him to turn his head in their direction. She reported she had the impression that he was not deaf, as Julie had suggested, and as I had wondered myself early on.

As his case manager, Inge's contribution included her own written observations of Ruffin while he worked with Emily and the other members of her group. She credited him with having "an emerging ability to initiate social games with an adult, as evidenced by his starting and continuing a ball game with Jack," and noted that "while working with the psychologist, Ruffin was able to transition from activity to activity without too much difficulty."

By working patiently, it was possible for her to complete the *Early Intervention Developmental Profile* to assess Ruffin across several developmental domains. Although written in cheerfully positive terms of what Ruffin was able to earn or demonstrate, by using simple subtraction it was easy enough, and devastating as well, to convert Inge's report into measures of delay.

At his 40 months of age, Inge had assigned Ruffin the following scores: Perceptual and Fine Motor: 28 months (a 12-month delay); Language: 24 months (a 16-month delay); Social and Emotional: 28 to 31 months (a 9-to-12-month delay); Gross Motor: greater than 35 months. Inge judged Ruffin to have been "cooperative throughout the assessment process," suggesting that her screening team had captured an accurate assessment of Ruffin's true abilities to perform.

I realized then; this was what was meant by "pervasive developmental disorder." Ruffin's delays were *pervasive*: over a wide array of domains of interest to his evaluators and educators.

Certainly, I found Inge's further depictions of Ruffin recognizable enough. He *could* jump with both feet together, and momentarily balance on one foot. No, he couldn't pedal a tricycle. He hadn't had much opportunity to do that. "He did not appear ready to attempt hopping." Finding this in her long report and needing a light moment, I had to chuckle to myself, Ruffin, not yet a rabbit.

Inge observed that Ruffin enjoyed manipulating objects, and he was adept at taking objects apart. Yes, I reminded myself, I would need to warn whoever taught him at school, "Watch out!" And, for his tantrums and meltdowns. But Inge had noticed the warning signs for herself. "At the end of the afternoon, Ruffin began to exhibit signs of overstimulation through increased running and louder vocalizations; however, he did not become unmanageable. At the conclusion of the staffing, his mother stated that Ruffin had been exceptionally cooperative during this evaluation process." Yes, thankfully! I credited this in great measure to Ruffin's recent treatment with Dr. Rimland's B-6 and magnesium with DMG. Otherwise, I seriously doubted whether Ruffin could have engaged in any testing at all.

Despite Inge's continuing adherence to Piaget's relatively irrelevant paradigms of typical development in her thinking about Ruffin, I liked her as a person, and admired her as a trained observer and a straight reporter. I had given Inge as detailed a description of Ruffin's behavior at Julie's as I could, saying he was more of an observer, engaging mostly in solitary or parallel play, but providing at least one instance of his engagement with a younger boy. Inge reported all that, suggesting that Ruffin's interest in younger children could provide him with an opportunity to use his emerging language skills. That sounded hopeful — or wishful . . .

Early on, though, this plan of Inge's seemed to beggar common sense. Was it appropriate to depend on a younger, disabled, also developmentally delayed classmate to help Ruffin teach himself to talk? I felt Ruffin needed a jump-start on language, with intensive one-to-one adult instruction to help him catch up. Ruffin's problem, as I saw it, was that he wasn't developing — language or other important skills — with other children, disabled or not.

But Inge and her group were more of a mind with Sue in Iowa City, and all too ready to offer what it was they had to offer. "These results, observations, and parental concerns indicated that Ruffin would benefit from receiving early intervention services.

Emphasis should be placed on strengthening his language and social skills, along with specific safety issues. While addressing Ruffin's language and social needs, it will also be possible to monitor and strengthen his concept development. It would be appropriate for Ruffin to receive these services in an early childhood special education (ECSE) classroom setting."

And, how exactly, I wondered, would emphasis work? And how would it be possible to strengthen his concept development by monitoring it? By just watching? But for me to ask how, raised the question of educational methodology. Bridgewater's and Sue's recommendations represented the ordinary best practices in special education of the time.

It was unfortunate that Ruffin's classroom teacher, Meg Holub; his local principal and special education director, Nan Hobbs; and Bridgewater's locally assigned speech and language pathologist, Kim Pope, were not in attendance at this first screening. They were not yet part of Ruffin's working educational team because, of course, this first meeting represented a separate, early evaluation stage, which did not include any of the people who would be assigned to teach him.

Dr. Caldwell had ordered an MRI of Ruffin's brain. In doing so, he explained his personal, research focus was on tuberous sclerosis, tubers of sclerotic tissue in the brain seen in young children and usually diagnosed with an early MRI, being one of the only known causes of autism he might either confirm or rule out in Ruffin at the time. I agreed that Ruffin could undergo the procedure, hoping this might help us all learn more about the cause of Ruffin's developmental delays. My private insurance would cover it. So, Ruffin's MRI was squeezed into the schedule at the ungodly hour of 6:45 in the morning on August 3rd.

I called ahead and planned to arrive the late afternoon before this appointment, so Ruffin and I could check into a hospi-tel room high up near the intensive care floor, where he had been incubated just after being born. He and I needed to spend the night there, because it would be unlikely I could get Ruffin up, get him decently dressed, get us both out of the house, and drive an hour up the Mississippi on a narrow two-lane blacktop in a rush of morning commuters in time for our appointment.

Midmorning, just before we needed to leave, I ran to capture Ruffin to sit him down. I wanted his attention, so I could talk to him about what was going to happen. I managed to get him onto my lap and held him tightly. He was facing away from me, but I could dip my nose into the warm dustiness of his hair and whisper into his ear as he squirmed and strained to slip loose.

I tried to make it simple. Concrete. I told him just what would happen most immediately. "We're going to take a trip in the car." I could tell, he sensed this was my serious voice. His whole body stiffened. Something in his routine was about to change, and he was not pleased.

"A long ride. To the hospital. And sleep there." Whatever this meant to him, he did not like it. It was not what he wanted to do. He let me know by kicking and screaming. A serious, wailing tantrum ensued. I hoped no one would come to the door. I wouldn't answer it, or the phone, if it happened to ring. Ruffin twisted away from me, up the stairs. A hard object came whistling down. I retreated and waited.

When Ruffin had settled back into his own room, lining up his little cars, I slipped quietly upstairs to pack a few things to stash in the hatch behind the backseat. Then, I went back for him. I said, again, trying to address him as a person, as the person he was, "We're going to take a trip in the car. A long ride. To the hospital. And sleep there." More kicking and flailing, renewed screaming. This was it. We needed to get going to be sure we arrived between the morning and afternoon rush hours. I gave up and lunged for his knitted blue blanket to roll him into, making a quiet, stiff column of his legs, binding his fists and arms to his heaving sides. This left his red and wailing face under a sweaty cap of unruly hair to let anyone who might have glimpsed our few steps out the front door to the car know — I was not trying to dispose of a small corpse in broad daylight.

I had wrapped his blanket so tightly, it took some effort to bend him into his car-seat. Once he was strapped in, I loosened the blanket a little. I wondered how I could get him out of the car seat, across the hospital parking lot, and through the revolving door of the entrance, but I couldn't dwell on that now. Maybe I could think of something while I drove through the immense, whispering cornfields. A mile or two out of town, Ruffin subsided into exhaustion. I could hear his steady breathing from the back seat. Which meant he wouldn't be likely to sleep much tonight. Maybe we could still arrive before the medical library closed, so I would have something to read.

The rest of the hour's drive passed peacefully with the river sparkling to my left after we passed over the rattling deck of the bridge at Lansing into Wisconsin, past the herons wading in the scuds of waterlilies in the backwater sloughs, past the waterside power plant, past the waterfront bars, and slowly through the one small town with its hypervigilant local cop.

When we arrived, Ruffin was still sleeping, heavily. Thankfully. It was easier than I had imagined loading him up on one hip, quietly checking in and out of the medical library. For the night's reading, I chose *The Encyclopedia of Autism Spectrum Disorders*, a heavy blue single volume the size of my *Oxford English Dictionary* two-volume set. With the huge unwieldy book under one arm, I shifted Ruffin carefully so he wouldn't wake up, re-slung our overnight bag of clothes over the shoulder of the one arm winged out over the book, and we waddled off to our blissfully air-conditioned room. I laid Ruffin on the bed, closed the door, and settled in with no further reason to venture out until morning, because I could order in — hospital food.

The small, pink slip of instructions for his MRI under sedation warned me Ruffin was to have nothing by mouth after midnight. I was not to give him anything. No bottle. And I was instructed to have him sleep from 11:00 that evening to 4:00 in the morning. Much easier written than done. As I had expected, Ruffin woke up soon enough and ran most of the night in circles — *Ninga, ninga, ninga* — running in patterns on the floor, up on his toes, until about 11:00, and then got up again, running, at 2:00 in the morning. By dawn, my hope was he might collapse, sleep again, and not need sedation for his MRI. In any case, it would be impossible to miss our appointment.

Whether he was awake, running and chattering, or asleep, collapsed on the carpet, or lifted back onto the bed, with his sweaty head on a pillow, I sat in our room's single chair under a lamp. I read all night. The *Encyclopedia* proved to be one chapter of scientific literature review after another, abstracting and citing all the then-published peer-reviewed academic psychological literature about autism from 1943 on, including many references to the original descriptive papers of Leo Kanner (1943) and Hans Asperger (1944).

I managed to learn quite a lot: about autism over time, about autism world-wide, about autism as distinguished from uncomplicated mental retardation, from Down syndrome, from tuberous sclerosis, from the effects of fetal alcohol syndrome, from Rett syndrome (mostly in girls), from fragile X (mostly in boys), from heavy metal poisoning's transient but similar behavioral symptoms, about categories and subtypes of autism proposed and decomposed through autism's relatively short but tangled history of academic wrangles, and critical reviews of all the various competing diagnostic instruments, checklists of behavioral and intellectual functioning, and verbal or non-verbal communication assessments.

By morning, Ruffin was dead asleep, and I was giddy from lack of it. Enough to need a nap during the procedure, so I could drive us safely home.

In his consultation, the day after the MRI, Dr. Caldwell described Ruffin's MRI images and explained Ruffin's thinning of the corpus callosum these had disclosed. "Where you and I might have an eight-lane superhighway running between and connecting the two halves of our brains, Ruffin has something a bit more like a narrow, dirt path. But, since he is still a very young child, Ruffin's corpus callosum has yet to be fully myelinated — its nerves are yet to be fully insulated by myelin's fatty sheaths."

Okay, I thought to myself. Electrical impulses shorting out.

"Usually, the process of myelination continues, with full myelination being reached in late adolescence or early adulthood."

So, I wondered, we might reasonably hope the function of his corpus callosum could improve over time? I comforted myself with the thought that the brain is plastic, remembering little magazine stories out of *Readers' Digest* about children born with half a brain who functioned normally.

Dr. Caldwell made a throat-clearing noise that brought back my attention, so he could explain that Ruffin did not have tuberous sclerosis, reminding me what that was, how it was associated with autism and often complicated by epilepsy, and reminding me this was his research interest. I realized that it would be really bad news if Ruffin had tuberous sclerosis, but he didn't, so this amounted to good news. I suspected Dr. Caldwell realized that this meant Ruffin was not a candidate for his own ongoing research. We moved on to discuss Ruffin's early fall downstairs in his walker, and what tests might be needed to rule out any other risks of epilepsy.

It's going to be okay. Everything's going to be fine, I told myself. My parents were on their way to Iowa, to help, and were expected to arrive in two days' time, from North Carolina. I could collapse for a day then if need be.

I always saw my mother as a capable person. As a child, I was glad she ran my life. As a young woman, I would say to myself, as a mantra of self-encouragement, your mother could have run General Motors.

As a solo practitioner in a rural county where paying clients were often thin on the ground, I continued to write poetry or make translations of difficult poets when I had trouble reading them in their originals. Before Ruffin was born, I had wandered off the legal reservation for weeks or months at a time, headed to writers' conferences and workshops, and taught poetry in the schools for the local arts council. Every year I re-read *Anatomy of a Murder* and hoped to catch a court-appointment to some interesting case I could write about later.

By early-August, while my parents were visiting, my mother and I were able to sit down together to write out a joint list of our questions for Ruffin's special educators at his upcoming IEP meeting, and for the medical evaluation team at Gundersen. Many of these questions reflected my mother's concerns as a teacher trained at Tennessee's Peabody College in the early 1950s.

Is Ruffin to adjust to the world, or will his world be adjusted to him? How fast or slow should he be exposed to new things? Should we try to stop Ruffin's tiptoeing? With heavier, stiffer, high-ankle shoes? Would it be okay to let him enjoy barefoot tiptoeing? Was there a way to train Ruffin to be less destructive of property without affecting his mechanical abilities and interests in the disassembly of items? We had questions about eating, vitamins, tantrums, his dislike of hugging. We had questions about screen time. Could computers help teach Ruffin? Visually? With auditory rewards? By removing human interaction as an interfering barrier between Ruffin and interesting subject matter? To our long list of questions, I added copies of the literature about the three *Edmark* computer programs Ruffin had already begun using at home.

Some of my mother's and my questions were meant to learn who among the local experts shared the knowledge that she and I now shared about autism. Our questions represented my parents' and my own concerns about the low levels of expectation for children with autism that seemed to be accepted all too readily. I felt keenly my obligation to be an effective, exceptional parent. I expected someone in these large professional groups to know the answers or be interested in finding them out.

My father had brought some of his fishing gear — in case Ruffin seemed to be ready to go with him. Was there a nearby pond? Seamus knew where one was, and drew a map during the time he sat with us for supper. But, my father and Ruffin never went. Ruffin didn't seem ready. And, it was hot, a little too hot for good fishing. That's what we all agreed.

My parents were familiar with Ruffin's more difficult behaviors and the safety risks, having taken care of him earlier, during the several weeks of my *Ezzone* trial. After I ran down all the recent evaluations and results of the MRI, we all agreed Ruffin wasn't much different than when he had been two.

Seamus agreed. He was very agreeable with my parents whom he had met in the hospital several days after Ruffin was born. That had been an emergency, yes.

And, the three of them had met again, briefly, when I moved into this Victorian, this lovely house in Seamus's hometown, just before the big trial, when they had picked Ruffin up. Yes, Seamus had been in the courtroom for those opening arguments and could tell my mother all about them.

Unlike my father, Seamus was a master of small talk, very charming with my mother. He complimented her mashed potatoes and ate a couple of helpings. Ruffin wouldn't touch them, despite my mother's urging.

Seamus asked me, "Doesn't he like mashed potatoes?"

Our child doesn't like mashed potatoes, I thought to myself, and managed to hold my tongue.

Gundersen's autism clinic had mailed me a schedule of seven new appointments for October 4th and 5th. A school records release was enclosed to sign so Ruffin's special education evaluation could be shared with his autism clinic's medical team. Gundersen had already copied their appointment schedule to Ruffin's principal, Miss Hobbs, so his local educators could participate in the resulting, final medical staffing, scheduled for the late afternoon of October 5th. It looked like the educators and the medical professionals were planning to work hand in glove. I hoped so.

I sent a copy of my signed release to Miss Hobbs. Then, based on what I had learned about autism, I let her know, "We look forward to accepting your earlier invitation to visit school soon. I'd like to bring Ruffin by and show him his room, the location of the bathrooms, and where he might be eating, so he can become familiar with these locations without being overwhelmed by stimulation from too many other people."

Also, to Ruffin's teacher, Meg Holub, I passed along medical questionnaires for her and the Bridgewater speech and language pathologist assigned to Ruffin so they could fill them out after observing him during his first month at school. I copied all these for Inge at Bridgewater, and all my cover letters with my signed releases back to the autism clinic, trying to move things along and keep everyone in the loop.

Who knew that a copy machine would prove to be among the most essential equipment in caring for a child with autism?

CHAPTER FOUR

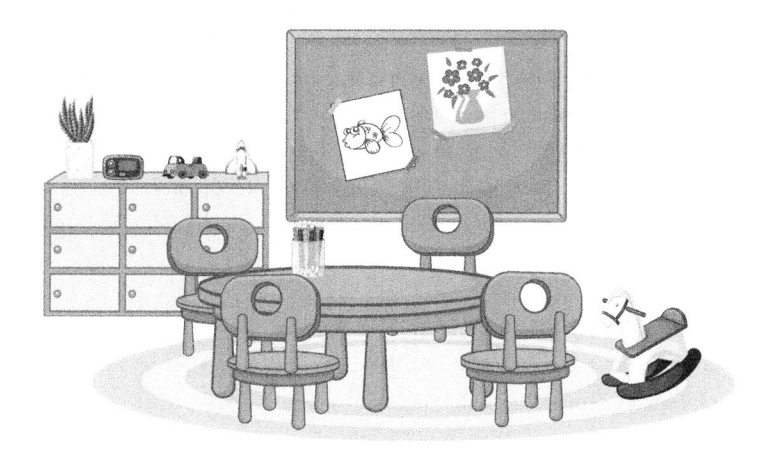

FIRST IEP

I smoked the house up with burning toner, copying all Ruffin's early medical records, and gathered other materials — including a video of an Indiana preschooler with PDD, very like Ruffin, working in his classroom with his teachers. In my anxiety, I assumed the mask of the-mother-from-hell to anyone tasked to help Ruffin, but this was my reflexive habit: to prepare, prepare, prepare.

No one taught this essential discipline of trial practice at law school, where the parsing of appellate opinions was the ordinary run of the legal curriculum. Preparation and filing were what I learned after law school by working through embarrassment, by walking into a courtroom for my client's single opportunity to be heard and finding myself to have been insufficiently prepared.

I had learned to prepare or be prepared to lose.

Absolutely fundamental to any success was Filing 101 — if I couldn't put my hands on it, I didn't really own it. I had learned. Nobody wanted to watch me scrabbling to find a particular piece of paper at any table, whether counsel table or IEP table. Not my client, not my trial partners, not my judge, not even opposing counsel.

I kept in close touch with Inge. Who on Ruffin's IEP team planned to attend Ruffin's early October autism clinic staffing at Gundersen? Since I had run up on the concept of "wrap-around services," I asked, "What can you offer to help Ruffin develop skills to go with me to stores, restaurants, and libraries?" I invited the school nurse to make a home visit to observe me and Ruffin. I wanted his educators to know how precious a child Ruffin was to me and our family — when every child is precious, no one more than another, to his or her teachers.

And, I had been slow to appreciate how necessary it was to put aside my professional ambitions to focus on Ruffin. At the time, some of my professional obligations were exceptionally demanding. With one of my long-time trial partners from our earlier *Ezzone* case, I had agreed to represent a school superintendent and his supporters in the far western part of Iowa. He and they had objected to his being let go by their remarkably lawless school board after thirty years' service. The resulting bench trial — a trial that did not involve a jury, thank goodness — eventually required 128 days of highly contested hearing before the judge ruled in our favor.

Having succeeded in my plan to enroll Ruffin in special education, I found myself suddenly uneasy that I was going to lose him now, lose the opportunity of raising him in my home. I became acutely aware that I had just agreed to send my three-year-old, who could not speak, to a large and busy schoolhouse. A wave of fear swamped my enthusiasm to follow through with this — even if it were the best thing for him.

Since he had become increasingly and embarrassingly difficult to manage at home and out in the community, I was afraid that Ruffin would misbehave at school. To help his classroom teacher, I described a few of my experiences of trying to manage him. "Unless I have been hurt by surprise — by Ruffin dropping a large object on my foot, for example — I have not yelled at him. I do not spank him. Ruffin used to irritate me a great deal by whining this spring. I sat him down and taught him to say, 'Help, help, please' to me when he wanted something. He was less frustrated, and so was I." I re-thought some of what I had been doing as discipline. Time-out did not work well. Ruffin did not settle down in a few minutes. It took longer. By the time it worked, he had become self-involved in his "babbling." I did this only when I felt *I* must have a "time out."

It had become harder to distract Ruffin once his interest flowered. Explaining shortly in advance what was going to happen, in very discrete steps was beginning to work, especially if I could get him to shake hands on it, even reluctantly. I *thought* Ruffin responded to praise from me. Other rewards seemed artificial. Food or treats — as bribes — these I dismissed as aesthetically disgusting. Not that it mattered. Ruffin didn't seem interested. I struggled along in relative ignorance of the effectiveness of all rewards in shaping human behavior, as the great tool of all employee and team management.

I wasn't feeling well. I was sick. I called Seamus for help.

"I'm having one of my spells. Could you pick up medicine on your way over?"

Seamus knew what I meant. Sometimes I would be talking and laughing, and a wave would move into my head, from the side — like a migraine, but without the headache — but with nausea and a quick trip to the bathroom.

"Benadryl and Imodium, over the counter," I reminded him. I told Seamus, no, I didn't think I could get out the door. No, I didn't need to go to the doctor.

Looking up from the mouse under his palm, Ruffin could see I was sick. From my end of the conversation, he echoed. "Medicine. Doctor." These words had come up many times before in his life, when we had to go in for his ear infections. When I shook my head and tried to smile, he ran to get one of his little trucks to give me as a present. Here he stood — ready to offer me comfort — when I cried. As I did so often now, having not ever much cried before in my life, or rarely. Seamus didn't care for this new behavior of mine, or for any whining, or my getting sick, or bringing up anything about autism, or my losing my temper with him and quarrelling. But, yes, he would come.

"You need to keep this stuff on hand, in your medicine cabinet. You know this happens to yourself."

Yes, sometimes, it happened when I was worried, when I couldn't solve a problem.

Like any parent, I had waited for my child to learn to speak and to listen. Given the results of the recent Bridgewater evaluation, I might have waited too long. Now, something was really wrong. At home, Ruffin had a fair command of the language he needed to make requests and to give me directions for meeting his needs. He wanted to know "What is it?" and "Where is it" very frequently. Not much interest in "Who is it?" Using the same exact, brief phrasing did work with him, whether he was learning to communicate or whether he was communicating by rote. At home, with me, Ruffin could respond to most of my simplest directions. His understanding of this sort of language seemed good enough, or he was a very adept guesser. As it turned out, Ruffin was a very adept guesser.

The medicines began to work. I considered Ruffin's more spontaneous, empathetic reaction to my crisis. I had often wondered before, how could Seamus and I, Julie, and his educators, all of us help Ruffin to learn that other people have their own lives, their own thoughts, and that he could share their thoughts as well as their actions? So, he would not always just be demanding something? Could the ability of children with autism to easily intuit the spatial perspective of another person be used to include the emotional perspective of another — say, by labelling an appropriate emotion, and having Ruffin "pretend" to be sad, happy, angry, or embarrassed?

These questions went right to the heart of the "theory of mind" deficit in autism, and I continued to wonder about them — as I continued to search for who else might have been thinking for years about these sorts of questions and might know exactly how to help Ruffin — without manufacturing a crisis.

At about this same time, Ruffin was just beginning to make observations about himself. For example, on the monkey bars at the park, "I am a monkey" while hanging by his hands. Ruffin liked to pretend to be different animals, a frog, and a bird frequently. He liked to pretend to be a scary animal and pretend an attack. It was a controlled, pretend attack that did not get out of hand. When I asked, "Where is Ruffin?" he pointed to his chest and said, "Ruffin lives in here." He pointed to mine, and said, "Mommy lives in there." These events and his instances of insight and pretense were memorable as Ruffin's one-offs, never terribly frequent. But wasn't this hopeful?

And this? Recently, Ruffin and I had been playing with a mother and baby kangaroo. They had been a gift from my youngest sister, Susan, last Christmas, of no interest to him then. I had taken up the baby and given him the mother. I began talking, pretending to be baby-Ruffin, doing all the things he did repeatedly, and saying all the things he said repeatedly. Ruffin responded for several minutes by playing the part of me — his mother. He responded to all my requests with the right "pretend" actions, and with spontaneous, appropriate remarks.

He really liked this game. We went on and on, and I ran him into the ground to let him experience what it was like to continually respond to his repeated demands. When he got tired of responding, he got a blanket and covered the kangaroos up to let me know he didn't want to play anymore.

Still, I felt I *was* learning. I could tell structure helped. "Structure prevents behavior problems. Structure stimulates learning." Being kept busy helped Ruffin, I thought. "Learning may be greater in independent-work settings, rather than in noisy, confusing groups. A single attending adult's active presence and attention, prompting and praising is important to laying a foundation for good future social behavior and communication."

Following these and other general suggestions harvested from Dr. Michael Powers' book had changed and come to guide nearly every interaction I sought with Ruffin. I rarely approached him now without thinking through my approach in advance. Because these suggestions had worked, I continued to use them, and offered them to Ruffin's educators.

No, Ruffin could not be left to figure out what was going on and what was worth attending to in groups. "Without structure, a child with autism may withdraw in groups even as small as 7 to 11 students." It was good that was going to be the size of our district's new ECSE class.

"Behavior problems may signal a given task is too difficult. For the moment. Go back to an easier task. End on success. Always. Task-analysis is crucial to the structured teaching of clear, consistent objectives in small logical steps." With Ruffin, that worked. "Eventual social integration with typically developing peers requires certain basic skills in the child with autism be pre-taught and requires careful planning and structure."

What else motivated Ruffin to talk? He wanted to be with us, his family, I thought. We could always call my parents. The technology of the phone would attract him. I called him over to watch me punch in the number, and then put the phone up to his ear so he could hear my mother answer and call my father to pick up the extension.

"Extension," Ruffin echoed — a new word he likely did not understand.

I could hear my mother asking him simple questions, "How are you, Ruffin?" "What did you do today?" to which he offered no response.

Then came her own news, "Today, I swam in the pool." "Today, Papa went fishing," to which he offered no responding news. After a minute or two, he handed the phone back to me. He was tired of this.

So, my parents and I began our visiting, our ruminations over Ruffin's autism. Before he had echoed as he did now occasionally, hadn't Ruffin communicated very well with gestures? Some of them were remarkable for their grace, beauty, and accompanying facial animation. My parents recalled such incidents, much commented on by family and strangers. I lived in this sort of hopeful memory, too, with my wishful thinking. Sometimes, I felt, it was all that sustained me.

Now, I reported, hopefully, "Ruffin's echolalia seems only to be immediate, not delayed." That is, it was limited to his parroting back words I said to him, or that he heard, but only shortly afterwards.

Ruffin was standing nearby, watching me on the phone, looking up — wanting something, I could tell.

"Do you want a cookie?"

"Cookie."

No, his echolalia had yet to elaborate and crystallize into many longer mega phrases uniquely connected to favorite bits of movies, song lyrics, or remnants of his own early experiences used to communicate in a way opaque to any listener not present at the creation — a type of behavior described by Kanner and Asperger in their early, classic papers of the 1940s. I was worried this delayed form of echolalia could develop in Ruffin as a downstream effect of his early communication delays if he were not taught to talk properly.

To my parents, I chattered on, "Ruffin understands the proper use of pronouns: you, I, and it. I've heard him use them occasionally, and correctly, in sentences about himself and me." But this represented my own wishful thinking, again, upon the rare instance. I told them about Ruffin at the park, and his pretending again with the kangaroos.

"Be sure to let Susan know," I asked my parents.

"Be sure to let his teacher know," counseled my mother.

"I will."

That night, I made a list of every word I could ever remember Ruffin having said repeatedly, with regularity — perhaps with understanding: "Wet, dry, mine, yours, yellow, hurry, wait, stop, let go, flying, upstairs, downstairs, go get, I show you, what is it, walk, eat, all gone, open this, close that, help."

In the morning, with Ruffin watching television, I worried, too, about Ruffin's eye gaze, his misplaced attention to the background of pictures and videos, and his failure to develop a more typical childlike focus on the narrative foreground of the story and its characters. Ruffin seemed more attentive to the background of videos and movies, picking out background objects, always his favorites: horses, trucks, and trains. He was enthralled by trains, sirens of all kinds, police, fire, ambulance, tornado warnings, chimes, doorbells, and church bells. Hearing any of these attracted his immediate attention and interrupted any other activity. He was also drawn to blinking lights, flipped light switches repeatedly off and on in our house, and seemed to be attracted by signs showing letters or numbers. Well, I might be imagining that.

Somehow, I felt anyone teaching Ruffin should be both encouraged by and warned about what I thought of as his personal peculiarities. "Ruffin does interact with things or events in odd, nonfunctional ways. We, Seamus and I, and his grandparents thought he was so creative. It is sad to think of this behavior as a symptom."

I was recalling a morning when I had opened the door to Ruffin's bedroom and found his crib disassembled into what looked like an open handful of pick-up sticks around his fallen mattress. Ruffin was not there. In how many nights, I wondered, had he unwound the metal bolts, their nuts, and washers, and then drawn out the several rods that were supposed to hold this crib together? Downstairs, I met a waist-high web of string in the pantry passageway off the kitchen. Ruffin must have walked from doorknob to doorknob to cabinet door to doorknob to cabinet door — every one on the first floor.

In the middle of this web, I found Ruffin sleeping — but there was no advance possible toward him.

I had to admire his construction, and to laugh with relief. But it would be a weekend morning's work to undo this. The sound of my scissors woke Ruffin and there was a tantrum. Ruffin's resistance was stronger than any I had ever met. I didn't think I could get the crib back together without help. We would need to wait for Seamus. When he walked in that afternoon, I told him. I took him upstairs and showed him, saying, "I hope he won't repeat this." I was afraid that he would. Ruffin liked to repeat any activity he discovered by himself. "I don't want to repeat this." Certainly not to anyone outside the family — not to anyone at school.

"Well, it might be time to think of buying him a toddler bed," Seamus suggested.

"What's that?" I asked.

Now that Seamus had his tools out, Ruffin was intrigued. Together, the two of them fixed a broken box fan, an event Ruffin remembered thereafter every time he glimpsed my screwdriver in our junk drawer. If something were interesting to Ruffin in the first place, he never forgot. Holding up his saw, Seamus reminded Ruffin of the tree they had cut down. Ruffin remembered that. Seamus asked if he remembered feeding the rabbits and the chickens. Ruffin remembered the big dog. I hadn't heard about that. I hadn't known to ask.

As for my vision of Ruffin's future, I shared what I hoped for at the time, and what I thought his educators would want to hear. "I feel comfortable with the choice to send Ruffin to you for a full school day. It was encouraging to see Ruffin talk with you and co-operate so well with all of you during the early August assessment. It makes me confident that you can reach him. Regardless of Ruffin's IQ test, his IQ of 50, or moderate mental retardation, I'd like to give him the best opportunity and strongest push toward learning to read and do math."

And, I may have lifted more than just a corner of the blanket dampening my fears about Ruffin's long-term future. "To read there is an expectation of post-pubertal decline is saddening. To read that even in adolescence, those with autism are still remarkably unable to match gender and age to appropriate behaviors and contexts, is dis-heartening." This had struck me as an alarming echo of Dr. Caldwell's prognosis that Ruffin would be unlikely ever to marry. "The milder degree of Ruffin's symptoms, his language, affectionateness, activity, hopefully his IQ, and your skilled intervention all make me hopeful for his progress. However, it is sad to learn that independent living and economic self-sufficiency are possible 'only for a very few.'" I was quoting Dr. Powers, but then it seemed more hopeful to close on another passage I had copied out of the *Encyclopedia* the night before Ruffin's MRI: "'The brightest of the passive autistic children, because of their amiability, as well as their useful skills, may manage fairly for normal children.'" This was my most fervent hope for Ruffin, and my goal I wanted to share with his educators.

I had other specific questions for Ruffin's educators — about speech therapy, about integration, mainstreaming or inclusion, about summer services and parent education, about my observing or volunteering in the classroom, about discipline there, and about how we would measure Ruffin's progress.

What I failed to appreciate was that Ruffin's and my first year in special education was our local school district's first year in special education, too. Our school board had been persuaded by Miss Hobbs that providing special education services closer to home might offer a savings over the earlier arrangement of busing children over to Decorah. The district had an obligation to save its taxpayers money. This was why Ruffin could attend school in our town.

Since my parents were back in North Carolina, where my father was still working for IBM, Seamus suggested I consider hiring a friend of his, a local woman, Rose Ward, to come in daily to clean up the house a bit and cook dinner. And keep me company, I imagined, so he need not always be expected to drop by. Ruffin's odder behaviors had begun to unnerve Seamus, more and more, all through last winter and most of the spring and summer. Certainly, all my obsessive talk and uninterrupted reading about autism since the July diagnosis unnerved him and seemed to put him off. There didn't seem to be much I could do about any of that now. I just felt overwhelmed on every side, and at every turn. So, I agreed, yes, Seamus could bring Rose by.

Rose was an early blessing in our upended lives. Tall, lanky, with a brown bowl of hair that resisted ever going grey, she was an awkward heron of a woman, long armed and flappy. The youngest of a brood of a dozen raised in Minot, North Dakota, she had moved to our town, when she got married. Divorced by then, still devoutly Catholic, the mother of a grown and long-gone daughter, she kept a small, messy house of her own, cleaned mine sloppily, broke things, chipped the porcelain of sinks and toilets, and was, at best, an indifferent cook.

Blustering in from her shift work as an order-picker on the button-factory floor in our river town of Lansing, she was never silent, not for a single moment. When Seamus dropped by, to check in about suppertime, he and Rose could swap small talk for a solid hour, over the hissing grease, gossiping about their wide mutual acquaintance, the running soap opera on Rose's factory floor. Her unrequited crush on her boss. Her grumbling over the other women on the floor determined to trip her up so she stumbled or fell, or who snuck cards of stapled buttons out of her orders behind her back, so her orders were returned by customers and made her look bad.

Ruffin and I sat at his computer, working through nouns and verbs, prepositions, and numbers, dragging and dropping squares, rectangles, and triangles, building virtual houses or churches. I called, "Seamus, come look."

Rose rattled on then with no listener, alone in my kitchen. For a hot meal of anything, to have Seamus feel comfortable here, I let her endless small talk wash over us, wash everything else away. Rose would be with us, until Ruffin was almost seven. I came to appreciate and depend upon her welcome appearance, and her undemanding stream of self-absorption.

Four days before school was set to begin, an assembled group of us — Ruffin's IEP team — were shepherded out of the commodious air-conditioned office, around a tiled corner, down a hallway, and into a very summery-warm and very-new-just-that-year ECSE classroom. Inside, a low table was set with tiny wooden chairs appropriate to a group of preschoolers. Not my size, and not a comfortable size for our stately woman-principal, Miss Hobbs, who steered herself and the group of us like an ocean liner. She also served as the special education director at the local district level.

Although I had carefully assembled thick Binderteks of medical records and treatment information — representing all I had learned so far about Ruffin and autism, and all the questions I had — it was immediately clear from the size of the chairs, ours was planned to be a short meeting. Which it was. Of mutual dismissal.

Ruffin's first IEP which issued from this meeting was a brief document on thin pink carbon paper, missing its first page, and mailed to me later. The educators in attendance that day were Inge, Emily, Miss Hobbs, and Ruffin's classroom teacher, Meg Holub. The speech and language pathologist Kim Pope who had been assigned to Ruffin was not present. A faint memory remains of delivering her copy of my Bindertek later, awkwardly.

Not that I ever witnessed it, but Ruffin's classroom teacher, Meg, had scribbled to catch up with the earlier evaluation findings of early August. Obviously, there had been a meeting before our IEP meeting — some meeting of the Bridgewater team, with Meg catching up, and without inviting me — anticipating that Meg would know somehow how to teach Ruffin and that I, as Ruffin's mother would agree, gratefully.

At the meeting I was invited to, I looked over to study Meg. She was tall enough to be particularly uncomfortable seated on a toddler chair, and her heavy, honey-colored hair weighed her head down as she bent over the handful of papers that Inge passed her. When Meg looked up in my direction, I could see her face was thin and worn. She was obviously nearer the end of her career than the beginning. Hopefully, then, she would be patient with Ruffin, and kind.

The IEP's second page began with the ritual statement of Ruffin's present levels of educational performance (PLEP) — the sound of a flipped pancake, nicely brown on the side listing his strengths, stippled on the other side with bubble-holes of his weaknesses. In this instance, a fair summary, and based on someone's careful reading of my recent notes and Bridgewater's early August evaluation.

This PLEP provided a foundation for three annual teaching goals, each of which was broken down further into three or four short-term objectives.

As to every annual goal and short-term objective, I was named as a person equally responsible to see to Ruffin's learning, along with Meg, and her aide, Ella Meyer. The speech and language pathologist's assignment was limited to the achievement of language goals, and Kim was excused from any responsibility to increase Ruffin's playfulness. No methods, teaching procedures, or suggestions were offered in the document to me or to anyone else about how to make any of this progress happen. Progress was assumed to arise out of the ordinary best practices of a self-contained ECSE classroom, described to me in our meeting as "watered down Head Start." Progress would be evaluated by Meg's observations, as she might choose to chart them.

One of Ruffin's objectives would be to "verbally identify the basic emotions of happy, sad, mad, and angry at appropriate times 85% of the time." I already knew from my reading that this was an especially difficult task for young children, and even older adults, with autism. It was difficult to teach, and often required one-to-one direct instruction.

Very cynically, at this low moment, as truly a mother-from-hell, I murmured to myself, how lovely it was to know the educational authorities considered sadness and anger to be appropriate emotions at times. At least I had known better than to come out with any of this at our face-to-face meeting and make it worse for Ruffin. I sat and listened on my toddler chair. I had contained myself. It had been uncomfortable. I had managed to hold in my outrage. Helpless, I had gotten through it. With the product of that shockingly brief meeting now in hand, I felt sad, angry, dull, and utterly demoralized.

When I tried to discuss how I felt about this meeting with Seamus, he said the same thing my mother did. He often did that. I suppose it was one reason why I fell in love with him. They were both easy-going, practical people. I reminded myself, you need to give the school a chance. You'll be getting free childcare.

Thankfully, though Ruffin and I lived in town, within easy walking distance of Ruffin's classroom at the elementary school, because he would have to cross a busy state highway of hurtling bulk milk trucks, long aluminum trailers of livestock, pigs, and cattle, Ruffin would be provided the related service of *portal-to-portal transportation*, from home to school and back in a stubby school bus dedicated to students with disabilities.

The legal justification for his educators offering Ruffin special education instructional programs with support and related services was also given. "Ruffin needs the help available from the self-contained ECSE class to reach his potential. He will be receiving speech and language therapy with a focus on increasing his expressive skills."

Again, there was no focus on increasing *receptive* language. No use or mention of computers. No arrangements for the administration of his special vitamins, or DMG. No parent training. I was willing to do my part to help teach Ruffin and wanted to know how. Despite my overriding dismay because of this meeting and this thin plan in writing, I remained eager to begin.

CHAPTER FIVE

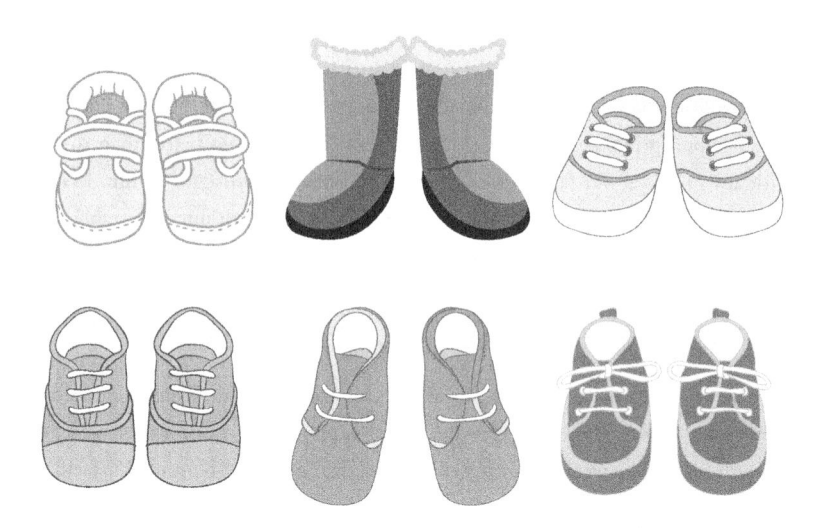

SCHOOL BEGINS

Ruffin began school August 29th. His classmates were five boys with various milder disabilities, and two visiting girls from a classroom across the hallway pointed out to me by Miss Hobbs, as also new that year — for "the severe and profound." Whenever I could, I took Ruffin to school and picked him up. He was too little, and without language, too vulnerable to ride a bus safely, even the stubby bus, although I needed to let him try because I had to have him ride over to Julie's daycare whenever I got stuck in late afternoon hearings or might be driving home from several counties distant.

That first day, though, I carried Ruffin in with a spiral notebook in which I had written, "Mrs. Holub and Miss Meyer, Ruffin's blanket is in his backpack. He went to bed about 9:30 last night. He knows he is going to school. We talked about your names and the bus. This weekend Ruffin rode on a tractor. He also fed rabbits and chickens." On Seamus's farm. He nearly always took Ruffin on Sunday afternoons for several hours. I needed them to make last-minute preparations for Monday's early morning motion day, to have my papers in order when my cases were called, beginning at 8:30 when the travelling judge arrived in town for the day. I might have any number of arraignments or sentencings or probation revocation proceedings or default divorces to prove up, with the same sort of motion day on Tuesday the next county west, and the same on Wednesday the next county south.

I suggested to Ruffin's educators that we could encourage Ruffin to open conversations if we sent notes back and forth about what had happened recently at home or school. The notebook I handed Meg on Ruffin's first day began a warm, daily exchange. The moment I walked out the door, Meg had run up against some of Ruffin's personal rigidities.

"Mary Jane, first hour, Ruffin would not take off his boots to put on shoes. I made the mistake of telling him no toys until boots off. Sorry. We *almost* got him to carry the boots to his locker on a toy truck, but at the last minute he figured us out. Later, we had a group time, which he participated in very well, attended to everyone's turn and appeared eager to have a turn. After that, we ignored the boots."

To which, I offered some commiseration, "We have two new pairs of shoes Ruffin picked out. He won't wear either one of them. Just barn boots!"

Meg stumbled across something of a solution later. "We put out his shoes and hid his boots during his nap and Ruffin let me put his shoes on afterward. He didn't even seem to notice all day."

Since Ruffin and most of his classmates were young enough to still have toileting accidents, I also warned Meg early on, "About Ruffin's change of clothes, Ruffin has one definite eccentricity. He has a 'princess and the pea' problem with tags and labels in the neck and waist of new clothing. He will or may say 'scissors' to ask you to cut the tags and labels out and won't put on dry clothes until they are completely free of labels and tags. It is okay to cut the tags and labels out of the new outfit I brought you. Sorry, I forgot."

When Meg let me know, "He's been tugging at his left ear some during the day. You may want to watch it," I was grateful. "Thanks for watching his ears. I'm getting my own ear examination instrument and our pharmacist is going to teach me how to use it. We need to practice at home so Ruffin will let his doctors examine him."

Also, on the very first day of school, Meg had raised another thorny issue. "Lunch, I need to talk to you."

About lunch, I replied, "At daycare, Ruffin is a fussy eater. He won't eat hot dogs, French fries, or junk food. He likes any fruit and almost any vegetable, for example, carrots. He likes lean meat. He can have anything off the lunch menu that is fruit or vegetable. I agree, you should try new things first. He won't starve. Somedays he eats, somedays not. His nutritionist at Gundersen tells me his is normal enough three-year-old behavior. Ruffin needs to stay away from artificial colors and flavors. I make an exception for special treats that are being shared around a group of kids for social reasons."

I didn't want Meg or anyone else in our town to think of me as overly politically correct or rigid. Ours was a very conservative community.

Meg remained persistent in brainstorming ways to get Ruffin to eat with her group at school.

"We've decided to put some of his own food from home on his tray before we bring it in, so he doesn't think he can have extra food if he refuses what's on his plate. That way we know he has something he will eat without having any concern about his refusing lunch."

By using this technique, Meg succeeded in getting Ruffin to eat corn, carrots, and applesauce.

Then, Meg raised the next problem.

"We've been trying to get Ruffin to use hand sanitizer right before lunch. He hates it, but with all these children sharing toys, we feel it's important. I have been squirting it on my hands and rubbing it on him. He hollers, but I tell him, 'Wash it off' right away and he settles down immediately. Does he use bar soap at home? I can try that instead."

Right, Ruffin would not use soap at home.

"Ruffin hates the feeling of soap! But he likes to be clean. Take him to a mirror and let him see the dirt. At home, he likes to wash with water in front of the mirror. Then I use the word 'Better.'"

All these small issues represented different examples of the sensory sensitivities I had read about as common in young children with autism. Throughout the fall and winter, Ruffin's eating, sleeping, toileting, changing clothes, and whispering at school proved to be inconsistent, unpredictable, and mildly but recurrently troublesome. Meg and I continued to write and talk often to report back and forth to problem solve together to keep school a positive experience for Ruffin.

I had been worried about Ruffin riding the bus after his first day of school. Julie warned me Ruffin had looked very startled when put off the bus. By the time I came to pick him up later, I saw no ill effects. He was playing with a little girl and didn't especially want to go home.

In the car, I tried to talk about school and the bus.

"You're big enough for school, Ruffin."

I got a nod, and an echo out of him, "School."

"Big enough to ride the bus," I added.

Another smiling nod from Ruffin, but no echo.

He had enjoyed school, then. He was happy.

Stopping to pick up milk from the convenience store, with Ruffin struggling to bring me two gallons, I got another echo. "One is enough."

"One."

Back in the car I tried asking about the long cloth tunnel at daycare. "That was scary, wasn't it?" but we weren't there. Ruffin didn't remember. It had been a long day. He was tired.

By the end of the first week in September though, I was able to write Meg, "Julie says Ruffin was very proud coming off the bus today. His status at daycare among the other children has risen on account of his arriving by bus." And, by the next day, "This afternoon Ruffin said 'Goodbye' to his bus driver when prompted by Julie. He also made a spontaneous remark to her which included her name and pleased her very much."

Even Meg's aide, Ella, joined in writing in our notebook on occasion. "During lunchtime today when Ruffin was eating, a piece of celery got caught in his throat, and out loud he said, 'Get that out of my mouth!' and then he proceeded to take it out and threw it on the floor and said, 'Yuk.' It was pretty cute."

I was encouraged. I responded, "Glad to hear Ruffin is talking out loud. He has spoken out loud in other emergency situations." I was remembering an earlier time at daycare, after he began vitamin therapy, Ruffin had yelled 'Watch out' to other children who were too close to the edge of a step. To Ella and Meg, I suggested, "When Ruffin whispers, try saying 'Talk out loud.' He will then speak louder. We have talked about 'loud' and 'soft' and whispering. I say 'loud,' loudly, and 'soft,' softly, when I address this."

Meg replied, "Today, he echoed out loud, 'Hi, Ruffin,' when he came in and we greeted him."

Again, this pleased me, and I offered more encouragement. "I think that if Ruffin echoes a greeting like 'Hi, Ruffin' you might want to try saying, 'No, please say, Hi, Mrs. Holub,' and when he echoes 'Holub' which he probably will, say 'Better.' This is a word he understands."

At home I tried to praise Ruffin whenever he spoke out loud. He was still whispering some at home. In the morning, when he came in to wake me, he knew to whisper, but even then, I would say, "You can talk out loud." And, when he could sense I might say "No," to something he thought he needed — a glass figurine off the shelf, my favorite fountain pen of worked sterling over black lacquer that I used when translating — he would also whisper. "No, talk out loud," I would say and prompt him to respond twice before moving on. This whispering was a babyish form of getting me to feel sorry for him and relent. Whenever I got a loud response, I praised Ruffin ecstatically, and granted his request if possible. "Ruffin," I had wailed, as he dropped my silver pen deep in the fins of the hallway radiator. I knew where it was. Seamus had some tool to fish it out. Later though — because here came the bus.

And because this sort of simple thing seemed to work with Ruffin, I found myself becoming more and more consciously, a budding behaviorist.

While Ruffin was in school, I spent several hours meeting with the parents of two older children with autism who lived near our town, and the mothers of two brothers and a little girl from two neighboring counties. These families formed the core of a local autism support group that met irregularly, aiming for once a month. Each family struggled with different issues since every child with autism seemed to present differently. There weren't that many of us. We usually met up for pizza, to commiserate and swap stories about our children, our various experiences of frustration and rare success.

From these families, I learned about several nearly nonverbal movies starring live animals as main characters that had a unique appeal to a great many children with autism. After a brief trip to the library, I settled Ruffin on the sofa and we tried watching *The Black Stallion*, about a boy and a horse surviving a shipwreck. Ruffin stayed right with it and seemed to enjoy it. This was the first "story" I had seen Ruffin follow and be concerned about. It had almost no dialogue — very visual. Ruffin "narrated" some parts, saying after me, "Horse hurt," "Scary water," 'Scary snake," "Climb rocks," and 'Swim."

Later, we watched another film recommended as a favorite of several other boys with autism, *Otis and Milo*, which I found very wooden, a perils of Pauline plot starring a cat and dog, just one peril after another, all of them dreadfully mild. Ruffin laughed all the way through at each surprisingly wrong turn. The other parents in our support group had said their boys had just adored this film. Ruffin certainly did.

He continued to be enthralled by *Otis and Milo* and *The Black Stallion* and mentions of these two movies littered his home-school notebook throughout the fall. They were both valuable in teaching Ruffin how to follow a narrative, a story over time, and in establishing talk about cause and effect, and in teaching Ruffin the names of a few emotions by offering my comments for his immediate echo. I was alert by then to every word Ruffin spoke, and to what triggered him to speak.

With Ruffin in school, I had time to set up more activities on Ruffin's new computer. Just after Labor Day, I let Meg know, "Ruffin played with *Bailey's Book House*, identifying letters, and then made and printed a story." Every week, Lois Fergus from the Y would send us a package from Cedar Rapids. "Look what's here," I would say as Ruffin walked in the door off the bus. "Do you want to open it?" Ruffin would set to work. This was something he could do. "Scissors?" "Well, let Mommy do that part, okay?" And Ruffin would tear the brown paper wrapping away to find the colorful box of the newest computer program inside.

This time it was *Grandma and Me*. Perfect, I thought. We could talk about it on the phone, too. Ruffin knew where to find the computer disc inside, and how to slip it carefully into the right horizontal slot. It was up and running, and Ruffin would be busy for the better part of a half-hour. He found episodes and features in the programs that I never discovered — because he tried every possibility, persistently. He found a few things he particularly liked, and did them repeatedly, but he did move on steadily without perseverating on any one thing. He didn't get "stuck."

Over the next weekend, Ruffin played *Grandma and Me* for several stretches. He discovered how to get into the Japanese language version and found that hilarious, maybe because I couldn't understand the language. As he clicked the mouse on a character and the character moved — danced, flew a kite, swam, jumped — we talked about the verbs.

Ruffin had no problem moving the cursor around the screen with the mouse. He discovered he could double-click to get into different programs. He learned how to exit and enter among three different programs, easily. By mid-September, Ruffin began exploring his newest computer program *Sammy's Science House*. This program was more challenging because it required Ruffin to "point, drag and release" the mouse. After my demonstration, he did this with good success. He enjoyed it, and I watched, cheering him on from over his shoulder, as he did well on a sorting game. He liked the movie game, which seemed designed to construct an ongoing narrative. As always, he tried all the games.

Daily, Meg and I continued to share developments and events in Ruffin's life, probably because they struck one or the other of us as unusual. Meg let me know, "We pretended today. Ruffin had a toy car, so I sent him to the store to get something. He drove the car across the table to the puzzle, which we said was the store, and brought the car back. He made several trips for things I 'forgot.'" To which I replied with real admiration, "Thank you for inviting Ruffin to pretend. How clever of you to forget so many things! Ruffin gave me his name tag, saying, 'Put on neck, Mommy.'"

Of course, I told everything to my parents. I mentioned little things to Seamus when I could get a word in edgewise around Rose.

Then, just before Labor Day, Meg reported that Ruffin was having trouble sharing. "Ruffin didn't want to let his classmate have the green tractor although the other little boy had it first. I had to take his hands and remove them, but he was readily distracted to help Ella vacuum. Later I made sure he had a turn with the tractor, so he knows everyone gets a turn. Ruffin seemed pleased when we made sure his classmate gave him a turn." In a typical nursery school, a child might be asked to leave had this behavior failed to get better. Ruffin had the impulse to share *sometimes*.

At home, a nine-year-old girl whom he knew well visited and wanted to play with Ruffin's computer. Ruffin let her have a turn. When he wanted it back, he said, out loud and repeatedly, "My chair, please." He was home. He knew this little girl well, Danielle, the daughter of the couple from whom I had bought our Victorian.

When Ruffin returned to school after Labor Day, Meg let me know, "Ruffin's classmate, Ruffin and I discussed what happened with the green tractor. I'm not sure how much Ruffin understood, but I wanted to try." I seriously doubted that Ruffin understood much — not with his severe receptive language delay and his difficulty recalling past events with other people. At the time, I wondered just how big a tantrum Ruffin must have thrown earlier, and worried.

Based upon some early videos Sue had suggested, I tried various activities at home as a nascent, untrained behaviorist to see how Ruffin might respond. To make an adventure of it, with Ruffin holding my hand, we walked down Main Street, past the bank and the post office, past the hardware store — which Ruffin found hard to pass up — past the jewelry store, and the bar, to the five-and-dime where we could buy construction paper. Since he could see we were buying something interesting and colorful — for him — Ruffin was well-behaved in the store. We came home. I cut out 4 different shapes in 5 primary colors. Then I put down the largest piece of each color and handed the 3 smaller pieces of each color to Ruffin, saying "Put it with blue." Or "Put it with yellow," if I had handed him yellow. He liked this game that just required him to match the colors. He was unable to spontaneously name them, but he was good at matching them — just as he was good at those matching games on his computer.

Then, Ruffin tore the mouth off a face he had made at school, and gave it to me, saying, "Over," and turning it upside down. I pointed to it, laughing, and said, "Beard." I was thinking of Seamus, who had one. We taped the mouth back on the face upside down. We talked about sad and happy. Then put the mouth back on as "happy." Finally, we assembled a picture board for Ruffin's weekday: bus, school, bus, Julie, Mommy's car, home, supper, bath, and bed. Ruffin recognized the bus, my car, and home right away. Using the pictures, he was prepared to take, and calmly took, a bath. And seemed pleased with his clean hair.

Worse was when I needed to warn Meg that Ruffin would be tired. He often woke up mornings well before dawn and had been up for hours — talking and rehearsing his sentences before the bus arrived. Early in September, he came into my room, crawled up on the bed, wanting a tummy and back rub, reaching out to use my hand as a tool, and seemed to feel ill. He wanted some water, was very affectionate, but then made some explosive babble and struck out hard, fell immediately into a short, deep sleep, then came wide awake, asked for food, ate, and went back to sleep with just a little talking to lull himself.

Was this striking out hard and falling into deep sleep a fit? Except for that brief episode, his talking that night was in coherent sentences — most of them as instructions and in two "voices:" "Put that down," "Come here," "Stop," "I go get it," with replies of "Okay," "I coming," "Okay," "I have it."

Ruffin's following-directions work paper Meg sent home to me showed his roughly scribbled coloring within and widely beyond the boundaries of its pre-drawn circles. Her notes on his paper indicated these circles were scribbled over after Meg had shown him another student's paper, meaning that Ruffin required visual support for verbal directions. This showed his weakness in receptive language, in understanding what was said, as foundational to any success in expressive language, in speaking with meaning.

At this point, I began to wonder if all this special education was anything more than glorified babysitting. Safe enough. Paper games, and picture boards. As I thought about them, they all seemed more appropriate to nonverbal children with autism, like most of the children whose parents I was coming to know. However, Ruffin *could* speak, as Seamus had pointed out. He could *echo* what he heard. None of these games and pictures seemed to be an effective means of teaching Ruffin to talk or catch up to his typically developing age-mates. Whatever the parents of older children with autism were doing, I began to realize that Ruffin being in school, being safely watched for the day, meant I needed to take more time for reading and research to look for better answers, for Ruffin. Seamus wasn't doing any research himself. That had never been his strong suit. He was deeply interested in history, but his graduate studies in that subject had foundered on the requirement for disciplined research.

Throughout the remainder of August and early September, I lay on my bed upstairs to plunder all the resources from the back pages of my new sacred texts, my new Bibles: *Negotiating the Special Education Maze: Children With Autism: A Parent's Guide*; *The Handbook of Autism and Pervasive Developmental Disorders;* and from the notes of my long-distance calls with Sue. In those days before Amazon, I launched a raft of letters to order all the books mentioned in these sources or by her as being more narrowly focused on autism. Having already found the vitamin and DMG information in the current issue so helpful, I ordered every available back issue of Dr. Bernard Rimland's *Autism Research Review Internatio*nal newsletter — now helpfully archived online — and his early prize-winning book.

I read every night, and all day. As I read, I threw each arriving book to one side of my bed, or the other: good books, ones that seemed sound science, to one side, for re-reading later; silly books, about how your child just needs our colored lenses, suggestions for sitting on the floor together with your child, playing with his or her feces if necessary — all the quick, complete, and apparent miracle cures, to the other, far side — as a waste of money. There had been a lot of nonsense written about autism.

When I asked, my longtime trial partner readily agreed to summarize the earlier depositions I had taken of the school board members we were suing for our clients, the superintendent and his supporters. We weren't scheduled to be back before the judge until mid-November. A murder trial came up. Our judge let us know he would be busy with that. I had to answer the phone, of course, to keep on top of the cases for my local clients. That's what my bedroom extension was for — that and the late-night calls from jail, after an arrest. But, until I found a better answer for Ruffin, I referred any new inquiries, every possible new client, to other colleagues.

On the near side of my bed there remained a thin scatter, three books I judged worthy of re-reading:

Bernard Rimland, Ph.D., Navy psychologist, father of a son, Mark, *Infantile Autism: The Syndrome and Its Implications for a Neural Theory of Behavior.*

Dorothy Beavers, Ph.D., chemist, mother of a son, Leo, *Autism: Nightmare Without End.*

Catherine Maurice, Ph.D. in French literature, mother of a daughter, Anne-Marie and a son, Michel, *Let Me Hear Your Voice.*

Were I reading now, I might add:

Gary Mayerson, J.D., lawyer, father of a son, *How To Compromise With Your School District Without Compromising Your Child* and *Autism's Declaration of Independence.*

Shannon Penrod, mother of a son, *AUTISM, Parent to Parent: Sanity-Saving Advice for Every Parent with a Child on the Autism Spectrum.*

All these were authored by observant, intelligent, and clearly loving parents. These, I would re-read mindfully, highlighters in hand.

Seamus and I seemed to be driven apart by Ruffin's strange behavior for the first time ever in our relationship. It crossed my mind he might have found someone else to see. This was a problem I couldn't do anything about. I knew better than to raise any argument with Seamus about where he had disappeared to recently — for as long as a week or more. He had farm animals, and a new night-shift factory job across the river in Wisconsin. A long commute. He needed to sleep sometime, during the afternoon. Seamus loved to run around, here and there, in and out of everyone else's business; to auctions, to livestock sales, to exotic animal swaps, to cut grass in cemeteries, to right and repair headstones. He was a fully social creature. So, I took my solace in reading. It was hard enough for me just to get Ruffin up every morning, dressed, fed, and out of the house. Only then could I retreat to my second-story bedroom and read, among the briefly brilliant leaves of boulevard trees sweeping my windows.

Re-reading Rimland's early prize-winning book, I came to appreciate how definitively he broke the back of Bruno Bettelheim's elaborately embroidered Freudian fantasies about autism, tales woven out of Bettelheim's boundless narcissism. Eventually, I ran across a 1997 biography of Bettelheim, *The Creation of Dr. B: A Biography of Bruno Bettelheim*, by journalist Richard Pollak, whose brother with autism had been ill-treated by Bettelheim. Dorothy, too, described how she was plagued in the 1960s when Bettelheim's 1967 book *The Empty Fortress* had appeared and as a result her co-workers had suddenly began to exhibit cold, hostile feelings towards her when "cooperation and friendship had existed before." As late as 1988, Catherine had been more than a bit pestered by her French in-laws' reading "the ever vigilant and feverish Freudians." Both Dorothy and Catherine agreed with Bernie regarding the lack of any meaningful help from the Freudian psychoanalysts of Bettelheim's school, or their speculations about autism and its origins. Joining in their scorn of the psychoanalytical, both Freudian and post-Freudian, I found myself reading much more pragmatically.

Autism: Nightmare Without End by Dorothy Beavers was written in the 1960s when there was nothing to be done about autism. When there was no known cause and no known cure. When autism, then often mistaken for schizophrenia, and its early diagnosis were rare. As I read her story, I found much to take warning of, and much to take comfort from, in her warm, wise, frank, unsparing witness to her life with her husband and Leo.

Most importantly, Dorothy offered me the comfort of knowing that my passing temptation to commit suicide after doing away with my own child, was hardly unique. Dorothy pointed out other pitfalls and dangers. She advised avoiding becoming a total recluse — as if I were not already one by my writerly temperament, bound by the confidences of others I held in my profession, and by long-standing personal circumstance, having accepted my arms-length relationship with Seamus as it was. Before Ruffin was born, I had admitted to myself, it worked for me. No socks to pick up, no hamster-wheel of three daily meals, none of the irritations presented by two sets of unchangeable personal habits. Just brief joy, great swathes of time to work, to write and to read, to travel and to publish, to laze or to walk. But now I couldn't seem to recapture any of that joy. I felt a sharp pang of envy for Dorothy's supportive and loving husband, even as she herself felt the two of them lived "a fragmented life."

Also, easily recognizable in Ruffin were the signs and symptoms that Dorothy described in Leo — aggression, pain insensitivity, initial suspicion of deafness — which helped me put away any temptation to run after a second, dissenting diagnostic opinion. And, love was present, resonantly, in Dorothy. "But I think in our case the tragedy went even deeper. Leo was our only child, and we had waited ten years for him." So, love was not enough. Fair warning.

If a young child's home environment didn't cause autism, then what did? Since the mid-1990s, an increasing incidence of diagnoses on the autism spectrum has been reported by the Centers for Disease Control — now 1 in every 36 young children — up explosively from the reported incidence in the mid-1990s, of Ruffin as the rare 1 in 15,000 births.

Under pressure from organized parent groups, sometimes with funding raised by parents, given the constraints of government funding for fundamental research, science is beginning to pick up the pace of autism research, into brain research, brain imaging, the sequencing of duplications and deletions in parts of the genome essential to neurological development, into environmental exposures as triggers and into epigenetics, the study of changes in organisms caused by modifications of gene expression rather than alteration of the genetic code itself. Answers are beginning to emerge.

Current thinking on the causes of autism suggests there may be various genetic susceptibilities, triggered by various epigenetic or environmental insults. But none of this research or speculation has helped much — certainly not by leading to any effective non-behavioral treatment.

That there might be some genetic link was strongly suggested early on by many published twin studies, with which Dorothy was familiar. It is predominately males, especially first-born males, who are afflicted with autism or severe genetic disorders. Girls are far less likely to have serious genetic defects than boys.

Given the early reports of transient autism symptoms with heavy metal poisoning, now confirmed by recent findings of high residues in shed baby-teeth, given that Kanner's and Asperger's classic papers on autism had their roots in Germany and Austria, I paused to consider Seamus's own history. A combat veteran of the Vietnam War, and a brown-water Navy man, he was heavily exposed to Agent Orange sprayed over his swift boat as it traveled widely through the Mekong Delta.

My pregnancy took place in rural Iowa, among corn and soybean fields of monocrops rendered virtually weed-free by heavy applications of chemical pesticides, running off into all the little streams, leaching into rural wells like my own.

And, as with Dorothy and her husband, both Seamus and I were older parents: I at thirty-seven; Seamus, at forty-four. Recent research suggests a small risk of autism with older fathers, as there has long been a known risk of Down syndrome with older mothers. But did I have the time, or inclination, now, in this rocky patch, to blame either Seamus or myself? No. Instead, we and Ruffin had precious little time to get on top of our immediate problems, and none to waste on any inclination to blame.

I was led to take a deeper dive into the autism treatment and research literature than Ruffin's doctors and teachers, because — together with Seamus, or not — I was Ruffin's mother. These professionals would eventually return Ruffin to us — maybe just to me — in the end. Fairly or unfairly, I had no time to waste on uninformed professionals and underpaid non-professionals who might compound what were our real difficulties with useless outrages. By now, both common sense as well as the best published, peer-reviewed scientific psychological research I had read so far suggested that any treatment for autism with a fair chance of success was bound to take more than an hour a week of any therapy.

Surprisingly enough, it took extraordinarily little time for uninformed or sub-standard treatment to ingrain poor behaviors which all too quickly became self-rewarding to the child and then, became difficult to un-teach or extinguish. Even today, a Medicaid-funded near-minimum wage respite care worker or sitter or teacher or teacher's aide untrained or unskilled in good behavioral practice might do a young child with autism more harm than good, and might amount to less quality care than Dorothy's 1960s-era solution of seeking help from the Society for Prevention of Cruelty to Children in order to hire a full-time licensed practical nurse to care for Leo during his first five years while he was able to continue to live at home.

Throughout this early period, I kept close to my heart Bernie's and Dorothy's abiding message, "It was not the professionals who helped us (it was ourselves, together with other parents)." Dorothy had noted that "operant conditioning seems to have the most promise in teaching autistic children. Dr. Loovas from UCLA is one of the major proponents of this technique." From my series of TEACCH volumes, I knew *Lovaas* was the correct spelling. Ole Ivar Lovaas, Ph.D.

Lovaas had come to the United States from Norway, as a college exchange student to study music, in the 1950s. He had come to Luther College, where I had taught creative writing, briefly as an adjunct, to an area where immigrant Norwegians had settled, in Decorah, Iowa. I had practiced there, my first decade as a lawyer. Norwegian was still spoken in the Social Security Office. It was just over twenty short miles from where Ruffin and I lived.

Eventually, Lovaas had settled into a long and controversial career of psychological laboratory research into autism at UCLA. There, he and his graduate students developed techniques of operant conditioning or behavior modification to teach children with autism — to talk.

His early research was not without controversy, however, resulting from his early use of aversives. For patients *in extremis*, in the late 1950s Lovaas had used electric shock to treat those developmentally disabled children and adults who engaged in extreme self-injury such as eye gouging, eardrum piercing, and head-banging. Such self-injurious behavior had put their parents to harder choices than I ever faced, having caught Ruffin's autism early before these extreme behaviors developed.

Despite the noise and unpleasantness around this issue of aversives, I could see Catherine and her husband Marc had managed to come to a reasonable treatment decision for their two children. "In our home program, however, no therapist ever used any physical aversive. The most restraining thing we did was to keep Anne-Marie in the chair when she would rather have crumpled to the floor, although some people would consider that very aversive indeed. After all, the sessions were going to be in our home. Surely, we could have some control over what went on under our own roof."

Aversive practices were largely abandoned by Lovaas and later behaviorists as they developed the techniques of *extinction* — a disciplined, strictly objective practice that attention be given rewardingly by the therapists, parents, and caregivers when, and only when, a disabled person was, momentarily or accidentally at first, *not* engaging in self-injury. Undue attention given to any unwanted behavior ran the risk of increasing the occurrence of unwanted behavior. Everything, everything was a behavior. To be watched, encouraged, and rewarded if good; ignored and extinguished if undesirable.

In making my own decisions for Ruffin's treatment, I considered, too, how clear it was that without being able to learn, Ruffin might remain permanently subject to other, severe risks common to children with untreated autism — jumping out of a moving car, climbing an electrical or water tower, or lighting out across a cornfield. I found it difficult, as most parents do, to think of disciplining a child with disabilities, whom we may suspect has no real grasp of the concept of punishment, whether intellectually or morally. Still, at desperate junctures, I considered cutting off the electricity to Ruffin's room to put an end to his staying up all night.

Lovaas himself described his 1987 research: "According to our data, 47% of the autistic children we treated before the age of three-and-a-half attained normal intellectual functioning and passed first grade in a normal school by the age of seven. Recent follow-up data, taken when the children we treated averaged thirteen years of age, showed that their treatment gains were maintained and that their cognitive, emotional, and social functioning still appeared normalized."

Lovaas's prescription for successful treatment of autism was: one-to-one direct instruction, 40 hours per week, for 2 years between ages 2 to 5. In practice, a rotating team of therapists delivered one-to-one instruction, each working in about 40-minute sessions, because providing the instruction itself was exceptionally demanding and rigorous and required careful data collection while interacting with the child. Of course, the child ended up working the longest and hardest.

In 1993, Lovaas's research outcomes for his recovered group looked like the kind of results I was willing to gamble for on Ruffin's behalf: average IQ, mainstream schooling, and socially indistinguishable behavior from age-mates by his early teens.

Throughout the mid-1990s, parents like me around the country and around the world began trying to mount programs of early intensive applied behavior analysis (ABA) treatment and instruction, with each family making determined, often isolated efforts to translate Lovaas's published laboratory research into our homes. These were isolated, fragile family efforts, because special educators or state departments of education were unlikely to read, much less take to heart, peer-reviewed scientific literature written in academia. Surprisingly, to those of us, just naïve parents wandering into these embattled arenas, research psychologists did not publish to school psychologists. The two psychological disciplines and literatures did not communicate with each other.

From 1993 and on into the following decade, controversies about Lovaas shifted to arguments about whether other researchers or behavioral practitioners would ever be able to reproduce Lovaas's claimed, long-term results. School districts facing parental demands for more effective special education practices in autism, and reckoning up the costs of these parental demands, remained quick to seize upon the lack of published replication by other researchers as a reason it would be "inappropriate" for parents to ask public schools to offer a Lovaas program of instruction to their children.

But, by 2005, Lovaas's results *were* replicated by other practitioners, and again showed that 47% of children could achieve normal functioning and go on to succeed in regular education without assistance; 43% could make significant progress, but continued to demonstrate language delays; and, sadly, 10% would make little to no progress. When the U.S. Surgeon General then issued opinions supportive of early intensive ABA, these continued to fall on deaf ears. Professional educators don't subscribe to the opinions of the U.S. Surgeon General either — not when they already have their own established literature, customs, best practices, and comfortably accepted constraints, as well as national organizations of school district defense counsel ready to charge them hundreds of dollars per hour to defend their comfort zones.

Now that the early lack-of-replication argument has become groundless, and the U.S. Surgeon General has weighed in, school districts need to get cracking. Future behavioral and educational research into autism ought to be refocused on how to reach the 10% who make little to no progress, and on why this may be so. Why do some cases of autism remain intractable? How, if at all, can clinicians distinguish the outcome of subgroups in advance of treatment and intensive special education — a triage function? Why does it *not* seem "appropriate" to offer each child with a new autism spectrum diagnosis an early, intensive ABA intervention, to probe for whether a robust or significantly good response might arise in an individual child?

This does not happen because it is hard and tedious work to mount an effective, intensive early intervention, a sad commentary on the slow advance of effective autism treatment and advocacy. The greatest challenge to addressing autism continues to remain in translating treatment protocols from behavioral laboratories into family homes, into public schools, group homes, job-coaching and sheltered workshops. As always, it falls first to parents to make the best judgments for their children, based upon scientific evidence in peer-reviewed published research.

CHAPTER SIX

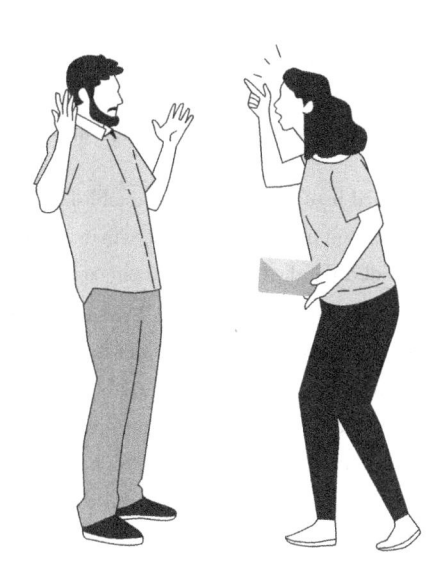

ASKING FOR LOVAAS AND AIT

I had read enough by the end of August to hope that Ruffin's provisional diagnosis of PDD-NOS was encouraging, similar enough to the diagnoses of other children who had recovered in the first books I had been reading. Finding the 1987 and 1993 Lovaas academic studies buttressed my hope.

I ordered a set of early Lovaas instructional videotapes, and *The Me Book*, Lovaas's own early manual of behavioral treatment. These materials seemed old, and not to contain nearly enough information to translate Lovaas's results into my home. But they were helpful to me as an emerging behaviorist, and when I came to recruit my home treatment team. Later, Catherine Maurice, Dr. Gina Green and Dr. Stephen C. Luce's book, *Behavioral Intervention for Young Children with Autism: A Manual for Parents and Professionals* became available.

On September 1st, I reached the crowning entry in the back pages of my autism resources: *The Catalog of Catalogs*. If you had a child with autism in the 1990s, this was how you shopped when you couldn't get out the door, when you couldn't get in and out of a store without a meltdown, when you really needed shoestrings or bottles or new rubber nipples or diaper-pins, or even a new pair of heels for court. Perfect. I would order it, so I could order myself a full collection of mail order catalogs. No, Sears was *not* enough! I found myself laughing, my first deep, unguarded laugh since Ruffin's diagnosis.

The same day, I returned Inge's materials about establishing a "special needs" trust for Ruffin's lifetime care, as a person unlikely to be able to manage his own finances. I assured her that Ruffin loved school. I thanked her for her help, and for responding so quickly.

Inge let me know that Kim, the SLP whom Bridgewater had assigned to deliver speech therapy to Ruffin "had me restate objective 3 for the expressive language goal. She wanted it to reflect her belief that Ruffin would be using more complex sentence structures than just adjective-noun-verb combinations." This represented a change in Ruffin's IEP made without prior notice to me as his mother, and my input and consent, as required by federal law. But, hey, it raised the educators' expectations for Ruffin. No harm, no foul.

As for my request for Bridgewater's financial contribution toward the cost of the upcoming autism clinic at Gundersen, Inge was on top of it.

With my permission to refer Ruffin, Inge also sent a handwritten note to Bridgewater's local autism resource team (ART) member Dot Gordon, a speech and language therapist based in Decorah who was part of Sue's state-wide autism support network. "Mary Jane White is very open to you observing in Ruffin's classroom." Inge suggested we all meet there September 8th.

Her typed referral form was a bit more cautiously worded for the record. "The mother would like assistance applying some of the language and play strategies she has been reading about. Please meet with the mother and classroom teacher. Transitions to and from community settings have been difficult. Can the autism resource team (ART) assist with addressing these issues?" No mention, of course, of any receptive language concerns, since the educators had left that matter unaddressed in Ruffin's IEP. No concern expressed that Ruffin failed to fall within the autism spectrum. And "language and play strategies" was hardly an accurate description of the intensive Lovaas intervention I had researched.

I kept Meg in the loop, brought her up to date on my recent reading and thinking, suggesting she read Catherine Maurice's book, and offering to loan her the Lovaas videotapes. "Inge is familiar with Lovaas's name. Perhaps you are too? I've seen his name repeatedly in the literature. Maybe he is legit? Do you have an opinion?" Meg offered back, "I've heard the name Lovaas but have not read much. I'd be interested in your videotapes and books. Not much time right now but things should settle soon." Undeterred, and unsympathetic to the demands she faced in organizing a new classroom, I continued to press, "Please let me know when you are ready for the Lovaas tapes. I'll bring them over. Can I pick up some things from you? Do you know where I can get or borrow some photographs of emotional faces?"

I continued to be alert to every word Ruffin spoke and its triggering context. Walking out of Julie's daycare, that afternoon, Ruffin said "square," but didn't point or indicate why he said that. I looked around, up and down the street. There was a square or nearly square window in the house across the street. Hadn't Ruffin been using squares in his computer program *Millie's Math House* to build mouse houses? Hadn't we been playing with colored squares of paper? I looked at the house, stooped down to Ruffin's level on the sidewalk, pointed, and asked, "House?" Ruffin replied, "Square house," putting our two words together.

In early September, just a week shy of two months since Ruffin's diagnosis, I approached Inge, and Ruffin's school psychologist Emily Knight — this time asking for what I firmly believed should be his appropriate education and calling their attention to his entitlement to "support services" and "related services," two completely open-ended federally mandated categories of special education. I asked that Lovaas's methods be considered to educate Ruffin. I offered to share the materials I had gathered, citing all the supporting academic research.

My letter to the two of them rocketed by fax over to Jack Wallace in Bridgewater's Decorah office with cover notes from both Inge and Emily expressing their widely differing personal reactions. "Tom, if you haven't seen this you might want to read it. What is the status of Part C funding? Inge. P.S. Dot Gordon of the autism resource team (ART) is going this Thursday to visit Ruffin's classroom." Helpful. Professional. Neutral.

Emily to Jack, "ENJOY." Unprofessional. A bit snarky.

In less than a week, Jack had faxed my letter up beyond his own paygrade to Mr. Montague in Elkader — with his own covering comment, "Here is the letter we just talked about on the phone."

What else had I sent for the educational authorities to enjoy? A copy of Ruffin's E-2 questionnaire and the report on its scoring from Dr. Rimland's group in San Diego. Bernie had reported back to me that Ruffin was the 19,325th child whose parents or teachers had sent in a completed E-2 questionnaire for scoring. Ruffin had been given a -5-behavior score, a 0-speech score, for a total score of -5.

Bernie's explanation of Ruffin's scoring at -5 was, "The scores on Form E-2 range from -45 (lowest) to +45 (highest).

"The average score on Form E-2 for a child diagnosed as 'autistic' by professionals around the world is -2."

In his early effort to collect a large volume of data to be subject to analysis by using computers, Bernie was ahead of his time and imagining beyond the capabilities of computer technology available then.

Today with the completion of the Human Genome Project, genome wide association studies over sets of DNA meta-bases and data mining of blood samples of children diagnosed with autism are undertaking the task Bernie envisioned. But progress remains slow, confusing, and uncertain, with multitudes of suspected autism genes having been identified for future investigation.

Bernie had added another helpful note to the form reporting Ruffin's E-2 score. "A word about PDD: several years ago, the American Psychiatric Association (APA) introduced the concept of PDD as a broad umbrella-like label for describing children with autism and related conditions. The PDD label has proven very unsatisfactory, in many respects, and has been frequently criticized by knowledgeable professionals and researchers in both the U.S. and Europe. The APA is very much aware of this criticism and is in the process of revising the procedures it recommends for diagnosis of children with autism and related conditions. It is hoped that they will drop the PDD label, inasmuch as it has added much confusion to what is already a complicated and difficult problem."

Since Ruffin's diagnosis in mid-1994, the process of revising the DSM-III's diagnostic criteria has tumbled through two more iterations, producing the DSM-IV and the current DSM-V. Issues of the *Spectrum's* online newsletter provide continuing, clear, journalistic accounts of how these further iterations roll on with their attendant confusions, the splitting and lumping of autism categories as determined by contentious committees with all the attendant social fallout — perhaps inflating the Centers for Disease Control's U.S. statistics of prevalence, but more likely, in the case of the newest DSM-V — constricting the eligibility of persons with autism and their families for needed financial and social supports and services by measures as high as 50% to 60%.

Is the latest fiddling with diagnostic criteria good government policy? As a taxpayer funding supports and services, you might think so. Is this good public policy? If you have a family member with autism, you might agree with me that it is not. Bear in mind that taxpayers already contribute millions of dollars for each untreated child with autism who grows up to be an adult with autism — most with the same chance at a normal lifespan as anyone — millions of dollars for each person with autism for so-called lifetime "sheets and eats" support in the form of federally mandated special education, Social Security Disability, and Medicaid.

The relatively smaller investment of $100,000 could easily provide a couple of years of intensive, early ABA intervention for every young child with autism. A home-based Lovaas program delivered to each child before kindergarten might well reduce the financially dependent adult population with autism by 47%. The functioning of another 43% might well improve, stabilizing their placements over their lifetimes. Better outcomes for these two groups might very well produce sufficient savings to fund more effective fundamental research into how to help or support the remaining 10% of the population with autism who so far fail to respond to intensive early ABA intervention.

Back in 1994 I had another project in mind, too, which led to my making another request of Bridgewater. "Several local parents have expressed an interest in obtaining auditory integration training (AIT) for their children with autism." These *exceptional parents*, as we called ourselves, had been reading about and discussing AIT. The treatment took 10 days — 2 30-minute sessions each day — to train the ears and brain to hear all frequencies of sound at the same level of intensity, so vowel sounds might no longer overpower the consonants. As a poet, this made some rudimentary sense to me. I had always thought of vowels as the sounds of singing, cut by the consonants, as the signifiers of meaning in speech.

I alerted Inge and Emily, "AIT will be the subject of one of the talks given at a medical conference at Gundersen on autism in early October. We have located a person who has the equipment and training to provide this service, who would be willing to come here and treat our children next summer, in June."

As a $500 auxiliary one-time treatment, I thought it might be worth adding to the core Lovaas home-based program I hoped to organize for Ruffin at home. As a group of parents, we didn't want much, but we did need some specialized help from a local audiologist. "We would all need and want to have three audiograms done on each child — before treatment, mid-way through treatment, and after treatment — to document whether the treatment has helped. Could you two or Bridgewater be of any assistance in helping to provide the audiograms?"

I concluded by asking if funding might be available for our trying Lovaas and AIT. I hoped with all the special education conferences our special educators attended, someone would take an interest.

Over Labor Day weekend, as my early September letter ricocheted around Bridgewater, the September-October 1994 issue of the Autism Society of America's newsletter, *The Advocate* arrived in Saturday's mail, featuring a front-page lengthy interview with O. Ivar Lovaas, Ph.D. Here was more about Lovaas's thinking behind his academically published results.

Because their nervous systems are incredibly different from those of typically developing children, children with autism do not learn well from the ordinary environment. The average family environment in which we raise typically developing children evolved over thousands of years to meet the needs of typically developing children. But Lovaas thought that the ordinary environment didn't engage the child with autism. It passed such a child by. "It's neutral. So, you have a child with little or no experience. Even though he's living in a rich family environment, it's not a rich environment for him." How to address this mismatch? Lovaas broke it down, simple as one, two three. "We created a treatment program that would make sure the autistic child was always learning. We taught the children at home; we trained parents to work with them, too. Each child in the experimental group received an average of 4,000 hours of therapy over a course of 2 years or more. And these children made dramatic gains."

I wanted to know: how normal would the resulting normal be? When the children averaged 13 years of age, Lovaas had third-party psychologists — blind to any early diagnoses — try to separate his precious recovered lambs from a confounding herd of perfectly normal teenage goats. None of these psychologists noticed any difference between the children who had a history of early childhood autism and those who had enjoyed normal development.

Originally, Lovaas's procedure to decide which child entered intensive treatment and which child would be relegated to a control group was planned to be a coin toss — the gold standard for scientific research — akin to a new drug trial, say, for childhood leukemia. Given a new drug, or a sugar pill placebo, it would be possible to remain unaware of what your child was receiving as a human research subject. But it would be impossible to remain unaware of whether your child was receiving 4,000 hours of therapy for his or her half-a-chance at recovery.

So, the gold-standard of a double-blinded research study was doomed from the start, as Lovaas himself readily acknowledged. "It didn't work out because the parents said they would strike." No parents would voluntarily allow their child to be put in the control group where he or she would receive almost no treatment at all. Lovaas had been forced to move to a first-come-first-served principle — that had been approved by the National Institutes of Health, the funding agency for his studies. Lovaas also agreed to give control group children some behavior therapy — but it was always less than 10 hours a week. So, the parent revolt had produced an interesting comparative-dose experimental design.

As I thought about what Ruffin was receiving as therapy during his ECSE classroom week, I began to wonder how much of Ruffin's instructional time was being eaten up on the bus, waiting in line for lunch or for his turn in the bathroom, trying to nap, going out for recess, going to the library with the kindergarteners, waiting for his turn to try a task or to speak, during all the time Meg and her colleagues needed to safely corral their two classrooms of disabled — including some very fragile wheelchair-bound — children? And, when most of the day every Friday was devoted to the long, time-consuming round trip to Decorah for adapted physical education and swimming? Both of Lovaas's control groups had received best-practice special education in California. That spoke to my earlier wondering about whether what Ruffin was getting in school might amount to no more than glorified babysitting — and rang alarm bells!

Lovaas estimated that about 30% of any random sample of children with autism would be described as "high-functioning." Yet only about 2% of all children with autism grew up to live independently. "What happened to all those other high-functioning little children? Obviously, they did not make the progress people expected." I found this chilling. What happened to them, I wondered, those promising "high-functioning" children? Did the failure to intensively intervene early result in even a "high-functioning" child *acquiring* mental and functional retardation?

And I learned: Ruffin's IQ of 50 was not too low for this. His measured IQ was no reason not to do what I wanted to try. Lovaas observed, "The only truly strong predictor of recovery we found was the child's skill in verbal imitation at the end of 3 months of treatment. Ninety percent of the kids who learned verbal imitation at the end of 3 months of intensive treatment reached normal functioning. The child who starts out the fastest, remains the fastest. The fastest learners — and this may not be the child with the highest IQ going in — do the best."

Lovaas explained what he meant by "verbal imitation:" "The children who achieved normal functioning became echolalic within 3 months; they like to echo adults' speech." Ruffin already had this foundational skill of verbal imitation. Even his early August Bridgewater evaluation team described him as echolalic.

I needed a way to watch, to measure, how fast Ruffin was learning. He learned quickly, I thought.

Returning to his first point, Lovaas concluded, "We help build behavioral variability in children with autism, which increases their ability to adapt to new environments. We taught the children how to pay attention, how to imitate sounds, how to understand what people were saying to them, how to use nouns, verbs, pronouns, prepositions, and other abstract language. We taught them how to play with toys, to show and receive affection, to relate to another child. We taught them everything. We had to teach everything because we found that the autistic child needed teaching in everything."

Later that afternoon when I handed Seamus my highlighted copy of *The Advocate* to read for himself, he was doubtful and unimpressed. "Mary Jane, this is ridiculous! How could we possibly teach him everything?" I wished Lovaas were here to answer Seamus himself, because it did seem formidable, if not impossible.

That same Labor Day weekend, the newest issue of Bernie's *ARRI* also arrived, with his personal editorial: "Intensive early behavioral intervention: a letter of support."

My early September written request for Lovaas therapy for Ruffin was already pending. Later, as I went in to inspect Ruffin's thick educational file I found both *The Advocate's* interview of Lovaas and Bernie's long editorial filed between my letter request — with its enclosure of Schopler's article from his book about preschoolers with autism — and the school authorities' later response.

Our parent group met again to discuss plans for auditory integration training (AIT). Meanwhile, mid-level administrator Jack Wallace at Bridgewater had been surveying his team and had received back an article about AIT from a recent edition of *ADHD Report*, which he faxed around to Inge and the autism resource team (ART). It was a why AIT won't work "consumer beware" article, not shared with me at the time, or with any of the other parents in our support group. It might have been nice to have had it to pass on to the medical professionals at Gundersen who were looking into AIT too and planning to offer it to children with developmental disabilities in residential care in LaCrosse.

The article Jack circulated quoted the cost for AIT at $1,200 per child. Our little group was being offered the service at $500 per child. But maybe all we were being offered was a bargain for a hoax.

At the time, I continued to have concerns about Ruffin's hearing that I shared with Meg. "I'm glad Ruffin seems to enjoy music at school and can manage a fire drill. Maybe he will not suffer a painful sensitivity to noise. I do think there are two types of hearing problems Ruffin may have: 1) He can't seem to locate me in the house by the sound of my voice. If he and I are lost to each other, he calls and calls, but looks in every room, until he sees me, with no clue apparently as to whether I am upstairs or even downstairs; 2) The whispering or loud phenomenon: An explanation I've seen of this in the neurological literature is related to a subtle hearing problem in which the different frequencies of sound are first 'heard' at varying, rather than roughly the same, levels of intensity. So, some sounds (vowels) overpower and drown out others (consonants). Also, the child may hear himself, his own speech, at an odd or varying volume with no perception that he is whispering." I asked Meg if Kim had any information, or an opinion.

But just then, I needed to work for two days. Two days straight: One full day to round up witnesses and prepare them to testify. One full day in court. Then, suddenly, but not predictably, under the pressures of preparation for trial, the matter settled out of court to my client's satisfaction. "Thank you," said the woman who was raising three children, a tenant who had rented a furnished apartment — with a refrigerator that had fizzled. The landlord would honor his written contract; a new one would be bumping up the staircase that afternoon on a furniture truck. "Could I pay you, little by little, every month?" That would work. As Ruffin stepped off the stubby bus after his day at school, I melted, from both the onslaught of love and my exhaustion.

The moment Ruffin was down for the night, I reached into his backpack eagerly, day after day, to see what Meg might have sent or written. Ruffin had drawn two nearly-identical scribbles for Meg, who dated and labeled them — "was a face, then 'dirty hair.'" Something Ruffin said? If so, pretty funny. More about scissors, more about a storybook Ruffin made and proudly put on his classroom's bookshelf. I found myself suddenly looking forward to being free to visit Ruffin's classroom myself the next day to meet his classmates and make the day's snack for the group. Meg reminded me, "Dot Gordon from the autism resource team is coming tomorrow afternoon."

Ah, yes, I remembered Dot. I had gotten a call a couple of days earlier from her about visiting us soon at home. But she was uncertain of her own schedule and couldn't offer me a firm appointment. She had yet to come or call back.

But Meg had more to offer. "Today during opening I asked each of my students if they had a name. When I asked, 'What is your name?' Ruffin answered, 'Name — Ruffin,' in a loud whisper. I could hear it from the back of the group." Just what I wanted to hear — Ruffin *was* echolalic, maybe even more than just echolalic — responsive? According to Lovaas, he had a 90% chance of recovery. I could relax. I could sleep.

The next morning, I drove Ruffin to school. We parked in the busy lot near the line of buses dropping dozens of children off into the nearby chaos of the elementary school playground before the opening bell. With Ruffin in my arms and his backpack slung over my shoulder, I waded through all the small children to the heavy steel door that opened onto an equally chaotic hallway of scurrying teachers. A maintenance worker pushing his wheeled mop bucket away, stopped to secure it in a closet. Turning, he brushed his hands together — been there, done that — and looked up in my direction. What was I doing here? I was a stranger, so I smiled and explained myself, that I would be going in and out today.

Handing Ruffin over to Ella in Meg's room, I went back for my ingredients and the bread machine to start the fresh buttermilk-maple bread Ruffin would be offering today for snack. Meg pointed me to a counter with an outlet, at the back of the room.

I watched the other five boys in the class arrive — one nearly blind, one not able to walk very well. That didn't keep either one from smiling or screaming and grabbing. After a period of free play, Meg and Ella corralled them into a seated circle for their first group activity — rhythm band and singing. Two larger girls arrived from the severe and profound classroom with their accompanying aide and squeezed into the circle. Instruments to make noise, to bang and to tinkle were passed out. I could see Ruffin, imitating the others, right along, participating fully with gestures. But he was not saying or singing a thing. At one point, he covered his ears and grimaced.

Still, I saw this as an improvement on his behavior with groups of other children. The imitation, at least, seemed promising. The research I'd been reading stated that the ability to imitate was predictive of good progress. I stayed through PE and lunch, until the group of boys went down for their naps. As I left, I whispered to Meg, "I would say Ruffin talks almost non-stop now at home, while still speaking rarely at school. You probably don't want him talking non-stop!" I laughed quietly. She smiled and whispered back, "He seemed to do a good job paying attention and staying with a task." I went home to check my answering machine but planned to come back. It was a little tricky to get the hot bread out. I didn't want Meg or Ella to burn themselves, as I had when I first tried to figure that out.

Dot and Emily were there observing Ruffin when I returned to help serve snack. Meg kept me busy. "Here's the knife. There's the butter. Why don't you serve the children?" When I did, Ruffin was having none of it, wouldn't touch his. When he slid it away, another boy grabbed it. "Mom!" Ruffin wailed. I couldn't even manage six preschoolers at snack. Ella stepped in to help. I was never introduced to Dot, nor approached, nor engaged by Emily either.

At the day's end, I reached into Ruffin's backpack and pulled out our notebook. "Thanks for bringing in your bread. Ruffin cried a little when he realized you were gone, but soon got into activities and was fine. He showed Miss Hobbs the bread machine."

As it turned out, I hadn't seen everything. I had missed Miss Hobbs's visit. Certainly, I missed its significance. I didn't put her visit together with Dot and Emily's visit the same day. I failed to envision the group of them visiting together in my absence or assessing Ruffin behind my back.

As a result of her visit with Miss Hobbs and Emily, Dot had written in her autism resource team (ART) report:

1. Ruffin is verbal and interacts with adults.
2. He was able to move from one activity to another during class time without incidence (sic incident).
3. He did repeat words and phrases of the teacher at times, especially upon being questioned. He was able to respond to suggestions and make comments.
4. He whispered most of the time but used an appropriate voice during interaction in a small group.
5. It appeared that Ruffin is in an appropriate educational setting.
6. His behaviors and actions were not considered to be significant, and a diagnosis of autism would be questioned.

This written report of her observations — of her open quarrel with both Dr. Caldwell's medical and Bernie's E-2 checklist diagnosis — was not shared with me until nearly two months later.

Despite my missed observations and my reservations about school, I was happier, as Ruffin became more talkative at home during every activity. He found me in the tub unable to help him. "I go get another shirt. I be back." He began using plurals at home, making regular note of any object he saw in pairs by saying "two lights," "two legs." Anywhere there were two of anything, I would point them out, offer Ruffin the name of whatever they were, and wait for his exclamation. I thought Ruffin's range of affect — whether on the happy side or the angry side — was growing, and that his voice was taking on a greater range of expression in the presence of the emotion arising from each discovery. But, if he ever missed a vitamin dose, he could not do this.

Nothing to do now but wait. Heat was still dissipating from the painted boards of the porch. Having kicked my heels off long ago under my desk, I could feel it rising around me as I stood there in my stocking feet, rechecking the mailbox. The sky overhead was washed clear of stars by the lights of town. No clouds or thunderheads on the horizon. No relief. It felt too late in the season for all that. Too late in the evening to call my parents back East. There had been nothing on my answering machine. Nothing was pressing. For the moment, I thought I had enough money, so that was a good thing. I could keep reading and trying new things with Ruffin. A pickup without headlights turned into my driveway. It was Seamus. We were going to have a nice time. It turned out I had a lot to share with him.

After Seamus left, Ruffin was up all night, a Friday night fortunately, until Saturday morning, just as it had begun to brighten on the eastern horizon. Then, inexplicably, he slept most of the rest of Saturday morning. So, I did, too. Saturday evening, we walked across Main Street to the pizza parlor, where Ruffin was well behaved but didn't eat. Ruffin's unpredictable sleep and wakefulness continued to make it difficult for me to work, to know when I could tackle housework and shopping. I needed to follow his lead, and did what I could manage in the cracks, during the times he suddenly crashed and slept. Over these last three years, as far as sleeping through the night, I might as well still have been caring for a newborn. Except that when he was awake, Ruffin also needed focused behavioral teaching of language, self-help, and social skills. He wasn't a sponge. He needed careful parenting.

Having read Lovaas's *The Me Book* and having watched his early videos and by trying what I could on my own, I was beginning to see some success. Settling him on the couch, I tried reading Ruffin a book of opposites and he did well with some of these concepts and words: push-or-pull — he confused these but associated both with movement — until we came up with the right hand gestures, an open palm for "push," a closed fist for "pull." Empty-or-full, Ruffin knew and used these words all the time. He had seen them in his chocolate milk bottle. In-or-out, was something he knew, and was easy. Up-or-down, again this confused him until I could shape his hand so he would have a finger to point with. It still didn't seem to get much better. Thick-or-thin seemed beyond him. But whole-or-broken, now that got his attention. Front-or-back and over, he could say and used with understanding. Big-or-little, which I thought we had talked so much about, still meant nothing to Ruffin. First-or-last — this was too hard for Ruffin, not surprising, I told myself since "day" and "night," two words he often echoed, meant nothing to him as a sequence, nor had either word anything to do with sleeping. Many-or-few were easy. Heavy-or-light and together-or-apart seemed within reach. Left-or-right: no clue. That was okay. I didn't know that one either.

Done with that, Ruffin wanted to read his alphabet book, saying, "I do it," meaning he preferred to read by turning the pages and naming each pictured noun, or if he were stumped ask, "What is it?" I thought I was hearing "I do it" a lot more often — when peeling carrots, re-booting computer programs, or opening crayons.

Out of books then, and too late to go to the library, we spent the middle of the night going through all the mail-order catalogues that had arrived, identifying each person as a "boy," "girl," "man," "woman." Every woman was a "mommy." We identified items of clothing: shoes, socks, furniture, and towels, whatever. I found that Ruffin could learn the name of almost anything he had encountered before. Around the house, Ruffin was using "this," "that," "here," and "there" correctly and frequently, saying, for example, quite functionally, I thought, "Put in there," when directing me to put batteries in the flashlight he carried with him everywhere.

We also began playing a body parts game regularly — elbows, eyes, cheeks, chin, and ankles — Ruffin *seemed* to know them all.

But Ruffin's persistent whispering and odd syntax remained mysteries that continued to flummox me in my attempts to teach him. I had only middling success with "I can't hear," while cupping my ear, needing to prompt Ruffin at least twice to move him from whispering to talking out loud. Ruffin's word order was idiosyncratic. "On blocks, wheel" seemed to mean "The tricycle's wheel is caught on the blocks." "In wagon, bottle" and several similar sentences drew my attention to a location first and then to some object, putting the natural subject of the sentence last.

I reported all this to Meg and asked, "Do you have any insight into what this means developmentally? I think it's good, but strange." Mostly, I simply felt helpless at times to keep the balance right for Ruffin, or to manage to get any sleep for myself.

Ruffin had spoken out loud to Julie and the other children in daycare rarely, and only at her prompting. When I modeled, "I love you, Julie," Ruffin echoed, "I love you, Julie" to Julie. She was pleased. Her strong face had melted into a smile that rose all the way up into her eyes, and then she scrabbled in her jeans pocket for a tissue.

Riding home, Ruffin unlocked the car door himself. He had a new lock and key fetish. Suddenly, he loved locks and keys of all kinds. It was possible to tempt him out of the car by promising he could play with his computer and watch some of *Otis and Milo*. But, once we were inside, he looked through our family photo album, asking me, 'Who is it?' repeatedly, pointing to the human figures in each photo. He did notice background items, but always paid some attention to the people, too. I found this promising. After he tired of the photo album, he went into his backpack and dug out the popsicle stick figures Meg had him make at school. He told me they were grandma and papa. I took one in my hand, and then grandma sent papa to the store for chocolate milk and many other things she "forgot."

Finally, in mid-September, I was called into school to meet with Dot and Inge in Meg's classroom. After Inge introduced her, the first thing Dot told me was how excited she was to have been appointed to our local autism resource team. She confided that she knew little about autism but seemed anxious to assure me — she would be learning. She asked to borrow my TEACCH volumes, and I told her she could come by the house if she wanted to pick them up. Then the three of them let slip that they had just attended a meeting about Ruffin. Likely, this was when Inge, Emily, and Jack had met to sign the answer, already travelling to me by snail mail and unmentioned at this time — to my request that Lovaas and auditory integration training (AIT) be added to Ruffin's IEP.

In her written report of our encounter, Dot recorded my personal concerns as Ruffin's mother: as a safety issue, Ruffin didn't know his name, address, or phone number; he was whispering at school when he sometimes spoke in a normal tone at home; he echoed the last part of my questions, without answering them. I wanted to know when she thought Ruffin would be ready for regular — rather than special — education. Dot let me know that I could expect her written report shortly.

When it finally arrived much later and long overdue, in early November, it laid out the school authorities' plan, probably as originally developed at that meeting about Ruffin to which I had not been invited. Emily was going to administer the *PEP-R* to Ruffin with the assistance of another school psychologist who had attended the training on how to do this. Kim was going to video Ruffin so she and Dot could analyze his echolalia. Sue would send me information about auditory integration training (AIT) and the autism society. Not so much as a whisper about early intensive ABA intervention as developed by Lovaas.

In mid-September long before Dot's report arrived, I got Ruffin's educators' response to my own requesting Lovaas and AIT. Dear me, they had addressed me by my given name. "We are also interested in continuing to provide an appropriate program for Ruffin. We value your ideas as we do those of other parents of the many children we serve."

"Darling, let this be a reminder to you," I minced in my fury before Seamus as I paced the powder blue carpet of my dining room office. "You are trespassing on our area of expertise. And, as a further reminder: As experts, we are terribly busy, and have other students, too." He was trying to talk me down.

"They *have* other students, too."

I stopped in my tracks. "Just listen to this: 'In order that all on the team share the same data, we have taken the opportunity to share your correspondence with them and other Bridgewater administrative personnel.' That means, 'Let this be a warning. Hereafter, you may expect to find all of us on the same page.' With a quick flip to the second page, I showed Seamus they were all there: Inge, Emily, and Jack signing the letter *Sincerely*, and copying it to Meg, Kim, and Miss Hobbs, and even to the special education nurse, Grace, and to the school district's nurse, Caroline, to Bridgewater's audiologist, Kara, to a Bridgewater sector coordinator someone, to Mr. Montague, The Man, and his Right-Hand Man, LaVerne Mosher, 'Moe.' "Not an ally left to me among them," I fumed to Seamus. "Not a single open avenue of appeal or maneuver. They've grouped up against me — against Ruffin."

"You really need to calm down, here, Mary Jane," Seamus warned me.

I handed him the letter, pointing, "This is the worst. 'We are already aware of some of the research you have presented, and we are looking into some of the remainder. Some of the methodology may not be appropriate for Ruffin, in that it is designed for children more seriously involved than he.'"

"Well, that sounds like good news . . .," Seamus ventured, before I cut him off, reexplaining all Lovaas's research and results.

Of course, it became much easier to understand their concerted refusal after Dot finally sent me her written report in early November of her classroom observation of Ruffin made back in early September. "His behaviors and actions were not considered to be significant, and a diagnosis of autism would be questioned."

"What about the other thing you were so interested in?" Seamus asked, trying to get off Lovaas as a sore subject between us.

"They say here," I said quoting, "'Because auditory integration training (AIT) is not widely considered a best-practice treatment, and it has not been definitively researched, it is not a therapy endorsed by Bridgewater.'"

"Well, you asked. They said no. That's that. They've given you their advice and made their decision. You're not going to get what you wanted."

"Oh, I get it. I write these same sorts of letters myself all the time, this pablum. 'Again, as we continue to provide an appropriate program for Ruffin, we do appreciate your interest and we, too, will continue to keep abreast of pertinent research.' How else do you imagine I read this, Seamus, — other than that *I* am being *im*pertinent?"

Seamus wasn't tuned in to my sarcasm. He hated it.

"Think, before you rock the boat."

"I know," I said. "This is my free childcare."

Then Seamus asked, because he knew he needed to know — just as my mother did, "What are you going to do about it?"

My mother had also asked, "How much do you think it will cost?"

"I don't know," I had told her. "Maybe a lot." Echoing what I had told Seamus, I said, "But it can't cost Ruffin his chance, even if it's only a half-chance, of recovery."

This was what I wanted to do. And I did not need anyone — not Seamus, not even my parents — to detour me into peripheral topics, such as how I might need to take care of myself and give thought to my own needs, or anyone else's. By then, I was certain that autism could become a serious, lifelong problem for Ruffin and for me — so I had better get moving because it looked like I had a lot of work to do. After reading all those books and studies, after asking politely and having been brushed off — all my naïve expectations of professional help fell finally by the wayside.

CHAPTER SEVEN

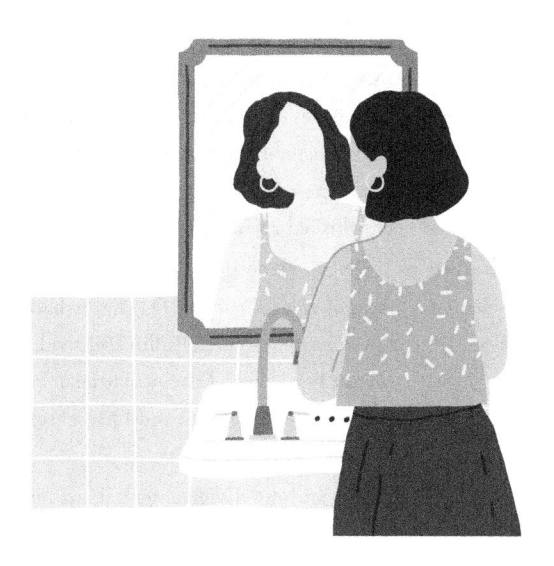

WHAT DID YOU EXPECT?

While I struggled with the arrival of the school's refusal letter, Gundersen's autism clinic had added a follow-up appointment with Dr. Caldwell in late September, and an audiology appointment to Ruffin's schedule in October, early in the morning. Ruffin and I would need to get out of the house before dawn for a long day likely to end at the hospital late in the afternoon — with another hour's drive to struggle home through rush hour. Other appointment-time changes had Ruffin scheduled for cognitive and speech and language pathology testing in the midmorning or early afternoon. And there was a bright yellow slip to remind me. "Due to liability concerns, parents are required to provide adult supervision for their children during the staffing."

There was no question of Seamus making this trip with us. His new factory job required near-perfect attendance. Missing two days' work was a firing offense there and at Rose's warehouse — at all the off-farm jobs within driving distance. I understood that. I had represented many clients who had been let go on that account, and then been denied unemployment benefits. Having been in the practice for over fifteen years, I had enough chair-side equity to be able to re-schedule all my upcoming hearings around Ruffin's two days of appointments.

Nor could Seamus justify asking for time-off, since — to protect him from any financial responsibility for Ruffin's prolonged stay in PICU — I had entered no name for Ruffin's father on his birth certificate. The moment I woke up after my C-Section, hospital social workers were at my bedside — afraid their state might be on the hook for the probable quarter-million-dollar hospital bill that Ruffin and I represented. I had yet to hold Ruffin, just glimpsed him once, reaching into his incubator from my gurney to touch one foot before I had been whisked away into recovery.

I told the social workers to leave me alone. I had private insurance. As for who Ruffin's father was — that was none of their business. Dr. Wyatt had been standing there with them, ready to tell me he *thought* — since Ruffin had made it through the delivery and the first night — he might live. He and the pediatrician expected Ruffin's stay would be long and expensive. It was, I remembered; and I had gotten through that. I could get through this now.

At this rocky moment of Seamus's and my disagreement about my continuing to press the school district for expensive experimental programs and services, I imagined he would want no part of spending two days at the clinic. I didn't even ask him. I didn't want to ask, beg, cry, or have any more discussion about it.

So, I walked down Main Street to recruit our local Presbyterian pastor, Dr. David Hansen, to watch Ruffin the first day, if need be. He already planned to be visiting parishioners at the hospital and was the parent of two small children with cystic fibrosis. I hardly needed to explain. He got it. Then I was able to recruit Renee's mother, Ruth, from our autism support group to cover most of the long afternoon staffing period the second day. She was willing, and certainly experienced in managing a tired, cranky child with autism, which, by that time of the day, Ruffin was highly likely to be.

On an early morning in mid-September, Meg and I met for our first parent-teacher conference. Although she was Ruffin's teacher, our personal contact had been limited to brief, early phone calls, the short IEP meeting with her professional group, and our back-and-forth notes written to each other trying to keep Ruffin afloat in school. Because Meg had the closest day-to-day contact with Ruffin, I wanted to know her better.

All the toys lying around her classroom seemed to be missing parts. The stuffed animals in her room showed a generous amount of lovingly applied grime. Meg caught me noticing. These were personal items that had once belonged to her children.

As I met other special education parents coming and going from the two classrooms — Ruffin's, and across the hallway, Amy's for more severe and profoundly disabled students — we agreed to do what we could to remedy this. We asked Meg and Amy for a complete wish list of what would be useful. Then, we parents met up to shop for these items from the thick, bright catalogues they lent us. Using our credit cards recklessly, we ordered as much as we could.

Technically, of course, everything we supplied became the property of our local district, like the donations from the music boosters and items bought by the sports uniform and equipment support group. These authorized, organized groups had long been warmly embraced, celebrated for their generosity, and photographed with each contributor's name included in the carefully composed caption in the local newspaper Seamus brought me to read when he was done with it.

"I brought you the paper," Seamus said, as he always did, that evening when he pulled out a stool to sit at my kitchen counter. Slapping his hand down on its surface, repeatedly, in sheer excitement at his love of being here, back in his own hometown. Usually he wanted to talk politics, the Vietnam War and its aftermath, or tell me about his sisters and their large Catholic families, or he would offer to critique my latest opening statement. He was the best shadow juror I knew. No one had a better finger on the pulse of our little community. Several of my recent verdicts proved it. Tonight, he wanted to stay for supper, and learn what might be new with Ruffin.

"When I bring you the paper, you should read it," he told me. "I learn something new every day. You can always learn something reading the paper."

I was gathering dirty dishes into the sink. It had been spaghetti and crusty buttered French bread, Seamus's favorite and something Ruffin would nibble, one thing I made well this day of the week Rose took off.

I jumped on Seamus's second mention of the paper to ask, "Will it upset you if our names are in the paper? Ruffin's and mine?"

"It wouldn't be good," he warned me, letting that hang in the heavy silence. "Nothing about this is going to be any good. This is going to cause trouble."

At first, I misunderstood and was confused. Being in the newspaper might be an unnecessary embarrassment. Before Ruffin arrived, I had heard what Seamus's view was about disability: a private calamity, a suffering to be borne by a family at home, in silence, as an unending duty to be borne quietly, with everyone connected to it being an object of unspoken, unspeakable pity.

"No!" He was irked to be misunderstood. "Your *gift* will cause trouble. At school. It will come as an embarrassment. I can see you don't see that. I know all those men on the school board, in town."

Seamus was a "Ridger" from the close-by but outlying West Ridge Irish Catholic original patent settlement, land still owned by a tight-knit original group of intermarried families. They raised corn and bred horses, and their sons had been drafted in disproportionate numbers before the selective service had adopted an impartial birthday-based lottery — by these men whom Seamus knew — the Protestant downtown merchants and the few Catholic bigwigs then on all the town's boards, the school board, the economic development board, and back in the day, the draft board.

I was ready to dismiss all this as more talk about the draft when Seamus spelled it out for me. "None of them will appreciate your stirring this up, just causing trouble. With the other parents. You'll hurt them, the other parents, and their children, too — and Ruffin — trying to be smarter than anybody else, just trying to be a hero. You need to stop. Keep your head down. Stay out of the paper."

End of discussion then. There was absolutely no danger of me or any of the other *exceptional parents* appearing in the paper, like the music boosters. I was worrying about nothing. So, I thought Seamus was worrying about nothing.

The following Monday afternoon I picked Ruffin up from school to meet again with Meg and Amy and several other parents to discuss the larger purchases we could not afford. I was grinning from ear to ear and waving a simple, long white, postage-free envelope containing $500. It had turned up in my mailbox on Sunday. I told the story, breathlessly. "End of the day, I went out on the porch to tuck outgoing mail under the back of my mailbox. Then, I noticed that someone had slipped this inside. It was as thick as my stack of outgoing mail and had my name on it. Look, no return address. No note."

The cost of the list had been approximately $5,000. We ordered what we could. With the $500 of unexpected donation, we could challenge the community to try to raise an additional $2,000 by asking for a match to our gifts so far. That seemed a fair ask. This call for help would spread the word about the new special education classrooms.

I confided to Meg, "I hope you and Amy do not get any flak for 'ordering out of school.' If so, I am happy to make clear that this was my initiative." To this — to Seamus's concern the school would be embarrassed — Meg replied, "I don't think we'll get flak. I hope not, and thanks for the offer of support."

We never learned who made the $500 donation, but we couldn't leave our single, anonymous donor go unacknowledged, so Ruth and I put a thank you ad in the paper. We wanted our community to see us and our children — that we were here, among them.

Miss Hobbs mailed us a note, postmarked the same day the paper came out. "Thank you for the donation of monies for purchasing materials and supplies. I am thrilled with our new programs and teachers. It is even more exciting when parents are positive and involved partners in the process." Nice enough, but the note was the size of a business card to slide into our wallets under our maxed-out credit cards. Seamus, who knew his own community in ways I never would, gave me a stern look, and after what he meant to be a meaningful pause, said, when he had my full attention, "What did you expect?"

Saturday morning, I wrangled Ruffin into the car and drove over to Decorah to take our video camera in for repair. Ruffin was fascinated, wandering the aisles of the camera store. At the counter, I rented a replacement to make videos at school for the autism clinic evaluation at Gundersen. I was hoping to ask Meg to video some class time she thought might be helpful for his medical evaluators to see. No, I cautioned myself, I needed to see what happened there, and see that it got recorded. Business was still slow from the summer when no one ever bothered to sue. It was too hot, and people were too busy outside for any real disputes. I had no motions or hearings scheduled on Monday, so I would just alert Meg that I would be bringing the rented camera in midmorning. Then, I would set it up to run, and stay the day to observe. With my mind racing ahead to Monday, I tried to propel Ruffin past the party-supply store, and of course, he had a tantrum. One balloon, it seemed, was not enough.

"Two hands," Ruffin argued, looking up at me, with his head cocked, as he waited for my ruling. He was adorable, and resembled Seamus in ways it would be impossible to resist. Here was Seamus's easy carriage, his squared shoulders, narrow hips, perfect nose, even his dark eyes that narrowed as they sparkled in my direction. And, Ruffin hadn't made a bad argument, I thought.

Two balloons, then, and we crossed Water Street, passed a toy store of no interest to Ruffin, and walked calmly enough into Ruby's where, fascinated by his balloons, Ruffin sat quietly, while I ate. Then, another tantrum outside Ruby's, another tantrum in Radio Shack, over their display of balloons. During lunch, the party store had decorated every store in Decorah with their balloons. Irritably, I thought, what an inconvenient promotion. This could have been a relaxing trip without the balloons.

With his balloons bouncing gently against the roof of the car over his car-seat, we headed into the countryside of weedy meadows and high, ripe corn, not yet dry enough for harvest. We had an invitation to visit friends for the afternoon. Horsewoman RoJene Beard with her short, dark curly hair and wonderful laughter was a long-time friend from my first decade of practicing law in Decorah. In midlife, she had just finished her own teacher-training. Chance was her third child, the first with her new husband, John, a welder, beef farmer, and local politician. Chance was about a year younger than Ruffin.

With RoJene's help, Ruffin mounted a horse for the first time — not a bit scared. Maybe it hadn't been his first time. Maybe, he had ridden with Seamus. Wouldn't Seamus have mentioned that? Probably not. Horse riding had its risks, as Seamus knew. He thought I was overprotective, his opinion, not a secret. Now, I would ask.

We drove home in the dark, along the white gravel roads, and then Ruffin was up all night well into the dawn's half-light. I got him up again for Sunday school and church, which we couldn't miss, since this was the Sunday Pastor Hansen planned to include information about Ruffin's autism in his sermon. In our pew, Ruffin behaved so well, the pastor's message must have seemed a mystery to the congregation, or unnecessary, at least that morning.

Sunday afternoon, Renee, one of the girls from Amy's classroom, and her mother Ruth came to visit and play. Ruth checked out the rented video camera and gave me a quick lesson in how to operate it correctly. Later, Seamus took Ruffin to visit the trout hatchery where they lured the fish with dog food and then caught them by hand, played in the park, and went out for pizza, while I caught a nap. With no work, with a bare desk, I caught a nap.

When Seamus brought Ruffin home, together, we gave Ruffin his bath. "No splashing — water like the fish swam in," he said, waving his hand back and forth in the air above Ruffin who was seated in the tub. This bath was a remarkably calm experience. We were headed toward getting Ruffin settled in bed early. Seamus told me all about Ruffin's afternoon. Yes, there had been a pony, earlier, that Ruffin had ridden.

I had news to share, too. "Ruffin is pointing. He saw an airplane in the sky behind the house, ran in, got me, pointing, and said, 'Mommy, airplane, airplane.'" This was the first true episode of him pointing. My speculation offered first to Seamus, later to my parents and then to Meg — might Ruffin's pointing be a development and extension of his computer "pointing" experience of moving the cursor?

The school district agreed to videotape Ruffin's activities in Meg's classroom in mid-September, as a way of offering the school's input into the medical multi-disciplinary team's effort at Gundersen. Their videotape segments showed Ruffin picking up toys at Meg's direction, throwing them hard into plastic bins, either carelessly or angrily.

Then, Ruffin with his classroom group at circle time playing a group game, "I am name, or have some feeling," and his group singing *Bunny Foo-Foo*, a narrative-repeat song with nonverbal imitation, and finally, art with Ruffin showing a mild tactile defensiveness with glue and using both his hands in assembly work.

In none of these video segments from school did Ruffin utter a single word. Nor did anyone individually prompt him to speak or sing with success. Instead, Ruffin was encouraged by hand-over-hand instruction, to express his feelings with primitive signs, either rubbing his stomach for "happy" or repeatedly scrunching up his fingers in front of his face for "grouchy."

At home, Ruffin suddenly developed what I thought was a new self-stimulatory tic, digging into his cheek with the hard knuckle of the first finger of his right hand. When I reached out to interrupt this behavior, my touching Ruffin triggered a tantrum. The next time I saw Meg, I warned her that this new tic seemed to have developed and recounted what had happened at home.

"No, you see, we've taught him a sign for apple," Meg informed me. "For him to ask for 'apple,' to let us know that's what he prefers here for snack."

"Why teach him sign?" I whined. "I thought we agreed in his IEP you would be teaching him to talk."

"Actually, no. We teach him to *communicate*. Sometimes learning to sign is easier to teach, and easier for him to learn. We can hope it might scaffold him to talk . . . . Just a few primitive signs . . . not like he's deaf . . ."

The expression on my face, of fury, had stopped her cold.

"In his IEP, you agreed to teach him to talk. If you're going to teach him sign language here instead, you need to let me know *every* sign you teach. At the very least. So, we don't have any more of these tantrums at home. If you think this is a good idea, you'll need to teach me everything, too. You know, so *we* can communicate . . ."

Meg was disappointed, even frightened by the acid vehemence of my reaction. Even I was caught off-guard by it, as it rose so unexpectedly, so viscerally, I felt nauseous. Time to take a break.

I excused myself to find a restroom.

On this issue of teaching Ruffin to talk, Meg and I were obviously not communicating very well. And I regretted it. But, as I leaned over the low sink in the little girls' room, off the hallway full of other students' talking, I wondered, "How can anyone imagine the fleeting movements of sign language would be easier for a child with autism to follow? Who imagines a child with autism would even notice them? Any more than speech that also passes quickly and disappears into the air? Both so unfixed in their fluid forms — signs and speech — with no way to pin them down, to hold them in mind and puzzle them out?"

It was ridiculous to waste time on these efforts at signing. Ruffin was not being taught anything approaching American Sign Language, the culturally rich language of the deaf. These were meant to be "just a few primitive signs," as a "scaffold." I imagined Ruffin marooned high up on a scaffold, with no ladder down into the world. Who, in the end, was going to know what Ruffin was saying if this was how he was going to be taught to communicate? Who would ever be able to reach him? Just his teachers? Just more special educators and caretakers?

The worst — what turned my stomach — was that I sensed I was being cut out here. Not just cut out of his education, but out of Ruffin's whole life and future. I threw up, ran water in the sink, wiped my mouth, and walked quickly out of the schoolhouse.

I had been talking on the phone to Sue about mounting a Lovaas program for Ruffin. She told me that Dr. Lovaas's 1993 co-researcher, Dr. Tristram Smith was teaching at Drake University in Des Moines and helping the family of an eight-year-old girl in Waterloo with a home-based program. So, I called him and learned that he was not very well and would be leaving Iowa soon to accept an academic research appointment at Washington State. But he referred me to Dr. Doreen Granpeesheh in California, recommending her as a fine clinician and his fellow graduate student who had also studied with Lovaas. Tris just didn't have her current phone number handy.

Then, I called Bernie in San Diego, to discuss Ruffin's recent E-2 score. I was in considerable distress at not being able to reach Lovaas himself. Bernie was on top of the great demand that was rising from parents around the world who were reading Catherine Maurice's book. When I shared my disappointing news about Tris, Bernie enthusiastically seconded his recommendation of Dr. Granpeesheh, and gave me the phone number of her California-based practice group, the Center for Autism and Related Disorders, (CARD). I called Doreen, and she sounded kind, and wicked smart. Later, when I met her, she was remarkably easy on the eyes, and persuasive, blessed with a set of social skills not very often to be met with. Very quickly, she and I scheduled one of her senior supervisors, Evelyn Kung, to come for a two-day assessment and training workshop with Ruffin, at our home in Iowa, in early November. I had until then to gather and employ my front-line, home therapy team.

I told Seamus as soon as I saw him. He hugged me and said, "I'm not surprised. Don't you always get what you want?" Then, I called my parents, and they offered money. "Hold on," I said, "I might need it later. I have what Dr. Granpeesheh needs for us to be able to start. My share of the *Ezzone* verdict should be coming in soon, after the appeal this fall." I was still flush, for the moment.

Back in July, I had even considered buying a larger house, a stately, massive home, built in 1913. It was full of cracked stained glass and woodwork that would need stripping. Located on a quieter side street near downtown, it would be easier to drive in and out of, than my Victorian right out on Main Street.

I asked a local decorator, Donna Schmidt, to come with me to the realtor's showing because she loved old houses — having restored and decorated my Victorian. I had bought it from her and her gifted carpenter husband, Kevin, when I moved to town with Ruffin. She brought her daughter Danielle, to keep an eye on Ruffin, so we could talk. I told the realtor, and Donna, "I am interested, but I need to sleep on it. One night is all, I expect. I should get back to you both tomorrow — no, it'll need to be the next day." I had to correct myself, because the next day was the day Ruffin and I had an appointment with Dr. Caldwell and Ruffin's PICU follow-up team at Gundersen.

When he didn't hear from me, the realtor called.

"Ah, no, I won't be taking the house. Sorry, it's beautiful, just what I want, but a family medical emergency's come up. You know, suddenly."

When Donna called, I gave her the same reason, and maybe because I was talking to another woman, my voice thickened, and I burst into tears. Still, I was embarrassed. I knew Donna, but we weren't close. We had been doing business together. She had been excited about the prospect of taking on the massive house with Kevin for me. If she had been disappointed, she hid it well, and let me blubber.

Throughout the remainder of the summer, Donna continued to be in touch. I called her, or she called me if I let too long pass, and we would talk. Aside from my mother, she was the one other person who seemed genuinely curious about what I was learning about autism. From doing business with him over the years, she knew Seamus well enough to know exactly how little support he was likely to offer Ruffin and me with this new diagnosis. With her experience, at her distance, she had Seamus pegged as sentimental, and not very responsible. I thought of him as a beautiful dreamer, damaged by the war.

Donna and her close friend, Lisa Murphy, were having to commute daily, and every other weekend, to LaCrosse, making the two-hour round trip to work for no more than minimum wage. They supervised residents during overnight shifts in one of the group homes there for disabled adults — exactly the sort of place I never wanted to be forced to place Ruffin. The dangerous winter driving season began around Halloween in Iowa. So, I asked Donna if she and Lisa would like to give up the commute, and work for me with Ruffin instead, after school, every day and on weekends. I would raise them on whatever they were earning in LaCrosse.

It would mean their attending two days of paid training soon. And, before that, I'd like to pay them both to read a couple of books, watch some videos, and spend some extended time with Ruffin to get to know him better. If they read the books and had concerns, or if they didn't care for what they saw on the videos, they should speak up, and I would keep looking.

Donna called Lisa, and they agreed to read and watch. Just that easily, I hired two experienced mothers, two friends, two wonderful women to be Ruffin's therapists. And, as playmates, Ruffin would have Donna's two children, Danielle, about ten, and Matthew, about thirteen, and Lisa's three children, all also older than Ruffin. Older children were who he seemed to relate to best.

Donna was part-Native American, half-Norwegian, with blue eyes and brassy blonde hair around her round and friendly freckled face. A large presence. Jovial. Commanding in a rough, but warmly evolved way. Her good friend, Lisa, was smaller, quieter, more distant than Donna, as deeply rooted in our small community as anyone, a long-time, trusted daycare provider. But when Lisa smiled into the face of a child, her nose wrinkled, and her eyebrows winged upward like a bird leaving a branch. Neither had any experience in special education.

Now Seamus was curious and agreed to attend Evelyn's training workshop, as my third trainee. He was still working nights at the time, across the Mississippi, but committed to spending the entire training weekend with us.

So did Rose, who agreed to cook and wash up.

So, they were my village.

In late September, although it would stir up trouble, I needed Dr. Caldwell's advice. I didn't want to put Ruffin through the ordeal of a difficult Lovaas CARD program, and spend money like water, if he and I would be working uphill against any rare form of intractable neurological, genetic, or metabolic defect.

While I was inclined to gamble on a CARD program with Dr. Granpeesheh, I needed to rule out as many difficulties as I could before laying down large on the table and rolling all our dice — both Ruffin's time and all my money. If Ruffin's condition were a progressive neurological disorder, I would rather spend what money I had to keep Ruffin comfortable, and to arrange to enjoy and spend all the time I had with him as happily as I could manage.

In my letter, I listed the various disorders and syndromes that I wanted Dr. Caldwell to rule out. I also wanted him to know I appreciated his early July diagnosis, and his blunt frankness. "Your provisional diagnosis of PDD-NOS has been most helpful to Ruffin. It has improved his life to be in school, for me to understand his symptoms and where they may come from and has helped me focus on what therapies may help."

With Dr. Caldwell and his autism clinic colleagues, I also shared my letter to school conveying my request for a home program of applied behavior analysis (ABA) of 40 hours per week of one-to-one language training for Ruffin. I described his educators' negative response as being "conclusory and not documented by any evidence or citation to any medical research or educational literature." Family resources were available for me to hire home tutors, and to have an appropriately trained person instruct them in CARD's ABA methods. Did they know anyone locally who might be interested in training as a tutor and working with Ruffin? What I planned was that my home tutors would work in coordination with the concepts being taught by Ruffin's teacher. I credited the group setting which Ruffin enjoyed in his public-school program to be of some value toward assuring his "social" development. And, it was true, despite my real concerns that Ruffin's public school special education was inadequate to teach him to talk, I felt that it did have some "social" value, and that Meg was doing the best she could.

To our next appointment, I would bring three brief videos: Ruffin at home, talking; Ruffin at school, working and whispering; Ruffin at Julie's daycare, not talking. Were the computer programs Ruffin was using, that had been developed for pre-school and developmentally disabled children, the "functional equivalent" of ABA discrete trial teaching?

Finally, I pleaded to the medical group for Ruffin and myself, as I would in any court, for any client. "Recovery from autism is possible, but infrequent, of course.

"Ruffin is my child. It is my responsibility to choose for him. And it's my money.

"Catherine Maurice, who succeeded in recovering her two children from autism, is my model. She read everything. She confirmed the diagnoses of her children with four different assessment groups. She tried everything, with her eyes wide open, and with undaunted curiosity. She sought help, and she hired help. She got ripped off. Emotional, she fell prey to charlatans. She did find something that worked for her children.

"If Ruffin and I are not as lucky or fortunate as Catherine Maurice and her children, I do have reserves of resigned acceptance. But I would like to keep them in reserve, for the time after I have gone down in the flames of public failure, after I have not gone 'gentle into that good night.'"

In late September, the patient coordinator for the autism clinic called. The clinic had not received their questionnaires back from Ruffin's teacher or his speech and language pathologist. I went to school to round them up and took a moment to read all the comments written in by Meg and her aide, Ella. With growing horror, I began to hyperventilate — their comments were an echo of Ruffin's behavior in Julie's daycare, and of everything we had learned about him back in early August. No progress had been made in nearly a month of school.

The next day Kim administered the *Peabody Picture Vocabulary Test, Revised* to Ruffin. Her assessment was the same as Ruffin's expressive language score in early August. This testing represented Kim's establishment of her own baseline for her direct speech therapy with Ruffin. I wondered if it might have been her response to the concerns raised at the earlier meeting at Bridgewater.

What did Kim think about intensive Lovaas instruction for Ruffin — as a child with autism who needed to understand speech? I thought he could learn to speak, even if it had to be by some means that typically developing children did not need. But, since Kim had never attended any of Ruffin's meetings with me, I didn't feel able to ask.

Meanwhile, I continued to call up and down the ladder of Bridgewater administrators, and called Sue again, about auditory integration training (AIT), angling for pre-treatment, mid-treatment, and post-treatment audiograms, and other assessments for the children of our parent-group. Nary a nibble. No interest, no help.

With the school authorities and me buffalo to buffalo over my request for Lovaas instruction, I needed to open another avenue of support, to try to recruit other allies. On my desk was an ominous, unattended-to denial of benefits notice from Prudential for Ruffin's latest Gundersen visit. The insurance company wanted a diagnosis and prescription for any further occupational therapy from Dr. Thompson, Ruffin's neo-natal pediatrician, team-leader of Ruffin's PICU treatment team since his birth. This was the first time Prudential had balked at covering Ruffin's medical care at Gundersen, or with our local family doctor. My focus shifted to a more pressing problem — the limitations of private insurance for mental health coverage would fail to cover the costly, early intensive treatment that might benefit Ruffin now.

I felt I was doing everyone else's job for them — and beginning to resent it. But I choked back those feelings to express the gratitude and the hope I would have preferred to feel. I closed my latest plea for help to Ruffin's doctors, "Thank you for all your efforts on Ruffin's behalf. He continues to bring great joy to his family, especially as we see him pick up and begin to make forward progress again."

CHAPTER EIGHT

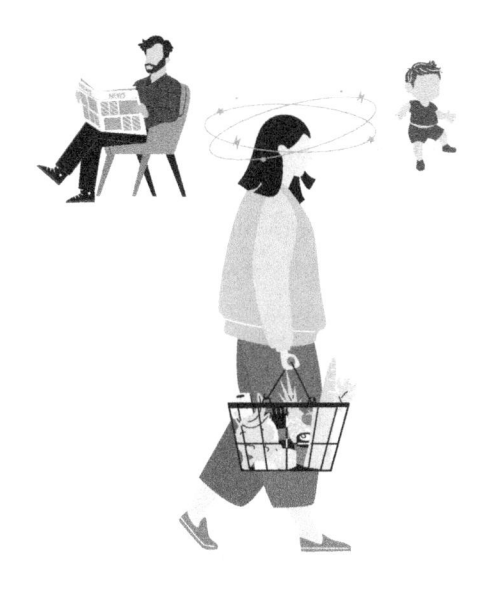

WHAT DO YOU THINK?

Ruffin and I spent a long weekend in Iowa City with RoJene and her friends there. Unsurprisingly, he had several tantrums: leaving Hardee's ball trampoline; in a large, nice but noisy restaurant when he couldn't have what he wanted; on the bank of the swollen river — when I wouldn't let him go up to see closer, or throw in a stick like the other, older children. He was up from midnight Saturday to dawn, and up Sunday night from midnight again. RoJene's friends, a couple with three children, were concerned that Ruffin would wake them. RoJene got up with me and made tea. We talked. I told her everything, including my plans. She listened. The stiff night breezes shifted and blew hard rains, dampening the sound of the river running past the small cabin where we all had tried to bunk down together.

The next day, without any more sleep, Ruffin was in and out of several stores, playing well in the group of five children, Chance, a younger boy, and two older girls. We had quite a good time despite all the rain.

I shared all of it with Meg. And, because I knew she planned to read *Let Me Hear Your Voice* over her long weekend, I wanted to know, "Tell me, what do you think of Catherine Maurice?"

I was on the phone with Dr. Carol Reed at the autism clinic. Ruffin's medical team had just met to decide how to respond to my many, written questions, which she let me know, in no uncertain terms, were "overwhelming for all of us." Oh, I thought to myself, rather meanly, and just how overwhelming do you imagine autism is? For me, and Ruffin, and Seamus?

She continued to press in on me. "Based on the nature of your questions, particularly of Dr. Caldwell, I need to ask you directly if you think we are what you're looking for to help with Ruffin's near future?"

Quickly, I moved to offer reassurance. "No, we've all gone to a lot of work to prepare for the upcoming appointments. I don't want to cancel them. I want to hear what you all know and might learn about Ruffin."

Then she "wanted to be clear," as she had obviously been tasked to be, "about what it is we do, and what we don't do. We can offer suggestions about what Ruffin needs. And direct you to other resources. For example, I've talked with Bridgewater's school psychologist Emily Knight, who could administer Ruffin the *PEP-R* to advise you how to meet Ruffin's needs."

Somehow, I didn't care for that idea. "No."

Dr. Reed sensed she wasn't going to budge me. "We can have a preliminary meeting before the end of September. To answer all your questions would cost a lot of money. Remember, our conference room is on the third floor. We'll see you there."

I tried to raise my request for ABA training and auditory integration training (AIT).

"Sorry, I'm on a tight schedule," she interrupted.

I had lost her attention. "Okay, then, see you in a couple of days!" I tried to be the cheerful I wasn't, before letting her go.

Over the last week of September, Meg charted Ruffin's response to her teaching objective that he use a noun with a verb. She was getting meaningless echolalia, and nothing when she tried prompting him with a picture. During that whole week she heard a single spontaneous question, "What's he doing?" and a single spontaneous answer, "Mamma hug."

While Ruffin was in school, I drove an hour up the Mississippi with all the leaf color reflected in the by-waters, for an hour-and-a-half long preliminary meeting to plan Ruffin's upcoming full autism clinic evaluation with Dr. Reed and Dr. Caldwell. We talked a bit about having a speech and language pathologist Mila Sokolov evaluate Ruffin, even though she had recently retired.

By the end of the meeting, our exchanges got to be productive and extremely amiable. The Gundersen group might have finally gotten my number — just throw books and information at this rabid woman, and she will stay busy, happy, and quiet for a little while.

I felt so light-hearted walking out of our meeting that I went shopping in LaCrosse for an hour — not for anything, just looking, for nothing. I realized I hadn't been in a mall since just after Ruffin was born, when I had left the hospital for an hour to go to a recommended high-end department store to buy preemie-sized onesies and hit the toy aisle for any doll-clothes that might work for a baby boy. I was disappointed there were not many outfits available for boys, or for boy dolls.

Having Ruffin changed my life in all the usual ways that having a child changes anyone's life, but Ruffin having autism had upended my life in much more profound ways. My life had become so narrowly focused on autism, Ruffin seemed to have moved out on the periphery, his face circling me like a small, pale, and waning moon. Seamus swooped in like a comet on his elliptical orbit. I couldn't keep track of him either.

Now, I felt oddly overwhelmed by the wealth of selections spread out before me on the shelves. Who needed six types of garden hoses, more than two pairs of shoes, more than fourteen brands of canned tomatoes, crushed, diced, with and without salt, or garlic, basil, or oregano? It was hard to focus on anything but autism. I felt unable to choose, unable to take advantage of this rare opportunity of being in a larger city to buy a single, solitary thing. Everything looked like an unnecessary luxury. I kept passing everything up.

Then, I stopped by school and got Ruffin. That night he sat through *The Story of Ferdinand* with complete attention and absorption — and with apparent understanding. Earlier, we had only examined individual pages in detail and only gotten through a few before he lost track of the story. He remembered and performed the whole little *Bunny Foo Foo* story song routine with me. He reminded *me* when I "forgot" to have the fairy come down.

In late September, Ruffin and I had our second visit with Dr. Caldwell, who breezed through my lengthy list of mid-September concerns. He offered me an additional information resource, *Focus on Autistic Behavior*, another Pro-Ed publication that I could subscribe to, and suggested I might reach out to Luther College in Decorah, or to the University of Minnesota, or the University of Chicago.

We discussed a sleep-deprived EEG he had scheduled for Ruffin in mid-October to rule out seizures, and to address Meg's and my shared concerns about Ruffin's recent staring spells. He handed me a little record form to keep at home and one to send to school for anyone there to record these spells or any other suspicious mental blank time or troubling events that might be suggestive of seizures. From visiting with their parents, I knew several of the other special education students experienced seizures regularly and that Meg, Ella, and Amy were all experienced in recognizing and reporting them to their parents.

The cost of repeat chromosome studies Dr. Caldwell quoted seemed high, and not to be of any therapeutic value now. He agreed to test Ruffin's serum lead and magnesium levels, which later proved to be normal.

Then as I sensed his patience wearing thin, I handed Dr. Caldwell copies of Lovaas's two academic studies, and their published peer-reviews. I offered to pay him for his time to read them and then tell me whether they were "junk science." I wanted him to read them as an expert, just as if he were preparing to be an expert witness in court, and then visit with me. He understood, and readily agreed.

As we were going out the door, he commented that Ruffin seemed to have more potential than he first thought during Ruffin's July appointment, when he had given me Ruffin's autism diagnosis. That lifted me up a little. Maybe some of what I was doing was working, some of my focus on reading and researching autism was paying off? Maybe what Meg was doing at school was helping, more than I expected or knew? I was sure the vitamins were working, because anytime Ruffin missed them, there was trouble. The computer was helping, too. I was going to get to be a good mother. I wanted to believe that Ruffin had quite a lot of potential. I wanted all my family and Seamus to believe the same and be proud of Ruffin, and to feel certain that I was a good mother.

I delivered the other copy of my materials to Dr. Thompson's office, outside the PICU, where he was busy with new babies. Then, Ruffin and I headed back home down the river. I talked to Ruffin about what we would be doing tomorrow, trying to get him excited. "We're going to see some big horses."

"Horses," Ruffin nodded, as we passed a scattered few in a roadside pasture.

We were going to a draft horse sale that Saturday. This happened once a year when the Amish gathered on the fairgrounds for an exchange auction of their field-working horses — golden Belgians, Percherons, black as coal and slick as a ribbon, Clydesdales, and Friesians — their tractors.

It was raining but not enough to dampen the feeling of this gathering. From our hatchback parked among the pickups, Ruffin and I wound our way through a pasture full of buggies and tethered horses, each draped in a green, blue, or occasional pink blanket. These were the solid colors of the Amish.

"No," I told Ruffin. "These are not the horses we've come to see."

As Ruffin and I walked into the metal shed of the arena, the women and older girls were cooking behind a counter of card tables piled with bowls of mashed potatoes, finely diced green pepper and radishes and Doritos that had been broken into a fine dust. The Amish called this a haystack supper — mashed potatoes and anything you cared to pile on, with milk or coffee to drink, and homemade ice cream after if you had any room left for dessert. Maybe Ruffin would try a bite of mine.

He and I climbed up in the stands around the arena to the highest plank — to eat and watch the proceedings. Clerks were slapping numbered stickers on the back haunches of the horses being registered for sale, and then the handlers, waving white flags on the end of their sticks, up and down, hurried each one along. The biggest horses — the ones that stood over seven feet tall — were fearful of that bit of moving cloth.

The Amishmen stalked about in their black felt hats, barn coats, and homemade denim pants, looking nearly alike, and kicking up sawdust as they conferred over this or that horse, flipping through the sale book. Then, the microphone came on and the first horses began prancing into the arena. The auctioneer began his warbling babble.

Ruffin began to squirm a little, so I put a hand on his leg, and said, "Hang in there, little buddy. This is going to be good."

Then, Seamus sidled in next to us — so Ruffin sat wedged safely between the two of us.

The first colt sold for the price of a small new car, and the next, a filly with a pedigree went for the price of a new pickup.

"That one is really flashy," Seamus poked Ruffin, and then pointed to what remained to be seen of her — her tail — as she was led out to her purchaser.

Meg had written me a note that I wriggled out of my jeans pocket to hand to Seamus over Ruffin's head.

"Read that," I said, a bit smugly.

"You missed this by a few minutes last Thursday; there were boxes in the office for us! All the *Constructive Playthings* orders arrived. And today another shipment of books came. It was like Christmas!"

"Ha!" Seamus said as he handed it back to me. "This — this is like Christmas!"

Most of the new Gundersen examiners attended a late-afternoon October 5th staffing to summarize their results, as I did, with Ruth sitting in the waiting room with

Ruffin, who was tired and distracted after two days of being tested and prodded and prompted and played with and challenged to do this or that.

From school, Meg attended and scribbled notes while my mind raced.

From her scribbling, it was Kevin Josephson, M.S., a genetics counselor, a chipper young man, all blonde moustache and fly-away hair, and thin-lensed flashing glasses who presented first, with all his negative laboratory findings, and his eliminations of all known genetic causes of Ruffin's developmental delays. Josephson also briefly mentioned the MRI findings of "thinning of the corpus callosum," explaining he was standing in for Dr. Caldwell, who was unable to join us.

Then, it was Dr. Carol Reed, the medical-educational specialist, who looked her professional, experienced part, with her short, stylish blow-cut, above large and lovely eyes, as she presented her general opening summary by describing Ruffin's current center-based, self-contained school placement. "Center-based" meaning Ruffin received his educational services at a schoolhouse, in a more intensive form of early special education delivery, well-beyond the usual brief in-home visits from travelling therapists. "Self-contained" meaning his class did not join other students in the lunchroom, and that most services were brought into the room.

Then Dr. Reed turned to Meg and Ella's concerns in the areas of speech and language, motor skills and social skills, and their specific questions regarding programming recommendations. Although I had already read their observations on the forms I had collected and passed on to the autism clinic, and even though Meg was sitting right there beside me, I was still taken a bit aback. The two people spending the most time with Ruffin so far at school had concerns, and specific questions regarding programming recommendations. It seemed clear enough, we all had reason to be here.

Dr. Reed recounted Ruffin's history for the group. "Medical developmental information indicated that Ruffin has a history of respiratory distress at birth with periods of apnea and bradycardia. He was previously assessed by Emily Knight, school psychologist, in early August. Her report indicated that he was 'significantly delayed.'"

Then, she called on the next presenter, Dr. Irwin Ladd, a child and adolescent psychiatrist, who cleared his throat, ran his tongue over his teeth, thoughtfully, and began, "Ruffin is an extremely interesting young man."

The day before, after Ruffin's actual time alone with him, I had been startled as Dr. Ladd emerged from his examining room with the stuffed puppet of a shark on his hand. He spoke oddly enough, just like a psychiatrist, as he greeted me. "Ruffin seems to like this one best, maybe it reminds him of his mother . . . ." He reported to me then, just as he said now to everyone assembled, "Ruffin has many of the characteristics of children described as being autistic. On the other hand, he has many characteristics that do not fit into this diagnosis in the classic sense."

It was clear that his unstated reference was to classical autism, or Kanner's syndrome. That was how I heard him, how I interpreted his remarks. I wondered how Meg might be hearing this, but it wasn't possible to ask or interrupt, since Dr. Ladd was on a roll.

"For example, Ruffin has echolalic verbalizations, but will maintain eye contact more than is typically seen in an autistic child. He has no specific transition object but will play appropriately with some toys. He allowed me to help him play with a toy and was interacting. He answered questions that were very simple. Sometimes these answers were echolalic in their form."

"There is no evidence of delusions or hallucinations."

Good, I thought.

Then, Dr. Ladd let loose a thunderbolt, out of the blue.

"Intellectual testing shows Ruffin to be in the mid-80s range."

Wow, 30 or more points to the good from Emily's earlier *Bayley* score of 50. True, there was a lot of uncertainty in intellectual testing in very young children. But 30 and more points in a scale of 100 was, as Ruffin himself might say today, an awful lot of noise in the data. And, dear me, not good, a lot of egg on Emily's face. I could just imagine why Dr. Ladd, and Dr. Reed's written summary had failed to recite Emily's number, her *Bayley Scale* 50, her underassessment, but had reported her findings in their measured, forgiving characterization that Emily had given of Ruffin: "significantly delayed."

Which, of course, Ruffin was — being very significantly delayed in his language development.

Meanwhile, Dr. Ladd continued to opine. "At the present time, descriptively, Ruffin's behavior fits somewhere into the PDD-NOS category, although it certainly seems that Ruffin is more affectionate and has some better language functioning than one would expect of a truly autistic child. It is possible that he does have a serious language-based learning disorder or that he is developing into an Asperger's type syndrome. Time is going to be necessary for a more formal diagnosis."

Wasn't that just clear as mud? For me and for his educators, Dr. Caldwell's little diagram had been so much clearer.

But, in that moment, I felt deeply and calmly delighted. The thought sailed slowly through my mind, if Ruffin were to develop into an Asperger's type, he would be right at home in our family of IBM and INTEL electrical engineers, my father and brother who struggled so mightily with their spelling. If Ruffin could just learn to learn, just learn to talk, wouldn't he be well on the way to slipping back into place, back into all the promise of the perfect baby he was when he was born? Wouldn't he still grow up into the little boy I had imagined? The one I had longed to have? That his grandparents and Seamus had expected me to deliver?

Finally, Dr. Ladd concluded, "Various medicines were discussed with Ruffin's mother at the time of the staffing and are not recommended at this time." That medical-record sentence didn't touch his and my actual discussion. From Meg's scribbles, Dr. Ladd's suggestions had included Prozac to improve Ruffin's language and behavior, fenfluramine to produce a better quality of relatedness, and Benadryl or chloralhydrate to regulate his sleep cycle. I feared the toxic potential of every one of these off-label uses of prescription drugs for young children with autism.

"No," I said, repeatedly, to Dr. Ladd's every suggestion for medication.

None of this was going to clarify matters for Ruffin's educators. Judging by their earlier letter, brushing off my own suggestions, they were already confused and ready to take advantage of their confusion to curtail Ruffin's educational potential and threaten his disability entitlements. I glanced over to see how Meg might be taking all this. She was able to read my face well enough, and shook her head, as if to say, "Not impressive."

I still felt uneasy. Dr. Ladd was going to be trouble.

The next presenter was Dr. Patricia Kondrick, a neuropsychologist who had written me back a detailed letter about what she planned to do in her testing of Ruffin. Her sharply chiseled features were set in a broad, round face, small nose, small mouth, and small deep-set eyes below thin brows encircled by a great fall of curling red hair.

"Ruffin was seen for intellectual assessment and a *Vineland Adaptive Behavior Inventory*. A school-based evaluation had been completed previously.

"As part of that evaluation, he was given the *Bayley Scales of Infant Development, 2nd Edition*, and I have reviewed those test results." A flat, merciless sentence.

I vividly recalled the day before. Dr. Kondrick had been retesting Ruffin after 25 days spent in his ECSE classroom. She and her assistant tested Ruffin, while I sat behind a one-way, mirrored window to watch, but not cue, nor distract him.

"Ruffin entered the test environment very quickly and willingly. He has learned appropriate social pragmatic skills and upon introduction, refers to me as "Hi, friend."

Ruffin was no better at catching new names than I was. There were ways he was more my son than Seamus's, and surely this was one of them. Seamus knew everyone, and the names of everyone's forebears back to the pioneer generation and their counties of origin in Ireland, the same way he knew the lineage of every piece of horseflesh in the county.

Through the heat of the afternoon, Dr. Kondrick's voice wafted back, "He was quite attentive to my instructions. He worked well and looked to me for additional instruction. He also looked to me for evaluation of his performance. On problem solving tasks, he demonstrated beginning skills, evaluation of his work, and made steps to self-correct his productions.

"When task directions became too complex for him and the mean length of utterance exceeded his ability to comprehend, he merely echoed back the last word I suggested. He demonstrated good ability to benefit from repetition and demonstration."

I remembered watching, too, like a hawk. Ruffin's back had remained turned to me, with Dr. Kondrick and her assistant facing me, exchanging quick and then ever quickening glances between them as his responses clearly exceeded their initial expectations.

"On the *Wechsler Preschool and Primary Scale of Intelligence-Revised,* he earned a Verbal IQ of 74, estimated Performance IQ of 86, and estimated Full Scale IQ of 78 (7th percentile), which placed his overall level of ability in the upper end of the borderline range."

Here were the new numbers. Somehow, Ruffin had been able to complete this standardized IQ test for 3- to 7-year-olds. Somehow, he had bobbed up out of moderate mental retardation to the borderline of normal intelligence.

I was acutely aware, too, that by testing above IQ 70, Ruffin had passed the presumptive cut-off mark to move into the danger of full criminal responsibility, including the death penalty, even execution as punishment for any later misunderstood or strange behavior resulting from his autism. From my legal studies, I knew that IQ 70 was a tricky spot, neither able, nor unable, responsible, but not really very responsible — IQ 70 was unstable.

Above IQ 70, Ruffin also passed the presumptive cut-off mark that would forever extinguish his eligibility for Social Security Disability, a possible funding resource. Ruffin had just lost a lifetime of financial support. It would be more important than ever that he have his chance to learn to talk, to catch up, and to run loose in the universe.

Dr. Kondrick had more to offer. "He gives a strong performance on tests of non-oral problem solving."

Yes, I thought, but he needed to learn to communicate, to understand and use language, to talk.

As Dr. Kondrick went on to explain how she found Ruffin to have a variable IQ profile, her explanations resonated with my earlier reading and research on autism. Marked variability between verbal IQ and performance IQ was often seen in children with autism. So-called splinter skills might be found in such children, isolated savant skills — odd things they did better than nearly anyone else. I caught my breath, caught up again in wishful thinking.

"The performance tests variously assess attention to visual detail, visual motor integration, and perceptual construction skills."

Yes, I thought, as I listened eagerly. I could have regaled this group with how Ruffin was fascinated by those early learning computer programs, styled like Lovaas's discrete trial drills, with their brief animated rewards. But, I listened silently as Dr. Kondrick continued.

"This profile was notable for a marked degree of variability across those performance subtest scores. Such variability is nonspecific and is seen in individuals with attention deficit disorder, learning disability, and organic brain syndrome. The pattern of performance suggested that there were select abilities which were age appropriate or better."

I had tried not to read too much into yesterday, into the examiners' momentary loss of their poker faces. I had sensed professional excitement rising and bubbling throughout the first long day of testing, but the full significance of the standard IQ and other testing results, the information by the numbers and their portent, didn't strike me — didn't floor me — until this day's meeting.

The day before, while Ruffin worked on, someone else had needed me for a *Vineland* interview. This assessment tool was familiar to me, from reading Catherine Maurice, ". . . a screening test for developmental maturity . . . . Anne-Marie was functioning at about a one-year-old level in her communication and socialization skills (with better motor skills) . . . . This uneven pattern of development reflected the common profile for autism . . ." — just as it did for Ruffin.

Dr. Kondrick rolled out her numbers to the group. "Ruffin earned an adaptive behavior composite standard score (SS) of 82, age equivalent of 2 years, 9 months. This reflected earnings in the following skill domains:

- Communication — SS of 85, age equivalent of 2 years, 7 months
- Daily Living Skills — SS of 76, age equivalent of 2 years, 4 months
- Socialization — SS of 88, age equivalent of 2 years, 8 months
- Motor Skills — SS of 99, age equivalent of 3 years, 4 months.

"Our findings suggested adaptive behaviors in the home were in keeping with his performance on standardized measures of intelligence. Expectancies of him in the home, therefore, appeared to be appropriate."

So, by Dr. Kondrick's numbers, I measured up as a good mother to Ruffin as a child with disabilities. This meant a great deal to me, because by now I suspected there were a lot of people who didn't really think so.

During the next presentation by Dr. Reed, Ruth slipped in with Ruffin to let us all know she needed to get home to meet Renee's school bus, so Meg kindly took mercy on Ruffin, who was beyond bored and cranky, and moved down on the floor with him to entertain him, to quiet him. He eventually fell asleep on the hospital's grey industrial-grade carpet.

"Ruffin was given the *Psychoeducational Profile-Revised Developmental Scale*." This was the *PEP-R* that Sue had suggested to me in late July. As Dr. Reed explained, "This scale measures a child's performance and interaction with various objects as well as behavioral responses in the areas of imitation, perception, fine motor, gross motor, eye to hand integration, cognitive performance, and cognitive verbal skills, with an overall developmental summation score. Ruffin's gross motor skills were measured in a limited space, and it is anticipated that this subtest can be expanded through the public schools, where he can be viewed in a comfortable, familiar setting and hopefully, a much larger testing environment."

Meg looked up from where she was seated on the carpet with Ruffin, and nodded, as Dr. Reed continued to report her surprisingly good results.

"Scores for Ruffin were very age appropriate, except for verbal skills at 26 months. Other scores ranged from 37 to 48 months, with his chronological age at 42 months."

Yes, I thought, repeating my own mantra to myself, he needs to learn to talk. We needed to teach him to talk. But this was not my turn to talk. Everyone there knew what I wanted- — to try a Lovaas program — but not one of them would speak to that possibility. I made myself go on listening in the close, warm room.

"Ruffin's performance was quite striking for his level of attention and cooperation. He also did not resist transition or changing of activities. He did echo me frequently.

"He identified the basic shapes of a circle, square, and triangle. He also matched color blocks with color paper swatches. He engaged in some representative play by making a house of blocks in the waiting room. This was observed informally.

"He identified, using picture representation, familiar objects, matching the object to the picture and identifying its function such as a comb, cup, toothbrush, etc.

"He demonstrated social routines spontaneously, offering a 'thank you' when I offered him a toy."

"He sorted objects by shape with prompting."

"He, he, he," Dr. Reed's references to Ruffin were pounding through my memories of yesterday, were pounding through my brain. Yes, of course, he can do all that.

"He did not demonstrate any particular tactile defensiveness.

"He used his right hand primarily for fine motor tasks such as coloring. Many positive observations included his looking to me for reinforcement.

"He was able to move from one activity to another without the negative behaviors that frequently accompany children with PDD-NOS.

"He followed directions easily, imitated, and interacted with me.

"He demonstrated knowledge of cause and effect and showed an ability to learn from his mistakes. Bubbles that he placed in his mouth produced a definite negative response from him and he did not do this again.

"He played symbolically with a set of puppets of cat and dog, having them chase one another around.

"His attention was quite adequate throughout the examination."

With that conclusion, Dr. Reed came to a brief stop, and looked about the room as if to check whether everyone was getting all this.

With Dr. Reed, yesterday, I recalled, I had also been welcome to watch Ruffin's testing. "It should be noted that his mother was in the room while he completed these tasks, and to the best of my observation, did not negatively influence his performance, as he was aware of her presence, but he did not become distracted nor seek her out in a manner that would have disrupted his performance. Overall, Ruffin's developmental score was 36 months with the range of variability as noted previously. There are many positives noted on today's examination that suggest prognosis for continued improvement is good."

The day before, we had lunched at the hospital cafeteria, then hurried on to meet the audiologist, David Palm, Ph.D., who stepped in for a few minutes to report to the afternoon group.

"This 3-year, 6-month-old boy was accompanied by his mother for evaluation of his hearing. According to her, his last ear infection was in August of this year. He is currently on no medication except vitamin B-6 and magnesium as part of the treatment for his behavioral problems. He does show sensitivity to sound, particularly sirens, whistles, and bells. He gets very agitated when this happens. His audiogram was obtained with very little difficulty. He conditioned nicely to pure tones and responded well within normal limits from 250 to 4,000 Hertz. His speech thresholds were at 15 in both ears.

Discrimination was judged to be adequate bilaterally. Tympanograms were reasonably flat on both sides."

I had found Dr. Palm friendly, and open to our parent-group's interest in experimenting with auditory integration training (AIT).

Now, he reported to the group, "I had a long discussion with Ruffin's mother. We discussed an AIT study currently underway with the Chileda residents. The data collection should be completed by February and if you would like to call in March" — here, Dr. Palm turned to me and nodded, smiling warmly — "I should be able to tell you the results. I do not recommend follow-up with a hearing test unless Ruffin develops some symptoms, like fever or pain."

I had learned the day before while visiting with Dr. Palm that Chileda was a residential treatment home in LaCrosse, where children with autism who were unable to live at home were placed in care. Dr. Palm and Dr. Ladd, among others at Gundersen, served all the children growing up at Chileda.

When I had offered Dr. Palm Ruffin's most recent Bridgewater audiogram, he scrawled me a little note to show the school authorities that I had followed up promptly on their recommendation, and that Ruffin's hearing seemed to be normal.

Late in the afternoon, we finally got down to brass tacks when the speech and language pathologist, Mila Sokolov summarized her findings.

"This young boy presents with deficits in both language comprehension and expression of more than one year secondary to a diagnosis of PDD-NOS. Progress is reported to have occurred over the last several months. . .. he is just starting to say 2- to 3-word phrases that are occasionally spontaneous but continues to have elements of delayed or mitigated echolalia."

I began to feel hopeful that Mrs. Sokolov had a good handle on Ruffin's problems.

Meg left Ruffin sleeping on the floor and returned to a grown-up seat at the table. She looked exhausted. Both she and I could have used some cold water, or coffee.

Mrs. Sokolov, however, was just getting started. First she detailed all Ruffin's prior language testing. Then, she described examining his mouth. To my astonishment, the day before, Ruffin had allowed this strange old lady, as grey and kind as a Russian babushka, to examine his mouth.

"Observation of the oral speech mechanism indicates structures capable of supporting speech. Ruffin was heard to make a variety of speech sounds that were developmentally appropriate. There were instances of occasional unintelligible speech, but this was a result of running echoed phrases together into 'mega words.' There is no history of difficulties with chewing, swallowing, or choking on foods. Ruffin is described, however, as having food preferences, including chocolate milk at all meals."

Finally, Mrs. Sokolov reported on her own testing.

"To assess Ruffin's language comprehension, I chose to administer the *Reynell Development Language Scale*, which assesses the ability to understand language that gradually increases in length and complexity. Ruffin achieved a raw score of 27, with a corresponding age equivalency range of 2 years, 5 months on the 'old' norms and 2 years, 1 month on the more current norms."

Here, she broke off to explain briefly how the *Reynell* had just been re-normed, since children nowadays were expected to be more accomplished than in the past. They were exposed to so much more and were expected to develop more quickly.

"Ruffin was able to follow some one-step directions but had difficulty with pointing to objects when given their function. When items became more difficult, he began repeating the questions.

"My informal observation of Ruffin's skills indicated that he was able to understand some simple directives and was beginning to play appropriately with toys even to the point of some 'pretend' play.

"Eye contact was good throughout most of the evaluation and behavior and cooperation was judged to be very good.

"Only toward the end of the session when Ruffin was obviously tired, did he begin to refuse to comply with requests. His mother reported that this was close to a time that he rested, and it was obvious that he was trying to indicate to us that he had 'had enough.' Even to the point where he took all of the toys out of the toy box and curled up in it with his stuffed toy."

Yes, Ruffin had been struggling to get over his cold and had seemed suddenly tuckered out, on the point of collapse. We were approaching the tail-end of a long day. I was concerned Mrs. Sokolov wouldn't get a good test of Ruffin's abilities or an accurate measure of his disabilities. She had decided then to continue with Ruffin the next morning when she administered the second half of the *Reynell* and another language test.

We were treated to another long roll-out of numbers, numbers I would study carefully later. I promised myself, I would learn to understand them, disentangle the *receptive* scores from the *expressive* scores, and figure out what they meant and how they meant something, or promised something, or threatened something for Ruffin.

"The expressive language portion of the *Reynell*, which assesses language structure, vocabulary, and content, was administered. Ruffin achieved a raw score of 23, with a corresponding age equivalency of 2 years, 2 months on the 'old' norms and 1 year, 10 months on the more current norms.

"He was able to name objects and pictures and was heard to speak in single word and some word combinations. He could not, however, relate content in pictures nor were his vocalizations extensively spontaneous. Many of them were echoed or, to some degree, repetition of 'practiced' phrases or dialogues.

"*Gardner's Expressive One Word Picture Vocabulary Test-Revised* was administered and yielded a raw score of 12, with a corresponding age equivalent of 2 years, 9 months, and a standard score of 86. It is noteworthy, however, that this was a naming task only, and did not reflect the more complex aspects of language."

At last, Mrs. Sokolov offered us her recommendations.

"It is recommended that Ruffin continue to receive speech and language therapy with emphasis placed on increasing spontaneous vocabulary to include action words and modifiers and increasing language comprehension relative to concept development and following more complex directives. Some additional specific suggestions which can be modified to meet Ruffin's needs will be sent in our written report."

I became quietly frustrated. Modified exactly how? That was the advice I was looking for, and that Bridgewater was paying for, to get out of this two-day ordeal to help Meg and Ella address their concerns. I couldn't believe how furious I was feeling, but as I stared into the glass of the hospital window at myself — there I was — as angry as the sky at sunset, as the sun went down on our long staffing.

Mrs. Sokolov concluded with a smile in my direction, offered kindly enough, as encouragement. "Ruffin is a bright and engaging young boy who appears to be making some gains in language in a relatively short period of time."

Well, no, as a writer, I would hardly choose the characterization "bright" to describe "borderline" intelligence. This was more pap, baby food in the mouth. I wanted to spit, or vomit as I had in the little girls' room at Ruffin's school.

And, no, Ruffin did not really appear to be making some gains in language in a relatively brief period of time. His language development by whatever measure, continued to lag behind his age and other developmental domains by as much as 18 months — by a year and a half's worth or more, by a measure that amounted to nearly half of his life. Ruffin's sliding descent into deeper language delay might have ground to a halt over the last few months. He might be holding steady, but he was not catching up. No one in this conference room except me envisioned Ruffin ever catching up. No one here really knew any sure way to help us. No one knew how to help Ruffin gain any traction in mastering language.

Meg and I, Miss Hobbs, Mr. Montague, and our family physician Dr. Olson were mailed a full written report later with Mrs. Sokolov's suggestions, the ones we should "modify for Ruffin individually."

As I considered all her fairly standard ECSE classroom techniques and best-practice speech and language pathology recommendations, flavored with a recognizable touch of Schopler's low-expectation outcome TEACCH methodology for autism, and as tweaked by Dr. Barry Prizant's suggestions with which I was already familiar, I felt tired, disappointed, and incredibly sad.

Bridgewater's money had resulted in no specific recommendations for Meg, Ella, and me about how to teach Ruffin to talk, and no answers whatsoever to my questions about using intensive ABA as developed by Lovaas. This controversial subject was not addressed anywhere in the collective recommendations.

"We recommend that both the family and teaching staff avail themselves of the literature available in the Comprehensive Child Care Center Library relative to PDD-NOS and autism, to enhance their knowledge base to help direct the focus of his educational program."

This medical team thought the school authorities and I were doing the best we could be expected to do with Ruffin. If we wanted to do better, we were remanded to Gundersen's medical library.

CHAPTER NINE

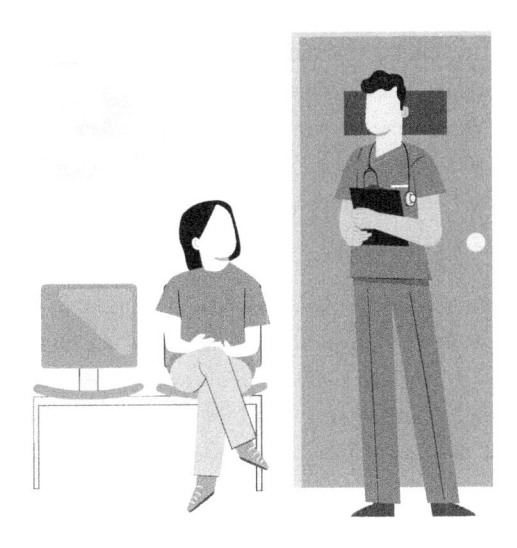

A NEW PRESCRIPTION

Fall had always been my favorite season, but this fall I was watching cold molasses move — just barely — anxiously biding my time until early November when Evelyn Kung was due to arrive from CARD. I invited Meg and anyone else from school to come.

"The training will be 'hands-on.'"

Ruffin and I made another morning journey in early October up to Gundersen for an EEG that Dr. Caldwell had ordered for Ruffin. Fog blanketed the river. Ruffin pointed it out as, "Smoke." I told him it was "Water smoke, called fog." He replied, "Cold smoke, fog," which I thought was smart, making a mental note to share this exchange with Meg, with Seamus, and with my parents.

It was difficult to glue electrodes to Ruffin's head, but Dr. Caldwell assured me his technician had gotten a good result, with no findings of any concern. Another relief.

There was still a lot of glue in Ruffin's hair. It didn't all come out with shampoo. I would need to use some nail polish remover to scrub it out before sending Ruffin back to school. I called Seamus to come over when he could, to hold Ruffin — so I wouldn't get that in his eyes accidentally.

Dr. Thompson, Ruffin's PICU pediatrician complimented me on my "Herculean effort to garner the best possible outcome" for Ruffin but deferred to Dr. Caldwell and the autism clinic for any advice. Any answer was enough to encourage me. So far, Dr. Thompson seemed the closest person to an ally I had, so I asked him to intercede with Dr. Caldwell "because I need a written prescription for Lovaas therapy for insurance purposes before early November."

Meanwhile, Ruffin was having trouble at school, getting in the water to swim. His Luther College student-instructor reported that Ruffin had reacted saying, "No water," repeatedly in the locker room. He wouldn't put his swimsuit on either or let her try to do it. The two of them had walked in *to look* at the pool. Ruffin wouldn't relent, so she had taken him to join another group in the gym. Meg went to get them back. She didn't give Ruffin much choice. "We're going to watch the kids swim." So, Ruffin watched a few minutes before it was time for the group to get out. When it was quieter, Meg put the ends of two foam pool-snakes into the water, so *they* could "swim." Ruffin was able to toss one in and pull it out, going right up to the edge of the water. He splashed his shoes and pants, which, of course, bothered him. Meg's plan was to put Ruffin's swimsuit on next time, or just take him in the pool with his clothes on, or in his pull-up diaper. I packed the extra change of clothes she asked for, since it sounded like she was determined to keep trying.

The next Friday, I put Ruffin's swimsuit on as his underwear, and suggested, "Expect a huge thrashing tantrum of resistance for several minutes. Just work through it; but get some help, for safety. You might get a calm after the storm, and then grudging acceptance. Splashing play will stop if he is praised when he stops for a moment. You might get this same series of behaviors once or twice, as we did at home with his baths. After the worst outburst ever, Ruffin completely turned around on taking baths and now asks for his baths, or gets in my bath uninvited, or runs his own bath without asking, or if he's up at night, wakes me up by trying to run water for a bath. He loves baths now. Same as with soap, the problem we had before, I guess."

I also showed up on a future Friday at the college — to volunteer — and to monitor Ruffin's reactions. The pool was brightly lit, noisy, and full of splashing college students preparing to teach special needs children, all bussed in from several area-wide schools — a much more challenging environment than our cozy bathtub at home.

Saturday morning Ruffin and I went fishing with Donna and her children. We drove out a county gravel to a bridge over a small stream running through a pasture. We planned to have fun — but with a purpose. Could Ruffin learn to fish, so he could go with my father in November? We had our troubles. With Donna bending over him, Ruffin managed to hook a worm, make a cast, and caught the fishhook on himself. It was okay. Donna had Band-Aids in the glove box of her van. When Ruffin caught a fish — that surprised him. It surprised me, and certainly pleased Donna. Donna's boy, Matt, showed Ruffin, "Now, you need to throw it back."

After that Matt and Ruffin threw big rocks off the bridge, because as Matt explained, "It makes a bigger splash." That spooked the herd of horses that were watering underneath. "Time to go," suggested Donna, "before someone shows up."

Sunday morning, I dropped Ruffin off at Sunday school so I could work. His teacher there reported he sang with the group for the first time and enjoyed chasing two other children. He had echoed some words for his teacher. When we came home, he played ball with the neighbor's grandchildren, but had trouble sharing and taking turns. There seemed to be too many boys in the group for him. I went out to bring him in.

"Look," I told him. "We need to hurry." Seamus had called and asked us to meet him over at The Pond's sugar bush. They were serving pancakes and sausage. Out we went and saw more horses there — at work, pulling trailers loaded with dozens of recycled white plastic sheetrock buckets full of sap. Seamus lifted Ruffin up on the wooden bed of a trailer so he could peer in at the rocking liquid. "Put your finger in, now in your mouth, like this." Ruffin did, and then we were off to watch the men stirring, with the vapor rising off the wide shallow vats.

Back home, watching *The Black Stallion Returns*, Ruffin made several spontaneous observations using subject-verb-object sentences: 'Boys ride camels,' 'Horse running,' 'Horse splash' and made clear to me that his computer printer needed fixing. Looking through his face-picture dictionary, Ruffin pointed to "happy," "sad," and "mad." He used "happy" and "tired" to let me know how he was feeling. And said, "Mommy happy," since I was.

I hoped Ruffin was tired and would stay down for a while. I had about half a night's worth of unfinished work on my desk — a couple of guilty pleas for drunk drivers, a burglary arraignment, a new stack of reports on foster placements and family reunifications. I had examinations to outline for another landlord-tenant dispute. Before I sat down to my computer with my highlighters and boxes of colored tabs, I put water on for more coffee. I had to be in the courtroom Monday, Tuesday, Wednesday and possibly Thursday in four different counties.

Monday after school, Donna, and Lisa — my therapist candidates — began working with Ruffin on the computer and prompting him to talk while reading books. They were drawing on what they had been able to learn from reading *The Me Book* and by watching the early Lovaas training videos. Donna had brought Danielle, too, for her to play with Ruffin, but they encountered several tantrums over taking turns and sharing. Still, Ruffin hugged Lisa goodbye, even after he had been angry with her earlier. Then Ruffin went to spend the night with Donna and her family, while I headed off across three counties to trial. Thankfully, I was home by late morning, the dispute having resolved itself by negotiations at the courthouse door.

I was trying another case the next morning and a third on Thursday. I hoped to get to school Thursday afternoon with a snack, and to install the rest of the computer programs there for Meg.

Friday, Ruffin spent some time after school sorting through Donna's collection of buttons of assorted colors and shapes: bears, bells, irons, and tiny scissors — preparing for a trip Seamus had proposed. We were going to the grand opening of the new addition to the Lansing button factory where Rose worked. There we were able to see many more buttons, the broken factory machines that had punched pearly blanks from fresh-water river clamshells, along with the new factory machines that stapled the newer plastic buttons to colorful cards. With Seamus holding one of Ruffin's hands, and I holding the other, Rose showed us the long aisles where she walked between metal shelves of marked cardboard bins to pick her orders. We had cake and shook hands with the newest CEO flown in from New York.

Back home, Ruffin replied in response to my question, "Who drives the car?" "Mommy drives car." "And who rides in the car?" "Ruffin riding." After Seamus left, Ruffin and I continued to work on verbs by having the computer's voice speak them while showing the animation of each action. I had Ruffin echo each verb and mime the actions: swimming, jumping, climbing. He seemed to enjoy this.

Later, while Ruffin was up in the middle of the night it seemed all his wires had suddenly connected. He was talking in complete 4- and 5-word sentences, commenting on everything in sight, talking about school and past events and coming events. This was remarkable *and* it was the middle of the night. He was in a great mood, too. "I wake up," "Ruffin is tired," — not true, but he didn't know the word "not" — "Ruffin is cold," "Mommy, shut the door," "I want pants." He correctly answered several times when I asked, laughing, "What is your name?" "What does the cow, pig, chicken, horse say?" When I asked him to, he correctly mimed walking, running, swimming, and jumping. He used several verbs in his spontaneous sentences. He talked about driving a bus, riding in a car, also about trains and trucks. He was really on a roll — and said, very distinctly, "I like school."

Meg charted Ruffin's progress the third week in October on her educational objective that he respond verbally to "What do you need?" On most days, he didn't respond to the question. He would only say what he needed in set situations, such as going to the bathroom. This was hardly a good report. I wondered, *why* wasn't Ruffin talking at school?

We were getting ready for Halloween. Ruffin was saying, "Trick or Treat," as an echo after me, and we were practicing knocking on doors, using several finger puppets: pumpkin, witch, Frankenstein, and vampire. We practiced walking the streets by walking to the public library to return books and work puzzles there and jump from orange to white concrete squares at the entrance. We worked on "stop" and "look" for cars before stepping into the street. Ruffin seemed to remember both "careful" and "wait."

Before supper Ruffin helped Rose with some of her factory piecework — pulling buttons off cards to make 'hash,' a mix of out-of-fashion buttons for export while I jotted a note to Meg that I thought Ruffin was beginning to do very well with questions which can never be answered by an echo, like "What does the cow say?" "Moo." (not an echo) as compared to "Do you want a banana?" "Banana." (an echo).

Toward the end of October, I took an entire day to review all Ruffin's files to prepare Donna, Lisa, Seamus, and myself, Evelyn Kung, and Dr. Granpeesheh at CARD, as well as anyone from the schools who might want to attend training during Evelyn's upcoming workshop visit. I drew on the IDEA model of writing out Ruffin's present levels of educational performance (PLEP) — the same pancake model — nicely brown on one side, stippled with holes on the other. It would be important that everyone on Ruffin's educational-therapy team be in the loop about what Ruffin could do for any one of us, so we could each expect Ruffin's best performance, across all environments.

On the bubbling side of the pancake, as a list of continuing problems for Ruffin's home-and-school teams to address, and resolve, I listed several, so I could keep track later how and when we resolved them, if we did.

"Sleeping at night and taking a nap. An afternoon nap and considerable physical exercise are associated with Ruffin's best nights of sleep. Absence of a nap and relative inactivity seem associated with late night or midnight waking." I was still using dimethylglycine (DMG) in the morning and withdrawing it after noon to help regulate

Ruffin's sleep. Napping happened at school, as did PE. Ruffin's sleep problems were resolved for the most part by the end of November.

"Tantrums when asked to share or take turns. The best solution seems to be to work through the tantrum when enough adults are available or remove Ruffin from the situation when not enough adults are available." Ruffin was strong for his age, and extremely determined to get his own way once he was decided upon it. This problem, too, was better most of the time by the end of November.

"Turning off all lights in the house, regardless of the wishes of others and regardless of what they are doing. Is this a signal, copied from school, that he wants a nap or rest? If so, we should try to respect this need." By sharing information, this problem was resolved by the end of November.

"Won't swim. The best solution may be to take him into the pool despite a tantrum which may last the entire first swimming session, maybe 20 minutes." Twenty minutes was a long, long time for a tantrum, especially in public. By the end of November, Ruffin had gone into the pool twice with Meg, crying. I thought that had been brave of them both.

The next afternoon was Seamus's turn. Ruffin and I went out with him to the exotic animal farm — one of Seamus's favorite places in the county. A large barn had been converted into a covered area for picnic tables, with horse-jumping barrels set out for trash — Ruffin was quite taken with those. A small counter-kitchen served sloppy joes, chips, soft drinks, and the sorts of elaborate brownies and bars I was familiar with from church suppers. We tried sitting Ruffin down for a snack. That didn't work, so I picked up our food and we tried walking around the petting zoo. That worked better, and I nibbled Ruffin's brownie, while Seamus guided Ruffin's hand over the low fence to the head of a pygmy horse. "He'll like it, if you scratch him between the ears." That was a long sentence, but Ruffin understood the gesture and scratched the tiny horse in the right spot. Donna and her family arrived later. There was going to be a live band and a dance. It was a big crowd. Seamus and I got to dance.

Saturday morning Ruffin and I went out to eat breakfast without incident. In the five-and-dime store downtown Ruffin identified colors of ribbon and yarn, and animal figurines such as pigs and cows. Ruffin was able to answer in non-echo fashion, "What animal do you see?" "Deer, donkey, goat, sheep, horse." He returned these figurines to the shelves without tantrumming — even an umbrella he wanted — when I told him his grandma would be coming soon to bring him one. Ruffin seemed to have latched on to color names and was using them as parts of repeated mega words: "black shirt," "black olives," "orange tag," "black pants," and identified red, pink, and orange in the store, as we picked out our Halloween decorations.

That afternoon, Donna, Lisa, Seamus, and I met to go over my notes, make plans and develop work schedules. Ruffin spent several hours later helping Seamus, unloading items from a truck, following his directions in caring for ducks, chickens, rabbits, and small kittens. They built a large bonfire. Ruffin was able to tell me about this adventure afterwards.

"Smoke."

Back home, Ruffin worked several puzzles, and talked as he did. His face, as always, was intent on whatever puzzle he squatted over, as he rarely looked up to address his remarks to me.

Donna called me as Ruffin arrived home from school to ask if we had plans for Ruffin to go trick-or-treating. Honestly, even with all our earlier practice, I wasn't sure he could, but, I responded, "Yes, we should celebrate." Why not? With this harmless small-town ritual of childhood.

Donna asked, "So, does Ruffin have a costume?"

"Not yet."

"What do you think he might want to be?"

"Good question."

"Look, Lisa, Danielle, and I need to go over to Walmart this afternoon. We could take Ruffin along. We could buy stuff so he could make his own costume working with us, as part of his therapy."

"Okay, sounds good. See you here in a few."

My doorbell rang. The four of us managed to get Ruffin out the door and into the car with the three of them. I cleared my law desk of everything I could accomplish in an hour. Then I lay down for a late nap.

My doorbell rang again and woke me up. It was Ruffin, back with Donna and Danielle, who looked a bit shell-shocked, a bit sweaty, both of them. Donna's bright hair was positively frizzy with humidity. Immediately, I knew why — I could see Ruffin running all over Walmart, or whining and protesting, under the bright, buzzing neon lights, among all the noise of shoppers and the general bustle. I had failed to warn them. It must have been awful. My reflexive but unuttered prayer came silently and unbidden, Donna, please don't quit. Please.

Donna handed me a folded yard of brown felt, two notebook-page-size sheets of red felt, and a small box of brass brads from which it was her plan that Ruffin make himself some fringed cowboy chaps and a little vest, using scissors and glue. Then, having explained the project she planned, and seeing that to leave these things with me and Ruffin was obviously hopeless, she and Danielle took back all the felt and little brass pieces, promising, "Ruffin still needs a costume. It'll be easier for us to make it at home. Ready before Halloween. See you then!"

"Thank you, thank you. See you!"

Donna was no quitter. Lisa remained along for the ride. Not until next Halloween, did Donna confess just how awful this Halloween costume trip to Walmart had been, how difficult Ruffin's behavior was to manage for two adult women, and Danielle along as their agile mothers' helper. Their harrowing visit to Walmart proved to be fortunate, because when Evelyn arrived to train us, Donna and Lisa were among the most keenly interested to learn. "How do we teach this child anything?" "How do we keep him out of a group home?" And most likely, "How are we going to manage to do what we've already signed on for?"

At least Ruffin slept soundly after his trip to Walmart.

Meg let me know, "I have worked it out and plan on being there for your training weekend." I replied, "So pleased you can come." And, truly, I was. Meg and her aide, Ella, now oversaw Ruffin and seven other disabled boys whose behaviors were as demanding as Ruffin's, if not more challenging. The two of them needed to implement and chart the other boys' IEPs, too, feed them all and themselves in their self-contained classroom, see to all the toileting, napping, safe arrivals, and departures, ready the class as a group to have PE, music, and library on time. I couldn't say they weren't working. Couldn't say they were ever wasting their time. I wondered, though, how much of Ruffin's time to catch up was being eaten up by a safe-enough environment that was failing to teach him to talk quickly enough to ever fully remediate his ongoing language delay.

Dr. Caldwell and I met again by appointment in late October. I asked if he had read the 1987 and 1993 Lovaas research and its academic peer review critiques. He swept his hair back, and assured me he had read both papers, and as scientific research, they were not "junk science."

"This is real, gold-standard science, and more than just statistically significant in the demonstration of the differences Lovaas's therapy makes, yes, longitudinally, apparently over the lifetime of children with autism."

I brought out a sheet of paper onto which I had copied out Dr. Ira Cohen's prescription language which had been used to support Catherine Maurice's and her husband Marc's insurance claim for funding their home-based ABA programs, revised into Ruffin's name.

I explained all this and slid it over to Dr. Caldwell. "Can you sign this for me? For Ruffin?"

He read silently for a moment, and looked up, over his wire-rims. "I don't think I'd be comfortable signing something like this."

I held his eyes, steadily, with my own. I had been reading and learning quite a lot about the power of eye contact since Ruffin's diagnosis. I echoed him, very, very softly, "I think if you don't sign something like this, I'm a trial lawyer, and I'd be very comfortable to sue you." No way was I pleased to be reduced to this, to have to threaten him, even softly.

No way was he pleased to have been threatened. He got up abruptly from the table between us, letting the door close heavily on his way out.

Dr. Caldwell had left my slip of paper behind. I picked it up, walked down the hallway back to the front desk, where I proposed to his receptionist, "Dr. Caldwell needs to sign this for my son but seems to have forgotten. I can wait here for it. I don't need to go anywhere, but I'd like to have it before I drive home today, back to Iowa."

She took my paper with a smile and walked it right back into the warren of small rooms and hallways and disappeared.

A half-hour later, she motioned me up to her desk, and handed me a sealed envelope. Inside, on Gundersen letterhead for the Department of Neurology, with his name there under his sub-specialty of Pediatric Neurology, and with Ruffin's name, his clinic number, and date of birth, Dr. Caldwell had written,

TO WHOM IT MAY CONCERN:

This letter is written at the request of Ruffin's mother. Ruffin is a three-and-a-half-year-old boy who carries the diagnosis of pervasive developmental disorder, not otherwise specified (PDD-NOS). He has been followed by me in our Child Neurology Clinic since July 12th, 1994 and was seen by the Learning Disability Section of the Comprehensive Child Care Center of Gundersen Clinic on October 5th, 1994.

Ruffin would benefit from an intensive behavior modification program. The program which Ruffin's mother and I endorse is the Lovaas method. There should be a high ratio of staff to child and the staff should be well-versed and specifically trained in the practice of applied behavior analysis and modification with autistic children as propounded by Doctor Lovaas. Daily records should be kept, and results plotted to analyze changes and reasons for success or failure. Parent training should also be an integral part of the child's therapeutic program.

Therefore, I would strongly recommend that the insurance company consider payment for training of three adult caretakers for Ruffin. Such training is available from the Center for Autism and Related Disorders in Encino, California. These people would apply their training to Ruffin in his home for 40 hours per week and for the indefinite near future.

Please contact me with any questions that you might have.

Sincerely,

James P. Caldwell, M.D.

I studied this second gift from Dr. Caldwell. I told his receptionist, "Please thank the good doctor." I was ecstatic, walking on air. Had any third-floor window been left open, I might have walked obliviously out, and gone plummeting to the pavement.

CHAPTER TEN

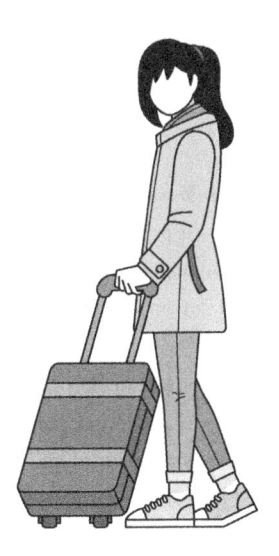

EVELYN

Ruffin trick-or-treated for about half an hour on Halloween, in the costume Donna and Danielle had made for him. He enjoyed the ritual of ringing the doorbell and holding his bag out and open. I enjoyed prompting and watching him from two steps back. At the far end of the four blocks of Main Street, Ruffin's interest waned. His haul of suckers, bright gumballs, candy-corn, and mini-candy-bars were of no interest to him. Still, he had done well. I was disappointed Seamus couldn't share Ruffin's first Halloween experience, but he needed his sleep now to be able to work third shift. I could dress Ruffin up again for him later.

The next evening, I left for Des Moines for our annual trial lawyers' association gathering to meet up with my *Ezzone* trial partners. Lisa would take Ruffin Wednesday night, and Donna Thursday night, as the first test of our new support system. I would be home by Friday.

I abandoned motherhood for two days of legal triumph. My trial partners, Mark Soldat, Don Thompson, and I had managed to scrabble to the top of the mountain. We were hoping to get support on the rehearing appeal to restore our *Ezzone* jury verdict of just over seven million dollars. We had a sideline meeting with members of the *amicus* committee — wonderful and important lawyers whom I had never met in my small-town, rural practice.

Chief among them was attorney Scott Peters of Council Bluffs, past president of the association, from all the way across the state, on Iowa's western border, on the banks of the great Missouri. The rehearing *en banc* of the appeal of our stripped-down verdict, our effort to reverse its deep remitter was pending, but here I was spilling my passionate story about Ruffin to everyone and anyone, especially to Scott, who although he had no personal connection to the world of autism was just an amazing listener — always the true polestar of a great trial lawyer.

Famed trial attorney and great mountain lion before the jury, Gerry Spence of Wyoming was our scheduled keynote speaker, and called Mark, Don, and me out by name — to come on down the center aisle for one of his hearty western handshakes that morphed for me into a full-bodied hug of congratulation.

I called Ruffin every night, but he didn't talk much, although he did echo, "Mommy back Friday." The night when Evelyn was due to arrive.

To reach us, Evelyn flew from Los Angeles to Minneapolis, then boarded a puddle-jumper, landing about midnight at the small regional airport in LaCrosse just ahead of some ugly midwestern weather. After a kerfuffle, with the airport closing on her for the night, Donna, Ruffin, and I located her, and were able to drive her out to our one and only cozy bed and breakfast in town.

Evelyn was tiny, slender, with shining black hair, obviously tired, dragging a single small roller-bag. But, from the moment she identified and introduced herself, it was clear, she knew a great deal about a great many children with autism, more than I knew by reading, or could ever know by reading. She had worked all day before flying and needed sleep. She dozed off in the close warmth of the slow-moving van. Donna drove us more than two hours back, through a storm of ice and snow that slanted through our headlights and crusted the outer rimlands of the windshield. It was a little early for this first blizzard. Had Evelyn any idea of Iowa weather, or the Midwest? I worried that she hadn't brought the right coat, or boots.

Early Saturday morning was pandemonium, with everyone who had been invited arriving on my porch at once. No worries. There was Evelyn, with a rested head on her shoulders. She seemed energetic, still, and quietly authoritative, at turns, both engaging, and professional. Dark turtleneck, comfortable knit pants, flat shoes, ready to work.

I was pleased to introduce her to Inge and Meg, who both planned to attend all weekend — on their own time. Ruth would be videotaping and learning all she could, as Dr. Granpeesheh had agreed. She was setting up our freshly repaired video camera on a tripod. Rose would be cooking. Seamus, Donna, and Lisa arrived, shedding coats, boots, headgear, and scarves, each finding a seat on the couch in my den, or on the matching loveseat, until everyone was gathered in an "L" surrounding Evelyn and cornering Ruffin. We thought we were ready. But was Ruffin? There was a small, metal-legged wooden chair for Ruffin, something Seamus had picked up at an auction.

It was clear as she began speaking that Evelyn had met, known, and actively treated more children with autism than anyone else present in the room. Inge was scribbling notes, and curious. Meg was attentive, too, her head bent under her heavy honey hair, and then lifting it again to watch. Evelyn explained autism. She explained the working, practical principles of behavior modification. Then she started right in with Ruffin, explaining what she was doing to assess him, to learn what he could do, and to learn what he did not yet understand.

Ruffin was not happy to sit in his chair. He protested and tantrummed. Evelyn hooked her legs around the metal legs of Ruffin's small chair. He had no possible escape. There was no escaping Evelyn, her brief commands, her praise, her tummy rubs and laughter. There was no place for Ruffin to look, except at her, twist as he might to slip away, or look my way, or to Seamus for rescue. He was screaming. It might as well have been bloody murder.

Evelyn commented that Ruffin was as strong as any three-year-old she had ever seen. Seamus sat up with a certain pride. It took Seamus and me both sometimes, to wrestle him into compliance. Had I not been prepared by my reading, by my watching Lovaas's early videos, I might have been very upset with Ruffin, or for him. But I wasn't. I felt confident. Evelyn was doing everything I had seen Lovaas do on his early videotapes.

In a rather brief time, Ruffin calmed down, began to look at Evelyn, eye to eye, at her request, and to work to earn the reward of escape, to come to me — Mommy — for his hug. Then, everyone, Donna, Lisa, Seamus, Inge, yes, and Meg, too, took his or her turn copying Evelyn, working to establish their own instructional technique.

I was ridiculous, trying to prompt Ruffin to say the word hippopotamus.

"Himolopolus," Ruffin garbled the word, which was obviously too long for him.

Evelyn caught my eye. "Say, 'No.' He needs information he's not right. A single 'No.' Clearly. Just once. Okay, now, you try again."

Evelyn prompted me to build the long word backwards in chunks, starting with "mus." "Get 'mus.' Then 'potomus.' Give praise."

I offered to Ruffin, "Say: mus."

"Mus."

"Good job!" Hug.

"Say: potamus."

"Potamus."

"Say . . ."

And Evelyn interrupted, "He needs praise."

I stopped. I offered praise, then, "Say: hippo."

"Hippo."

I offered praise.

Then Evelyn called a halt, "Now, take a break!"

Over two days, over a dozen hours, everyone took many turns with Ruffin, on the hot seat, with Ruffin working harder than any of us. Donna was a natural, a rock star. Lisa, surprisingly solid, in her own quiet way. I continued to be ridiculous. I doubted Seamus would ever do any of this after today. He was more physically inclined. As Ruffin and we all learned to say, "Take a break!" Evelyn worked in more information about autism, about what we could expect of Ruffin during this course of intensive behavioral treatment — in little bits.

But it was surprisingly hard work, and not as simple as it looked: to plan what to ask Ruffin to do next; to make a written record of his every response; to end, always, on success; to manage a 40-minute session of several different forms of discrete drills and trials, across differing content and activities, some of which were easier or more difficult for Ruffin, some more inherently rewarding than others he also needed to master.

With hands-on practice, we all got better at this. With information. With "No." With praise. With Evelyn.

That first morning, Evelyn had filled one of my Binderteks with a brief list of seven basic drills. Overall, we needed to maintain Ruffin's compliance and good behavior, so he could focus and attend to learning what we had to offer him.

First, we would teach one-step instructions using brief commands, "Sit down, stand up, come here, hands down, clap hands, arms up, give me a hug, turn around, stomp feet, wave," etc.

We would work to have Ruffin master only one or two contrasting commands at a time, in each session. Mastery was explained by Evelyn as: Ruffin performing the action correctly for every one of us, anywhere he might be. At first, if Ruffin did not understand a command, we would physically move his body as we would like him to do, and then demonstrate with our bodies so he could imitate us. The goal was with practice, practice, practice, for Ruffin to be able to follow and discriminate among spoken commands without any physical cue or clue, using just his ability to understand spoken language.

Once Ruffin learned several actions on purely verbal command, we would chain two mastered actions together: "Turn around and jump," and teach with the same procedures of prompted physical movement, then demonstration with our own bodies for Ruffin to see and imitate. All this was really a receptive language drill, designed to instill in Ruffin a firm understanding of how spoken language worked — as communication between people.

Before we would expect Ruffin to speak expressively, we would teach nouns, receptively, by asking him to "Touch X," while presenting two highly contrasting three-dimensional objects.

Once he mastered touching the correct object, we would move to the more cognitively challenging task of touching a correct choice between the clean, clear presentation of two highly contrasting two-dimensional photographs.

We were going to teach Ruffin various shapes: circle, square, triangle, and rectangle using another discrimination drill, by placing two examples on the table between Ruffin and one of us as a therapist, saying only, "Touch circle," and letting Ruffin know, by saying, "No," should he touch the wrong shape. Clear the table of examples, reset the table, then physically prompt him, if necessary, to touch the right shape, praising even his seemingly accidentally correct or partial effort. Pretty tedious. As Ruffin mastered each shape, we would record the data and the date.

When he had firm mastery of touching all the right shapes, all the time, with every one of us, then we would change our brief instruction to "What shape?" in order to prompt Ruffin to say, at first maybe only by echo, the correct name of the shape, "Circle," until Ruffin had mastery to say the correct name of each shape, every time, with every one of us.

We were going to work to expand the length of utterance of Ruffin's verbal imitations, or echolalia, from simple sounds, to words, to short sentences, each prefaced by the same short consistent command, "Say."

We were going to teach the understanding of verbs of action, by presenting photographs of people in action and saying simply, "Touch jumping."

When he demonstrated mastery of understanding by touching, we would present the same photographs, asking, "What is he doing?" And prompt Ruffin to echo or say, "Jumping."

When he demonstrated mastery of understanding by answering with a single, salient correct *ing* form, then we would begin to prompt Ruffin to echo or say the brief sentence, "He is jumping."

As Evelyn prepared to leave, having gotten thoroughly acquainted with Ruffin and with all of us, she re-filled my blue Bindertek with her newer, more ambitious list of 21 drills, prepared in her attic bed and breakfast room overnight: Alphabet; Block Imitation; Categories; Colors; Emotions; Expressive Labels; Information; I See; Name Recognition; Nonverbal Imitation; Numbers; Opposites; Prepositions; Present Tense; Pronouns; Receptive Actions; Receptive Commands; Receptive Labels; Shapes; Verbal Imitation, and Play Activity.

Evelyn expected us to be able to teach Ruffin quite a lot over the next couple of months before she planned to return in early January. We were going to teach all the letters of the alphabet using a discrimination drill, placing two highly contrasting examples of different upper-case letters on the table between Ruffin and one of us as a therapist, saying only, "Touch A," and letting Ruffin know, by saying, "No," should he touch the wrong letter. Clear the table of examples, reset the table, then physically prompt him, if necessary, to touch the right letter, praising even a seemingly accidentally correct, or partial effort. Way tedious. As Ruffin mastered each letter, we would record the data and the date. And Evelyn asked us to remember to go back frequently to refresh and retest mastery.

When Ruffin had firm mastery of touching all the right letters, all the time, with every one of us, then we would change our brief instruction to "What letter?" to teach Ruffin to say, at first maybe by echo, the correct name of the letter, "A," until Ruffin had mastery to say the correct name of each letter, every time, with every one of us.

Then, we would teach and discriminate every lower-case letter.

So, that amounted to 26 times 26 or 676 separate discrimination objectives under a single one of our 21 assigned drills.

With each of the 21 assigned drills for Ruffin, we got specific written instructions of what we were to say. Exact, brief phrases, "Do this." "Put with same." Each brief command was coupled with Evelyn's exact written descriptions of how we were to present each task. We were going to teach Ruffin to think, and then to name, in categories:

food, furniture, clothing, farm and zoo animals, people, vehicles, appliances, fruits, vegetables, drinks, and then add more categories, but only one at a time.

I would spend many winter nights cutting category photographs out of a tumbling stack of mail-order catalogues and pasting them on large, white index cards, securing each category with a fat rubber band, to place in a travelling drill bag, stashed with a makeshift, otherwise tumbling tower of plastic shoeboxes from Walmart that travelled from our house to Donna's house to Lisa's and back — always with Ruffin.

Evelyn ordered a red and blue Tiny Tikes table and chairs for Ruffin to sit across from a changing parade of us, each working as his therapist. We were going to teach Ruffin eleven colors in rank order, from easiest to more subtle: yellow, red, green, blue, white, black, orange, purple, pink, grey, and brown, in the same "Touch color" manner as we taught the alphabet, until we could ask, "What color?" and Ruffin could say to each of us, correctly, the name of each color.

When Ruffin did learn all his colors with complete mastery, a minor miracle occurred in our life at home. As Ruffin began his "uh, uh, uh, uh" grunting which I knew meant "I want" but which I knew I had no way of knowing what, I had him look at me, and when I knew I had his attention, then asked, "What color?" So, Ruffin said, "Red." And I would know to look around only for some red thing nearby to offer him. Even this rudimentary communication of color cut through his frustration and scythed down several of his tantrums before they flowered.

We were going to teach Ruffin happy, sad, surprised, angry, and scared. Back to more winter nights of cutting out pictures of people with those emotions on their faces, to paste onto cards. Eventually, we would say, "Show me happy," and expect Ruffin to respond with his face. Later, we would ask, "How do I feel?" while exaggerating those emotions on our own faces, until Ruffin could respond, "You feel happy."

Eventually we had dozens of sturdy plastic shoeboxes from Walmart stuffed with catalog photographs of common objects and emotional people on cards. Why not just flip through the pages of books, and ask him to point? Because even a single page of most books offered too much information at once, too much distracting background. One object, a single face pasted on a single white card, allowed Ruffin to focus and build understanding more readily, with less opportunity for error, more efficiently.

Every label or noun had to be mastered first, *receptively*, by Ruffin demonstrating his understanding by touching, before being introduced and mastered *expressively*, as a word Ruffin could echo and associate with his earlier establishment of understanding.

This *receptive* first, *expressive* second drill procedure promised to fill the empty echo of echolalia with true and useful meaning.

We would teach Ruffin his important safety and personal information, by brute rote echo because it might be essential, lifesaving even, that he be able to spit out a short, rote response to "What's your name? How old are you? What's your address?" He needed to be able to answer usefully if he were lost.

"When's your birthday? What color is your hair?' What color are your eyes?" "How are you doing?" He needed a little rote something to say to church ladies and people on the street who thought he was cute. He needed something to say to Grandma and Papa.

Asking "What do you see?" to prompt the answer "I see" when shown an object by a therapist was one way to practice joint attention, a way of learning to share minds with others, to begin to infer the presence and work of other minds.

I gathered photographs of everyone important in Ruffin's world, so we could teach first by touch to have Ruffin know, and then by echo to have Ruffin call everyone by name. Although it might have impressed Dr. Kondrick at Gundersen in early October, "Hi, friend" was hardly a universally acknowledged greeting. Some unfriendly people might even take offense.

We were going to teach imitation, at first nonverbally, as monkey-see-monkey-do, saying simply, "Do this," as we clapped our hands, raised our arms, tapped our legs, tapped the table, touched our heads, made whooping sounds by clapping our hands over our open mouths, stomped our feet, stood up, shook our heads no, nodded our heads yes, and anything else — fun! — we could agree on.

And we would teach more imitation of fine motor actions: pointing, opening, and closing our hands, touching our head, nose, feet, stomach, eyes, legs, ears, eyebrows, hair, knees, elbows, and ankles.

To teach Ruffin to speak and use the verbs he was working with in his computer program drills, we would ask Ruffin, "Show me eating." Then drinking, clapping, waving, etc.

We were going to teach Ruffin the use of the present tense by saying, "Do this," while miming an action for Ruffin to see and imitate. And when he did imitate, by asking, "What are you doing?" And continue to prompt his reply, at first, "I am clapping." Until it dawned on him, until we could see the light go on.

In the same manner that we taught the alphabet, we were going to teach him numbers.

And rote counting, as an exercise of auditory memory.

By discrimination drills, using three-dimensional objects, we were going to teach big and small, hot and cold, long and short, near and far, and fat or thin.

Using photographs, and later building blocks in relation to each other that Ruffin could manipulate to show his understanding, we were going to teach him a receptive understanding of the prepositions: in, on, and under.

After we taught body-part names, we were going to teach the difficult matter of personal pronouns, which children with autism and echolalia often confuse. With a heavy verbal stress or voice prompt on the differing possessive pronouns, we would say, "Touch *your* nose," for Ruffin to touch his nose. Then, "Touch *my* nose," for Ruffin to touch our noses.

To me, this was special education — as I had imagined it — as I had read about it with Anne Sullivan and Helen Keller, and with Laura Ingalls Wilder's sister, Mary, at the Vinton School for the Blind — yes, special education of the 1800s, in Iowa.

Mindful of Ruffin's experience during my recent two-day trip to the top of the legal mountain, I contacted Judge Stephen P. Carroll, my fine co-counsel and trial mentor, Mark Soldat, and our three opposing counsel to ask for a postponement of my appearance in the long hearing scheduled to resume for the school superintendent and his supporters. I briefly recounted Ruffin's diagnosis and the results of my research since mid-July, and my plan to give Ruffin a fighting chance, explaining that children who failed to begin proper therapy before age five were at substantial risk of further decline.

Then, I begged, begged, as I had never done in my professional life, for a delay on grounds personal to myself. "In all fairness to my son, I beg you to continue this trial for a period equivalent to the federal Family Leave Act. As a self-employed person, I know I am not entitled to this benefit, but my need and situation are no different from that of a court employee facing a family medical problem for which the act was intended."

Like most trial judges, Judge Carroll was most understanding, solicitous, and frankly protective of his court employees, his bailiffs, his clerks, and his court reporters, a bit more than he was for any of us, the legal advocates who appeared before him on our clients' accounts. I needed him to see me as in need of his protection, too. "Please be assured that Ruffin's problems have not materially affected my actual preparations for trial, since that preparation is mostly complete for all the witnesses, save one, assigned to me for questioning. I would be able to pick up my trial notebook and come to trial in the spring ready to proceed."

I was painfully aware that without the grant of some delay, I would need to be back in the courtroom by mid-November, for days on end, working several counties west of home.

That Monday afternoon, I opened Ruffin's notebook to read Meg's latest. She thanked me for Evelyn's workshop and explained how she was using Lovaas's techniques with Ruffin to encourage him to eat, and to teach another student to make eye contact.

Donna and Lisa got in their first true drill sessions with Ruffin that afternoon. He was upset at first but got into it. He could really do some things. Other things he couldn't do right away, but he learned fast how to do what he couldn't do at first. Ruffin told Rose immediately when she asked, "How old are you?" "Three!" very loudly, and proud of having the "right answer." Lisa prompted Rose to say, "Good job!" before she slipped out the door for home.

I had gotten a call from court administration that I would need to try a case. Two other disputing parties had suddenly settled. So, I would be up all night preparing. I was also trying to take Ruffin off his bedtime bottle, so this night was a disaster. Without his bottle, upstairs alone, Ruffin went into his first troubling episode in a long time. By the time I heard him, he was pretty far gone into his personal babble. I got him up. He wanted to "work in chair" then, but I had to get ready for the next day's last-minute trial. I brought him downstairs with me and put him on the couch where I could interrupt any babble immediately. I decided, since I would be taking his bottle away, it would be important to stay in the same room with him until he fell asleep. The bottle had kept his mouth busy, and quiet. We weren't completely out of the woods yet, but I felt confident we had found our path.

Ruffin was moving, or back-creeping into sleep problems again. I had weaned him down to a small bottle each morning and evening, to be certain he got his dose of vitamins and DMG. Hadn't he eaten rather well for supper? Olives, jello, and crackers — the olive juice as "soup," with some multigrain chips and a bite of rice.

Upstairs in therapy, he had worked on alphabets, emotions, expressive labels, the prepositions in, on, behind, and under with me, and then with Seamus. Later he had gotten under his blanket and said, 'under,' and 'I'm in the doghouse, arf, arf.' Pretty cute stuff, Seamus and I agreed. Seamus spent an hour roughhousing with him, and Ruffin really liked that. I was pleased to see Seamus enjoyed it. I thought Meg and my mother would both be happy to know.

But now it was midnight, and Ruffin was still up, very active — jumping, running, and pulling his train by its string around and around in circles. I was determined we were not going to have any problems with "babble" though — since I was going to keep him downstairs on the couch until he fell asleep.

I turned on the television to try to catch some late news. What was going on in the world? A woman had been elected president in Sri Lanka. To help Ruffin drop off, I turned to whatever the VCR had recorded off Nickelodeon. *Aahh!!! Real Monsters*. Here were Ickis, whom Ruffin mistook for a rabbit, Oblina, reaching down to pull stuff out of her stomach, and Krumm, who stank. They were attending monster school where they went to learn how to scare humans, from their teacher, The Gromble, with her four legs and high-heel shoes.

"Red shoes," offered Ruffin.

"Right," I replied wearily, praising Ruffin somewhat inappropriately in the British manner.

In mid-November, Meg and I met for another parent-teacher conference. She had silk flowers for me, as a thank-you, for including her in our weekend training with Evelyn. She confided in greater detail about how she had been using what she had learned from Evelyn to teach other of her special needs students in Ruffin's class. Then, she handed me a comb-bound flip notebook she had made herself so she and I would have a fresh notebook to continue to write back and forth to each other daily about Ruffin. It was decorated with drawings of cats. Over her weekend at our home, she had learned Ruffin and I kept two cats, Stripes, and Whiskers, who were important to him — as his "portable heaters" — because they were always warm, and because they purred like motors.

We discussed new goals to set for Ruffin; how to get his attention by saying his name, how we might begin to work on his concept of time, and on helping him understand and talk about situations and the functions of objects and categories by asking, "What do you do when? What do you do with a bed?" She let me know that Ruffin seemed to be doing better sharing with his classmates. We asked ourselves, "What else?" What a pleasure it was to work with her, and her gifts said she felt the same about working with me.

CHAPTER ELEVEN

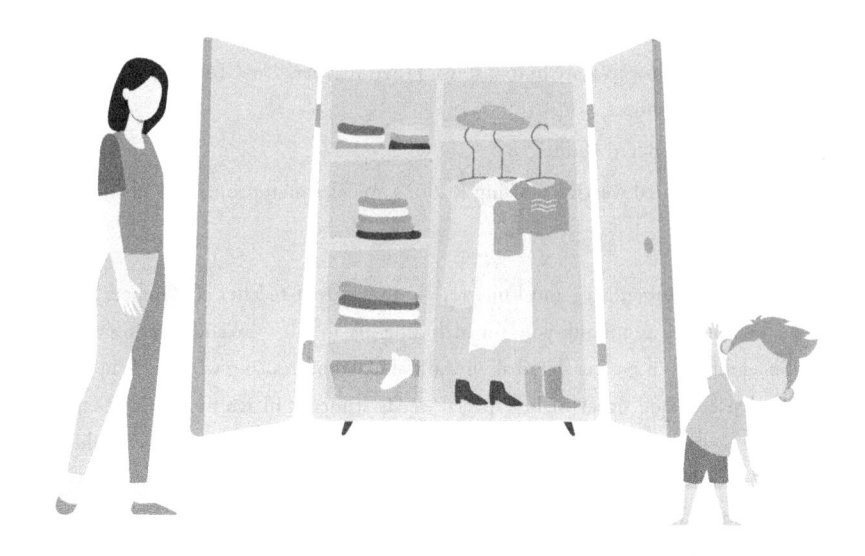

I LOVE YOU. I LOVE YOU.

On November 13th, I sat down to list *Ruffin's Expressive Vocabulary with Mother* to share with Meg and Kim, Dr. Granpeesheh and Evelyn, and all Ruffin's home therapists, Donna, Lisa, and Seamus. The population of nouns and other isolated words had exploded to 274 words. These were all words Ruffin had been exposed to in his new CARD program, his computer programs, including *WordWise Software* and *Talking Macintosh* software.

By the end of that week at school, Ruffin demonstrated mastery of three primary and two secondary colors, but not purple, although purple was coming. And, under *Other progress*, Meg had noted, "Ruffin is reading the names red, yellow, blue, green, and orange, but hesitates with purple."

I called for a meeting to write a new IEP. I wanted an updated and more challenging plan for Ruffin "incorporating his CARD program, computer work, and addressing

Ruffin's special need for education over the coming summer." Any day that November or December would work for me.

Ruffin found a metal part that had fallen out of his crib. He dragged me to our kitchen junk drawer and got out my screwdrivers. Then he went back to his crib, disassembled the necessary parts, slid out a metal rod, screwed in the missing part, re-inserted the rod, and secured the rod back with a screw he had carefully placed aside during disassembly. At times, when he couldn't exactly manage this, Ruffin directed me to help him. He seemed to be able to use a screwdriver very well. Amazing. It was a new feeling, a good omen, to see Ruffin as amazing. Not just good-looking, or handsome. In that way, he had always seemed amazing to me. But, in this way: competent. And, he had picked up a new phrase for saying "No" to me, for refusing: "Not today." Not that he cared for this phrase when I used it.

Seamus worked with Ruffin that Sunday using a *Numbers Wildlife Book*, and some number puzzles. Then he showed Ruffin how to use a tape measure. Together, Seamus and I saw the light go on as the two of them measured and counted the inches of a myriad of items. Ruffin was intrigued to learn that numbers *mean* something. Working together, the three of us took down his crib and stored it in the attic.

Ruffin could blurt out his complete address now. He did this for each of us in our home staffing.

Afterwards, Ruffin and I visited the Christmas tree walk at the fairground. It was warm enough neither of us needed more than a sweater. The sun brought out the smells of pine, fir, and cedar as we wandered, counting each tree, as we searched for the one Ruffin recognized — that Donna had decorated at her home to donate. Ruffin behaved beautifully, sat right up on Santa's knee, thanked him for his candy cane. When prompted, he told Santa what he wanted for Christmas. "Train." He must be remembering. He had gotten one last Christmas.

I received formal notice of an IEP meeting to be held on December 8th. I would take this as another opportunity to cajole, persuade, and advocate for Ruffin — to try to get the schools to help fund his CARD home program as a part of his free, appropriate public education (FAPE).

At the kitchen counter I was cutting apples for supper. Ruffin was upset when I cut the first apple. He wanted some tape to repair it and went to my law office desk to get it. It took a while, but he accepted a demonstration, and then an explanation, that this wasn't going to work. "Besides," I announced, "We're going to eat this apple!"

Then, Ruffin was up all night long, babbling with jargon. "A mystery," I mumbled to myself, "This child is a real mystery!"

Meg sent home a typed note about her Thanksgiving project — making whipped cream for pumpkin pie. The class had also tasted cranberry sauce, having read a story about cranberries the day before. Her note sent a brief, sharp pang of something akin to jealousy through me. How much I would have liked to be doing these things with Ruffin, playing with him, as the mostly-stay-at-home-mom I had worked hard to afford to be, keeping him home with me, and enjoying every day until he began kindergarten or first grade. I had wanted to keep him at home with me until he was seven, but he was a mystery, and my original plan had been, as I could see now, some sort of ancient Ozzie and Harriet sitcom-fantasy.

Over the Thanksgiving holidays, Meg and I worked independently of each other to rate Ruffin on the 20-page *Help for Special Preschoolers Assessment Checklist: Ages 3-6*. She and I saw Ruffin in different environments and from different perspectives. I gathered additional input from Donna, Lisa, and Seamus. We all found that what Ruffin could do was exploding.

At home Ruffin was into more exploratory mischief, smearing deodorant on the upstairs bathroom mirror, smearing white shoe polish on the downstairs hallway mirror, carpet, and wallpaper, scattering bath powder and tissues around the whole house. I needed to stay off the phone and put things up as I had never done when Ruffin was younger.

Also, Ruffin was trying to expand his observations with 2- to 4-word remarks, for example, about dinosaurs: "big tail," "big neck," and "big dinosaur." He began to enjoy "reading" to me — he liked the control. It had taken him a long time to seem to be taking after me. Seamus, for one, found it hilarious. The three of us were able to eat out two or three times without incident.

We had welcome visitors on Thanksgiving Day. RoJene and her son Chance drove in from the country. Ruffin showed Chance how to use the computer, giving him the mouse and directions — "Up, down, over here" — telling him where to move the mouse and what icons to click. Ruffin seemed proud of being able to teach and share. RoJene was amused and assured me that Ruffin was getting better. I took comfort in that. She was a trained teacher.

Ruffin even had a haircut. He allowed the barber to use scissors, comb, spray bottle, hair dryer, and clippers. Donna and I had given Ruffin a model — Donna's son, Matt, who went first. Ruffin got right in the barber's chair for "Ruffin's turn!"

To prepare for our upcoming IEP meeting, I shared the *Help for Special Preschoolers Assessment Checklist* with Ruffin's IEP school team and his home team, Donna, Lisa, and Seamus, along with a letter I had written to Dr. Granpeesheh and Evelyn about Ruffin's progress, reporting everything Ruffin was doing to generalize his learning from each drill, and including information Meg had passed along about what Ruffin was able to do now in school.

We videoed Ruffin's work at home to send to school. "I'd like to see some of Ruffin's CARD drills and skills incorporated into his IEP, so that his work at home continues to be generalized to school."

I had finally been able to observe Kim, Ruffin's speech and language therapist, working with Ruffin, playing a bingo game with another student. I was pleased to see Ruffin responding verbally to her question "What is it?" and to see Ruffin doing fairly well at taking turns and offering help to other players — both to the adults when Kim and I played "dumb" and to his classmate.

Ruffin's vocabulary of nouns and verbs was really picking up, but his ability to structure sentences and conversations had not improved a great deal. "Is Ruffin using his full vocabulary at school? If not, why not? Do you have any suggestions for a sentence-building program for him at home or school? The *Laureate* computer program I've ordered has been delayed in production. Is there something else we could use to help him put sentences together?"

Overall, Ruffin was making good progress. He was not losing any more ground and I hoped that he was beginning to make up some of his 16- to 18-month language delay with all his hard work.

But, according to the assessment, I was still babying him on eating, drinking, dressing, and tooth brushing. I promised myself to work harder on these areas at home. He was doing significantly better for Donna, Lisa, and Seamus. And I wanted suggestions about places where Ruffin could get hard physical exercise indoors for the winter. Was there a gym open anywhere?

I let Meg know, "Donna Schmidt is going to attend Ruffin's IEP meeting with me. She will represent the CARD team, as she has put in the most hours with Ruffin." As Ruffin's parent, I could ask anyone I liked to come to his IEP meetings, whether as an outside expert, a notetaker, or just for simple emotional support. That was federal law.

About this same time, Seamus brought Ruffin a small trampoline and he grew to love it as an indoor break. Donna and Lisa liked it, too, since it gave them a moment to scribble their data into Ruffin's drill-book. On weekends, after his CARD drills, Seamus continued to take Ruffin for several hours at a time. The two of them worked with Seamus's animals, feeding, watering, and doing farm chores. Ruffin was quieter with him, but Seamus found him much more cooperative. It seemed normal enough to me.

Ruffin was learning better at school, carrying what he learned there into his evening hours after school and drills, into Seamus's barn, and into his life with other people. I was hopeful in every conversation with my parents and mailed them our latest videos so they could see for themselves and let me know what they thought.

"He seems to have really perked up," my mother observed.

"He's learning fast," I said. "That's important."

"Do you think he might recover?"

"Maybe," I said. "Not everyone does."

Then they checked, "Did I have enough money?" I thought so. His special education was supposed to be "free." I was having a meeting soon. I would be asking the school to pay their fair share.

On November 30th, in the middle of the night, I heard Ruffin grunting, "Uh, uh, uh, uh." I woke up into a dark grogginess. His pull-up had failed. He had wet the bed. That woke him up. I found a fresh pull-up and dug a clean set of sheets out of the upstairs linen closet. Ruffin wanted to help make the new bed, ducking his head, as he tucked in the corners. He wanted more blankets, all the blankets in the closet. I looked down at him, and suggested firmly, "One is enough."

"Two is enough," Ruffin said, smiling up at me, and reaching in, up on his toes. As he often was, he was very chatty in the middle of the night.

I said, "I love you, Ruffin."

"I love you, Mom."

It came spontaneously — and struck my head like a hammer. This was the first time I had ever heard Ruffin say this. I was painfully aware as the recognition flooded me, that he had never said this before, and now suddenly he had. Suddenly, I found I needed a tissue. "Ruffin, do you think you could find me a tissue?" No, there weren't any left, except in the wastebasket clotted with baby powder. "How about some toilet paper?" Ruffin trailed a long tail of toilet paper into my bedroom. He knew what it was. He knew where it was. And he could see what I needed it for, too.

When he was warm and dry, when I finally let go of him, he had slipped back to sleep. I found myself wide awake in my bed beside him, dry-eyed and restless, with nothing to read, nothing to write, no one awake whom I could call now, just waiting impatiently for the sun to come up. Here, this far north, in November, it wouldn't be up early.

With Ruffin at breakfast, with Ruffin at his computer, I scribbled a short version of that night's story first to Meg. "This morning, I wonder if the very rudimentary exchange of greeting drills in his CARD program, when he must use the name of a person he addresses, somehow helped him along? I have said to him hundreds of times, 'I love you, Ruffin,' and I wonder if he didn't finally turn the sentence around in his mind?"

With the sun finally over the horizon, I planned to call Seamus, call my parents again, call Evelyn, tell Donna, and have her pass the word to Lisa. Tell Rose. For the first time since July's diagnosis, I felt we had a fighting chance to catch Ruffin up on all his earlier, measured delays. We could teach him to talk, teach him to learn for himself, whatever he might want to learn for himself. With all of us working together, with Ruffin working the hardest of any of us, we were sure to see him turn himself loose into the universe.

Meg let me know, "At lunch Ruffin cried not to have to taste pears. Is he texture intolerant?" I responded with a hopeful observation. "At home tonight, Ruffin pointed to our notebook and said, 'Ruffin cried, eating,' referring in all likelihood to your pear incident." He had remembered — and he wanted to report his feeling.

Then, Ruffin tugged at my hand, wanting to go upstairs and work on his CARD drills. He and I started with his favorite block assembly drill. Working behind a simple cardboard blind, I assembled my set of blocks into a towering or sprawling pattern before removing the blind in an *ah-ha* moment of magical reveal. Provided with a set of blocks of identical shapes and colors, Ruffin would then focus on assembling an exact copy. As he worked, Ruffin talked quite a bit in longer phrases, narrating everything as he did it. "I climb, I reach," and "I can't." He also used the word "bigger," his first comparative, and used it appropriately to compare a couple of loose tinker-toy sticks — one *was* longer. We had a couple of conversational exchanges of 3 and 4 turns as he made appropriate short answers or comments indicating that he was listening carefully and understood where our conversation was going. Really, it seemed wonderful.

It didn't just seem wonderful, it *was* wonderful. Although to me Ruffin had always been the perfect Gerber-faced baby of my dreams — my 100% chance of a 2% chance of my ever having one — now the mind behind that perfect face seemed to be moving and gaining traction. Ruffin was learning something new every day, some novel word or concept, some way of being in the world of others, beginning to make up the developmental delays that were all too obvious last summer.

I felt as if I had clambered up the crumbling talus of a small mountain and could rest for a moment and contemplate the prospect of Ruffin's continuing development with some serenity. But, no, all the professional resistance I had encountered and had worked my way around left me feeling unsettled and restless. I put my feet down beneath my law desk, listened to the whispers of the wind and watched the lightest snow fall over our small Iowa town, out the window beyond my green and flickering computer screen.

Dr. Caldwell needed to know the prescription he had written seemed to be working. "Ruffin continues to do well with his CARD therapy which you prescribed. He now counts to 10 by rote. He is beginning to understand the concept of counting and quantity. He offers a variety of spontaneous remarks: 'I love you, Mommy.' and 'I eated all my cereal.' 'This one is bigger.' He can offer his name, age, my name, and street address in answer to appropriate questions. He can name 11 assorted colors, 6 different shapes, copies an assembly of up to 12 blocks exactly, uses several prepositions, shares more readily with others, and does well in games that require him to take a turn. His vocabulary is growing very rapidly. We hope that a *Laureate* computer program *Micro-LADS* will help him in learning to speak in more complex sentences."

But then, I pressed on past my simple summary. I couldn't help myself. I pushed, I offered, I advocated. "Within the next week or so, I will send a blue Bindertek up to place on the shelves of the autism clinic library, containing those items which have been of the most use to me with Ruffin. I'd like it to be available for loan to parents of newly diagnosed children like Ruffin, together with a video that begins with the sequence you used to diagnose Ruffin last July. It goes on to show his present work, his classroom work, our CARD training workshop, CARD drill sessions with lay therapists, and Ruffin in more naturalistic settings through November." I offered him a complete video record of Evelyn's training weekend, too.

I couldn't help myself. Was I growing a bit rabid? Why not just relax? Why couldn't I? And just enjoy Ruffin as he was clawing his way back to us? And Seamus, as he seemed to have resumed visiting Ruffin, and me, with renewed interest? And the frequent phone calls with my parents back in North Carolina who were eager to hear any good news?

The news from school was better, and better, bit by bit. Ruffin was counting aloud in school during his exercises in physical education, eating well, and walking safely to the local grocery and back to school on the classroom caterpillar rope. He shared a crust of his bread with Meg's classroom aide Ella when she asked. He was even speaking up on occasion. "At lunch, the name of a classmate was mentioned, and Ruffin commented that boy was 'Not here.' When asked where his missing classmate was, Ruffin knew, 'Kindergarten.'"

All our news from home seemed good, too, better, and better, bit by bit. "When Ruffin came in from the bus, he announced he had been to school. He said a full spontaneous sentence to Lisa, 'Donna has gone home.'"

Early in the morning on December 2nd, I made another brief video of Ruffin in what his clinicians and educators called "a natural setting" — our den at home, while preparing him for his upcoming visit to the dentist. It would be his first. We had been offered an appointment to see Dr. Michael Funk, a pediatric dentist who served children with disabilities at Gundersen in a setting where the full range of anesthesia was readily available, if need be. I had been fearful of what we might face as Dr. Funk approached Ruffin's mouth, knowing Ruffin's strong protests early-on to bathing, swimming, haircuts, and earphones.

With Dr. Funk taking his time — a long time actually — with the assistance of two other people to help steady Ruffin in the chair, and by using brief sentences to tell Ruffin what would be coming next, he was able to complete his examination. This included the insertion of a device necessary to hold Ruffin's mouth open so he could have his teeth examined and then cleaned with a noisy rotary device full of sticky, pink paste.

Ruffin sailed through his first dental appointment — although he was drenched in sweat afterwards. I had to mark that as progress. Dr. Funk assured me that despite Ruffin's continuing attachment to his baby bottle, full of chocolate milk to disguise the bitter taste of his vitamin and DMG doses, he had no cavities and Dr. Funk had no other concerns. Because Dr. Funk was so kind, I continued to bring Ruffin to see him regularly through the next summer.

As we walked out of the glass lobby of the dental clinic through the revolving door — that fascinated Ruffin, of course — I felt we were walking on air. Ruffin was walking beside me, without balking, except to examine the door. And wasn't that natural enough for a young child to be curious? For Ruffin to just be holding my hand, and looking around quietly, but alertly.

Even the temperature had risen to the point that all the week's earlier snow had melted away. It was hardly cold enough for more than a light jacket. To me, Ruffin looked cool and collected now, well past the experience of his appointment, jaunty in his plaid flannel coat and matching flat cap, like some cross between the warring Scots and the Irish — as he was — as a cross between Seamus and me.

There was no great rush to hurry back home since this was a Friday. No court. Our judges rarely held court that late in the week. Ruffin and I might as well spend the rest of this sunny winter day up north in the big city and see what we could see, and see all we couldn't see, much less shop for, back home in Iowa. We dropped into Chucky Cheese for a treat. With all the lights and noise, I didn't imagine Ruffin would like it, but he surprised me and loved the cavernous place, and seemed eager to try out every ride and game. We wandered about waiting for our pizza to arrive. I told our waitress I would keep my eye on our table, but did ask her, "Would you please come get us while it's still hot?"

It helped that we had arrived at noon on a weekday when there weren't so many other children and their families there. It was not like Ruffin had to wait or share. While he explored the game floor freely, he threw three tantrums, none of them too bad, nothing I couldn't cover for with our waitress. Hot pizza was too delicious, and too expensive here to walk out on or leave uneaten on the table.

As Ruffin began to tucker out, we visited a bookstore, and I quickly picked out a newer computer program for him — *Broderbund's Tortoise and the Hare*.

Our local autism support group held a business meeting at my home-office the next day during school. We were hoping to complete auditory integration training (AIT) over the coming summer. Since neither Gundersen nor the schools were interested in offering this service to any of our children, it would be our own experiment, by our own design, with our consent, and at our own expense.

Although I had invited her to join us, Inge had been a surprising no-show. As a consultant, Inge had never been tied to any classroom schedule, free to come and go, as far as I could see. She had been comfortable enough visiting my home for our early November workshop, so I was puzzled. With the opportunity of meeting up with so many parents of the children whom she served, with all of us gathered conveniently together, I wondered why she would fail to show. I wondered what was up.

Ruffin arrived home and reported that he had "pizza" for lunch too. He was beginning to offer more spontaneous comments to Donna and Lisa, and to show them affection with hugs and kisses. He readily identified "Teacher Holub" and "Meyer" for us from pictures Meg had sent home to add to his drills. He was able to blurt his birthdate.

A three-year-old neighbor girl wandered over for the afternoon. After I called her mother, she and Ruffin played and talked together, mostly chasing and romping, but using puppets and soft animals as characters. Ruffin said, "I like girls." He seemed to have discovered several sentence structures to use. "I like this," "I have that," and "This is not that," and made deliberately wrong answers as a teasing joke, laughing.

He did well on a new drill of "your" and "my" when we asked him "Touch *my* eye" "What are you doing?" "I'm touching *your* eye." Or "Touch *your* foot'" '" What are you doing?" "Touching *my* foot." We were also using "her" with the neighbor girl present for the same drill. This was hard and confusing for Ruffin at first, but soon he reached about 60% accuracy. Ruffin's teacher Meg and I continued writing back and forth, happily, beneath all the administrative radar.

By my reaching out again, Dr. Caldwell and I were back on guarded letter-writing terms. He had offered no comment or acknowledgment of Ruffin's recent developmental gains, or of my offers to share information. The advocacy I had directed his way must have been ill-pitched, falling into the depths of a bottomless, dark pool without so much as a plunk or a ripple.

This was all a brief calm before the latest storm on the horizon, Ruffin's second IEP meeting, scheduled for the next afternoon. A call from Bridgewater's regional nurse broke into my mental rehearsals over what might happen then. Ruffin's vision was a bit near-sighted, at 20/25, and he might need glasses should it deteriorate to 20/30 or 20/40. I was thankful to know, but unsurprised. Everybody on both sides of Ruffin's family wore glasses. Myopia was a readily accommodated disability in the modern world, although, as I thought about it, it could have been a dangerous one in our early days of bringing down the mastodons.

At home, my phone rang again. The local district's nurse, the second nurse on Ruffin's IEP team, was checking in to update Ruffin's health history. Ruffin was now 40 inches tall and weighed just over 38 pounds. His immunizations were all current. By calling me in advance and filing a written report, she and the first nurse could both duck out of attending tomorrow's scheduled IEP meeting credibly enough. The upcoming issues at stake didn't fall into school nursing's particular bailiwick anyway, and who would want to waste precious, professional time meant for serving children by sitting for hours on the sidelines at an upcoming sabretooth catfight?

The morning of December 8th, before Ruffin's afternoon IEP meeting, my phone rang again. A strongly accented voice greeted me. "This is Ivar. You wrote me a letter." When I didn't, when I couldn't seem to respond, he prompted, "Is this you who wrote?"

He was calling about my early request letter to the schools. I had copied him, in hopes of what? Scaring or embarrassing the authorities? Now Dr. Lovaas, Dr. O. *Ivar* Lovaas himself, was calling to chat.

"Yes, this is Ruffin's mother."

"I could help, if you like, by sending you copies of some of our papers from UCLA. Would you like that? Someone at school could read them."

"Please, yes, although I have your 1987 and 1993 papers already. I would like that. I'm a long distance from a good medical school library."

"I thought so. Where is this town in Iowa? Near Decorah?"

"Yes."

A chuckle, and Dr. Lovaas recalled, "You know, I was a foreign exchange student at Luther College there? In the sixties. In music."

"I know, I remember, I read your interview in *The Advocate* from October."

"Then, you know." And Dr. Lovaas quickly dropped the subject of his past for the present. "There's a professor there now, in the psychology department, Dr. David Bishop. Let's check your address and I'll have him be in touch and send you a film. Someone at school could look at it."

"I know they need to learn a lot. And so do I."

He assured me of Dr. Granpeesheh's and her senior therapist Evelyn Kung's credentials in detail, since he had trained both at UCLA, and encouraged me to stay in touch with them frequently, at least weekly.

My own immediate concern about that afternoon's IEP meeting surfaced. "And, I need to find money, you know, not stop on that account."

"Ah, yes, that's been a problem. We've been working on it here in California. I could send you copies of some of the . . . What do you lawyers call them? The legal opinions? The rulings? In our favor. In favor of our parents. We've been testifying."

"There are rulings? Any favorable rulings?"

"Yes, Ruffin's mother. And you, you are a lawyer, there in Iowa?"

"Yes, I am. A trial lawyer, you know, the kind who would rather go to court than sit home in the office."

"Then, I'll have someone here in our lab collect them up, all the rulings, and send them to you. You use them, then, in Iowa."

"Yes, I think we need them here. We can use them."

I ran down a brief account for him of all the other families I knew who were trying to mount home-based, intensive early intervention programs in Iowa. Throughout our conversation, I found Dr. Lovaas abrupt, but extremely kind and helpful, encouraging about Ruffin's home program, and pleased by Ruffin's early, robust response to treatment as I rattled my way through the details I had gathered for that afternoon's meeting.

In closing, he invited me out to California to attend a conference for parents and professionals that would be convening in late January in Los Angeles. I left for Ruffin's afternoon IEP with courage in my heart and loaded for bear.

CHAPTER TWELVE

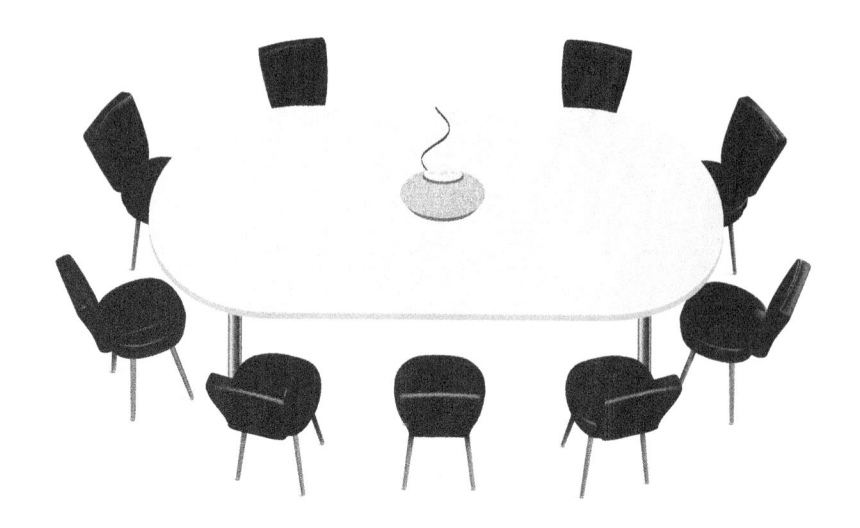

A MID-WINTER IEP

Donna and I unbundled from the cold, excited by Ruffin's progress at home and hopeful of working with Meg and Inge's support to get some of Ruffin's CARD program and his computer work incorporated into his fresher, morning hours at school. To accommodate Sue Baker's attendance from the university in Iowa City, we were all gathered closely around a speakerphone, set on an adult-sized conference table in a windowless, climate-controlled room tucked behind Miss Hobbs's office.

Meg began by passing around her handwritten notes of the annual review of Ruffin's earlier August IEP goals, stamped with a reminder that none of this was due until next August — some nine months into the future. Ruffin had already met all his first year's early social interaction goals with both his teachers and his classmates and had met all his early functional and imaginative play goals, especially with puppets.

Yes, I thought to myself, with Worm and Sheep. Worm was a flowery blue fabric tube stuffed with polyester fluff I had sewn to nestle Ruffin into his car-seat as a tiny preemie. Now, at three, he used it as a toy, whipping it up and down in waves and dragging it behind him on our staircase. Sheep was a gift from Seamus, a stuffed toy that Ruffin carried to school or daycare.

Over my reverie, Meg continued. Perhaps because of Evelyn's emphasis on teaching receptive language first, Meg wanted to include some new receptive language learning goals in this revision of Ruffin's IEP — proposed to run for a wildly off-kilter "school year" from this December to next.

This was all good news. Donna and I exchanged glances. I let my eyes say, "All okay by me."

Then Meg passed around her handwritten present levels of educational performance (PLEP) and began reading it out. "Ruffin will play interactively with other children without adult guidance. These are mostly 'chase' games, and the variety and type of his peer interactions needs to increase."

When I offered my observation that Ruffin didn't play "dress-up" or "teacher" yet or participate in other activities by pretending to be someone else, Inge assured me that those were activities more typical of 4- and 5-year-olds.

Oh, okay, I thought. We had time to teach him.

Meg continued, "Ruffin responds verbally when asked 'What do you need?' almost all the time. He rarely calls us or verbally asks for attention. He places himself in a position so he is close and can make eye contact, then waits for us to ask what he needs. He needs to request attention verbally."

Yes, I thought, as Meg went on speaking. He must seem a bit too shy.

"Ruffin will participate in teacher-structured turn-taking games or activities. He needs cues for his turn but waits patiently."

Yes, I thought. We want him to be polite.

"He uses non-traditional objects to represent traditional objects and participates in peer-directed imaginative play. He uses words with peers and staff to label, request, and make refusals on a regular basis. He can and does make choices. He will use labels for emotions when presented with photos showing happy, sad, and angry."

Donna and I exchanged glances again, both of us pleased to hear that Ruffin must be generalizing into Meg's classroom some of what he had learned at home.

"Ruffin is beginning to use phrases and sentences but needs to continue to improve this skill. Current testing reveals these needs and accomplishments: He can name 10 colors; count to 10 by rote; name 20 body parts; name 4 shapes; his fine and gross motor skills are within age range."

Donna, Lisa, Seamus, and I had been working hard over the last month for Ruffin to learn these concepts, together with the language for them. Now Ruffin had other opportunities to be asked for this information and was generalizing these skills into his classroom.

In her final points, Meg covered what she and I had discussed at our recent mid-semester parent-teacher conference when she had surprised me with her thank-you gift of silk flowers. "Ruffin needs to learn to answer comprehension questions and questions about the functions of objects. He continues to show resistance to giving up a toy to let another child have a turn. He needs to increase his ability to comprehend time."

Then Meg turned to Emily to present Kim's contributions. Kim was absent, again, just as she had been for Ruffin's first IEP meeting. I had been hoping this might be an occasion to get to know her better. But I listened eagerly, and saw Donna turn to listen, too, as Kim's handwritten notes were passed around, and Emily began to read. "Ruffin has basically met all his speech and language objectives. Currently, he has very good articulation skills. The only misarticulated sounds are all well within developmental norms for a child of his age. He has a little difficulty voicing the /z/." I was pleased with all this. Ruffin must be hearing well enough, despite his long history of troublesome ear infections, and must be listening to all of us, since he was able to echo most of the sounds he was offered.

"Ruffin is always talking in a loud voice now, not whispering."

Yes, I thought. He must be feeling comfortable there, at school, and with Kim.

Donna shot me a quick glance that said, she knew I knew she, too, knew about Ruffin's loud voice — it was there on our late November videotape we had just mailed out to California to Evelyn and Dr. Granpeesheh.

"He is responding better to questions daily. I get very little, if any, echoing in response to questions now. Ruffin has made great strides using many verbs now, including the *–ing* present tense. Other verb tenses are emerging."

I made a quick check with Donna, who spoke up. "We have a drill for that, and it seems to be working."

Emily's reading of Kim's report continued over Donna's unacknowledged interruption. "Although I have not attempted a retest of Ruffin's basic concepts, he is gaining there as well. He is naming most of the colors and is able to follow simple directions easily."

Donna and I didn't interrupt again, but we were grinning, back and forth, all the way through to the end of Kim's written report.

"Turn-taking is starting to greatly improve also. Pronoun usage is emerging. I hear him use 'I' frequently and have noted usage of 'her' and 'him.' Plurals are also emerging.

I have heard sentence constructions of up to 7 or 8 words. Example: 'I watch a duck, TV, Mommy near.' 'Her is a Mommy, Mommy is Mary Jane White.'"

Then, Meg and Emily passed around Kim's newest handwritten speech and language goals and her proposed short-term objectives to reach them. I found them disappointing. They struck me as unambitious as the first yearly goals Ruffin had already mastered in less than a semester, representing at most some isolated probes for developments that Kim expected to monitor.

When Donna offered to report on Ruffin's progress at home, she was shut down — quickly. When I took over, allowed to speak because I *was* Ruffin's mother, I was hurried along, surprisingly enough, by Meg, who appeared uncomfortable to have been assigned this task of mother-wrangler.

It was clear. Meg and Inge expected my assent to this handwritten plan, so they could make Ruffin's IEP all official again. Inge seemed more than a little stressed. I knew her well enough by then to be able to tell. I watched as she retreated into the safe and silent absorption of taking notes. She would be the one responsible for typing up the results of this tricky meeting and needed to be particularly careful.

When I brought up the question of adding Ruffin's CARD drills and his computer work to his formal IEP, by listing all his current computer programs and simply appending his drill book, Miss Hobbs cleared her throat with an aggravated, "Harrumph!" She shot Inge, who was startled, a meaningful look, so Inge spoke up. "Public funding for Lovaas programming is an administrative issue and so we can't decide this as an IEP team, not at this time, not in this meeting." Over Inge's voice which was by then thin and thready, Emily chimed in, "If Lovaas training only works for 47%, less than half of the children treated, there isn't much promise in it, or any reason to pursue it with Ruffin."

I was dumbfounded, and angry. During the worst moments of this meeting, on repeated cues from Miss Hobbs, the three of them, Emily, Meg, and Inge, set to work on me, suggesting that none of these Lovaas drills were necessary or even possible to do at school, and that to put a 3-year-old on a computer was ridiculous.

I appealed to Sue over the speakerphone. She remained quiet as a church mouse, making no contributions of substance, offering no opinions, and evading all direct questions by begging off that she had never met Ruffin in the flesh. I had no way to make eye contact with her as I recounted my own enthusiastic follow-up on her better suggestions to me, including Lois Fergus's YMCA lending library of computer programs for children with disabilities and Dr. Rimland's vitamin and DMG therapy. Not even lavish praise would draw Sue into anything more than listening. It dawned on me —

Sue was monitoring our meeting — she, too, like Meg and Inge, was powerless, with no administrative authority to commit anyone to provide services or funding.

Our meeting slogged on to the line at the end of the form for summer school or extended year special education (EYSE). I advanced my view that Ruffin, as a unique individual, as a child with autism, would need an educational program this summer and cited two Iowa state rules by number and letter part.

Miss Hobbs shot Inge another time-for-you-to-speak-up-again look. "Public funding for summer programming is an administrative issue and so we can't decide this as an IEP team, not at this time, not in this meeting." Inge was parroting illegal nonsense then, on cue. I said so.

Miss Hobbs was unable to contain her impatience with my pettifogging insistence on the federal and state legalities. "No child routinely qualifies for EYSE. It's for children with brain injury or stroke, for children who qualify. EYSE is paid for by us, the school district, not Bridgewater."

I shot back, "So, you'll pay for it for Ruffin? Because he needs it. He *needs* his CARD program to continue year-round, as prescribed by Dr. Caldwell, Dr. Granpeesheh, and Evelyn. His development will be at risk if it is interrupted."

She offered me history. "Last year we had a program run by the local group home provider for disabled adults, but it was just for our more severely handicapped children through a funding source they receive." Donna was horrified by this mention of a group home and was quickly growing red and sweaty under the freckles over her face. She had been working hard to prevent this ever happening to Ruffin, and all her efforts with him seemed to have been dismissed here.

Then I began to argue more calmly and forcefully, with emphatic patience, with the right legal word. I spoke up for myself and for Donna. "Well, that doesn't sound to us like it would be *appropriate* for Ruffin. Our goal is to keep him from ever living in a group home for the mentally disabled."

Miss Hobbs looked pained and replied with equal measures of honey and vinegar. "Ruffin has already made such wonderful progress. I can't see that he will need it either." I wanted to scream. Here was her disagreement offered in the form of condescending agreement. But it was not the time or place to scream, and I didn't.

Miss Hobbs was frustrated, but I would not discover how frustrated she was until the summer two years later when a memo she circulated describing this early meeting surfaced in the loose file of one of Ruffin's school nurses — who had failed to discard it. To me then, her memo read as Miss Hobbs venting and explaining the situation to our superintendent.

But, even without reading Miss Hobbs's mind or her secretly circulated memo, I realized we had gotten as far as we were going to get. She and I were buffalo to buffalo. I insisted that Inge mark the cover page of the IEP to show that further EYSE review was needed, not because, as she had written at first, "Issues have not been clarified," but, as I dictated, "Issues have not been resolved."

After the meeting broke up, Inge walked Donna and me outside around a brick corner. There she slipped me the phone number of a colleague of hers, Marion McQuaid of Heartland AEA, a special education region near Des Moines. Marion wanted to talk to me about Ruffin's CARD program. I took her name and number and followed through with a long call, answering all Marion's questions, addressing all her concerns, encouraging her interest, because I thought — foolishly, as it turned out — that if Heartland adopted a CARD program into an IEP for another child, that might help me get one for Ruffin.

I asked Inge for a typewritten copy of the IEP the school authorities had proposed because by then I was weary of all the nineteenth century word-processing, all the illegible handwriting.

Finally, before we walked our separate ways that afternoon, Inge encouraged me to keep writing my letters, because it was a violation of federal law for there to be no one at the meeting with the authority to offer me answers or commit resources. I looked her in the eye and said, "Yes, I know."

Donna and I doubled back together and bundled Ruffin out of Meg's classroom. The three of us headed for my house, where Donna put Ruffin through his paces, while I answered the never not-ringing phone, calmly counseling my clients, "Let's make a plan."

Ruffin and I ate dinner with Rose. Then the three of us braved the cold and dark, drawn to the brightly lit, outdoor St. Patrick's nativity pageant: the animals, the traditional angels, shepherds, and wise men. Ruffin petted all the donkeys and brushed the snow off their backs. He knew them because all of them belonged to Seamus.

Then Ruffin bathed. He let me gently wash his hair. I read to him until he fell asleep. Still not the time or place to scream. Meg's gift of silk flowers caught my eye, the ones she had given me at our fall parent-teacher conference. I would never be able to sleep with them in my home. I snatched them up, closed the door on Ruffin, crept down two flights of stairs into the darkness of the basement where I tore Meg's silk wildly to scattered bits, screaming, and screaming, to let myself feel and regret with naked keenness the weakness of my carefully cultivated but powerless allies: Sue's politic silence, and Inge's and Meg's forced betrayals. Primal scream therapy must be something more sophisticated than my raw untutored attempt. Afterwards, I found myself painfully hoarse. I was also utterly weary. I wasn't sure I felt any great relief. I sure couldn't talk.

Still, the next morning, I wrote to Meg, "Thank you for your support and thoughtful contributions to Ruffin's IEP." And why wouldn't I? She was the one administratively powerless person who cared most closely for Ruffin, day in and day out. She was not my enemy, nor the decision-maker as to what would or would not be offered in Ruffin's IEP. As Ruffin's parent, I needed to advocate with someone else, somewhere higher-up — over her head and mine — who seemed not to have been present at yesterday's meeting.

Since I couldn't talk, I got busy, writing a third widely circulated letter of request, supported by video clips of Ruffin, the next in a long, tedious exchange of letters and videos throughout the spring and following summer.

At the keyboard, I recalled dragging my yellow highlighter over Dorothy Beavers' opinion from the 1960s when she was raising Leo. "Parents should also be permitted to bring in their own private doctors and consultants to help determine the best course of study and treatment." I knew from my legal research that this permission had already ripened into a requirement of federal law. Parents could bring independent medical opinions and assessments to IEP meetings, and those needed to be considered, although the school team was free — at its legal peril, of course — to reject or discard them.

Recounting that I had asked Prudential to cover 80% of the cost of Ruffin's CARD program, I cited all the reassuring provisions of the *Code of Federal Regulations* that required insurers to help pay for services provided to a child with a disability while attending school.

I toted up the exact costs of Ruffin's home therapy so far. I needed to know how much money I needed to seek in reimbursement, and how much money I needed to ask for to complete the full two years of treatment prescribed in late October by Dr. Caldwell. The cost of Ruffin's home therapy provided by Donna and Lisa then was about $430 per week. Were Prudential to pay their fair share of 80%, the public-school funding I needed would be about $86 per week. For a full two-year program, I would need $6,880 — or $8,944 were I left to provide two years of summer school, at home alone. And there would be bills for CARD's services and Evelyn's travels.

I set out Ruffin's and my case, citing chapter and verse to the federal law, the IDEA, and the IDEA's implementing *Code of Federal Regulations*, and to Iowa state statutes governing special education and its implementing *Iowa Administrative Code*. Every state had at least these four layers of rules that were required to mesh and needed to be read together carefully to understand the peculiar workings of each state's special education system.

Beyond those, there were administrative proceedings' due process written rulings, state court rulings and federal court rulings on their appeals, with similar cases often decided quite differently, depending on what federal appellate circuit in which a family might reside. Ruffin and I lived in the notoriously conservative Eighth Circuit.

I tried to be both cautious and inviting since I was a newcomer to this area of law. "This letter reflects my preliminary thinking, offered as a resource, and is designed to offer you my view of the available pathways to get to our common goal of providing Ruffin a free appropriate public education (FAPE) without substantial dispute." Because I knew Iowa Protection & Advocacy Services, Inc. was already representing at least one other family with a young child with autism, I hoped my independent legal research from my remote corner of the state might be helpful to share with them.

I posed the questions crucial to Ruffin as an individual, as he had a right to be considered under the IDEA. "Have we got the right mix to help Ruffin reach his potential? Is it best educational practice for Ruffin to undertake his most demanding academic-like work in the afternoon? Who are the professionals who could most reliably advise us? This is our joint responsibility to Ruffin, although by rights I may feel it more keenly than you, who have both the responsibility to decide, and control of the public resources."

Then, I turned to the matter of Ruffin's upcoming late January second-opinion evaluation appointment at the University of Iowa Hospitals and Clinics' Department of Child Psychiatry which served children with diagnoses on the autism spectrum from every part of the state.

Because I was beginning to fear litigation might become inevitable, I closed this, my third letter of polite request, "If, and only if, you find yourself blocked from going down each and every one of the pathways I propose, this invites your written and documented formal reply so the issues we must resolve can be accurately framed."

I waited a couple of days for my latest wave of snail-mail to crawl out across the school district, through the various Bridgewater offices and out to the state educational, legal, and political offices in Des Moines before picking up the phone. Somehow Miss Hobbs's point had failed to sink in — that our *local* school district was primarily obligated to commit financial resources for Ruffin's education. Certain that Inge was powerless within Bridgewater and in her role of consultant to Miss Hobbs, I went looking all over in the wrong direction, appealing to her superiors, Jack Wallace and Mr. Montague, instead of engaging directly with my local district superintendent and school board.

CHAPTER THIRTEEN

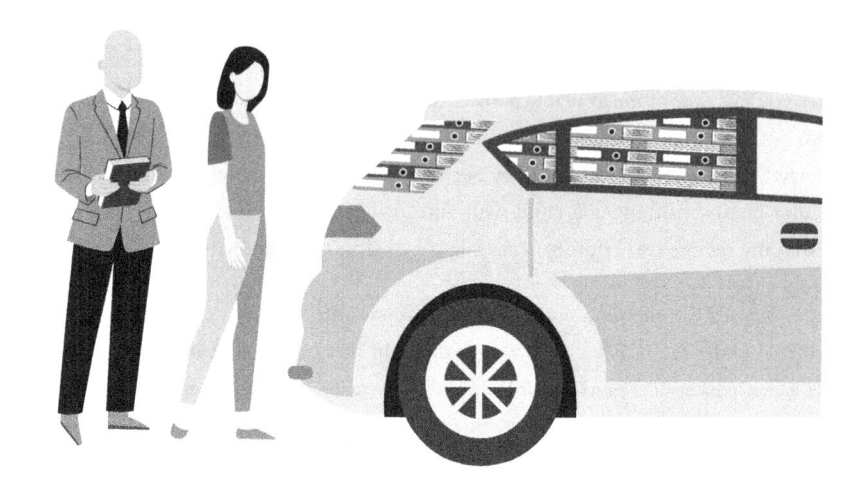

CURT

In mid-December, I re-read all my polite request letters of September, November, and early December, and reflected — by looking at myself in the downstairs bathroom mirror — that in myself, I did indeed have a fool for a client. Although Ruffin was continuing to learn, to develop and improve, I was getting nowhere with my rabid researching and writing on my own time and diving headfirst into debt. I needed some dragon-breath from someone with greater experience in special education law and advocacy — from someone who knew all the players on the special education field so their ears would perk up — if he so much as whispered.

So, I called Iowa Protection & Advocacy, Inc. in Des Moines, hoping to talk with attorney Curt Sytsma. I was lucky to catch him in. He came on the line as a sonorous, but very warm voice. I couldn't imagine what he must look like, but I was immediately curious.

From a family whom Tris had been working with, I had heard how Curt worked quickly and elegantly, often to mediate, or to settle. He was well-acquainted with the higher administrators within the state department of education, the university professors of special education, the political appointees, and all the various career professionals. He had cordial relationships with his adversaries, the handful of attorneys who represented local districts and area education agencies (AEAs) across Iowa. He had cultivated them, and valued them, as partners in reaching resolutions, case by case, and in suggesting and pushing through various reforms of wider effect.

It didn't take the two of us long to come up with a plan. At Curt's suggestion, I did a little follow-up letter writing to sharpen the focus of my requests. This and all my future correspondence clearly indicated it had been copied to Curt at Iowa Protection & Advocacy Services, Inc. — our school-whisperer with dragon-breath — Ruffin's new legal counsel.

That afternoon Ruffin told his first lie to me and Donna. She had asked who opened the Christmas presents. Ruffin had, while I was on the phone settling my Forest City case, I hoped. Ruffin told her, "Mommy did it." Smiling. Ruffin and I worked puzzles that night — the Christmas presents from his grandma that he had opened.

I was called in for a meeting with Inge and Miss Hobbs to identify those "critical skills" Ruffin had developed — the ones he might lose if he were not provided summer school. Inge showed me two expressive language skills that she, Meg, and Kim had identified to chart before and after the upcoming two weeks of Christmas vacation.

"This is what we plan to do."

"Well, understand," I responded, "that what I plan to do is have Ruffin continue to work intensively at home on both receptive and expressive language drills Evelyn has provided for him. Donna and Lisa are already scheduled to come over every day except Christmas and Christmas Eve. Ruffin, Donna, Lisa, and I will be working additional hours every day he won't be in school."

My plans to teach Ruffin at home were going to confound theirs for measurement at school. Miss Hobbs's mouth turned firmly down and white. Whatever, I thought. Go ahead, be frustrated. I am. At home we were not going to stop and let Ruffin drift for two weeks, certainly not to prove a point, not even to gain a benefit, and certainly not to accommodate a school experiment inviting Ruffin to demonstrate a relapse. I succeeded in keeping my mouth shut about it.

But, since our mini meeting was going sharply sour, I offered another idea. "During Christmas vacation Ruffin won't be spending all day with other children. Why don't we try to measure the effect of that interruption?" Inge thought this was not a bad idea and managed to agree with me before Miss Hobbs could insert herself to complain about the excessive number of meetings we were having about Ruffin, and the expense of organizing a summer school to benefit a single child.

"Our district simply doesn't have the funds budgeted to provide Ruffin summer school in the form of continuing his ECSE classroom, or his CARD program at home." With her greater experience in special education law and procedure, Inge knew this sort of individual cost-pleading was a bald violation of federal law, and so did I, as I glanced in her direction. Miss Hobbs was quick to read Inge's and my brief eye contact, and immediately began to backpedal. "Of course, if Ruffin is entitled to summer school, it will be provided somehow."

"Well," I said, "his entitlement is more likely to fall under the 'rare and unusual' circumstances of his autism diagnosis, as an independent legal ground under Iowa's regulations. 'Critical skills' measurements would be irrelevant in that case." Then, we were all just treading old ground, covered in our most recent IEP meeting. Our exchange devolved into something like a bad argument between spouses, with Miss Hobbs harkening back to what I considered ancient history.

"Really, I don't understand why you don't consider questioning Ruffin's autism diagnosis. As his mother. Some of us here at school do."

"I don't see how you can say that after my sending you his May to December video."

A December 15th meeting convened in my absence to advise Mr. Montague about Ruffin surfaced, as well as Miss Hobbs's complaint that no one at that meeting had seen his May to December video beforehand. In the anger that had driven my hasty video-dubbing, several of the tapes I had provided turned out to be blank. I promised to provide replacement copies.

"Look," I said, "I can't believe we are revisiting square one, but I'm willing to take Ruffin over to Madison, Wisconsin to see Dr. Glen Sallows about his diagnosis. I've already sent him Ruffin's videos, and our complete indexed medical and educational files to date. Dr. Sallows can offer us a second expert written opinion about whether Ruffin needs a CARD program, and if so, how many hours a week it should be, and whether his education should continue without interruption over the summer."

That was it. We were done. Miss Hobbs and I were mutually exasperated. Inge was stuck in the middle, reporting back to Mr. Montague and "Moe," "Today's meeting went okay, and another meeting is scheduled for Monday after school."

We were back to writing more dueling letters for the record. Inge's to me was in her dictated-to voice — echoing officialdom. "This is considered the Annual Review of

Ruffin's IEP thus indicating that a new IEP has been developed." More legal nonsense, since no new IEP could be developed without my agreement, my written consent on Ruffin's behalf. Inge knew that, and without noting the enclosure on her correspondence, she slipped in a pamphlet *Requesting a Special Education Hearing* which included contact information for Iowa Protection & Advocacy Services, Inc. — obviously, her quiet smoke-signal to me — seconding my own recent decision that it was time for me to invoke due process procedures for Ruffin.

My own next letter was addressed to the wider circle of all those to whom I wanted to advocate. Since Inge had asserted that a new IEP had been developed, there was no way I could let that stand on the educational record. I needed to be clear. "It remains my position that a new IEP has not yet been completely developed in view of the several unresolved issues I have noted in all my correspondence since early December." It also included a full read-out of the latest mini meeting with Inge and Miss Hobbs. By then I was writing over the heads of the school authorities for the eyes of a future mediator or administrative law judge (ALJ), state judge or federal judge — depending on how far up the legal ladder Curt and I might need to climb to reach resolution for Ruffin.

I offered five additional "critical skills" Ruffin had recently acquired to chart before and after his Christmas break — to be alert to their possible loss: Ruffin's interactive play with his classmates without adult guidance; his use of words with his classmates to label, request, and make refusals; his capacity to share or give up a toy to a playmate; his capacity to take turns with a classmate; his ability to sleep those eleven hours a night — as recommended by Miss Hobbs's early school year memo to parents — without medication which might compromise his cognitive abilities.

Sleep was a critical self-help skill. Ruffin needed rest to benefit from both his school and home programs. Meg and I had plenty of daily notes of the absence of this critical "sleeping skill" before Ruffin's home program began. Over the two-week holiday break from school, I kept careful track of Ruffin's sleep. He experienced five nights of wakefulness when he was up several hours in the middle of the night.

Over the weekend I had Ruffin home, working hard with Donna. After drills, we went to Donna's house to make wrapping paper with inky stamps — for Ruffin to re-wrap our Christmas presents. Ruffin came home so tired he went to sleep immediately, skipping his first dose of vitamins and DMG since late July. His behavior Saturday morning was difficult with a great deal of self-stimulatory tapping of objects and other repetitive motions. I scolded myself. I must *never* miss giving him his vitamins again. By

Saturday afternoon he was better and able to do artwork with Danielle, while Donna, Lisa, Seamus, and I held our staff meeting.

Ruffin dressed himself for bed and again in the morning, except for his socks, which were tight. He searched now for tags in the back of his underwear and his pants to put them on the right way around. Life had become increasingly normal, more like I had always imagined it could be.

As we watched *Old Yeller*, Ruffin looked up from my lap and said, "I like story." During the film, I tapped his shoulder to ask him, "What is so-and-so doing?" and Ruffin replied with the verbs he knew. He was scared during the scary parts, and when the dog died, asked, since that puzzled him, "Where did the dog go?"

Seamus dropped over to spend time, and together we assembled Ruffin's Little Tikes worktable and chairs. Although it wasn't really a normal family activity to put together a drill table, it felt normal, more normal than life had seemed for nearly a year.

I leaned back and let that sink in, as Seamus showed Ruffin what he knew about screws. "Like that, they need to sink in like that, all the way in."

Ruffin didn't know how to ask why yet but had looked over at Seamus inquisitively.

"So, they don't ever fall out on you."

I hoped Ruffin understood that. It seemed to me that he did.

Mr. Montague sent me a placating letter. But he made his limited interest clear. "As you know, I am particularly interested in knowing more about the use of Lovaas in the public schools and what portion of that service is the responsibility of the school vs. what portion is the responsibility of the parent."

At the same time, Mr. Montague reached out confidentially to a Dr. Hagen in Des Moines, by a letter which turned up later in my inspection of Ruffin's school files. "By now you have received the voluminous materials from Ms. Mary Jane White, attorney, related to her son, Ruffin, and the use of the Lovaas method with him . . . . Upon return from the holiday vacation, I will be contacting you for some technical and legal assistance related to this case. ... I do not, at this time, have enough information to ask appropriate questions about our agency's responsibilities related to the Lovaas method."

Ruffin and I made an uneventful trip to the single local box store to shop for socks, new boots, and the last few Christmas gifts. Then Ruffin headed upstairs to work with Donna, and Lisa later.

Just before Christmas, Ruffin began spelling his name and asking to have it written on any new possession. He was also responding, "I don't know," when he didn't, as well as when he didn't care to know, and "I can't do it," when he didn't care to.

Donna, Lisa, and I held an extended telephone conference call with Evelyn to revise Ruffin's drill book to include related, but more difficult tasks. Evelyn had our most recent videotapes of Ruffin working with each of us, as samples of his work on all his earlier drills. By reviewing them in California, she was able to coach each of us on improving the precision of our instructional technique — and she was able to write a far more challenging set of drills to keep Ruffin moving forward without boredom.

Just as Ruffin was released from school for Christmas vacation, all the snow-laden Iowa clouds broke open. He was home! He was home! And we — Donna, Lisa, Seamus, and I — were free to work with him as much as we were able to schedule. I depended on Donna and Lisa to implement Ruffin's home program of drills. Donna took the lead, and Lisa was happy to follow. The two of them worked out their own schedules between them, tried their best to keep good notes, swapped information back and forth as they passed each other on my porch, coming and going.

The two of them brainstormed without inviting my micro-management, leaving me free to work on funding, advocacy, and some time to enjoy myself with Seamus, and as a mother to Ruffin, after everyone else — they, and Rose — were gone for the night. The Christmas tree in its gold foil-covered bucket blinked in time to Ruffin's favorite carol, *Silent Night,* tinkling away at his press of a green button. He and Seamus had re-assembled last year's model train which circled its trunk, in and out of the ornaments weighing down its lowest branches.

By the end of December, Curt and I met in Mason City to firm-up the details of his representation of Ruffin and me. Curt was a tall man, with bright eyes, and a truly courtly demeanor. He was the single Iowa Protection & Advocacy Services, Inc. attorney who covered the entire state of Iowa for his government-funded agency, representing students with all sorts of disabilities. He was always on the road during the school year, driving out of Des Moines onto the small two-lane state highways in the snow to meet with parents and witnesses, to attend IEP meetings, settlement negotiations, state-supervised mediations, due process hearings, appeals into state and federal courts, and arguments in the Eighth Circuit all the way down in Missouri where those black-robed federal judges sat.

For our Mason City meeting I had loaded all my blue Binderteks into banker's boxes and hauled them out over the tailpipe of my small red hatchback. They contained all Ruffin's chronologically indexed medical records, all his educational records, all my correspondence, all our home treatment records, all the research, both psychological and legal, and one of my books — Catherine Maurice's *Let Me Hear Your Voice* — as a display of my organizational ability and my serious intentions. They were meant to show Curt at a glance that I promised to be a good client: the tedious, documentary scut work had already been done.

"Like a coloring book," was what I said. "This will be fun." Because nobody who litigated ever did it unless it also looked like it would be fun. Otherwise, litigation was just wearing — a long weary wrangle. But all my blue Binderteks settled snugly in their banker's boxes were overwhelming to Curt, I could see — as he seemed to sag.

I encouraged him, "Don't worry! You only need to take half of them back to Des Moines with you, you know, your copies."

As we visited over coffee, I learned how Curt came to his mission of practicing special education law. He had educated his son with dyslexia — grown by then, and a professor of philosophy at Victoria University in Wellington, New Zealand. Curt was clearly the proud papa, and there we bonded quickly over our love for our children. But I was also passionate, impatient, new to his area of the law, and by this time, utterly frustrated and confounded, determined, ready, and more and more inclined to be uncompromising, since no one responsible for Ruffin seemed willing to engage, much less compromise with me.

So, Ruffin became, formally: a vehicle. And I became: a client — as well as Curt's understudy in special education settlement negotiation — sometimes, reluctantly. Although Curt and I came to be, and remained, close friends and colleagues over the years, I doubt that he found me a very easy client to represent at first, because, although I was organized, with all my paper ducks in a row, I was demanding. I was forever writing letters, continuing to press those authorities responsible for Ruffin, and those widely beyond — stirring up all kinds of trouble, both good, and bad trouble.

And I knew — I promised myself — none of this advocacy, this troublemaking could ever come at Ruffin's expense.

Down in Iowa City, Sue had read my latest letter and watched my May to December videotape of Ruffin with interest. She picked up the phone to put Mark Monson, Western Hills AEA's clinical supervisor of speech and language services, in touch with me. Mark invited me to come speak for a two-hour slot at a mid-January autism in-service gathering out on the banks of Iowa's other bordering river, the Missouri. Mark expected a couple of hundred parents and special educators to attend.

What a different reception this was from ours so far in Bridgewater, and in our local district — where Donna was remembered as a student who seemed hardly likely to graduate. She had been told she wasn't and would never be college material. But then, I knew, she and I would never be recognized as prophets on our home ground. In our town, they knew us too well.

Finally, I thanked Curt for meeting with me and taking on Ruffin's case. Because autism needs a face, because every client should be familiar to his champions, I slipped a little two-inch by three-inch swap-with-friends copy of Ruffin's fall school picture into my newsy letter to him, knowing by then he was the sort of person who would call Joan, his legal assistant, into his office to share it.

CHAPTER FOURTEEN

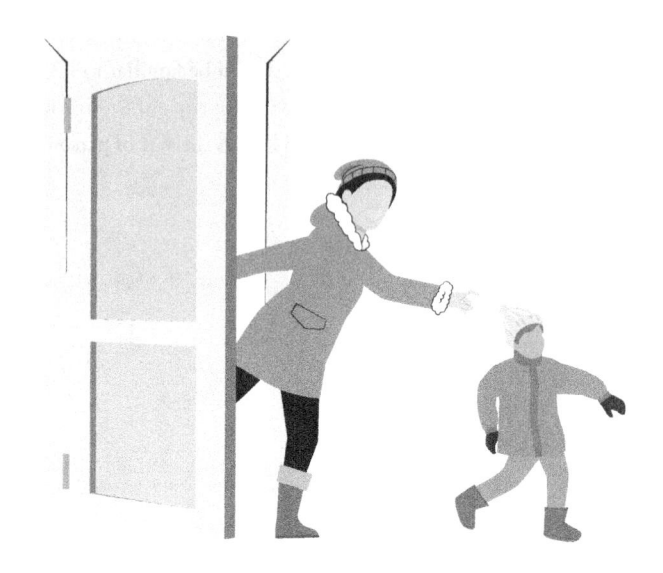

CHRISTMAS BREAK

Late in the afternoon on Christmas Eve as the sky darkened, a thick FedEx envelope arrived from California, from Dr. Lovaas's UCLA lab. Fresh copies of all his published research and all the California rulings supporting school funding slid out and covered my kitchen counter — just as Dr. Lovaas had promised. We would need these. Curt and I could put them to good use. I felt the arrival of his package as a mutual recognition of courage.

After his morning drills with me, Christmas Day ran along quietly — just Ruffin, Seamus, and me, our presents, and his train under our tree.

Ruffin had difficulty eating out on New Year's Eve. Although I had dressed him to be cute as a Lansing factory button, and although he was, with his little face — oddly as still as a doll's and expressionless — he seemed determined on something, on doing something not here. Unwilling to sit in his chair at all, he went wandering around, tapping this and that. We had left our meal uneaten. I heard a stranger whisper behind us, "What is wrong with that child?" as we struggled out the door into the cold. Ruffin missed the routine of going to school which usually helped tire him out. He experienced a few difficult days of uncontrolled babbling. I would need to hire more staff than just Donna and Lisa to manage over the summer.

But Ruffin knew all the letters of the alphabet, except "N" and all his numerals except 6 and 9 which he was like as not to mix up. As I counted it up for myself, since mid-July, Ruffin's pace was quickening, two steps forward, one step back — so much better than the other way around.

The New Year, 1995, dawned quietly, dampened by snow, with everything closed in town. But, Donna arrived, then Lisa, to work with Ruffin and keep him busy and engaged in drills for the day.

I was free to write to Mr. Montague to pass on the flier for Lovaas's conference and alert him. "I thought you would be interested to send someone from Bridgewater, perhaps Inge Nilsen who attended my CARD training workshop, or would like to go yourself." I was even bold enough to suggest he consider sending me as a parent-representative.

Then I devoted a couple of days in January to carefully marking up all the California rulings, coming to focus on a long, fact-laden California administrative law judge's ruling of 1990 in favor of Bernard Smith against his Union Elementary School District, and a February 1st, 1994, Ninth Circuit opinion, affirming a federal district court judge's review of the administrative ruling — all, fresh, new law, from a high federal appellate court, situated just below the United States Supreme Court. Although I was interested in the law, as a mother I was more intrigued by all the reported facts, test results, measurements, and assessments, searching down among the weeds to find both a roadmap, and more reasons to hope for Ruffin in the smallest details of Bernard Smith's development.

Having read the unanimous 1994 Supreme Court opinion in the *Shannon Carter* reimbursement case, and the later Ninth Circuit opinion in *Bernard Smith's* case, I knew that because I had money of my own to risk or spend, to invest in my child, I had choices: to front the cost of appropriate education at home, or even at an uncertified private school on the East or West coasts. I remained free to think outside the local schoolhouse box. I could dream, move, and travel to seek out what was appropriate for Ruffin. I was free to walk away.

But, should I choose to stand my ground to fight and win, other parents, my friends, and people whom I would never know, who didn't have the money to risk, spend, or invest, who were not free to move or travel, might benefit somehow — even if they simply stumbled onto some eventual ruling — they might at least learn about the possibilities for their child by reading the facts of Ruffin's case, as I had read *Bernard Smith*'s. With Curt's help, the risks of advocacy were worth taking. Mr. Montague and my local district seemed willing enough to go to the mat, and unprepared to engage in either real cooperation, or a pitched legal battle.

A brown padded envelope arrived from Dr. Bishop with the documentary Dr. Lovaas had promised me, *Behavioral Treatment of Autistic Children*. As Dorothy Beavers had noted in her book, and as Catherine Maurice had in hers, public dissemination of information about behavior modification had begun with early films by Lovaas, including this classic 1987 documentary. I found it well worth three-quarters of an hour of my time to break off reading law to watch it. I learned more about autism and its unsuccessful and successful treatment: what untreated autism looked like in older children and adults; why behavioral treatment worked; why it worked more readily with children who began treatment as early as possible; the long history of evolving behavioral treatment research, and more detail about Lovaas's own research throughout the 1960s, 1970s, and early 1980s.

I could see Lovaas and his graduate students at work with young children, extinguishing tantrum behavior, establishing eye contact, and then teaching language. I felt comforted to see them doing exactly what I had seen Evelyn do in early November with Ruffin, and what Donna, Lisa, Seamus, and I were doing now with Ruffin at home.

Lovaas's experimental work at UCLA underlying his 1987 seminal publication was reviewed, explained, and clearly illustrated with graphs. The late-stage introduction of children with a history of autism into mainstream public-school classrooms by kindergarten or first grade was shown. In the latter half of the film, five individual children were profiled — shown at diagnosis, and during treatment — fully illustrating the range of Lovaas's outcomes.

One child, Chris, with severe mental retardation, continued to make slow progress, but still lived at home as a teenager while continuing to prepare his good behavior and adaptive living skills for stable group home placement in his future.

Another child, Val, a child of color, with moderate mental retardation, still experienced language delay, but continued to live happily at home, preparing for work as an adult, assisting his father, as a tile-setter.

Three of the children, Ian, Scott, and Neils were presented as recovered, with their IQs having risen with treatment into the normal range and beyond. They were each shown talking with their family and friends about their college futures, when they would "meet the girls you marry."

Of these three, one, Neils, was being educated as gifted and talented. Unsurprisingly perhaps, he was most interested in STEM — science, technology, engineering, and math — the geeky subjects for the nerdy ones. In the segments showing him as a high school senior, Neils reminded me of no one so much as all the men in my family with their various engineering degrees.

Meg was typing a memo to Ruffin's educational file by early January to be copied to Miss Hobbs and Inge, but not, of course, to me. "I am writing this memo to clarify my position in relation to the Lovaas training offered by Mary Jane White. The training was at her instigation, arranged by her, and conducted in her home. She issued an open invitation to anyone who worked with Ruffin to attend and observe so that we would understand what she was doing for a home program." The rest was a long *mea culpa* to her superiors — which also implicated Inge.

Mr. Montague complained over the phone and admitted, "I tried to reach the psychologist at Mayo, several times. No success yet, but I'll keep trying. I haven't gotten around to calling Dr. Sallows yet."

"It's the holidays," I conceded. "By now, Dr. Sallows should have Ruffin's complete medical and educational file, including the long video you have."

"What I'd really like to do is be able to hear from the University of Iowa Hospitals and Clinics group after Ruffin's appointment there before we schedule the continuation of his IEP meeting. When is it, again, that he's going to be seen?"

"January 23rd," I reminded him, as I realized he was planning to kick the can further down the road.

"Yes, let me make a note of that."

"Well, did you get to review Ruffin's video, the one Dr. Sallows has?"

"I did."

"And what did you see, what did you think? Talk to me."

"During the classroom segment, Ruffin was relating well to his teacher, Meg. He did better at circle time than several of the other students."

"The girls, yes, at circle time, who were not attending very well, they were brought over to Ruffin's class from a severely and profoundly disabled classroom across the hallway, Amy's classroom. One of them, the older girl who has the most difficulty paying attention during circle time, is also a child with autism. I know her and her family from our local autism support group." Then, I stumbled a little, "I mean, thank you, for referring me."

"Humph." I heard a little scribbling.

"And bear in mind, Ruffin and I have spent quite a bit of time working together at home on his computer, on his joint attention skills. That, and his megavitamin therapy, the one we started in late July, Dr. Rimland's, seems to have improved his ability to pay attention. You know, since May, that first segment of Ruffin's video."

More scribbling.

"But I have to say, what struck *me* about the classroom segments of Ruffin's video was that although Ruffin was talking, using one and two words at home with me, as you can see in the computer segments filmed the same week with me, at school, Ruffin hardly spoke a word."

"Home and school are two different environments."

"They are. But I'm sending him to school to learn, you know, to talk. Like a person."

"We can't know what will happen. There are no guarantees. I'd like to video Ruffin in the classroom again before he goes down to Iowa City."

"Fine with me. I'll let Meg and Miss Hobbs know."

Then I launched into a full description and summary of Dr. Lovaas's 1987 documentary that Dr. Bishop had sent, winding up with, "I've ordered my own copy. It's the same documentary I mentioned to Jack Wallace before Christmas. Could I send you my copy when it arrives?"

"Sure." But I heard a suppressed sigh, which I ignored.

Instead, I pulled out my notes about Bernard Smith and launched into the details of a comparison of Bernard's course of development with Ruffin's, which Mr. Montague quickly interrupted by asking if I would send him copies of the Smith ruling and the Ninth Circuit opinion upholding it.

"Of course, if it would help. And, I have a November 3rd, 1993 letter authored by Dr. Lovaas I'd like to send you which addresses the question of what, in Dr. Lovaas's opinion, constitutes an appropriate intervention for a child diagnosed with autism. If it would help . . ."

"Sure."

"What I found most interesting was on page 2, paragraph 6."

Here, I heard more scribbling as I read out this passage for Mr. Montague, "'The majority of the 40 hours per week of one-to-one instruction, at least during the first 6 months of the intervention, should consist of remediating speech and language deficits (Lovaas 1977). Later, this time may be divided between promoting peer integration and continuing to remediate speech and language difficulties.' Doesn't that offer us some guidance for planning Ruffin's education?" I asked.

Mr. Montague offered no response.

I pressed on, foolishly, "I don't think three 20-minute speech therapy sessions a week, what is that? Sixty minutes, okay, an hour with your speech and language therapist Kim Pope working with Ruffin and two other students can be expected to remediate Ruffin's 16-month language delay. Lovaas training can, and may be beginning to do so, even though I can only provide him 28 to 30 hours of one-to-one instruction each week after school and on weekends."

Even more foolishly, but because I thought in his position Mr. Montague ought to know, I let this black cat out of the bag: "Meg told me that Kim had a full caseload last year and that she had not been relieved of a single one of those cases, even though she was expected to take on all the special education students moving back to Miss Hobbs's campus this year. That's thirteen special needs children, including at least one other with autism, besides Ruffin. That might be a lot to put on a single speech and language pathologist."

More silence from Mr. Montague. I had advanced too far into his agency's territory. We were done. I was back to writing letters aimed at decision-makers over his head.

Before I could write anything more, here came Ruffin, home from school in a great mood, very talkative. We headed out to the grocery store because we were down to our last banana. I asked him, "What will we do?" Ruffin was right there with the answer. "Go to the grocery store, get bananas." I was pleased, of course, but I said, "We can't go. Ruffin has no shoes." Ruffin replied, "I put on my running shoes," and headed for the door. My heart lifted, of course, but I said, "We can't go. Ruffin has no coat." Ruffin put on his coat, saying, "I have a zipper. Mommy's coat has no zipper." It was true, yes, it was true. Lately, I noticed, Ruffin seemed to love making this form of comparative observation. I felt we might as well have been flying to the store.

Back home with bananas, Ruffin watched his *Spot* and *Pooh* videos. I especially appreciated the *Spot* video's static background against which only the characters moved. Somehow this helped Ruffin focus. He could answer questions or make remarks about *Spot*, while Rose cooked dinner.

He and I played *Sammy's Science House* on his computer together before bed. I used his infatuation with the workshop feature to have Ruffin tell me, "This part goes on top" or "to the side" or "underneath" some other part. Later, I noticed Ruffin was very absorbed in the appropriate use of Legos, building complex towers with holes, "windows and doors," with a sense of symmetry. He appeared to look carefully for specific blocks with special attributes or colors.

That night as Ruffin slept, I prepared the long read-out letter of that day's phone call with Mr. Montague for Curt, enclosing my own detailed written comparison of Ruffin's and Bernard Smith's individual characteristics, their assessments before and after Lovaas intensive intervention, and the development of skills affecting their readiness for integration into a classroom of typically developing classmates.

Copying it widely, up and down the ladders of Ruffin's educational agencies, including Dr. Bishop at Luther College as the newest member of my advocacy loop, I closed my letter, "I sincerely hope that by providing this additional material you will be able to set aside any concerns about the public education agencies' responsibility to pay for a Lovaas program and integration into a classroom or other socially-appropriate group, to continue through this summer, in order to effectively remediate Ruffin's developmental delays, including, but not limited to, his very severe, continuing language delay."

With school back in session, I offered Meg a copy of Lovaas's 1987 documentary.

Afterwards, Meg had invited a junior high school student volunteer to drill Ruffin on 20 sets of mastered drill materials designed to prompt him to use verbs in full descriptive sentences with a pronoun — "She is riding" — which I had sent along to school. Ruffin was able to respond using the 20 verbs he had mastered — even though the untrained teenager couldn't possibly give Ruffin as clean or direct a cue as Meg or Donna, or as Lisa or I might do.

Meg crowed, "I'd say he has these. Kim wanted to do them, too!"

I was thrilled. "What a great idea to have a junior high schooler drill Ruffin in his areas of mastery. Is it okay for you to tell me who she is? If I need to structure Ruffin's summer without a classroom, I'd be interested to hire some of these students who have had some experience or have taken an interest in Ruffin to help."

Ruffin continued to work hard on his drills with Lisa and with Donna. We were working on pronouns and his first conjunction — "and." Ruffin was finding shapes everywhere he looked now, saying to me, "Your eyes are like the moon," and "My ear is a broken circle."

Outside drill time Ruffin was becoming useful around the house as a go-fer. He had gone to the pantry to bring me flour, gone to a drawer for a spoon, and brought me a washrag from the bathroom. This was a delightful change.

In a more formal note to Ruffin's educational file which she shared with me, Meg assessed that Ruffin had experienced no loss of the "critical skills" upon which his entitlement to summer school depended. I could read the handwriting on the chalkboard. As Ruffin's special educators saw it, no summer school would be necessary. No EYSE looked likely for Ruffin.

But Meg and I continued to work well together, hand in glove. She sent me her weekly charting of Ruffin's IEP goal that he correctly answer the question "What do we do with a particular object?" Ruffin was able to give appropriate answers: cutting with scissors, coloring with crayons, blowing into a tissue, and continuing to couple over a dozen verbs with dozens of everyday objects. Meg's own excitement sprang from her penciled note, "I think we've got functions!" I thought Ruffin seemed much more aware of what was going on in his world and how to talk about it.

Then Meg offered up the names of three junior high students who volunteered regularly in the special education classrooms to do CARD drills with Ruffin there, using the materials and routines he had mastered at home.

Time to rattle Mr. Montague's cage again. I had the 1987 Lovaas documentary to send him. He immediately asked whether I knew of any additional, independent research to support the efficacy of Lovaas's methods. He admitted that no parent with whom he had spoken had anything negative to say about them, and that all the parents he had spoken to reported good progress and said that they were pleased. I told him I had heard the same — since by then I had spoken to numerous families in California, Pennsylvania, New York, Virginia, Kentucky, Arkansas, Texas, and Minnesota.

Mr. Montague expected some of Iowa's nine AEAs or regional special education agencies would go one way on Lovaas, and some would go another — without giving any indication of which way he planned to lead Bridgewater. I let him know I would be speaking at Western Hills the next week, presenting Ruffin's case to that group, and invited him to attend or send anyone he liked from Bridgewater.

That seemed to rile him. He let me know in no uncertain terms that Bridgewater had no obligation to pay for Ruffin's upcoming University of Iowa Hospitals and Clinics evaluation — the very one he was so interested in having the results of to kick the can down the road.

Curt called to brief me on his two-day struggle with the governing board of his publicly funded agency. He had managed to persuade them and had just received the go-ahead to advocate statewide from a pro-Lovaas position, identifying Lovaas as an educational method more appropriate to young children with autism than any other currently available. This came as a welcome victory. Now Curt had institutional support to file a petition for a Lovaas family in Mason City. Joan would fax it over to me for review. I thought I might be able to read it that night — if Ruffin slept.

But that afternoon, right then! I needed to get off the phone to attend Miss Hobbs's principal's committee meeting to plan an open house at the end of the month and come up with some ideas for more regular events to invite community people into the schools. This is what I had been roped into after I had asked Miss Hobbs whether our district had a parent teacher association.

"We don't have a PTA. We have a partners-in-education concept," she replied.

It sounded like a company union to me.

CHAPTER FIFTEEN

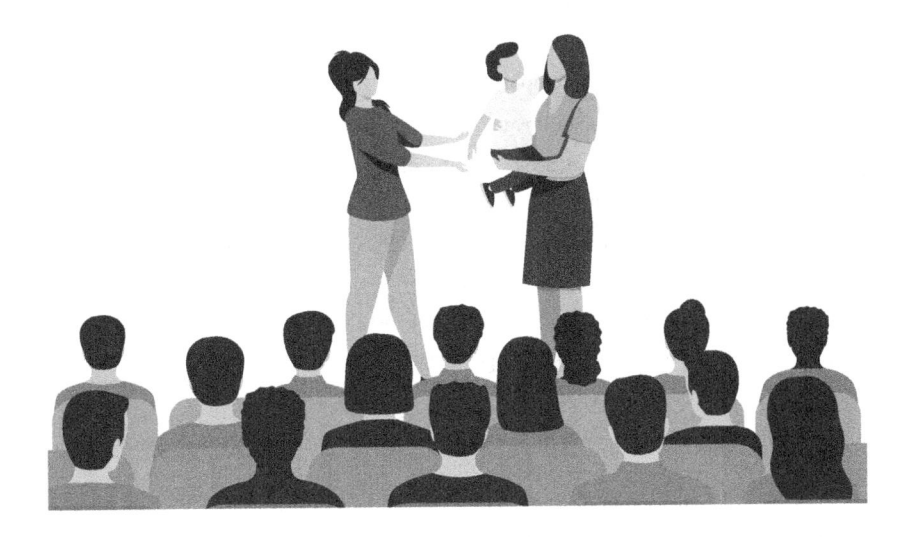

TIME IS OF THE ESSENCE

What *were* my questions for the University of Iowa Hospitals and Clinics (UIHC) evaluation group? I re-ran the hamster-wheel of gathering all Ruffin's previous information to send out again. "The public schools and I will need some objective measurements and assessments of Ruffin.

"We need to know:
- What educational interventions are appropriate for Ruffin?
- How much one-to-one programming does Ruffin need daily and weekly?
- When during the day — morning vs. afternoon — should one-to-one programming be scheduled?
- Who — teachers, aides, speech therapists, CARD therapists — should provide one-to-one programming?

- At what locations should programming be provided — school, home, community?
- How long should programming be provided — for 2 years, more, or less?
- What form of positive behavioral intervention program will meet Ruffin's individual needs?
- Is 60 minutes per week of small group speech therapy sufficient to meet Ruffin's individual needs?
- What parent-training component would meet Ruffin's needs?
- What mainstreaming or integration component would meet Ruffin's needs?
- Do Ruffin's individual needs and the unique possibility of his remediation by CARD programming require the provision of extended year special education?
- What computer programs would meet Ruffin's needs — *Laureate, Edmark, Broderbund*?
- What opinion can you offer on vitamin B-6, magnesium, DMG therapy? Can you check for appropriate dosage in any way?
- Is Ruffin's present programming inappropriate in any way?
- If so, please specify what improvements are necessary to meet his individual needs?"

I needed the answers to these questions for Ruffin. For litigation, Curt and I needed the answers in the form of written expert opinion rendered to a reasonable degree of medical and educational certainty. Ruffin's educators needed these answers, too — to learn. Having chosen to put my back to the wall, and litigate, if necessary, that was my view.

My doorbell rang the next day. I didn't much care for clients who dropped by without appointments. I left my desk, grumbling, annoyed at having to answer the door, and was surprised to find Inge on my porch, shivering in the cold. She wouldn't take time to step in, as she handed over several books about typical preschool development. Over her shoulder, she was keeping an eye on the street — Main Street — as she quickly let me know that Mr. Montague had just decided to send Kim and Emily to Lovaas's upcoming conference in Los Angeles. She thought I ought to go too, and explained exactly how I could apply for parent-training funds from Bridgewater to help with my travel expenses.

I told her I would be speaking at Western Hills in mid-January about Ruffin's case.

Then she was gone, as quickly as that. I understood immediately — she had left before anyone from school, or anyone in town could notice she had been here. I went back to my desk to wonder why. What did this portend?

Some drill materials I had sent to school — 20 more verbs Ruffin had already mastered and that we were using to teach him pronouns — came back with a note from Kim, suggesting that Donna, Lisa, Seamus, and I seemed to be getting out over her skis. "You will have better success if you stick to singular ('he' and 'she') first, then after that's accomplished or at least firm, add ('they'). We are working on *he* and *she* at school."

Next day, the phone rang mid-morning. It was the intake coordinator from the University of Iowa Hospitals and Clinics (UIHC) making the by now familiar, difficult, and wary "clarification phone call" she had been delegated to make. "No," she was in no position to discuss it. While charging me a small fortune, the powers above her had no wish to be drawn into matters of educational dispute about Ruffin.

There was also a letter from Prudential's Ms. Crews letting me know she was reviewing my claim for Ruffin's CARD program as a form of "occupational therapy" and that as soon as her review was complete, she would get back to me.

It was January. It was cold and icy. Everybody was cranky. It wasn't just me — but maybe it *was* me.

As I carried an armload of envelopes out to stuff on the top of my mailbox, my carrier walked up and handed me a large, manila envelope from Curt. Here were a dozen heavy, creamy pages — Curt's due process petition for the Mason City family. Curt had chosen to sue the local district, Northern Trails AEA, and the State — the Iowa Department of Education. He had sued all three agencies under both the *IDEA* and a related federal disability statute, *Section 504 of the Rehabilitation Act*.

The Mason City boy, a 4-year-old, had been born the month I became pregnant with Ruffin, so, he was 7 1/2 months older than Ruffin, and had been diagnosed with PDD about the same time as Ruffin had been in his development, at 35 1/2 months by a developmental pediatrician who assessed his development then at no greater than the 17- to 18-month level, amounting to a 13-month developmental delay — in that respect also similar to Ruffin. A second opinion from a licensed psychologist offered the family a diagnosis of autistic disorder. At 3 years, 6 months, the child had "the complete want of a spoken vocabulary and an inability to understand cause and effect."

His parents were offered nearly the same special education for him that Ruffin had been offered: 6 hours a day in a small group ECSE setting of 8 variously disabled students, 1 teacher and 1 aide, and 60 minutes a week of speech and language services, by an IEP team, which, like Ruffin's, had failed to include any recognized expert in autism, or any member of Sue's state-wide network of autism resource teams (ARTs). The local district and the AEA conducted no evaluation of the child of their own and failed to follow the recommendations of the family's two diagnosticians.

Lacking expertise, and ignoring medical recommendations, the schools offered a series of inappropriate IEP goals including demanding cognitive tasks and — as with Ruffin — expressive language goals in the absence of any receptive language training.

When the boy failed to develop speech, his teachers tried using a few simple signs to communicate with him — just as Ruffin's teacher, Meg, had tried early last fall.

Although the AEA advised the local district that their student needed much one-to-one assistance and a smaller classroom of 5 students with 2 teachers — effectively suggesting a drop back of the boy into a severe and profound disability placement — the local district kept him where he was without change.

The parents then sought out a further independent educational evaluation of their son at their own expense and hired a fulltime aide to go to school with him as recommended by their son's doctors, reduced their son's time at school each day by an hour or two, as also recommended by the doctors, to allow their aide to instruct their son one-to-one in their home. The boy would also have benefitted from occupational therapy to address his sensory integration issues.

Summer programming (EYSE) was denied, as was parent and aide training. The parents were forced "to undertake the difficult task of creating, at their own expense, an in-home program" by "massive self-education, the hiring of consultants, a major coordination effort, and the hiring and training of one-to-one educational therapists for 30 hours per week, and the boy began to learn and develop."

When the parents withdrew their son from school, the school authorities failed to tell them about their due process rights under the *IDEA* and *Section 504* and warned them — wrongly — that their decision to educate their son at home had "waived" any right for them to seek reimbursement or compensation from the school authorities.

Over the next summer at home the boy had learned all the upper- and lower-case letters of the alphabet and how to identify several basic shapes.

Late in the summer of 1994, Curt attended an IEP meeting for the family to seek the school authorities' best offer of a free, appropriate public education (FAPE). He and the parents were offered 30 to 40 minutes per week of speech and language therapy, no summer programming (EYSE), and placement for their son in a severe and profoundly disabled classroom, 4 days a week only, with no parent training — and no training for his teachers in the one-to-one methods that were helping him to learn at home.

On Curt's advice, the parents had rejected this school offer as inappropriate.

But "the stress, the time demands, and the inherent difficulties of staffing a home-based program in a small community" led the parents to live separately on a temporary basis, with the mother, the boy, and his little sister moving ahead to a new home in Lawrence, Kansas — selected for the sole purpose of providing an appropriate education for the boy in that university town. There, he continued to make outstanding educational progress while the father remained behind in Iowa to wind up his own medical practice.

"In fact, and in effect, the family had been driven out of Iowa by the state's failure to provide a free, appropriate public education (FAPE) for their child."

For these wrongs, the local district and the AEA were sued. And, as the agency having "overarching responsibility" the Iowa Department of Education was also sued. Discrimination was alleged against the boy "and other children with autism under the age of 6" by the state of Iowa failing to adopt or implement "effective procedures for acquiring and disseminating to teachers and administrators" significant information on early childhood intervention in autism cases "derived from educational research, demonstration, and similar projects."

In his petition, Curt had written, "In fact, highly significant research results produced by UCLA, Princeton, and other reputable institutions have neither been acquired nor effectively disseminated, and, as a direct result, the IEP teams for children with autism, including the boy, are not appropriately informed concerning that child's educational needs and options."

And I thought to myself as I read it — neither were Ruffin's.

To do justice, Curt sought an order of injunction to compel the Iowa Department of Education to distribute information about recent research results on the early education of children with autism, and actively facilitate the adoption of appropriate and promising practices for their early education.

Nor did he forget to ask for his attorney fees, as provided for by the "fee-shifting" provisions of the *IDEA* and *Section 504* — civil rights statutes — enacted by Congress to prevent discrimination against those with disabilities.

It was several hours' drive over the windswept, snow-covered prairie from our side of Iowa to the other, so Donna, Ruffin, and I bundled up, with our overnight luggage, our videos, and all my banker's boxes of blue Binderteks. We stopped on the way out of town for my coffee, chocolate milk for Ruffin's vitamin-bottle, and a full tank of gas for Donna's van. We were prepared to spend a long day on the road, sleep the night in the nearest inexpensive motel, and get to the speaking venue at Western Hills AEA early.

I was not exactly nervous, but for this audience I wanted to set out my blue Binderteks in a long bank on the table that supported a small podium, as a visually impressive, yes, even intimidating demonstration of the scale of the "difficult task of creating, at my own expense, an in-home program" by "massive self-education, the hiring of consultants, a major coordination effort, and the hiring and training of one-to-one educational therapists," as Curt had rightly described it in his newly-filed due process petition for the Mason City family.

Looking out over my thirty-foot long blue bulwark into the full auditorium of rising seats and shifting bodies, I wanted to say, and to show, how receiving a diagnosis of autism was not like getting a parking ticket. It was like being served an indictment for first degree murder, a large matter that arrested you, and stopped your former life in its tracks. When you looked down to read the papers you had been handed, there your child's name was — as the victim — unless you were prepared to react as quickly as possible, at the appropriate scale, and with all the necessary intensity to prevail.

I wanted to convey urgency, but it didn't take long before I settled into speaking more and more conversationally. I forgot the cameras, and the NBC film crew who had been invited. I had this jury, had their eye contact, their attention, their fingertip at the corner of an eye, their tears. Ruffin's video ran with bits of my stop and go commentary, and then Ruffin and Donna emerged from an off-stage door to applause and congratulation.

Right away I could see on Donna's face what this recognition of her accomplishment, her contribution meant to her, coming from a group of educators and parents, eager now for our answers to their questions. It was absolutely the right thing to have done to have brought her along to share in this. Ruffin was as adorable and well-behaved as any 3-year-old. He reached out to come from Donna into my arms.

It was time to tickle Mr. Montague again. I told him I knew that Bridgewater would be flying Emily and Kim to Los Angeles for the conference hosted by Dr. Lovaas. So, I wanted to go too, and asked for parent-training money.

"I reiterate my request that when we schedule Ruffin's IEP meeting all those persons whose authority is necessary to address his IEP issues be jointly present so that his case can be resolved without additional routing. It is not acceptable IDEA procedure to route Ruffin and me on and on to other persons and agencies, or back and forth between agencies. All the agencies need to be present, prepared to cooperate and coordinate, and with each agency represented by a person with sufficient authority to commit to providing services and funding.

"Time is of the essence to the law, precisely because time is of the essence to Ruffin."

CHAPTER SIXTEEN

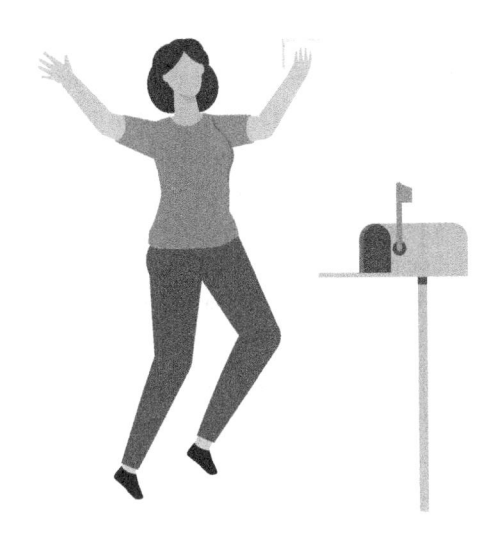

THE UNIVERSITY OF IOWA

Dr. Guy Norman, an educational consultant and the UIHC evaluation team leader began preparing for Ruffin's upcoming visit in mid-January. He called Meg and Kim at school, to learn what he could. By requesting copies from their medical records department of all the underlying clinical notes — including those taken during phone calls concerning Ruffin — I was able to read Dr. Norman's handwritten notes later, after he, Meg, and Kim had spoken to one another in confidence.

Meg had no questions or concerns for Dr. Norman. She was happy with Ruffin in her school program of a full 6-hour day, 5 days a week, with 7 other boys and an aide to help her and pleased with Kim's speech therapy pull-out for him a couple of times a week. As always, she noted Ruffin's excellent motor skills. "In the past, Ruffin has been in daycare. We will plan some integration with typically developing students for him next year." His autism was on me. "Mom feels Ruffin has autism (Gundersen has said PDD-NOS) and feels he needs Lovaas method instruction."

When Dr. Norman probed, the real problem surfaced. "We have written another IEP recently, but the mother was unhappy that it did not prescribe Lovaas." Meg's plan for Ruffin's future surfaced, too. "I would like to have Ruffin another year in my ECSE class with some regular preschool, and the next year after that, hopefully kindergarten and some special education."

When her hair was down with Dr. Norman, Meg owned up to having more trouble with Ruffin's behavior than she had been willing to share with me. Ruffin was screaming with refusal when offered food and upset with excess demands. He continued to toe-walk and was preoccupied with the sort of nonsense self-talk that I was familiar with from last May before Ruffin's diagnosis in July. It was clear. Meg didn't envision that Ruffin could or would run loose in the universe — or *ever* move beyond special education. Confirmed in my disappointments of early December, I was dismayed to learn the limits of Meg's frankness, her experience, and her imagination.

Kim confirmed that she was seeing Ruffin for three 20-minute sessions a week with other students. She continued to rate him a 3, or maybe a 2 ½, on the *Iowa Severity of Language-Delay Scale*. Ruffin had a fair amount of speech; labels and verbs were coming, with a few pronouns. Dr. Norman learned that she and the school psychologist were being flown to Los Angeles the next week for Lovaas training. Kim reported in air quotes, "Mom and 'therapists' work with Ruffin at home for several hours after school daily." She claimed she got good responses from Ruffin to her structuring situations to get him to initiate and respond spontaneously. He did echo when he experienced low comprehension, but she was not getting too much echoing anymore. Maybe because she had never attended any of Ruffin's IEP meetings, she claimed, "Communication with mom has been pretty positive and very frequent."

At home, Ruffin asked his first "why" question. He was upset when he found one of our couch pillows in a plastic grocery bag and asked, "Pillow in bag?" I gave him, "Why is the pillow in the bag?" to echo, and when he did, I answered, "Because it's broken. Mommy is taking it to be fixed at the store."

Within a day or two I got a surprising letter from Mr. Montague. It confused me, as perhaps it was meant to do. He thanked me for the legal decisions and assured me, "I have read both. I would hope that we are not making the same errors as the public agencies who are parties to those decisions did. We are sailing in some new and uncharted waters. I do appreciate your patience."

He expressed interest in both the upcoming UIHC re-evaluation and Dr. Sallows's expected second opinion. "I am particularly interested in his views related to the number of hours Ruffin might need of his CARD program in the home as well as those which might need to be carried over into his classroom milieu. This might be significant as we look at drawing up an appropriate program for him from both an educational viewpoint and a support service perspective."

I immediately called UIHC's intake coordinator to offer her a copy of Mr. Montague's latest letter — as an indication of the public-school authorities' shifting position. She wanted it, along with another copy of all the court rulings. Off they flew by fax to Iowa City, and to Curt in Des Moines — who promised to hand-carry copies to Dr. Hagen, the chief of the state bureau of special education, since he was already planning to see her about the Mason City family. He expected her to assign that case to Dianne Wilson for mediation.

I might have been less confused had I been copied in on Mr. Montague's memo of the same day addressed to Kim: *"Re: Research Article — Autism — Language Development (Ruffin White, and Others).* "Recently, I sent Jack in Decorah several court decisions related to the Lovaas method. These decisions were based on the fact that the local school district did not provide an appropriate program for the child with autism in question, therefore, the parents sought a private placement which was deemed more appropriate by the ALJ, and the district was required to pay for that program."

Mr. Montague hadn't risen to become the director of a special education regional agency by being the first hayseed to fall off a turnip truck. He could read the law well enough, understood it, and could distill it in writing to his subordinate. "As you read those decisions, you will note that there was a primary focus on language development in the programming. One of the expert witnesses in the New Jersey decision was not supportive of the Lovaas system. Attached, you will find a language program which is designed for children with autism by that person, Andrew S. Bondy. I forward it to you for your review and use as you deem appropriate."

Bondy's dense 19-page article about his *Picture-Exchange Communication System*, was one I was familiar with from the August 1994 issue of *Focus on Autistic Behavior*. His *PECS*-language program was perfectly appropriate for children with autism who also had *aphasia* and were unable to produce the sounds of language accurately without a long course of speech and occupational therapy to improve the development of the mouth's musculature and the workings of the vocal tract — not Ruffin's problem, since he produced abundant echolalia. Reading Bondy's article would be no substitute for hands-on-training in his method — any more than reading Lovaas's 1987 peer-reviewed academic research article would substitute for a long weekend visit from a trained practitioner like Evelyn.

I had been relieved to take a step back and let Curt take up the fight in Des Moines. Knowing Dr. Hagen well from their previous legal battles and settlements, he could make an appointment to walk into her office and negotiate away the embarrassing prospect of the state becoming subject to a court injunction that would require her to disseminate information about Lovaas programming. Curt offered to save Dr. Hagen the trouble — he could write something for her. Having roiled the waters, Curt came bearing all the oil to pour on them, and Dr. Hagen, who trusted him, was fine with that.

Writing Mr. Montague back, I couldn't help but crow a little because I was so pleased. Giving him the benefit of the doubt, I imagined he might be, too. "Ruffin's teacher let me know yesterday that he has already achieved one of his newly formulated short-term objectives: to be able to report the function of objects in response to the question, 'What is this for?' He was incapable of comprehending or responding to this type of question last October at Gundersen. Here at home, Ruffin has also met another of those newly formulated short-term objectives: complying with verbally complex 2-adjective, 2-step commands. So, when we do reconvene, we will need to formulate a more demanding set of short-term objectives for him than were offered in December. Wouldn't that be a great success to share in?"

CHAPTER SEVENTEEN

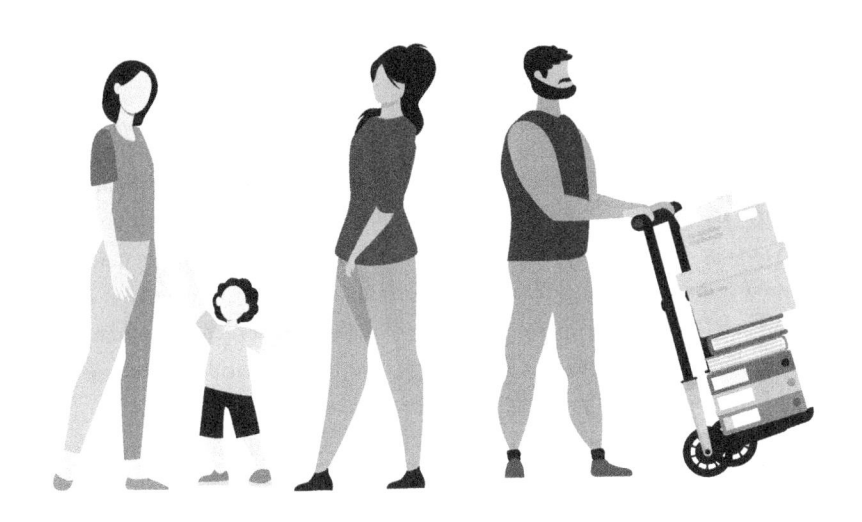

DOWN TO IOWA CITY

It was a measure of Ruffin's considerable progress that he, Donna, and I were able to organize ourselves and manage to get out the door before the crack of dawn to start our three-hour drive south to the university in Iowa City. But it was cold — not bitterly so, just a few degrees above zero. "Good," I chirped to Donna. "Too cold to snow or sleet." We could expect the roads, already plowed, to remain clear throughout the day until evening.

Seamus was coming today too, curious, having accepted the notion that Ruffin might have been suffering from something that seemed to be getting better this Christmas. Seamus always liked to visit Iowa City, where he had graduated with a degree in history. It would be good to have his strong arms and hand truck to move my heavy litigation boxes of blue Binderteks in and out of my car. I had Seamus and all these boxes with me, mostly as a show of force. I wanted this new evaluation group to take us — Ruffin, Seamus, Donna, and me — seriously.

After we wheeled off the elevator onto the clinic floor, the three of us were immediately separated from Ruffin. He was led away, down a long, brightly lit hospital corridor, escorted by two strangers, Dr. Norman, a tall man with a dark beard, and Dr. Betty Simon, a short, roly-poly figure with cropped grey hair.

Go, little one, I thought. Go strut your stuff. None of us would be allowed to watch, but it would be okay, Donna and I reassured each other. Ruffin wouldn't need us — not me, not Seamus, not even Donna, I thought. This visit was meant to be an acid test of Ruffin's recent progress.

Dr. Norman's account about our 3-year, 8-month-old boy began, "Ruffin started his formal assessment day working with Dr. Simon. He seemed a bit anxious for the first minute or so after separating from his mother but then calmed down quickly and was smiling and positive in his responses thereafter. Eye contact increased over time. There were a few unusual behaviors though. He did sometimes echo or repeat parts of directions and the last words that Dr. Simon spoke. This happened more frequently on demand tasks and more difficult questions.

"Most of Ruffin's time with Dr. Simon was spent completing the *Stanford-Binet Intelligence Test (Fourth Edition)*. Ruffin is at the young end of the range of children for whom this test is appropriate and is therefore at the bottom of the normative structure. This calls for a careful interpretation of the results." My own later research disclosed the young end of the range was 2 years, and that this IQ test was not considered particularly helpful in discriminating between mild and moderate mental retardation. Nor was it designed for testing IQ in children with learning disabilities. So, as far as I was concerned, it was a fine acid test.

"Today, Ruffin scored well into the average range with the following standard scores: Verbal Reasoning 95, Abstract-Visual Reasoning 89, Quantitative Reasoning 114, and Short-Term Memory 91. His composite IQ score was 97." A mere 3 points off the IQ norm of 100, up 18 points on his early October *WPPSI-R* composite score of 78 — and nearly whoppingly-double the early August *Bayley Scale* mental development index of 50 pinned on him by Emily. I didn't imagine we were completely out of the woods, but Dr. Simon's finding that Ruffin tested well into the average range of IQ was reassuring and encouraging.

Dr. Simon found Ruffin "unusually cooperative and attentive for one of this age" and "able to remain seated throughout." Usually, the administration of the *Stanford-Binet* took an hour to an hour and a half. Dr. Simon administered only 8 of the available subtests, omitting 7 others, so Ruffin's time sitting amounted to the better part of an hour — still quite a long stretch for him or any child under the age of 4 to work in a chair without a wiggle-break.

It impressed me that Dr. Simon's summary of Ruffin's previous assessments showed that she had reviewed Ruffin's earlier evaluations by Bridgewater and Gundersen with careful attention to detail, before offering her own results. "Ruffin's IQ factors are variable and feature an increment in quantitative reasoning, while abstract and visual reasoning is relatively reduced. Ruffin has unusually well-developed arithmetical skills. He was able to match the face of die, counts one-to-one correlation without difficulty, and was even able to complete the series '1, 2, 3, 4, 5, 6' where he needed to insert '4 and 6' with dotted dice."

Dr. Simon offered us a bit of sage advice, too, about future IQ testing. "As testing at younger ages is so frequently unreliable, a periodic reevaluation is strongly recommended to determine functional levels more clearly and to help in making recommendations for class placement. There should be at least one year or two between assessments to obtain the most valid and reliable results." By choosing to administer the *Stanford Binet* to Ruffin, rather than re-administer the *WPPSI-R* that Dr. Kondrick at Gundersen had used in October, Dr. Simon avoided any possibility that Ruffin might be too familiar with the test and over-perform.

That was Ruffin by the numbers, but I was also keenly interested to read the anecdotal embellishments, like this, from Dr. Norman, who got to watch Dr. Simon work with Ruffin. "He seemed interactive, although he rarely initiated. Ruffin tended to be perseverative at times and would use the same word to answer any number of questions. He did very well on the picture vocabulary tests, counting activities, and matching. He had a little bit of difficulty with some abstract-visual tasks, particularly with reversing or inverting designs." Dr. Simon observed, "Ruffin was an attractive, appealing little fellow who knew all of his personal information including birthdate, city, and state, and the parents indicated that he also knows his street address if he is asked in the proper way."

Ms. Clara Wilding, the speech and language pathologist who tested Ruffin later in the day, was very much less impressed. "Ruffin was able to provide personal information such as his name, age, town that he lives in, and so on. He was able to tell the name of his school and the name of his teacher. Many of these responses appeared to be delayed echolalia in response to a specific question that was asked of him. It did, however, indicate that he was understanding the questions."

"Ms. Wilding noted that Ruffin's speech was generally intelligible though he did have some articulation errors which were typical for a youngster his age. She also noted a fairly high pitch. He often echoed the last word of her comments and, especially, her reinforcing comments or phrases. He did not consistently attend to question forms. For instance, when she asked Ruffin how old he was, he responded 'Three.' When she asked, 'How are you?' he responded 'Three.'"

In her own written report, Ms. Wilding continued to be critical, even dismissive, especially of Donna, and inferentially of the Lovaas method of teaching language. "Ruffin has a limited range of inflection. He tends to sing information as opposed to speaking it. The majority of the prosodic elements of speech will need to be periodically re-evaluated as Ruffin gains more control of his language system and increases his length of utterance. At the present time, fluency is appropriate, but Ruffin is using short phrases. Volume, although appropriate at this time, will need to be looked at since Ruffin has a tendency to loud volume as opposed to normal volume."

I was unsurprised by her observations but dismissed much of this as carping. If Ruffin needed to sing for his supper or sing out his name and address as a long-memorized bit, better that, than he go hungry. Better that he sing his personal information rather than meaningless snippets of dialogue from a Disney video or remain lost should he wander away. I was pleased to hear that Ruffin was no longer whispering.

Ms. Wilding asserted, just as she urged us later in conference, "We would favor a program which does not include singing, odd inflections, and rhythm disruptions by unnecessary repetition. According to his primary trainer Donna, that is the technique that is being used for his training sessions. It is up to the individuals who are currently working with him on a frequent basis to determine which programming style they will be using. We are simply calling attention to the fact that that is the style we saw him using here and note that it may be difficult to unlearn those behaviors once they have been established."

She was really hung up on Ruffin's prosody.

"It was significant to note that he named each of these pictures three and four times in a sing-song giggly sort of voice which certainly distracted from his skills. He was not able to stop this behavior even though we attempted to structure him up for stopping on several occasions. It seemed like whenever we presented to him the material in picture form that he was to name, he used this particular style for naming."

Here I did take Ms. Wilding's point about certain ingrained behaviors being difficult to unlearn, and this was a matter Donna and I raised with Evelyn during her next telephone conference call with us, and over her later visits.

In assessing Ruffin's play skills, Dr. Norman continued to describe his opportunity to watch Ruffin with Ms. Wilding. "Ruffin did make spontaneous comments in identifying play items. He tended not to share things easily and on one occasion said, 'No, I wanna play with that.' Despite these verbal responses, he generally would share and was consistently cooperative."

Ms. Wilding's report was a bit more expansive. "In terms of following directions, we found Ruffin to be compliant to those that we had for him and to be understanding simple 'give me' and 'put away' type directions here. We did not need to use additional support or prompts or pointing out things that we wanted him to give us.

"As we asked for a turn, he remarked, 'No, my toy' and moved away. We acknowledged this by saying, 'Okay, you can play with this a little bit longer' and engaged ourselves in playing with another toy. We again asked for a turn with that particular toy, and he indicated again, 'No, my toy.' We found this to be particularly communicative since with other toys he was very happy to give turns and to share."

I was pleased with this account of Ruffin standing up for himself. He needed to do this in his classroom of so many other variously disabled boys — some with fairly challenging, sometimes even aggressive behaviors of their own — judging by Meg's comments and my own observations during my classroom visits.

I also valued the considerable detail of Ms. Wilding's informal observations of Ruffin's speech. "The longest utterance for Ruffin today was a 4-word phrase, but his most frequent utterance length was a 3-word phrase. His utterances tend to be 'I' type statements or information type statements which contain subject-verb-object. He is not consistently using plural markers, past tense markers, articles, 'is' verbs, and so on. At the present time, he is using the primary meaning-carrying words of utterances." I found all this very encouraging. Ruffin was using words as a form of meaningful communication. He was learning that language worked to carry meaning.

"In terms of question response, Ruffin is using 'yes' and 'no' and is making a response to some of the 'wh' questions. He was not always successful at 'wh' questions and was specifically having difficulty with inferential type 'if then' questions. He is using the strategy of a verbal 'um, um, um' and rolling his eyes when asked a question for which he does not have a response. That indicates then that he understands the task, but does not, at present, have the language formulation skills to be able to come up with a response or perhaps even the comprehension skills to understand the actual question.

"Ruffin is making 'I' statements as comments about the materials we were working on that he had some personal experience with. For example, as we looked at a picture of a snake, he commented, 'I like snake.' At another time when we were looking at fruit, he remarked, 'I like two bananas.' When he selected a car to play with which was broken, he commented, 'That's a broken toy, uh oh, Seamus fix that.' He did not seek my attention to deliver this information but delivered it to the room. He did not show me the toy that was broken but was simply commenting on that information as he identified it as being important.

"In terms of protest mode, we heard him use the word 'no.' We also noticed 'yes' type answers as affirmation, and he is also shaking his head 'yes.' We needed to prompt greetings, but once that situation had been structured, he was able to follow through on greeting routines."

Of course, there were still residua of Ruffin's autism. "On occasion, Ruffin was noted to line up like objects. He has some degree of aggressive play in that he is banging cars into other objects. He seems to particularly like playing with puppets and does have a routine script which he uses with them which generally has to do with asking each puppet for its name."

But there were clear improvements, as well. "During the time that we spent with Ruffin, he was interested in a variety of toys and seemed to enjoy playing with new toys and materials. We were able to teach him several different verbal routines easily and quickly as we played with various toys. We mapped language onto his play routine and made increasingly longer utterances. He was very comfortable with that system."

What struck me as I flyspecked her report was how remarkably focused Ms. Wilding was on the present and her own personal observations. She never referred to any of Ruffin's previous language assessments. She never made any attempt to assess his recent language development since Bridgewater's first evaluation of early August, or Gundersen's evaluation of early October. Her exclusive focus on her own "slice in time" seemed to blind her to Ruffin's ongoing remediation of his previously measured 16- to 18-month language delay — as compared to the 8-month language delay that she found during her own examination. A more longitudinally focused, comparative evaluation might have acknowledged that somehow — remarkably, and quite recently — Ruffin had developed language at a rate nearly double the rate of a typically developing child. This had also enabled him to demonstrate his IQ on a test designed for typically developing youngsters.

Dr. Norman summarized Ms. Wilding's formal speech testing. "During these testing situations, Ruffin also showed some tangential responses and specific difficulties in coming up with information or words or phrases that he wanted. When shown a picture of a couch or sofa, he responded 'watch TV.' When shown pictures of statues, he responded 'decorations.'" Yes, I recognized "decorations" as a word we had taught him for Christmas.

"On the formal testing work, his speech generally was at about the 3-year-old level." By pointing to 1 picture out of 4 in response to single words offered him by Ms. Wilding during the *Peabody Picture Vocabulary Test (R) Form L,* Ruffin earned an age equivalency of only 3 years, characterized by her as a "low-average" score. Likewise, he did well on the picture vocabulary test on the receptive portion of the *Sequenced Inventory of Communication Development.*"

At my specific request made during the final interpretive conference, Ms. Wilding provided exquisite detail in her written report — exactly what I wanted to be able to share with Evelyn and Dr. Granpeesheh. "The *Expressive One Word Picture Vocabulary Test — Revised* was attempted, but a basal level was not attained since Ruffin missed item number 6 which is 'watch.' He continually called that item 'clock,' and we were not able to elicit the word 'watch.' Consequently, we were unable to score this measure. As we looked over his performance on this naming of line drawings, we saw that he had some errors of association such as calling 'chickens' by the name 'turkey,' calling 'tiger' by the name 'lion,' calling 'fireplace' by the name 'watch the fire.'

"It was interesting to note that he did not, at this time, seem to have group nouns since he was naming all pictures which were presented to indicate category. For example, he named all the fruit pictures rather than use the group noun 'fruit.'" From reading Temple Grandin, I knew this failure to use group nouns — or even *see* items in terms of common sense categories — was typical enough in autism.

The *Sequenced Inventory of Communication Development (SICD)* also assessed Ruffin's comprehension and production through a greater variety of language tasks. "Ruffin scored a Receptive Communication Age of 3 years (an 8-month delay) and an Expressive Communication Age of 2 years, 4 months (a 1 year, 4-month delay)." This was the test Sue had recommended early on in July, and which I had specifically requested that Ruffin be given. Dr. Granpeesheh and Evelyn could use information from this test, with which they were familiar, to help fine-tune Ruffin's latest drill book from afar. This proved invaluable to all of us who were trying to learn what might be working in Ruffin's home program, and what we might still need to address in guiding his speech development.

Again, Ms. Wilding took extra time to write up exactly what Ruffin had passed, or missed, during this particular test. "On the receptive language portion, Ruffin was successful in selecting objects correctly from a group; responding to position commands: in, on, beside, and under by putting a block in the named position within a box; following directions and commands for movement; demonstrating an understanding of the function of objects such as 'show me what you wear on your feet' when offered a choice of 3 pictures; giving turns and understanding the idea of turns; identification of big and little; discriminating various noise-makers, but not the discrimination of those noise-makers in terms of low, medium, and high; identifying colors; following directions involving 2 objects, but not being successful when there were 2 objects and 2 actions.

"On the expressive language portion, Ruffin was successful in naming single pictures such as 'baby' and 'shoe;' he was not able to name a ball as a 'ball' since half of it was red and half of it was green and he continued to fail with each presentation even though those presentations were separated by time; he called the picture by the name 'red and green.' He imitated words, sounds, syllables, and multi-syllables; repeated 3 unrelated digits and 2 unrelated words; repeated a 4-word sentence and then repeated the last 4 words of longer sentences; answered very specific simple concrete 'what' type questions; and identified up to 5 of an item.

"It is specifically interesting to look at his comprehension of various question forms. The *SICD* does not look specifically at what, when, which, why, if-what and -then type questions. Ruffin is having difficulty on all but the most concrete of those questions. It seems appropriate as we present information to him and ask him questions that we be careful to use the form of question with which he is familiar and can be most successful.

"As we present other types of questions to him, we will need to give him some augmentation and support so that he can be successful in comprehension and then in formulation of a response. We need to be specifically careful with him in terms of inferential type questions and expecting him to be able to infer at the question level." I found myself quarreling a bit with this. I fully expected Dr. Granpeesheh, and Evelyn would know how to teach Ruffin to make inferences and reason his way through the world.

Then, Dr. Norman took Ruffin into his own testing office. "Again, he made a very easy transition and worked well throughout his time with me. He was a little avoidant of eye contact early on and when I controlled materials to present tasks for him. On a couple of occasions, he put his hands over his ears or shielded his eyes with his hands. He also had a little tendency to line up materials in his play with me.

"Other play was fairly limited with preferences for noise makers, pull toys, repetitive simple play with cars and other toy objects, coloring, and scribbling, and so on. He had an immediate and positive response to playing with hand puppets. These elicited much more language and affect from him than did other activities. He initiated verbal responses, named the characters, and carried on some pretend dialogs with me.

Most of Ruffin's time with Dr. Norman was spent completing the *Developmental Activities Screening Inventory — II*, a more non-verbal test of cognitive abilities. "Ruffin passed all the items on this instrument through the 2-year, 6-month level. This included tasks such as nesting cups, discriminating colors, stringing beads, putting together a simple 2-piece puzzle, and imitating some strokes with a crayon."

As Dr. Norman pushed on, Ruffin performed surprisingly well — well beyond expectations for his age. "Ruffin continued to have more positive and accurate responses than not on all the additional tasks going up to the 5-year-old items on this instrument. Among his positive or demonstrated skills were verbally labeling objects and pictures, finding pictures and materials when I labeled them, counting (rote beyond 10 and objects to 3), demonstrating the concept of 'one,' demonstrating the concepts of big and little (a little weak), categorizing pictures into groups (by animal, food, and people), making functional associations with pictures (e.g., an iron to an ironing board, a frying pan to a stove, etc.), matching pairs of printed numerals and words, copying a 6-block pyramid, stacking rings in order of size, naming colors, and completing a 2-step vertical paper fold (weak). Overall, he passed items worth 51 to 52 months credit on this instrument. That was greater than expectation for his current age of 45 months." I found this very encouraging. When Donna and I went over it together, she commented, "I'm not surprised."

Finally came Dr. Norman's own little anecdotes and observations. "On some additional informal tasks, Ruffin was able to identify almost all the uppercase letters of the alphabet for me. He was able to copy a circle, a cross, an X, but not a square or a triangle. He was very interested in drawing in general and took great delight when I drew a picture in crayon of him. He countered by drawing a big smile with two eyes above it, saying, 'That's mommy, girl.' At another point, he drew a line on the paper and labeled it 'I.' I drew a capital I, a lowercase i, and a picture of an eye beside his letter. I noted that each of these was an I. When I pointed to the picture of the eye, he looked at me, laughed, and said, 'That's funny.'

"No other perseverative or stereotypic behaviors were noted today in my session or observations. When Ruffin was very happy or overstimulated, he tended to jump up and down and clap." I found that hardly surprising. Our little one — up so early — was clearly missing the small trampoline he was accustomed to use at home when we would say, "Time now, to take a break!"

While Ruffin was busy, I was also interviewed and questioned by a resident physician in child psychiatry working with a social worker. We went over several parent questionnaires I had completed back in the fall when these appointments had been scheduled: *The Child Behavior Checklist*, the *Conners Parent Rating Scale*, and the *Autism Behavior Checklist*. Scoring of these instruments found Ruffin to have "a clear pattern of social difficulties and other significant behavior problems, including oppositional and stubborn responses, mild social problems and immaturity and some difficulty in compliance to others" and suggested that I had concerns about speech, eating, and other daily living activities.

In writing his report, Dr. Norman compared my view of Ruffin in the early fall to Meg's much later view of him in January by comparing our responses to the *Autism Behavior Checklist*. Meg saw Ruffin as having fewer autism behaviors than I did earlier. Meg's scores showed Ruffin to be "a little rigid, set in his ways, and likely to become overstimulated or wound up, but no clear behavior problem."

After Dr. Simon finished with Ruffin, she interviewed Donna, Seamus, and me as a group to administer the *Vineland Adaptive Behavior Scale*. Working from our answers toward a consensus view of him, Dr. Simon scored Ruffin with standard scores and age equivalencies: Communication 98, 3 years, 7 months; Daily Living 97, 3 years, 6 months; Socialization 79, 2 years, 5 months; Motor 108, 4 years, 1 month; and Adaptive Behavior Composite 93, 3 years, 5 months — an overall 3-month delay. Dr. Simon's scores on Ruffin's *Vineland* were extremely encouraging. In every domain — except socialization — Ruffin was catching up fast to his more typically developing peers.

The last formal stop on Ruffin's day was a physical exam and an interview and play session with Dr. Sharon Koele and Dr. Joseph Piven. In that play activity, Ruffin did prefer to play with materials by himself but would allow Dr. Koele to intrude. They, too, found Ruffin did much better at taking turns and interacting with puppets than he did with toys.

"On the physical examination, Ruffin was fairly cooperative. It was clear that he had practiced some of these routines and anticipated requests. On some other activities which were less familiar to him, he had a little more problem in complying or responding appropriately. He did also tend to become overstimulated during the physical examination and ran around the room a bit."

Ms. Wilding had noticed, too. "In the afternoon during the interpretative session, we also noted protest in the form of tantrumming behavior when things were not going to Ruffin's liking. During the time that we spent with Ruffin, he did not call our attention through verbal means or through a communication system to get our attention, but we noticed that he did do that with his mother in the afternoon.

"When he was wanting to leave, he approached his mother, grabbed onto her hand, using verbalizations, 'Come on, Mom,' and then eventually started to use gestures and tugged on her to get her to move. This was a nice progress of hierarchy which indicated his serious intent to have his way which meant leaving the area where he was uncomfortable."

Not so nice for me, as Ruffin's mother. There were no toys in the conference room. Seamus seemed embarrassed by Ruffin's behavior. But this was why Donna had volunteered to come along today — so when Ruffin tired without a nap, got wound up without a trampoline-break, or even descended into full meltdown — Seamus and I could continue to focus on the conference with the evaluation group as they presented their results and took our questions.

CHAPTER EIGHTEEN

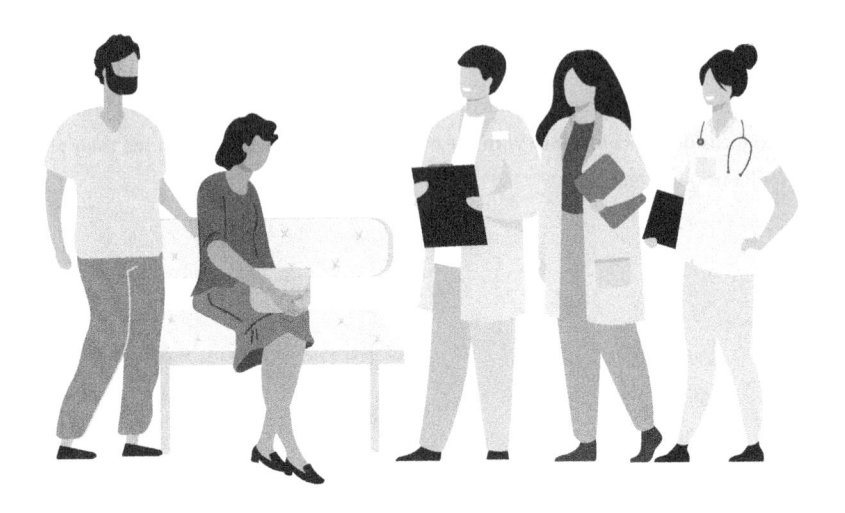

LETTING SEAMUS LISTEN

My first question was whether this group had reviewed Ruffin's May to December video? "Yes," Dr. Norman assured me, acknowledging it as an opportunity to observe Ruffin "in a variety of activities including some free time, computer-work, sing-along activities, and other programming with various adult trainers." He would not utter the name Lovaas.

Seamus's first question was whether Ruffin really had autism. Dr. Piven explained, "Ruffin continues to show the general symptoms of PDD-NOS based on the *DSM-IV* criteria. Asperger's syndrome was excluded as a diagnosis because of Ruffin's history of language delay, a delay which continues as measured today by Ms. Wilding." All this made sense to me, but Seamus wanted to know — did what the doctor said mean Ruffin had autism?

Dr. Norman interpreted, "His diagnosis falls on the autism spectrum. He has had problems in the development of language, in social interactions, and with repetitive and stereotypic behavior patterns, interests, and activities. But his symptoms in none of these areas are as severe as we would expect in the disorder of autism. In addition to his mild symptoms, we found today that Ruffin is quite a bit brighter than typical for children with his diagnosis. The combination of good general intelligence, a mild set of symptoms, and his rapid progress over the last half year, since summer, are very encouraging. You should feel very encouraged."

Then Dr. Norman turned to Dr. Simon. She reported her IQ of 97 for Ruffin on the *Stanford-Binet*.

Seamus looked over at me, and I knew what he was thinking. I had told him Ruffin's IQ was 50, that Ruffin was "moderately mentally retarded." Then I had told him later it was better than that, 70- or 80-something, "borderline." Of course, Seamus was puzzled. I asked Dr. Simon if she could explain how Ruffin's IQ measurements had changed from 50 on the *Bayley* in early August, to 78 on the *WPPSI-R* in early October, and now up again to 97.

Dr. Simon squared herself up in her chair and spoke with an air of confidence. "Ruffin's general intellectual abilities appear to be greater than those earlier assessments would indicate. It's quite likely his lack of receptive and expressive language earlier interfered with anyone obtaining a better performance from him on those two earlier occasions." Yes, it's hard to show what you know, I thought to myself, if you can't talk. I reminded myself, too, to keep my mouth shut, and listen. Let the others speak — especially in answer to Seamus.

Dr. Norman broke in again to support Dr. Simon. "It did appear to Dr. Simon and me, and all of us, really, that Ruffin was very cooperative, attentive, and comfortable in our testing situations today. It seemed as if his efforts were optimal." I didn't speak up to argue the point, but I remembered — every single evaluator from Bridgewater to Gundersen had claimed the same. "We, with our expertise, were able to reach him today."

All this satisfied Seamus. Donna was happy, too. She looked like the cat who had swallowed the canary — since all this new testing confirmed her personal conviction that Ruffin was as smart as a little whip.

Dr. Piven needed to leave early. "Any questions?" I asked about Ruffin's vitamin and DMG doses. Dr. Piven and Dr. Koele exchanged glances, and Dr. Koele tackled that one. "We don't see any reason for any medical treatments for Ruffin now. His attention and behavior are in pretty good shape. He does tend to have some of the difficulties that other youngsters with PDD share: wanting things his own way, becoming attuned to routines, preferring to do things himself or alone, wanting to direct others, and having difficulty expressing himself when he experiences stress or unhappiness."

Then, acting in his role as moderator, Dr. Norman excused the busier doctors, and moved the meeting along, by turning to me. "We know you've invested a great deal of energy and time to learning about autism and PDD, therapies and training, programming alternatives, and resources. We know you are active in a local autism support group. So, let's focus on specific programming and teaching goals.

"In general, we feel that the types of services and the training goals employed with Ruffin at this time both at school and at home are appropriate to his needs. It's clear to us that Ruffin is making good progress in his current situation. School programming and home and school teaching goals appear to be appropriate for Ruffin at this time."

Yes. I relaxed. It was unlikely the school authorities would find any comfort in this particularly inclusive conclusion, which Dr. Norman also committed to in his final report. The schools wouldn't find any expert witnesses to call *against* Ruffin from around this table. I didn't hear anybody here suggesting Ruffin be moved over into some partial replication of North Carolina's TEACCH program as Mr. Montague had been flailing about in his letters to me — much less a picture-exchange communication system (PECS) regime as implied in his concealed marching orders issued to Kim.

I pressed in for more, asking Dr. Norman if he could account for Ruffin's recent progress. "It's impossible for us to attribute Ruffin's improving course to any single aspect of the treatment or combination of the various aspects." Well, that left Curt and me with the Midwesterner's finest argument ever trotted out against precipitous change — if it's not broke, let's don't fix it.

Then Dr. Norman smiled and confessed, "We really had some anxiety at first about meeting your expectations in this staffing. We had thought it best we limit our evaluation of Ruffin to objective measures only."

I smiled, too, but asserted, "No, I am here to gather your recommendations about what is appropriate for Ruffin. I expect you to address that issue — since I will be paying you, you know, quite a bit of money."

"Fair enough," Dr. Norman conceded. "Yes. And, we'd like to get and consider Dr. Sallows's report from Madison, before we make any recommendations."

"Fine," I agreed. "I'm happy to share that with you. I expect it will be available soon."

Nevertheless, without waiting to hear from Dr. Sallows, most members of the UIHC evaluation team handed in their full, final reports the following day. If I had to guess, Dr. Piven and Ms. Wilding outranked or outvoted Dr. Norman — along with the long-term financial and professional interests of their clinic in serving school districts who usually engaged and paid for their services. Surely, as between parents and school districts, schools were their greater market.

Their reports went straight to the schools with a myriad of suggestions:

1. Ruffin is making good progress with his learning in all respects from what we can see. It does appear that general developmental preschool curricula and guidelines should serve to outline the overall goals for him until he enters kindergarten school-aged programming. This does not mean that he may not require some special techniques or methods from time to time, but he does appear to be ready for much, if not all, of the readiness curriculum generally intended for youngsters 3 and 4 years of age.

Dr. Lovaas had sent me a summary chart of his two-year curriculum. It was divided into various developmental domains — designed to cover them all eventually — by tackling each component skill of each domain in a sequence drawn from his years of clinical laboratory experience, as designed to be the most accessible to and most readily achieved by students like Ruffin.

2. We do see that some of Ruffin's skills at this point are rote and associational rather than functional. This is not unusual for youngsters who have newly learned materials and skills, and particularly not unusual for youngsters with PDD. To make the learning more useful and for these skills to generalize to new situations and maintain over time, people at home and at school will have to be sure to incorporate these new learning activities into real-life contexts and everyday functional activities.

Generalization, yes, I knew we were getting it. This would be something for Seamus and me, as parents, to concentrate our efforts on. Meg, too, saw that Ruffin got quite a lot of this type of opportunity — coming and going, eating and napping, playing and turn-taking, inside and out at recess. Check.

3. We would like to see Ruffin exposed to and integrated with more non-handicapped preschoolers. To make this programming most successful, Ruffin and the non-handicapped peers should receive some informal coaching about what they should be doing, how they should behave, how to fix problems, and so on. Appropriate activities might include social play groups where kids can share activities under the supervision of a skilled adult and have opportunities to try out and practice new social skills. Snack times, recreational games, role playing, or puppet play are activities to be considered. I will forward some additional materials regarding social interactions and coaching procedures for use with Ruffin.

I was pleased that Dr. Norman found Ruffin had the rudimentary language, toileting, and social skills to begin integration with typically developing children and that he would offer some thoughts about how to do this so I could run them by Evelyn and Dr. Granpeesheh. Could we do this as early as this summer, I wondered?

4. We want to give strong endorsement to learning through play and game activities. This is very important for all youngsters in this age group and will be particularly important for Ruffin to normalize some of the new skills he has and learn new skills and concepts in an entertaining fashion. There are several good resources for play and game activities. Some that stress the learning components are: *Kids and Play* by Joanne Oppenheim from Ballentine/Childcare and *Learninggames for Threes and Fours* by Joseph Sparling and Isabelle Lewis from Berkley Books (both in paperback).

Order books, check. Read for some ideas for a summer play group, maybe?

5. Ruffin is showing a good deal of interest in letters, numerals, and print information. We would encourage family and school staff to stimulate him in these areas without emphasizing direct instruction at this time. We would encourage adults to take advantage of informal opportunities to point out and to highlight print information and numeral or number information in the world around him.

With this, I disagreed. Without Evelyn's drills for direct instruction, we would never have been able to teach Ruffin his letters and numbers so quickly and so securely. This knowledge would be Ruffin's personal leg-up at school, so he could turn his attention to learning social skills and other information that might be delivered in groups. Now that he had his homework down cold, it would be time to go generalize and join a typically-developing group — his future, high school graduation class.

6. Ruffin needs a little more time than other youngsters to enter a new environment, pick up on a new routine, figure out directions and language prompts, and deal with unexpected changes than do most kids his age. When Ruffin must face something new or make a change, it is best to go about things slowly and carefully while giving him a chance to warm up to things gradually. As much as we can, we should build in bridges to make the new situation more comfortable and familiar. Ruffin should be given more control in choosing from options we present so that he can do things more in his own way. He should have the opportunity to look at and benefit from the models of others when possible.

This resonated with Meg's experiences of taking Ruffin swimming, as it did with many of my own: our previewing the empty school, our carefully planning his trips to the barber, the dentist, and our local doctor.

Because Ruffin had developed the ability to imitate by then, I was concerned that he not imitate the unchecked self-stimulatory behaviors of his variously disabled classmates, or the uncontrolled aggressions of others. This might be a hard issue to raise with the schools, but I came to think of this as a little ledge I could plant myself on.

7. Generalization and maintenance of skills is important. With training activities, we like to emphasize the "rule of threes." Once a basic skill has been taught and learned, we can be very effective in broadening the learning by involving three teachers, three differing sets of materials, three alternative activities, three different locations, and so on. This will ensure that learning is not rote or specific to any individual set of circumstances. This type of approach to training should help Ruffin apply his skills and abilities in new situations which he has not encountered yet or where he has not been trained.

We had Seamus and me, Donna and Lisa, Meg and Ella, Kim and the visiting junior high school students, home and school, Donna's house, Lisa's house, and Seamus's barn — all in accord with Evelyn's very similar advice about how to achieve generalization and maintenance of skills.

8. When Ruffin was a little slow to respond to something or did not seem to have adequate skills or information to proceed, we were very successful in giving him hand-over-hand prompts. We consistently asked to "borrow" his hand before we took it and proceeded. At times, this appeared to be a little uncomfortable and Ruffin would glance away but still keep the activity under surveillance out of the corner of his eye.

I could well imagine. Although we had used some hand-over-hand prompts early in Ruffin's home program on Evelyn's written instructions for some drills, by now Ruffin had easily moved to lighter prompts and to purely verbal instruction for most tasks. This suggested heavy-handedness struck me as a near-reversal of Ruffin's own early behavior of taking my hand to use it as a tool when he was unable to tell me what it was he wanted — pretty strange behavior, not to be encouraged or re-initiated, no, not as Ruffin might be moving into a group of typically developing classmates and be teased or ostracized for needing this form of instruction or employing this behavior when he wanted to share with his new friends.

9. In general, if there are situations where Ruffin is refusing or resistant, we would first back up a little in our thinking to make sure he understands the task and demands. Give him a chance to watch, begin again at an easier level, make the task more familiar or simplify it, and give him other support. If the resistance continues, try to give him options which will allow him to make a choice and build some control.

The ease and beauty of the drill book Evelyn had provided and revised periodically for us at home was that she had already deftly assessed exactly where to start with Ruffin, with what supports — so Ruffin's own experience with us was one of ready success and increasing mastery — without our having to waste time and energy on backing up in our thinking, and confusing or frustrating Ruffin into resistance.

10. In some situations, resistance can become more oppositional or defiant in nature. A simple technique that sometimes gets around this problem is called "behavioral momentum." The key here is to camouflage our intention away from the issue or oppositional situation by interspersing easy and pleasant directions or requests among things that will be more difficult or provoke resistance. A short paper on this will be forwarded to home and school.

Evelyn had shared this technique at our November workshop, and Donna and Lisa quickly learned which easier drills to offer Ruffin as a reward for tackling harder ones, or to offer him as a break from more difficult tasks. Yes, sometimes this worked like a charm.

11. For more serious and recurring problems of behavior resistance, adults need to have some clear means of informing Ruffin that there is a bottom line, that "the adult is the boss." Rather than talk about this to any degree, it is better to demonstrate it through gestures, pictures, other visual cues, and even through print or rebus print techniques. A rebus is a small picture symbol which carries meaning. It will not be long before Ruffin does tune in very well to print. He is already well tuned into pictures and other visual cues. We would begin linking pictures with print in this situation as well as at other points in his general instruction. The bottom-line response should be a visual presentation of the adult demand, request, rule, or direction. Further interaction with Ruffin should help focus him on these cues and to review them. These visual presentations often carry much more weight and leave less room for resistance, verbal refusals, or other fussing than would a typical verbal direction, rationale, or discussion.

Among the group of us working with Ruffin at home, Donna was the best at "the adult is the boss." Lisa and I were both softer touches. Seamus was particularly good with the nonverbal gesture as a firm direction.

Every good classroom should be full of visual cues, but beyond my early September trials of a picture board to sequence the events of his day for him, Ruffin had already come to manage without this accommodation.

Ms. Wilding's separate written report was more severely critical of Ruffin's functional language and of our home program than Dr. Norman's had been. "Formal tested language skills appear to be at the 2 year, 6 months to 3-year level. His functional language use, however, appears to be somewhat more between the 18- to 24-month level." This seemed to be her minority dissenting impression, or opinion. Ruffin's "functional language use," both his ability to understand testing and to respond to Dr. Simon offered no impediment to his ability to demonstrate his IQ at 97 — a score Dr. Simon had attributed to his language ability — or to work with Dr. Norman to demonstrate his non-verbal development well beyond his chronological age.

Ms. Wilding offered us several recommendations as well. "We support the fact that Ruffin is receiving direct speech and language services with Kim Pope. We have available to us a copy of Ruffin's IEP which was dated August 25th, 1994, and we see that he has goals for requesting help, answering questions, turn-taking, role playing, using words with staff and peers, identifying emotions, and increasing language length and structure skills. We support all these goals." Somehow, Ms. Wilding remained unaware that Ruffin had already achieved all these goals of his first IEP. An uninformed professional was no help to me as Ruffin's mother, but my lawyer's mind marked this lapse as fertile ground for any future cross-examination.

I had what I needed here on paper — fresh objective measurements of Ruffin's progress and detailed information I could share with Evelyn and Dr. Granpeesheh. None of these university hospital professionals could testify effectively against Ruffin in due process. Dr. Norman's conclusion that what was appropriate for Ruffin was what I had chosen for him — both school and our home training program — was helpful enough. I was frustrated I didn't get everything I wanted. I had failed to inspire any great enthusiasm for Lovaas's methods, but there were no recommendations for anything else, either. On balance, I thought I could live with it, pay for it — and, if necessary, have Curt litigate with it.

Other than his meltdown during the final interpretative conference, Ruffin's behavior on our trip continued to be exemplary. He was able to eat out at the hospital cafeteria and at a restaurant later. He enjoyed looking at mechanical cranes over the hospital construction sites with Seamus. At the hospital gift store we bought him a macaw bird balloon, so he surprised all of us by pointing out a real macaw in the pet store downtown.

CHAPTER NINETEEN

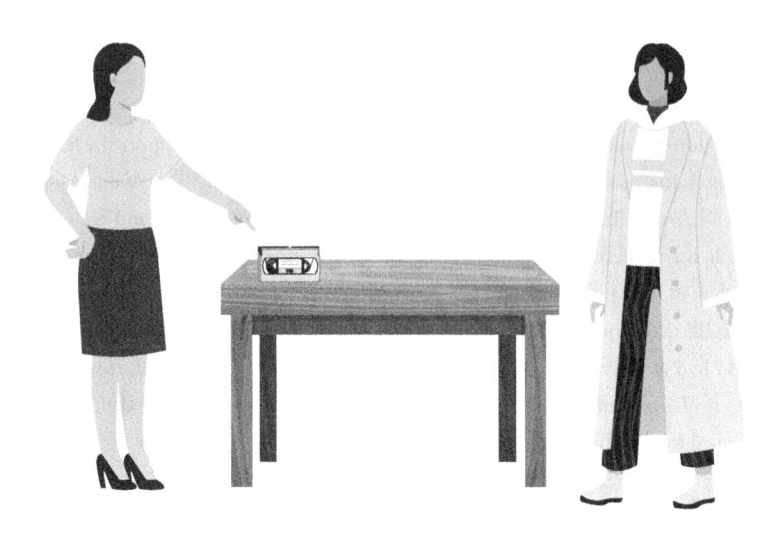

CARRYING COALS TO NEWCASTLE

Back home, Bridgewater speech and language pathologists bedeviled me. Dot Gordon — writing to me this time as the chair of the skills training council — how many hats must this poor woman have to wear? — snail-mailed me a memo that she had been unable to fax. Faxes *were* new-fangled finicky machines then. Enclosed was a raft of Bridgewater paperwork for me to apply for funds to travel to Los Angeles — so her council could meet with me after my return to consider my request. Just how well was this after-the-fact funding system working for parents without the money to front the expense of travel and training? I crabbed.

I must have been tired, because even Dot's grammar grated. I needed to "take a break." Or, as we used to say in the South of my childhood — I needed to "take a powder" — with Dot, as my recurring, personal headache. Wasn't she a speech and language pathologist by training? She must care about how the language was spoken, if not how it was written. Okay, so she wasn't an English major, a writer, a lover of literature, not that I knew. I didn't know Dot well enough to know whether she was anything like me — whether she might even have proved to be a friend had I met her at another time, in another place.

This is just paperwork, I scolded myself. You know you love it. And so, I quickly filled it all out, attaching a copy of the Lovaas conference flier and answering her questions, "Will you be willing to serve as a resource to other individuals and groups? If so, how?" I assured Dot that I would be delighted to offer a report of the conference proceedings and offer Bridgewater a do-over of the autism in-service presentation I had just given at Western Hills — the one no one from Bridgewater had bothered to attend. I needed to refocus on this as an opportunity I couldn't pass up.

Then I walked a block down Main Street to the bank and borrowed the money for a round-trip flight to Los Angeles, the conference fee, and a hotel room.

I called Bridgewater to ask them to turn on their fax so I could feed all my paperwork back to Elkader, as Dot had directed. In my follow-up call — to assure every page had come through safely — I was able to give Mr. Montague's personal assistant a brief account to pass on to him of what the UIHC group had offered us in their final interpretive conference.

My news tickled Mr. Montague back into activity. "Enclosed you will find the Lovaas video which you copied for my review. Thank you for sharing it with me." It seemed to have made no impression whatsoever on him — that's all I could tell from his polite note.

Then, without copying me, or any of his other colleagues or subordinates, Mr. Montague contacted the executive director of the Autism Society of Iowa inquiring about the "Lovaas method." I never found any evidence of any reply, one way or the other, but I was unsurprised. My own earlier brief contact during last summer with the Society — a state chapter of the national organization, the Autism Society of America, originally founded by Dr. Rimland and Dr. Lovaas in the 1960s to disseminate information about Dr. Lovaas's earliest research — had been disappointing. The people I reached there were unaware of their own organization's history, wary of Lovaas's research, and uninterested and unsupportive of my interest in it.

Later, from my *Me-List* friends on the internet I learned that many of them found little to no support from their local ASA chapters either. So, many younger families had begun to organize themselves as Families for Early Autism Treatment. Their acronym

FEAT expressed — as Curt did in his petition for the Mason City family — the sheer feat it was to mount a home-based Lovaas program anywhere in the early 1990s.

Mr. Montague had continued writing — another letter wanting to know — would the Mayo Clinic be serving as a replication site for Lovaas's research? "Mayo's involvement could directly impact our services to children in 25 school districts in Northeast Iowa, Bridgewater AEA." To me this read less as an inquiry into whether the Lovaas method might work than as a flag-waving warning. Don't you, Mayo, think for one moment you can invade the kingdom of Bridgewater. I never found any evidence of a reply — just as there was no invading army of certified applied behavior analysts and therapists gathering on the undefended Iowa-Minnesota border. Trained providers were in short supply — scarcer than hen's teeth across the United States and the known world. The only threat Mr. Montague faced was that Dr. Lovaas's UCLA clinic was providing services to a single child of a solitary physician at Mayo.

Still excited and wanting to relay all Ruffin's new scores directly to someone at Bridgewater, I called and got Emily, his school psychologist, who offered no real response to Ruffin's new "average" IQ. She didn't seem to be listening, reacting, or taking any notes — which suddenly infuriated me after she got me off the phone.

I threw on my long, down coat, pulled my L.L. Bean overshoes over my highest pair of courtroom heels, grabbed the copy of the 1987 Lovaas documentary and swerved down two blocks of packed snow and ice, into one of the reserved spaces at our local special education satellite office for Bridgewater — that couple of battered trailers cobbled together across from the junior high's blacktopped playground. I walked swiftly, intrusively in and directly to Emily's desk, tracking snow, determined to offer her this footage of recovered children, and to demand that she share it with Kim.

Holding it out to her, my cold hand trembled with suppressed fury. "You and Kim might want to watch this before the two of you take off for Los Angeles."

She stood up, irritated no doubt at having just managed to get rid of me, and snapped, "I don't need to see that! I checked that out back in September or October, whenever it was, we first wrote you back. No! Anyway, I just checked it out again . . ."

"Checked it out! From where?" I demanded to know. I was still furious, still standing there, in my long, dripping down coat. No one but me could know how my whole body was trembling.

"It just came over from Bridgewater's library in Elkader. Look," she said, pointing to Kim's desk.

I walked over, flipped the video cartridge, and stared briefly, disbelievingly, at a faded accession sticker — *Bridgewater*.

Emily walked up behind me, and I turned right back into her face, which failed to daunt her in the least. "When I watched that video this fall, I recognized Ricky and Pam right away. I studied those children, that same footage, back when I was in college. I've been familiar with Lovaas since the 1970s. We all were, and always have been. This," she said, brushing past me to place her index finger firmly on the cartridge, "is nothing new."

I was too stunned to ask: why if she had seen this 1987 video last fall, if she had studied and learned about Lovaas's research back when she was in college, why had she and Bridgewater withheld this information from me as Ruffin's mother when she knew I was so obviously desperate to help him? Why had she and Bridgewater actively discouraged my pursuit of this information and this form of schooling for Ruffin?

Then, I took a breath of the warm, close air inside this horrible trailer, stopped trembling with anger, and utterly deflated. It sunk in. Everyone here in special education already knew. All the rest of them, Ruffin's entire educational team, knew already. And they were going to let me know — when? I realized I was carrying the proverbial coals to Newcastle and slipped Dr. Bishop's copy of the documentary deep down into my coat pocket.

Just as quickly, my next thought flashed. Are the only people my "news" had been news to been other parents?

I stepped back and quietly brought up Dr. Norman's passing remark that Ruffin should be spending some of his time mainstreamed with non-speech-delayed students.

Emily responded, "Kindergarteners are the only students like that available here at school. We don't do that . . ."

"Well," I protested, "I know some of Ruffin's special education classmates are mainstreamed up to kindergarten."

"And they're *older* than Ruffin. But Meg and I have been discussing bringing a few kindergartners down into her classroom so they can get to know him, so they could help him in the kindergarten room. In a few weeks' time . . ."

I thought this — what Emily and Meg were talking about — was a terrific idea, if Evelyn and Dr. Granpeesheh thought Ruffin were ready for it. It sounded like Meg's idea, to get around Emily's own first knee-jerk negative we-don't-ever-do-that. My mind kicked calmly back into gear, as I thought how this conversation might indicate the school authorities were concerned that they might have a legal Achilles heel in the current program for Ruffin — no real mainstreaming, no real inclusion.

Emily had another idea to share. "And we'll need to think about using a communication board with Ruffin, so he could use pictures to make himself understood in kindergarten." I was appalled and couldn't speak up any better than Emily thought Ruffin could. In our town's own Irish American lingo, I was well and truly gob-smacked! For Ruffin to use a communication board would be a total social cop-out, and weird-looking to boot, especially to typically developing kids, and off-putting to adults in our back-to-the-1950s sweetly unsophisticated rural village. Ruffin could already talk and must be expected and prompted to talk, or he would just silently point.

But I let Emily's remark pass without objection because it seemed so stunning and stunningly uninformed, even as she moved on to crow about how she had been reading the *Bernard Smith* case Mr. Montague had sent her. "Ruffin is nothing like Bernard Smith. Ruffin is toilet-trained and can attend at circle time." It was true, my mother had toilet-trained Ruffin using M&Ms as his reward, months before he was ever diagnosed. And, yes, judging by the October classroom videotape, Ruffin did pay attention during circle time better than most of his special education classmates and way better than most of the severely and profoundly disabled students brought over to visit from across the hall.

I stood there. We were done here.

It would take Dr. Lovaas or whomever Emily considered to be the greatest god of psychology himself to make any meaningful impression on her. Certainly, I couldn't. But I suspected my ambush of Emily had allowed her true thinking about what was appropriate for Ruffin to surface. If he could sit quietly in a circle, he didn't need one-to-one intervention to improve his language skills, especially not when he could be managed, herded, and passed along using a communication board, or if he could otherwise make himself understood with gestures.

Then, I began to wonder, with Ruffin's new "average" IQ, if Emily weren't feeling defensive, or personally embarrassed at having hung a *Bayley Scale* score of 50 — the suggestion of moderate mental retardation — around Ruffin's neck back in August. She really had no reason to be embarrassed or defensive about that. It had come as encouraging news to me at the time. It was perfectly understandable, too, that examiners more experienced in testing children with autism like Dr. Kondrick at Gundersen and Dr. Simon at UIHC would be able to draw a better or higher IQ performance from Ruffin. In all my correspondence circulated to her, and even in my talk at Western Hills, I had carefully parsed this point to avoid embarrassing her.

But now I could peg Emily as an intellectual obstacle within Ruffin's IEP team. Today was not the day to confront her. I hoped that she and Kim might learn something in Los Angeles — surely, Mr. Montague must want them to learn something there.

The next morning, I sent Meg and Kim more sets of drill cards from which Ruffin was able to sight-read the names of various animals and clothing items, and then sort them into their correct categories. "With questioning, he should also be able to give more information about each item, including what color, how many, who wears it, and whether an item goes on a person's hands or feet."

Then, I confided to Curt, "Yesterday afternoon I learned a couple of things which very nearly broke my heart. They may also bear upon your requests for injunctive relief to have the courts order the state to spread the word about Lovaas as set out in your petition for the Mason City family." I gave him a full account of all Emily had let slip, disclosing my disappointment and my suspicion that any court injunction would just be "carrying coals to Newcastle." It seemed likely that all the special educators in Iowa already knew and had long known about Lovaas's methods. "I probably made the same foolish delivery in my address at Western Hills earlier this month."

It helped to share better news with Curt. "Still, all in all, my broken heart is singing for Ruffin's progress." I offered him a summary of what we had learned in Iowa City, and what Mr. Montague had just written to me. "When I get back from Des Moines, I would like you to think of ways which you feel the Lovaas home program can be reasonably and effectively married with the program in your local district. I am anxious to explore how we can find some middle ground as to how this can be most effectively accomplished."

Mr. Montague had addressed this latest letter directly to me — but not copied it to anyone else concerned. Could he be extending an olive branch to me, behind everyone else's back? I gave him the benefit of the doubt. But he might have been rushing out the door to Des Moines in a hurry to beat a blizzard or a sleet storm. The two-lane roads in and out of Elkader were hilly and steep, among the most dangerous anywhere in Iowa.

CHAPTER TWENTY

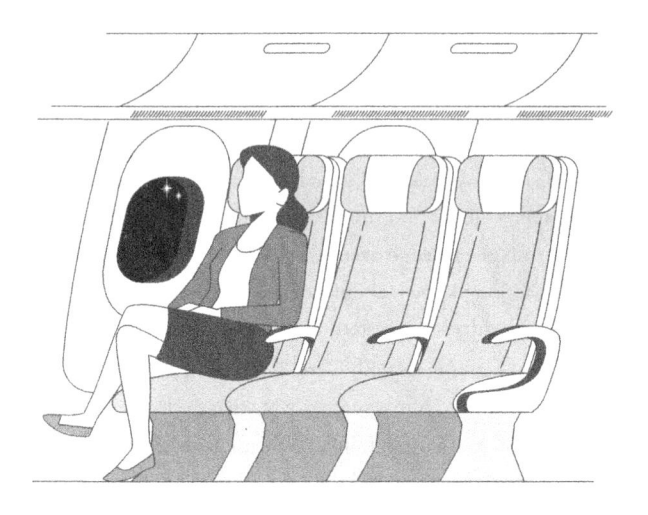

LOS ANGELES

A whirl of questions kept me awake on my night-flight to Los Angeles, as I peered out from my narrow seat deep into the starry, winter sky. What might have become of Ruffin, had I entrusted him to Emily and Kim, to Bridgewater's care and expertise? Would he have made his newly measured gains? Or would he be the little forever-star-of-special-education, limited to learning rudimentary signs, or lugging around a communication board with someone else's small selection of messages? Would he have become like the children Inge had spoken to me of with regret after Evelyn's workshop — who "have probably been damaged by our not using this earlier." Really, I fumed, I could run every one of these women down with a grocery cart, skinning the backs of their bare ankles. And I did, repeatedly, in my dreams, and thought nothing of it.

The plane's wheels hitting the runway jarred me awake as the sun came up. I gathered myself to get on a standing-room-only shuttle to the downtown Westin. The man crammed in beside me was carrying a huge television camera on his shoulder. He apologized as he shifted it from shoulder to shoulder and told me he would be filming an O. J. Simpson hearing this morning — juicy footage that would knock NBC's story about young children with autism out of any future line-up on Dateline.

I was able to scurry into the Westin's crowded ballroom, just as Dr. Lovaas and his clinic staff and newest Ph.D. students were mounting the speakers' platform in front of and beneath a couple of large video screens.

As I looked out over the crowd, I saw couples whispering, holding hands. Then a man's arm moved across the back of a woman's chair to cradle her shoulders. None of these parents seemed to have brought their children, either. I thought of all the other people — several times the size of this crowd — who were not here, who were at home caring for children with autism, some of them grandparents, anxious to hear some report of better news out of this conference.

I sat with the huge conference binder balanced on my lap, my red briefcase at my heels, and scanned the crowd for Emily's and Kim's faces, or for the backs of their heads. It was a large crowd. I didn't see them.

For the next couple of hours Dr. Lovaas spoke about his research with which I was already familiar, and demonstrated his methods, explaining the setbacks at first when he started treatment with adults and older children like Pam and Ricky, and his disappointment that when treatment was discontinued most gains were quickly lost. He explained how his early failures to produce lasting changes or improvements had led to his working with younger and younger children.

As he spoke, he illustrated his lecture by screening many video-clips from the early 1960s to the present, showing how he and his clinic's group had come to solve problem after problem in teaching language and more typical behaviors to young children with autism. Every clip was a reassurance to me that Dr. Granpeesheh — who was featured in many of them — knew what she was doing, and so did Evelyn, and so then did Donna, Lisa, Seamus, and I.

The mid-morning coffee break came up quickly. I glimpsed Emily and Kim seated together on adjoining stools at the hotel bar. They were still there, as the crowd settled back into the ballroom again, as I balanced my coffee, briefcase, and notebook on my knees, and leaned forward to listen again to Dr. Lovaas and his students recount their most recent interviews with some of the "recovered" children from their 1993 study. Data analysis and publication had taken years, so some of the original children from the

1987-1993 studies were then in their late teens and early twenties, attending college or just entering the competitive workforce.

There was a collective gasp from the crowd, from parents like myself, who had been told to expect their children were "likely never to marry," when Lovaas let loose with an anecdote of his dilemma when one boy from his experimental group whom he had invited back to Los Angeles for a follow-up evaluation and interview had called in to the clinic to ask if he could bring his girlfriend along to stay in the hotel room offered him. Would Dr. Lovaas and the others please agree not to tell his parents?

Sex! And deception! I thought. How typically human.

Time for lunch. Emily and Kim were seated together in the hotel restaurant. I stopped by their table briefly, to greet them, and ask about their flight. They seemed surprised to see me there, even worried I might try to join them. No, no, I thought. Not a chance. I was due to meet up with other parents to learn what was going on here in California with private insurance and school district funding before returning to the ballroom to watch Dr. Lovaas's students present case-study demonstrations and discussions for three young boys, and one little girl — reflecting the usual gender distribution in autism.

Another break with cold sodas was announced to keep us awake. Not necessary. By then my adrenaline was running full force. Two more case studies of young boys, and then an hour of lively Q and A. A good part of the audience consisted of interested schoolteachers, teacher's aides, principals, administrators, pediatricians, diagnosticians, and school consultants. Time ran over. The hotel staff loitered openly on the sidelines, impatient to clear the room.

I waited in line for my turn to offer Dr. Lovaas a brief hug, to whisper a thank you into his hairy ear and let him know I had been able to come. "Yes, Ruffin's mother, from Decorah," he mumbled in his confusion, as a great many people pressed in behind me to have a word with him or ask a question.

Just outside the door of the ballroom, I was overcome with exhaustion. I wanted my room. I wanted room service. I had no interest in seeing any other part of Los Angeles or any more of the Pacific Ocean than I might have flown over in landing.

Saturday morning our first speaker was Catherine Maurice. "Maurice" was the pseudonym she used to protect the identity of her recovered children, "Michel," and "Anne-Marie." I had my copy of *Let Me Hear Your Voice* ready for her to sign, as I thanked her, and reminded her about our earlier phone call, my asking who I needed to contact to buy copies of her book in bulk. I planned to give a copy to each of Iowa's special education regional libraries, and to some influential Iowa special educators Curt knew. She wanted to know would I keep her abreast of how Ruffin came along in his development and how matters continued to progress, or not, in Iowa?

Dr. Ron Huff and Linda Mayhew spoke about what parents needed to do to get a home-based program organized, and what steps to take to keep it running smoothly. They laid out the architectural plans for how to build your own village and fund it. I thought of the Mason City family and all the other Iowa families — each of us trying to build our little villages, our houses of straw in our isolated spots — but in touch now with so many other parents and others of good will.

At the late-morning coffee-break, I glimpsed Emily and Kim again, stepping off the elevator. They might have missed Catherine Maurice, so soft-spoken and inspiring. Could she have touched their hearts in ways I never would, or ever could?

The conference topics then turned to questions of how non-profits and physicians could help, and to replications of Lovaas's results at research sites in Norway and England.

For lunch I joined a conference-sponsored discussion again with many of my *Me-List* internet friends who were organizing local FEAT groups across the United States. We recognized each other's names on our nametags and connected faces for the first time to all the late-night, bare text we had exchanged. I passed a pen and legal pad around the group and managed to collect the snail-mail addresses of over twenty families.

When I re-entered the ballroom, Emily and Kim were seated together in a row half-way back. I slipped into a row behind them to watch them — their faces as they turned to each other, and away — to monitor their exchanges.

The afternoon hours were given over to two speakers, attorney Katherine Dobel, who had represented Bernard Smith and his family in their Ninth Circuit reimbursement victory, speaking on the topic "*What Parents Have a Legal Right to Ask from the School District,*" and attorney Mark Williamson speaking on the topic "*Working with the School Districts Without Going to Court.*"

Emily was scribbling furiously. Kim seemed thoroughly bored. Mr. Montague had sent the two of them here to learn something — this seemed to be it. Somehow, I didn't want to be seen again by Emily or Kim. I slipped out a minute early to the afternoon's cold soda break. I felt small for spying on them.

The final presentation addressed how to recruit staff. This perked me up to share how I had recruited Donna and Lisa as older women with group home experience whom I had found highly motivated by the goal of keeping Ruffin out of such placements. Other members of the audience discussed the difficulties of using judgmental family members, or young high school and college students who tended to become entangled in romances that competed with the efforts needed to maintain team cohesion — all the usual human resources issues.

Then, after exchanging safe-travel hugs with dozens of new acquaintances, I left to pack, and shuttle back to the airport for another night-flight. Even if it turned out I got no reimbursement, it had been worthwhile to come, I told myself, as I uncapped a fresh highlighter and began reading through the thick conference notebook of research and printed resources.

While Emily, Kim, and I were in Los Angeles, Dr. Norman had called Meg again, and she urged him to hurry up on sending the UIHC group's written re-evaluation of Ruffin and their recommendations.

Having been away for just a couple of days, the new things Ruffin could say were startling. He was using prepositions and articles. He and I played a pointing game with the beam of his flashlight.

"I'm pointing at the ceiling."

"I'm pointing under the refrigerator," on and on using all the concrete nouns he knew. He was really trying to keep up his end of our "conversation."

In the snowdrift of two days of accumulated mail, another letter had arrived from Prudential letting me know their review of my claim would take more time.

I let Meg know all about my trip to Los Angeles. "It was fantastic. I met lots of parents who were using home Lovaas programming, many of whom have it written into their children's IEPs. After seeing the UCLA demonstrations, our team is as good or better than any I saw, as our results would suggest. Also, the comment was made that the 'best' programming for a child with autism is structured activity — not all Lovaas drills, but carefully planned — for 'every waking moment.' We are close to that with Ruffin. And, 40 hours per week of Lovaas is 'appropriate.'

"The most exciting part of the conference was meeting the systems advocates and fundraisers who have succeeded in putting together a $300,000 federal grant for Maryland to provide reimbursement to all their parents who wish to pursue Lovaas home programming and a Sacramento regional special education authority that has a private fundraising project that reimburses all their parents and offers extensive information, training, and support to new parents.

"The other parents I met were a phenomenal group. As one might expect, all had financial means and great resourcefulness. All were willing to share and exchange information. All very committed people and not terribly whiney, very 'let's do this now' types."

Meg and I were able to talk more at a school open house that evening.

Right away, Emily had reported to Mr. Montague — a single page listing a handful of court cases with their legal citations and her notations of her understanding of their principal holdings — including the United States Supreme Court's *Shannon Carter* case on reimbursement, and the *Bernard Smith* Ninth Circuit reimbursement decision I had shared with him earlier.

"The two lawyers stressed to the group that Lovaas is the 'appropriate' not the 'best' free public education. If parents can document that progress at home is meaningful and progress at school is trivial, parents can push for payment of Lovaas.

"There is a case coming out soon dealing with summer programming (EYSE) according to one of the lawyers, Katherine Dobel, who represented Bernard Smith in California. There was such a case in Virginia, but she didn't give an exact reference. According to one mom from Texas, autism there is considered to automatically qualify for summer services (EYSE)."

That same day Mr. Montague wrote to me, enclosing a "list of items you wished to have addressed in your upcoming IEP meeting," all gleaned from my correspondence by "two of my staff." Interesting to learn — although Mr. Montague could handle the law, he was no detail man himself when it came to gathering the facts. Joy and whoever helped her had compiled an exhaustive list of my "asks," stripped of any supporting research or analysis, drawn from my five request letters written since early September. Mr. Montague asked that I review their list to "validate it" for him.

"There are some issues which are clearly outside of my domain of authority and must be directed to others. These items relate to the commitment of funding with 'state dollars' which are controlled by the Iowa Bureau of Special Education. I will be meeting with Dr. Hagen in early February and will attempt to seek some clarification on this." From his marginalia on Joy's list, Mr. Montague intended to ask Dr. Hagen whether Dr. Granpeesheh and Evelyn Kung of CARD could work under her direction as support personnel qualified to do applied research while consulting on Ruffin's IEP.

Within a day or two, Joan and Curt had a copy I had made them of the conference binder from Los Angeles. Curt was putting together a review of all the recent case law concerning young children with autism and their entitlement to a free, appropriate public education (FAPE), including their need for summer school (EYSE). He planned to boil his analysis down to a single-page grid — as a synthesis — and print a comb-bound 178-page booklet to include all the underlying rulings and decisions mapped out on his grid, together with all the supporting, published peer-reviewed academic research.

Curt called, eager to share the *Introduction* he had written for their booklet, and read it out over the phone to me, in his wonderfully sonorous courtroom voice. "The afterward in a 1994 book, *Autism, From Tragedy to Triumph* by Carol Johnson and Julia Crowder, is especially moving. It is a biographical essay written by the subject of the book, a young man named Drew who is a second-year college student and who is now considered normal in all respects. What is particularly interesting about Drew is that he was one of the patients with autism enrolled in Ivar Lovaas's Young Autism Program at UCLA in the 1970s.

"In recent weeks, the parents of no fewer than six children from different corners of Iowa have called our offices with remarkably similar concerns: Each pre-school child has been diagnosed as suffering from a pervasive developmental disorder or autism. Each of the parents has learned about the Lovaas method of educating preschool children with this diagnosis, and each is challenging a local school or AEA's failure to provide such education. In several instances, the parents have instituted or secured private educational services on the Lovaas model, and they are seeking reimbursement of their expenses from the public educational agency."

Mentally, I counted: Ruffin, Seamus, and myself; Noah and his parents Mike and Chris Foster in Davenport, whom Sue had referred to me; Michael and Susan Smith and two of their triplets in Brayton, whom other parents in our support group had referred to me; the Mason City family who had been working with Dr. Tristram Smith early on, and one more. Who was I forgetting? Ah, yes, the other family who had also been working with Tris.

"To date, only one due process action has been filed, but that one action is clearly the tip of an iceberg. Accordingly, the staff of Iowa Protection & Advocacy Services, Inc. has prepared this *Synthesis* to focus attention on the issue and to facilitate a rational, cooperative dialogue on the best approaches to resolving the concerns these parents have raised. To prevent bias in its presentation, this *Synthesis* contains verbatim copies of the primary relevant literature and of the primary court and ALJ decisions bearing on the issue. It is thought that a single-volume compilation of these resources should vastly facilitate discussion, analysis, and cooperation.

"In presenting this material, Iowa P & A emphasizes the fact that, under the Individuals with Disabilities Education Act (the IDEA), 20 U.S.C. Section 1400 et seq., the concept of an 'appropriate' education is not — and is not intended to be — static. An educational practice that is fully appropriate at one point in time can be rendered inappropriate by developments in educational research. For this reason, the IDEA insists that every state establish "effective procedures for acquiring and disseminating . . . significant information derived from educational research, demonstration, and similar projects." 20 U.S.C. Section 1413(a)(3)(A). The IDEA also requires 'effective procedures for . . . adopting, where appropriate, promising educational practices . . ..' 20 U.S.C. Section 1413(a)(3)(B)."

I was thrilled.

Curt had more good news. Dr. Hagen had agreed to circulate Iowa Protection & Advocacy Services, Inc.'s booklet, *Judicial and ALJ Interpretations of The FAPE Requirement for Pre-School Children with Autism: A Synthesis of Recent Developments* to all of Iowa's AEAs by February 10th.

Curt faxed me his one-page grid that compared the results of six cases — two from California, two from New Jersey, one from Pennsylvania, the *Bernard Smith* case from California and the Ninth Circuit Court of Appeals opinion, all decided between 1989 and 1994 — laid out across the top of his grid. Down the left-hand side of his grid, these five brief questions were posed: Which party won? Identified defect in program offered by school? One-on-one required or upheld? Number of hours required or upheld? Relief awarded to or secured by parents?

As an idea, and as executed, Curt's grid was brilliant. School administrators anywhere could take in the gist of his *Synthesis* at a glance — no need for any of them to be detail-people — since many of them were quite busy across a wide range of special concerns. The grid showed that the five most recent cases had all been won by parents. Only a 1989 case had been won by the school — but only after the educators agreed during due process proceedings to revise the child's IEP to address virtually all the parents' concerns.

The types of defects in school programming included: failure of the school programs to be systematic, intensive, and consistent, no one-to-one aide for the child, goals and objectives not really geared to the needs of a child with autism, and written by teachers not trained in autism, using a watered-down North Carolina TEACCH program of 10 hours per week, or by offering only 17.5 hours a week of schooling.

All six cases resulted in one-to-one instruction being required after due process proceedings. Five of the six cases resulted in full time or 40 hours a week of instruction.

The types of relief awarded the parents included: all the costs of their in-home program, including costs of experts, assessments, evaluations, aides, and the construction of a classroom in the family home, teaching materials, transportation, tuition at Dr. Lovaas's clinic, the cost of a second residence for the child and mother to attend Dr. Lovaas's clinic, attorney fees, the cost of continuing a Lovaas program for a future, second year, in-home counseling, parent training, and summer school (EYSE).

For the meticulous and those willing to dig into the supporting, academic peer-reviewed scientific literature, the booklet also included 75 pages of reprints of much of the research drawn from my blue Binderteks and the contents of Dr. Lovaas's Christmastime FedEx envelope.

Soon enough, Curt and Joan's new booklet arrived from the printers. My copy came with a thank you from Joan. "We feel this publication will have a positive effect for a lot of families across Iowa." I was sure it would — and equally determined that it would travel far beyond the borders of Iowa. I ordered copies to distribute to the activist-couples I had met in Los Angeles and their friends back home. I hoped distribution to this widespread group would pay off in many places for many families who needed this information to share with their own state's counterpart of Curt's agency, or with non-profit or local private legal counsel.

Curt agreed we should announce the availability of their booklet in Dr. Rimland's newsletter, *ARRI*, and in the several FEAT newsletters circulating in other states. I agreed to handle the filling of orders out of my office.

Meg had asked Ruffin to draw a self-portrait at school. He scribbled what he told her was "hair," completed two circles as "eyes," a long line with both ends curled up as his "happy smile," and three vertical lines below that he told her were his "bottom." Then, he drew a much more elaborate portrait of me, set up on two long legs with shoes — a detail Ruffin had noticed on another child's drawing and added to his own, saying, "I made shoes."

Meg also sent me her charting of Ruffin's IEP goal to make sets of objects up to 6 by showing him a numeral and asking, "What number?" and then asking him to count that many into her hand, and then asking, "How many blocks?" In just over a week, Ruffin learned how to do this, but still needed a cue to start counting blocks into Meg's hand.

On February 6th, Kim administered the *Preschool Language Scale-3* test of receptive and expressive language to Ruffin, who was then 3 years, 9 months, and 27 days old, and scored his auditory comprehension at 3 years, 4 months, his expressive communication at 3 years, 4 months, and his total language score at 3 years, 4 months. Granted, she was grading her own work with him — but by her own numbers —

Ruffin's language delay of 16- to 18- months measured in early August had shrunk to no more than a 6-month delay. Over the most recent 6-month period from August to February, Ruffin's language development had grown remarkably. In another half year, could Ruffin claw his way back to join his typically developing educational cohort?

Kim's score sheet was littered with notes of little things Ruffin had offered up during her testing: "That's a boy?" "Kids playing a measure tape." "Build the doghouse." "He is playing." "She is eating a cracker." "In blanket, keep warm." "Go to sleep." "Sleeping." "Girl's cat." "Cat's food." "Eat breakfast." "Wash off." "Dry off." "Put on." "Go get Mommy." "Cross the street." "Be careful, it's too slippery." "At home, Mommy's house." "Mom, I putting butter." "Seamus is sleeping in chair; Mom is reading newspaper."

Ruffin's new language was an open window onto his widening world.

CHAPTER TWENTY ONE

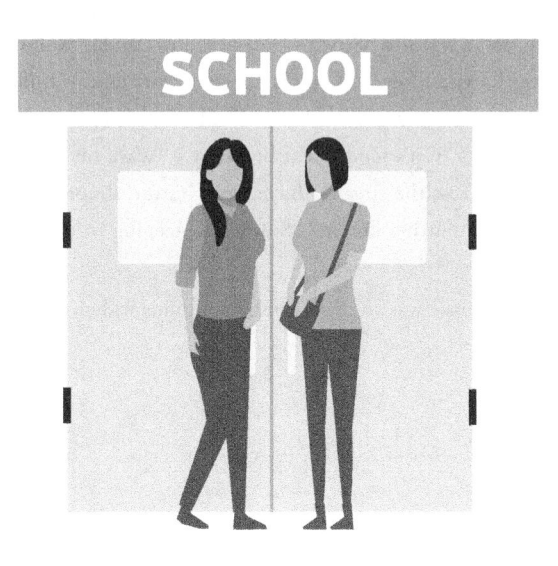

SEARCHING FOR THE MAINSTREAM

Inge and I began trying to find a mainstream or inclusion site for Ruffin with the two of us taking to heart Dr. Norman's recommendation that Ruffin was ready to learn from typically developing classmates. There were no public-school programs for 4-year-olds anywhere in our county. The closest public-school program was in the northern reaches of a neighboring county, a treacherous cross-country hour-and-a-half round trip bus ride — not a viable option.

But there might be a government Head Start classroom, and St. Patrick's Catholic School housed a small, private nursery school program that we might visit — but quickly, Inge warned — before their two classes filled up for next fall, usually by April. Only two dozen children would be admitted.

"We need to get moving," she urged.

We also discussed the possibility of creating a kindergarten language group for Ruffin to integrate with right there on Miss Hobbs's campus.

"That would require her administrative cooperation . . .," Inge said, as her voice trailed off.

As for Head Start, my income was too high for Ruffin to qualify. He would need to be admitted by documentation of his educational disability.

At home Ruffin was excited about repairs to the house next door. He reported, "Men are working hard. He is climbing the ladder. He has a hammer." And on and on. Ruffin wanted to know what they were building — by using the inflection of a question — "Building like a bridge?" He was delighted to have me offer him a special word: "Scaffold!"

I called Dr. Norman at UIHC to let him know I was expecting Dr. Sallows's report soon, now that he and I had completed a long clinical interview. Dr. Norman owned up to having jumped the gun and called Meg while I was in Los Angeles. He had failed to wait for Dr. Sallows's input as he and I had agreed, but there was no point in my complaining. The UIHC reports were already in the mail. The horse was already out of the barn.

We went on to discuss the mainstreaming issue. Dr. Norman encouraged me to look hard for such a group with a teacher or trained person who could set up interactions between Ruffin and his typically developing peers — preferably bright, verbal children his same age without articulation problems of any kind — because this type of company was likely to drive Ruffin to communicate.

Dr. Sallows issued his second opinion on February 10th. Since Ruffin had progressed more rapidly than others according to Dr. Lovaas's typical schedule, he seemed ready for exposure to typically developing peers. "The rationale for doing this is that average children are more likely than handicapped children to exhibit age-appropriate cues and expectations for age-appropriate behavior. If Ruffin can be helped to respond to these cues and expectations which require the prerequisite language comprehension and ability to change one's behavior, the peer group of average children will be able to shape his social interactions to be more and more like theirs are with each other."

He also recommended that Ruffin's educational program be "as close to year-round as possible" since Dr. Lovaas had evidence to show that cessation of treatment for as little as two weeks during the intensive phase could set a child back.

He addressed the issue of cost, too. "While such treatment is of course costly, the cost of long-term care of unrecovered people with autism, not to mention the emotional cost to the individual and his or her family, would seem to make treatment a bargain by comparison." I was reassured by Dr. Sallows's assessment that Lovaas programming was a bargain and hoped his second opinion would be enough to shake loose some money from somewhere — either from Prudential or from the schools — before I would need to turn to my parents.

Dr. Sallows's report slid out the fax to the widest circle of people whom I hoped to influence: Ruffin's IEP team, other educators, state administrators, physicians and evaluators, parents, autism societies and support groups, and politicians — along with a newly-published article from the February 1995 *Journal of the American Academy of Adolescent Psychiatry*, "Case Study: Deterioration, Autism, and Recovery in Two Siblings" *34:2:232-237* by Richard Perry, M.D., Ira Cohen, Ph.D., and Regina DeCarlo, M. D.

Into Mr. Montague's envelope, I also slipped Catherine Maurice's book, *Let Me Hear Your Voice,* for him to read before Ruffin's upcoming IEP meeting. I took care to connect the dots for him. "Enclosed please find a recent published medical journal article which describes the cases of the two Maurice siblings."

Evelyn visited us again in mid-February. Donna, Lisa, Seamus, and I had been pushing for complete sentences from Ruffin in all incidental settings, with some success to report. Evelyn reviewed our drill-by-drill daily notes, watched each of us work with Ruffin, and then assigned us *another* very substantially revised set of drills. We were going to teach Ruffin how to sound out words from the letters he knew, teach him to sing the ABC song — not to teach him his letters, but as a long auditory sequence to exercise his memory. Many of the new drills were less formal and involved less of the discrete trial format of clean, clear, repeated presentations of materials across a table.

The table drills we kept were expanded and elaborated. For example, we aimed to teach Ruffin as many as 50 functions of objects and expand his knowledge of shapes to more subtle figures such as ovals and diamonds. Several of the new drills were designed to give Ruffin practice in discriminating among the "wh" questions by building on his newly acquired knowledge of shapes, colors, and objects.

Other new drills were designed to help Ruffin with sequencing events and with his perception of time, of development, and of change. Others were designed to provoke and structure more and more spontaneous comment and conversation from Ruffin, by addressing him with more open-ended prompts, such as 'Tell me about . . .' Specifically, we were going to begin to teach Ruffin how to identify more subtle human emotions by showing him more evocative and perplexing photographs of faces and interpersonal situations.

Donna and I needed to drop everything else to gather and organize new teaching materials. And, since it was winter, indoors, in Iowa — Ruffin, Donna, Lisa, Seamus, and I, and all our children passed around a wicked flu during the remainder of February.

On February 14, using a large legible font, and leaving lots of white space for comment, I prepared a 38-page draft IEP for Ruffin and began to circulate it to Meg and Inge — an unwelcome Valentine, I knew. "Ruffin's CARD drill book will be updated as needed by video-telephone conferencing, and by another day-long visit from Evelyn Kung of CARD on Mother's Day. The costs of her transportation from California will be shared with two other CARD families."

From notes I recovered later from Ruffin's educational file, it was clear that someone — maybe some group gathered again in my absence — had read my long Valentine carefully, with Meg taking notes of objection all over it.

For many of my suggested goals and objectives, I had proposed that Ruffin spend time with both boys and girls, at or above his language level, with an adult who would facilitate interaction between Ruffin and typically developing classmates in both structured and unstructured activities. These terms had been repeatedly scribbled out.

I expected it would be a reasonable goal within the next year for Ruffin to improve his language skills to the normal range for his chronological age, that is, for him to fully catch-up to his typically developing cohort. This, too, had been repeatedly marked, "No," even as I had proposed IEP goals and specific short-term objectives to get there — as suggested by Evelyn and Dr. Granpeesheh.

Even more boldly I had proposed: "As assigned by Evelyn Kung of CARD, Ruffin will be able to master all language drills assigned by her. As a drill is mastered, the directions and materials will be provided to school for generalization with the ECSE teacher, speech therapist or classroom aide, volunteer, or student helper."

Of course, Meg and I were already doing this — well under the administrative radar, and with success — but there was strong objection to any assignments by Evelyn or CARD, or to the mention of any particular methodology in Ruffin's IEP. The dictation to Meg was: "We will work on concepts. We will consider generalization by our methods in class."

There was also evidence of strong objection to the incorporation of community trips, and written reports of outings taken by Ruffin with me and with his home therapy team as any part of Ruffin's IEP. There were repeated objections to acknowledging his home therapy team — or me as a parent — as any part of Ruffin's newest IEP.

Objection was expressed to providing transportation from Meg's classroom to any off-campus integration site, such as the little private nursery school that was housed at St. Pat's, about a quarter mile across town.

Whoever was reading or whatever group was meeting had stopped scribbling up my Valentine. On the back of a page mid-way through, in Meg's handwriting was an echo of her earlier written *mea culpa* to her superiors, "Document me as an observer at training. I do use some methodology. Classroom for generalization. No unusual techniques. Only use it (behavior modification), as one of many. Baseline in three days."

Whatever I was unaware of at school, I was encouraged by a letter from Dr. Lovaas's co-researcher, Dr. Tristram Smith, still in Des Moines at Drake University, to whom I had sent all Ruffin's earliest and latest written evaluations. "I agree with you that Ruffin has improved substantially, and I am very pleased by his development."

I answered his letter, by running down all the recent developments in Iowa, my presentation at Western Hills, and my trip to Los Angeles. Tris' contributions to Iowa had been crucial. "As a result of the groundwork which you must have laid with our state autism specialist Sue Baker somehow, a great many Iowa and regional meetings will address the issue of home Lovaas programming and how to make it available in the Midwest. Now, in Iowa, when our parent network learns of a newly diagnosed child (and Sue Baker usually tips them off by giving out one of our phone numbers), we send them a 500-page binder containing the most useful information we have found. As that information is digested and we hear back from the family about their intentions, we send along a collection of legal cases, and help the family contact a workshop group to provide training so a home program can get up and running."

Meg sent home Ruffin's latest drawing of himself — which showed remarkable improvement — a fully formed head with eyes and mouth, a clothed body with arms, legs, and feet. To me, it evidenced his growing self-awareness.

Donna and I began playing *Candyland* with Ruffin. He got the colors easily. We asked him "Whose turn?" to have him identify the right person by name. We also spoke in terms of "ahead," "behind," and "between" as the play pieces chased each other around the colorful cardboard map.

Ruffin knew his table grace by then and was working with Lisa's family to memorize the longer Catholic table grace.

I continued nattering on to Meg in cheerful ignorance because — with some rest — I was happier. Ruffin enjoyed spelling out words in books for me. He was coloring a drawing Donna had made of our house. When he finished, Ruffin asked me to turn the paper over and print his name on the back. He could tell me what letters I needed to write.

And I was wrestling the local Head Start bureaucracy. They had no room for Ruffin. Who took this kind of a "no" for an answer? Although Head Start had all the necessary releases, my copy machine ran hot and sooty to offer them all Ruffin's disability documentation. By late February, I had arranged an on-site Head Start visit. Ruffin would "be considered for placement if we have an over-income slot available this spring at the local center. He will also be considered for our fall enrollment, according to our eligibility criteria."

As Ruffin arrived home, here was Meg's charting of Ruffin's ability to answer what we called "situation questions" — "What do you do when you are cold, hungry, sleepy, sick, or dirty?" Ruffin was able to come up with one-word answers, "blanket, olives, bed, doctor, wash" and some phrases, "I go to bed," "dirty clothes, wash it off," "with water," "go to doctor," — all of which Meg had marked as "achieved to some degree."

Donna and I had conferred about the UIHC evaluation reports and Ms. Wilding's position of soft discipline — of letting Ruffin have his way — which we agreed seemed to lead to problems and Ruffin cutting up at the drill table, and Dr. Norman's position — that the adult with Ruffin should be the boss — which we agreed seemed to lead to better results. We decided that Ruffin responded better to firmness.

Meanwhile, for "the baseline," due in three days, Kim had administered the *Boehm Test of Basic Concepts Preschool Version* to Ruffin. This measured a child's performance in the mastery of concepts involving space and time. At 3 years, 10 months of age Ruffin tested much better on the *spatial* concepts he had been drilled on but was left at a total loss on the *temporal* concepts we had yet to include in his drills.

Over the phone, Dr. Norman and I ranged over the full UIHC reports in the context of Dr. Sallows's second opinion. I pointed out — using the UIHC report and Ruffin's drill book — that Ruffin was able to demonstrate the skills we had worked on at home using CARD's direct instruction, but that skills we had yet to tackle with him were ones he could not demonstrate and didn't seem to have picked up from the general environment.

"It seems to me," I explained to Dr. Norman, "that Ruffin learns through the small bottleneck of direct instruction, as if Donna, Lisa, and I are placing pea after small pea into the hard glass mouth of a Coke bottle. Once information enters, it is captured, but Ruffin is not a sponge."

We addressed the prosody issues that concerned Ms. Wilding so much. They concerned me, too. Evelyn was working on these with us.

A long discussion ensued about how other Iowa families were using various strategies to fund their home Lovaas programs. Because he was curious, I offered Dr. Norman a full update of recent developments, providing him copies of all our resources.

In late February, Inge and I visited the private nursery school and the local Head Start class, both housed in the same two-story yellow brick building at St. Pat's.

The private nursery school for 4-year-olds met in part of a converted gymnasium, in the basement. No windows. Also, no outdoor playground because the older playground equipment at St. Pat's failed to meet state department of education standards. Also, no computers. The little group met only 2 or 3 days a week, and only for half the day. Ruffin would need transportation between school campuses.

The children were a genuinely nice group, well-behaved, and under good control of experienced, qualified teachers. This group met the suggestions of the literature provided by UIHC, as urged by Dr. Norman, and in accord with Dr. Granpeesheh and Evelyn Kung. The program was not very structured, consisting mostly of "free play." It would offer Ruffin a true social opportunity. If he could swim when he was thrown in, that would be very encouraging. I was willing to consider this nursery school as a part of Ruffin's IEP. Moving him from environment to environment, from teacher to teacher, from group to group would promote generalization of his new skills, too.

Unfortunately, admission to this private nursery school was by lottery. Were Ruffin to be placed there, Miss Hobbs would need to cut a deal to guarantee Ruffin a slot. Could our school district offer some of the state money it received for educating Ruffin as a child with a disability to this little school as a contract provider of services? Inge didn't know. The educational materials and toys in the room were all well-worn. I thought some of Ruffin's share of state money could be put to good use there.

The Head Start program for 4-year-olds was in another basement room, with high, frosted windows. The room itself was extremely small, hot, noisy, and very crowded. There were several small play-stations along a narrow aisle. All the materials were dreadfully and commercially garish. No computers. The pipes running across the ceiling appeared to be insulated with asbestos. This class met 5 days a week, all day long — just like Ruffin's current special education class. But there were 15 rowdy children, attended by 2 staff members without college degrees or any teaching certification. They were "moms" who had been trained at the local community college in some early childhood education. Both seem devoted enough, but I was shocked by their extremely poor uncorrected grammar.

For half a minute I gazed in the mirror over the sink in the little girls' room and wondered if the person I saw reflected there wasn't just a snob. I shouldn't be so judgmental. I was relying on Donna and Lisa, and they were both just bricks — wonderfully effective and thoroughly dependable.

No, this Head Start room was wretched, completely unacceptable. The reverberating noise would have made it difficult, if not impossible, for Ruffin to process instructions from either teacher, or any language offered by the children.

And as Dr. Norman and Dr. Granpeesheh had counseled me, Head Start classmates were not likely to be an appropriate choice recommended for mainstreaming children with autism. Integration peers needed to be exceptionally social and academically able.

Yes, I chided myself, I was a hopeless snob.

I kept Meg in the loop. "Mrs. Pittman at the private nursery school seemed very intrigued with Ruffin and quite friendly on the phone. Have you met her? She has a Monday, Wednesday, and Friday afternoon class for a dozen 4-year-olds that might be good if Ruffin's name is drawn during the lottery for admission. If he came back to your ECSE to be integrated up to kindergarten on Tuesday and Thursday that would really require him to generalize his skills next year."

Meg reported she had been working for a couple of weeks on Ruffin's IEP goal that he tell her how many objects she had given him. Ruffin was just guessing and always guessing "3." She found him "extremely distracted while working on this task." That sounded to me a lot like Ruffin — when he was bored.

CHAPTER TWENTY TWO

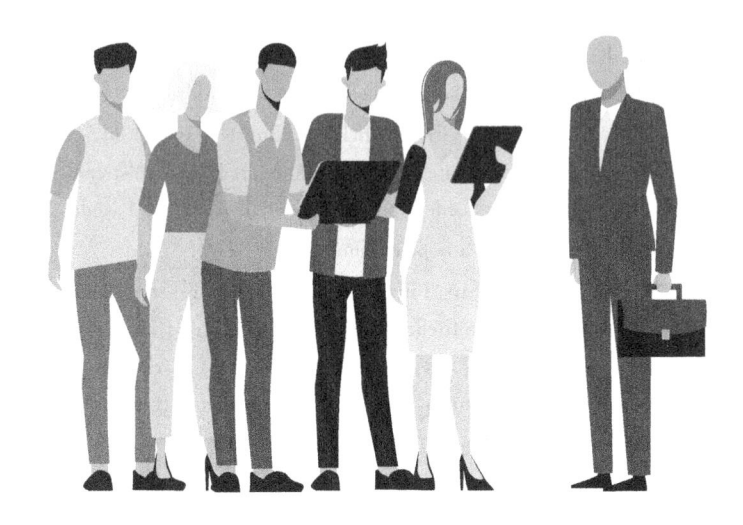

SPRING, AN UNSETTLED SEASON

My doorbell rang in the middle of the afternoon. The mail carrier had a certified letter I needed to sign for, written by Miss Hobbs — scheduling the continuation of Ruffin's IEP meeting for the morning of Thursday, March 16th, in the board room at the high school. It warned, "That date will meet the stipulated timelines established by Special Education Rule 41.17(8) (enclosed) regarding Extended Year Special Education (EYSE). If we do not meet prior to March 30th, we will not be in compliance with this rule." Miss Hobbs had not left Inge to write this — which sounded more like it might have been dictated or drafted by legal counsel.

But for the first time since Ruffin had entered special education, it complied with the federal requirement that I receive an advance list of the meeting's participants, an all-star lineup: Inge, Jack, Miss Hobbs, Kim, Emily, Meg, Mr. Lord, our local superintendent, Mr. Montague and his right-hand man, "Moe," of course.

I called Curt to ask him to come. He wanted to know exactly what Ruffin would need, and why. I alerted him, "There may be a bad problem about where to find children with whom to mainstream Ruffin. This has already been the cause of some friction between Miss Hobbs and me. There is no public preschool for 4-year-olds. Our local district is still in the planning stages — 2 to 5 years out."

I whined, "If Miss Hobbs started right now, couldn't she rent a trailer, hire a teacher, and share the wealth of instructional materials now available in the special education and kindergarten rooms — and start a program for 4-year-olds by next fall?" This was never going to happen. The Ocean Liner, Miss Hobbs, as I still saw her in my mind's eye, was not a nimble vessel. She didn't seem to cotton to me, or to my implicit criticism of her district's planning, or to my overblown sense of entitlement, or even to Ruffin's simple legal entitlement under the IDEA not to be discriminated against. For Curt, I anticipated the school authorities' argument: no 4-year-olds attended public school in our town, so how could Ruffin be discriminated against?

Then Curt and I reviewed the available St. Pat's nursery school and Head Start options.

"Evelyn suggested that Ruffin would benefit most from spending time with typical 5-year-olds from kindergarten — because 5-year-olds are more 'helpful' than 4-year-olds, more socially mature, and more willing to take a little one under their wings, especially the girls. The 'language gap' is not too great for Ruffin to bridge."

Then, like all my clients, I argued my case to my lawyer. "Why couldn't Ruffin do kindergarten twice? If he made no friends among the 5-year-olds and was simply the 'pet' of several talkative girls, he could go back the second year with his younger cohort and, knowing the routine and having his academic skills down cold, he could concentrate on social routines and making friends. If he did kindergarten twice, Dr. Norman thought that would be fine, because Ruffin would end up with his age-group by the second year.

"What I have heard is the school wants to keep Ruffin in special education in his present ECSE classroom. They would justify this placement by claiming that at least 3 of the 9 boys in his classroom now have more language than Ruffin. Some are 5 and 6 years old."

Bearing in mind Mr. Montague's quiet olive branch extended earlier — encouraging me to think about how to "marry" Ruffin's home Lovaas program with the school's offerings — I let Curt know, "We need to schedule Ruffin's more academic and demanding intensive drill work early in the morning. I can send Donna to school, and she is willing to work there with a small reverse mainstream group to include Ruffin. Evelyn spent her last day here with Donna talking to us about mainstreaming techniques she suggested Donna could use."

Of course, even with Mr. Montague and Mr. Lord attending, Ruffin's IEP team was bound to founder on the great rock of summer school or EYSE, since that would require paying their employees to work over the summer months. "Bridgewater and the local district are not going to offer summer programming to any of their special education students unless it is something along the lines of home tutoring, because the special education classroom is already leased to a private Medicaid mental retardation waiver respite care provider, so that private agency can run a 'summer activities' group for disabled children.

"This 'summer activity' is not EYSE, is not run by teachers or the school authorities. It is run by a local group home on grant funding, staffed by local folks and high school students who are paid about $5.50 per hour out of mental retardation Medicaid waiver monies each child has qualified for by family application and are required to contribute. Transportation is not provided. The program runs for 21 days and meets in the afternoon. There is no guarantee yet that Ruffin could be 'buddied' with a talkative child who might be physically disabled, whom Ruffin could help. And, as you know, Ruffin does not qualify for mental retardation Medicaid waiver funding."

What did I want for Ruffin? Ideally? And what was my bottom line? That was what Curt wanted to know.

"I want the school authorities to pay for 40 hours per week of CARD programming over this summer, to have Donna and Lisa available for that amount of time each week of the summer to work one-on-one with Ruffin, or with Ruffin and a small playgroup." If the school authorities were unprepared to offer this, I was prepared to provide it as "appropriate" — and to have Curt seek reimbursement.

Curt said, "Okay, we can try that."

For just a moment, I found myself looking up from the computer screen on my desk and longing for what had seemed a simpler time for me, an earlier summer of my own childhood, troubled by trivial matters, dark thunderstorms with lightning, and dragging magnets through curbside dust to collect iron filings.

Now, the why. Curt wanted to know *why* I was so incredibly determined to do all this for Ruffin now.

"All of us have worked so hard to help him improve. It's been wearing. I don't want to see him 'stall out' now in a less than challenging environment. Nor do I want any of our hard work undone by persons not knowledgeable in handling Ruffin, or by over-stimulating environments that would be overwhelmingly noisy and crowded."

And, as always, a lot of it came down to the money. "I should have a complete figure for my reimbursement claim by next week, with supporting copies of all my bills and receipts. I expect it to run between $10,000 and $13,000 for Ruffin's home program to date." As it turned out, that was a gross underestimate.

Curt asked that I pull all this together in writing. As an attorney myself accustomed to representing others with considerable difficulties, I knew even a long letter took far less time to read than conducting a long, rambling question and answer interview.

I let Meg know what I wanted too, in our home-school notebook, to share with Miss Hobbs. "I did not mean to get Miss Hobbs so very upset. The mainstreaming problem needs some legwork and thinking to address before the IEP meeting so there is a better answer then than, 'I don't know,' or 'We'll have to find out.' I don't want to sit through another meeting like early December, where Donna and I talk into the wind, and receive placating replies. I would accept the least expensive option rather than require a public preschool for 4-year-olds (which Inge says can't be put together in less than 2 1/2 years' time) or me starting a 4-year-old preschool in my home, remodeling at public expense, materials at public expense and certified staff at public expense. See *M. A. v. Voorhees Board of Education*. I slipped Curt's booklet into Ruffin's backpack with a yellow sticky note, "Miss Hobbs can keep this for a couple of days and read it."

"Your comment about Ruffin being able to come back to your class when not over at St. Pat's campus is very reassuring. If so, who would Ruffin spend his time with? 'Special' classmates or typically developing classmates, or what mix? What do *you* think might be best, given the UIHC reports, Dr. Sallows's, and your own observations?"

Like as not, the impatience of my tone had to do with Ruffin being up the night before. I needed to warn Meg. "He's not sick but is having very irregular breathing (breath-holding) and rigid posturing, sitting up. Hard to know what the problem is." I was fearful that Ruffin was returning to a pattern of night-waking, during which he would be very breathy, gasping or holding his breath. This odd breathing sometimes preceded his waking. During the day he was busy and able to refrain from behaviors like these, but they did emerge during these night-waking periods in the form of staring, blinking, focusing on lights, and some body-rocking. All this terrified me.

I felt better once the sun came up, when Ruffin was supposed to get up, and I softened my message to Meg, by adding, "He's building a 4-walled block structure now on his own, pretending to make a car out of a chair turned against the sofa. He stops and goes places, or pretends the enclosed space is a cave, doing all this by himself."

When the morning mail arrived, I heard from another CARD mom, a sunny handwritten note. "I gave one new parent the information about attorney Scott Peters — her AEA seems willing to talk and cooperate. Could you send me the name and number of the LeClaire, Wisconsin mother? Will talk to you soon!"

Chris Foster, a long-time court reporter, understood what I was trying to do as an advocate and was both my advocacy partner and my personal support, always with a cheerful shoulder to offer. There was another thank you note from a grandmother in Indiana. Turning to this sort of networking helped lift my spirits. All of us already knew each other's children had autism. None of us gave a rat's ass about confidentiality. I couldn't see that confidentiality had helped a single one of our children yet.

And, in the bottom of the mailbox, I'd overlooked another letter from Prudential's Ms. Crews prompting me to supply Donna and Lisa's "medical credentials" so she could reply to my claim.

No school, but I was invited to Head Start's open house. I skipped it. Ruffin and I didn't qualify. I had seen it. And I was too busy. Monday was the single motion day at our local courthouse, our all-day-long hurry-up-and-wait day for criminal arraignments, hearings on motions to suppress evidence by challenging the constitutionality of search warrants, sentencing drunk drivers and felons, mostly baby-burglars — my mental nickname for young men stealing stainless steel flatware out of the neighboring trailer for their new girlfriends — proving up no-fault divorce decrees and hauling those delinquent in their child support in for contempt, so the judge could tongue-lash them. This Monday, Donna, Lisa, and I were determined to make use of a snow day to have the two of them both do double shifts at my home with Ruffin.

While meeting with all the AEA regional directors, Dr. Hagen determined the state would remain utterly agnostic on all matters of autism methodology. The state would respectfully defer to each AEA regional director's decision to honor that most sacred cow lumbering around and branded 'local control.' Curt learned later, too, that this would be her steadfast leadership position.

When a slim letter did arrive from Des Moines, I tore it open. It was a coldly worded request, trusting that I would immediately correct my records to spell consultant *Dee Ann* L. Wilson's name properly. I cursed myself under my breath. Curt had already alerted me she was an especially important person in special education consumer relations whom we needed to persuade, and here I had relied solely upon my hearing, assuming she was a *Dianne*. I needed a private investigator's headshot whiteboard with colored yarn and thumbtacks to keep track of the structure of this far-away state department of education, just like, no, even more than Ruffin needed his set of photo drill cards to learn to call his classmates and teachers by name. Had I offended Dee Ann beyond any possibility of opening her heart to Ruffin? The phone rescued me from a backwash of regret.

It was Susan Smith, another CARD mom, calling from Brayton with good news about her two sons. I mouthed a silent thank you to Inge for slipping me Marion McQuaid's name and number back in early December, after our awful meeting. With her permission, I was able to share her latest news with Curt, and with attorney Scott Peters in Council Bluffs, who had an IEP meeting for the family he represented there scheduled for the day before Ruffin's.

Meg reported, "At nap Ruffin had a bloody nose — didn't say anything — must have just kept wiping it with his sleeve and blanket until we noticed. We are still working on getting him to say, 'Teacher, help!' I'm sending his blanket home for a wash." No way did I want Meg to feel badly about this. "Ruffin had a two-hour-long nosebleed Saturday morning, woke up with it bleeding again badly. The air is so dry. Glad it didn't bleed more."

With Ruffin having been up in the middle of the night again — his night-time waking pattern re-emerged as his and our schedules devolved to be far less rigorous as Donna, Lisa, and I each went down again with the flu. After a full school day, I made a new 20-minute video of Ruffin working with me, Donna, and Lisa on his newest exercises to send to Evelyn and Dr. Granpeesheh for review. It captured Ruffin in conversation with me at his upstairs drill-room window, describing what he saw and imagined, while the wind outside rattled the glass — "'Those birds wear snow to keep warm." It also showed Ruffin in conversations with his therapists structured around moods-and-emotions posters and sequencing cards used to prompt more complex cause-and-effect narratives.

I sent copies of this newest tape to Sue, Dr. Norman, and to Ruffin's educators to review and share. Specifically, I encouraged Inge, "Several other families in Iowa who are running home programs now are being asked by their AEAs and local school districts for permission to use video and other materials concerning their children at meetings which are planned for late March in Clear Lake and early April in Council Bluffs. I understand from talking to Dr. Tristram Smith that he will be speaking at these meetings." I asked her a question Sue had wanted me to ask. "Is anyone from Bridgewater scheduled to present Ruffin's case at these meetings? If so, would you please let me know who? I hope Ruffin's educators would plan to make some sort of presentation, and hope that Donna, Lisa, and I can provide any further information that might be useful."

With the parents' permission, I shared all the details of the public-school funding of another CARD family's home program by their local district and Heartland AEA with Inge. That portion of my letter was underlined, as Inge faxed it over to Jack.

I also asked Inge a few questions Curt needed me to ask. "If there are any documents that you or other members of Ruffin's IEP team are planning to present as his present levels of educational performance, and as proposed annual goals and short-term objectives at the March continuation of his IEP meeting, Curt and I would appreciate having a working-draft copy at least 3 days beforehand. I have previously provided you with my working draft of an IEP" — my earlier, unwelcome Valentine — "and hope you can extend us the same courtesy. I look forward to having a good, productive meeting in March with you and all the others who are coming."

Meanwhile, Meg and Dr. Norman were talking on the phone again, with him scribbling. "Meeting with Mom in mid-March to finalize the IEP. They are not going to offer Lovaas or summer school at this time. Will be integrating some Head Start kids before early April into Ruffin's class." None of this was shared with me at the time, or with Curt. Not by Meg.

And, not by Dr. Norman either, to whom I wrote in blissful ignorance, "It was a great pleasure to talk with you, and as I promised you, here is a letter of reply to your report. I know your team felt the heat of some challenge to a pre-existing allegiance to TEACCH and to more traditionally functional programs in my request for you to evaluate Ruffin. As I said to Dr. Piven, we need to make room for the possibility of excellence anywhere. That is the only way to see that it emerges everywhere. I was pleased with the quality and the detail of both the oral and the written reports. Your efforts and the efforts of every team member are appreciated."

At his request, I also sent copies of Ruffin's various CARD drill books to date, explaining, "These books describe the format for each CARD instructional drill which Ruffin has worked on. Summary sheets at the front show the dates he worked on each drill, with the therapist's initials. Behind each drill-format-page, we also keep pages of daily notes written between therapists to foster generalization, and to record other daily observations. These are the two sets of drills Ruffin worked on at home before coming to see your team in late January." I went on to explain the newest revisions of Ruffin's drill book from mid-February, and how Ruffin's program by then included less of the discrete trial format — which nevertheless remained the one surefire way of teaching him anything new.

Ms. Wilding's concerns about prosody needed to be met with a full written account to Dr. Norman of Ruffin's developmental history from his medical and educational file. "We are delighted to be wrestling with prosody issues. Ruffin could be mute, or unintelligible, but he is not. . ... We have found his classroom teacher's suggestion helpful — to speak to him in lower pitched voices of our own. He is just beginning to pick up some 'normal kid' inflections and expressions from other children, such as, 'Oh, my gosh!' (in exasperation), and 'I said' (argumentatively), and 'That's neat, Mom!' (with enthusiasm). Also, he is beginning to show bursts of emotional reaction: sobbing inconsolably over the departure of a friend, crying in reaction to an impatient correction, bouts of delight, excitement, and anticipation. Maybe these emotions will begin to find expression in his speaking voice as well soon."

Ruffin's fragile ability to learn remained dependent on how, and exactly what, he had been taught. "At the time of Ruffin's January examination, we had yet to address plurals, past tense, the use of articles or 'is,' and not many group names or category nouns or the discrimination of loud and soft noises. With his newest drill book, these language forms will be taught explicitly."

I wanted Dr. Norman to know my long-term goal for Ruffin as a person. "We are working very intensively with sets of sequencing cards — 2-card sets to 12-card sets — to help Ruffin work out time, self-care, developmental, growth, and weather routines. Maybe an early emphasis on these tasks will help him to avoid needing to use anything more than typical visual reminders we all use — lists, and the like."

Two days before the scheduled continuation of Ruffin's IEP meeting, Inge sent me a proposed present level of educational performance (PLEP), and a couple of pages of proposed goals and objectives, all of them focused on Ruffin's integration into a group of typically developing peers or "mainstreaming." The PLEP page simply acknowledged, "Ruffin's interactions with peers typically involve run and chase games or pretend games with stylized dialogue. He needs to expand his repertoire of play and conversational skills to meet this need." A single annual goal was proposed with four short-term objectives that he begin talking and engaging in pretend play with other children.

The final page was a typewritten note on school letterhead, signed by Meg — a memo to the parents of all the boys in her classroom about "A program update," describing a pilot program to incorporate "dual programming with the Head Start classroom a couple of afternoons a week."

Group-based goals paralleled the individual goal proposed for Ruffin. But the fundamental concept of the IDEA — that each child with special needs receive individualized consideration in the planning of his or her education — was sacrificed by offering the same group experience to all nine boys with widely differing disabilities in Ruffin's classroom. Each boy deserved to be considered individually as to his readiness, and the typically developing guinea pigs deserved at least a modicum of training on how to encounter each boy with some chance of social success. Certainly, the parents of these Head Start children deserved notice and a choice whether to volunteer their children for this special education role, or not.

Later, an unsigned typewritten note arrived, folded into Ruffin's home-school notebook. "We have been informed that it will *not* take an amendment to your child's IEP to participate in the integration program with Head Start. Your child will participate as part of our classroom program *unless* you *do not* want them to do so. Please sign the form below so that we have a record of your being notified that this program will be starting."

In my own mind, confusion reigned. What was it that I and all the parents of Ruffin's classmates were being asked to sign now? The individualized *mainstreaming* or *integration* requirement of the IDEA had been reduced by our local district to a "field trip" permission slip. I printed Ruffin's name in and scrawled my signature.

I had hoped that my advocacy for Ruffin might bring about better services for other children with disabilities. Maybe this represented an incremental increase in our district's awareness of the need for mainstreaming and inclusion for special needs students.

But a certified letter as notice of the IEP date, and now these dithering memos? The fine hand of some school legal counsel must be at work behind the scenes. I let Curt know we might expect legal counsel to attend Ruffin's IEP meeting.

"Good," said Curt, who was as pleased as I was hopeful. "Perhaps we'll have someone to talk turkey with, to get Ruffin settled."

"Why not be hopeful?" I replied. "So many good things are happening across the state. See you tomorrow evening, however late." We laughed ruefully together since it so rarely happened. "A good night's sleep beforehand, always the best preparation."

Curt and I puzzled a bit the next morning, at my kitchen counter, but not long, over all the tea leaves. We reviewed our list of what we agreed Ruffin needed before heading off in the warm spring morning.

All the people from school were seated in padded, swiveling boardroom chairs when Curt, Donna, and I arrived. No strange face who might be school district legal counsel — but then, his or her name would have needed to have been included in the formal notice of this meeting — so whatever the school authorities were paying for legal advice, it was limited to getting advice over the phone, not paying for early-morning travel over any long distance, even in our fine spring weather.

We sat, and I introduced Curt.

A printed agenda was passed around. Everyone shifted, readying to launch into his or her part in the long litany of the present levels of educational performance (PLEP), and proposed goals and objectives, before marching through the pages of the federally mandated state form.

Curt interrupted all this to propose that we simply offer opening comments to state our respective positions. In the absence of school district legal counsel, it might as well be a short meeting.

I set out what I wanted for Ruffin, and why. I passed out an itemization of $39,153.67 I had already spent on Ruffin's appropriate education through mid-February, including in that figure the cost of my gifts of teaching materials to Meg's classroom — since the IDEA spoke in terms of a *free* appropriate public education.

Speaking for the educators, Miss Hobbs asserted exactly what Meg had told Dr. Norman earlier: Ruffin had no need of Lovaas-type special instruction, because Ruffin's IEP and Meg's classroom methods of instruction already met the IDEA's standard of "appropriateness," and always had. Ruffin didn't meet either of the Iowa Rules' criteria for EYSE, or summer school. However, Meg would add a mainstreaming component to her classroom, because the UIHC had suggested that Ruffin seemed ready to encounter typically developing children.

I looked over to Mr. Montague to see if he had any intention of waving his olive branch, his proposed marriage of our home Lovaas program with what Miss Hobbs had to offer. He sat quietly, monitoring the scene, like a Roman statue with a Roman nose and wavy hair the color of fine marble. I wondered, "Is he sitting in as a powerless 'consultant' to the decision-makers here — Miss Hobbs and Mr. Lord?" Curt glanced over at me and saw I seemed confused about the lay of the land here.

Calmly and sonorously, Curt made his case that my expenses in mounting a home-based CARD program should be reimbursed, that EYSE should be provided during the upcoming summer, and warned that if I had to mount a home-based EYSE classroom of typical peers for Ruffin in the afternoon to supplement his continuing home-based CARD program, the school authorities should be prepared to reimburse all those expenses, as well as the attorney fees his agency would charge for representing Ruffin and me. He passed out copies of his comb-bound booklet of case-law and peer-reviewed research articles supporting his argument, and went over them, briefly and pointedly.

As he spoke, Miss Hobbs was making careful notes. But so was Mr. Montague — what Miss Hobbs had said meant that Bridgewater was going to be dragged in behind the local school district into a difficult and expensive mess.

Then — as Curt and I had agreed in advance would be our break-the-log-jam strategy — Curt offered that rather than all the reimbursement I might be legally entitled to, I just needed the funding to *continue* Ruffin's home-based CARD program.

After Curt nodded my direction, I spoke up. "I would be willing to cap Ruffin's CARD programming at 40 hours per week for 2 years' duration or end earlier — should Ruffin reach typical levels of functioning across all developmental domains, including language and socialization."

Miss Hobbs immediately rejected our proposal, but with a nod from Mr. Lord, she agreed to Curt's bend-over-backwards suggestion that the local district work together with Bridgewater to put the school authorities' final best offer for a free, appropriate public education (FAPE) to Ruffin in writing by late March. Curt and I would do the same. All parties would then review each other's plans and reconvene before late April to see if any amicable solution could be reached.

I agreed. We all needed to kick the can down the road in the absence of any local district legal counsel. Our written exchanges should begin to smoke him or her out.

Mr. Montague looked over at Inge who was scribbling frantically. I felt badly for her since I read his look in her direction as handing her the miserable assignment of wrangling Miss Hobbs and the remainder of Ruffin's IEP team around to some new offer I might accept.

So, the meeting ended, not with a bang, but with a whimper.

And with the certainty for me — a certainty I would need some time and reflection to accept — that I needed to drop any hope of easy settlement and dampen my efforts at any statewide advocacy to focus entirely on organizing an every day, day-long educational program for Ruffin at home this summer.

CHAPTER TWENTY THREE

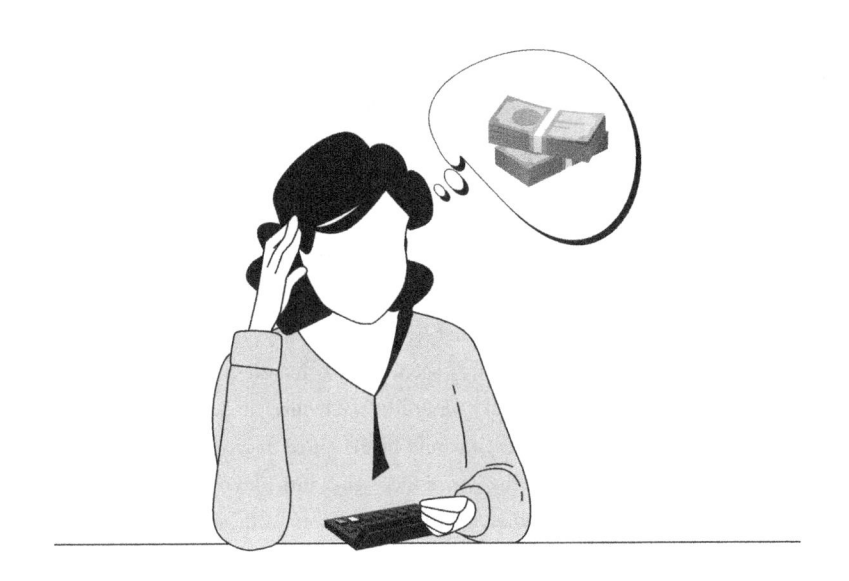

PREPARING. FOR WHAT?

I was on the phone to Prudential arguing most of the afternoon with Berna Crews and then up the chain of command to a Dr. Northrup. After I was well and truly frustrated, having blown my stack and sobbing, Dr. Northrup conceded that diagnoses on the autism spectrum were not excluded "mental illnesses" in fact or in law. Given Dr. Caldwell's prescription, she was not questioning the "medical necessity" of Ruffin's CARD home program. But Dr. Northrup was well and truly hung up on the fact that Donna and Lisa were not licensed medical providers.

At her request, I explained my claim to Prudential, adding additional supporting material, laying out the arguments I had been too angry to urge clearly as I had been reduced to tears. "This same medical service delivery pattern of workshop training of paraprofessionals and continuing supervision by video, fax, and telephone by a clinical psychologist is used not only by Ruffin's provider, CARD, but also by UCLA, Rutgers

University, the Bancroft School in New Jersey, Dr. Glen Sallows of Madison, Wisconsin, and Dr. Tristram Smith at Drake University."

And I warned that the refusal of my claim might result in a far greater claim. "Very similar methods of treatment are used effectively by the Princeton Child Development Institute in an institutional setting — at $35,000 per year. Therapists on the east and west coasts are typically paid $25 per hour. Ruffin's therapists are paid $10 per hour, quite a reasonable rate." I enclosed our video records of Ruffin's progress in which, as I asserted, "His improvement is obvious."

Ruffin arrived home from school wound up and tired. He slept early that evening, but then he and I were up a good part of the middle of the night, reading and playing, cooking and eating.

I was disappointed when yet another letter arrived from Prudential demanding to see Donna and Lisa's credentials. Curt's agency didn't handle private insurance claim disputes. It was too challenging to take on Prudential by myself. So, I called Scott Peters in Council Bluffs. Scott assured me he would be delighted, it would be his privilege, to handle this matter. "Just fax me the entire file." And, just like that, I did. Later Scott took on many such cases for other families of children with autism. As he steadily collected one letter after another conceding coverage, he would share his growing collection with the next insurance company to shame them into providing coverage for the next child's family.

Scott began wrangling Prudential by laying out for them with dates and details how Donna and Lisa were "now completely trained and qualified in the CARD method of applied behavior modification therapy, the only method nationally recognized by scientific study as well as case law, for the treatment of autism."

To Prudential's earlier objections that Donna and Lisa had "no license or certification," Scott countered, "None is available anywhere in the United States for training in this treatment procedure."

Then, Scott recounted, "In reviewing the history of correspondence and telephone conversations, it appears that your discussions with our client, Ms. White, regarding her expenses have been ongoing for almost three months. I have reviewed your policy applicable in this case. *There can be no question whatsoever* that this treatment is medically necessary, prescribed by a physician, and is not covered by any exclusion set forth in your policy."

Having set them out in detail, Scott toted up my claims of nearly $10,000 to date for payments made directly to Donna and Lisa. "Since these bills are currently out of our client's pocket and causing very significant financial hardship, I would request that she receive your check for payment of all these claims, minus her remaining deductible, not later than fifteen (15) days from today."

Donna and then Lisa were scheduled to work with Ruffin on his CARD drills that Saturday. I had the time I needed to write Curt the detailed letter he wanted about what Ruffin needed so he could prepare our cross-offer to Ruffin's educators.

First, I estimated my future expenses to be able to complete Ruffin's CARD program. Scott would need the same financial information to give Prudential for our future insurance claims, so I fortified myself with the thought that the adding machine and I would be setting out to bring down two birds with a single stone.

Because it was of equal or greater importance to me than money, I needed to document, both factually and legally, a high demand for money so that I could let go of some of it to buy as much language in any settlement agreement that would commit the public educators to change — so they might come to embrace Lovaas's proven methods. I didn't want to hear about another young child with autism going down the drain. Any mind is a terrible thing to waste. I could not let anything like that rest on my conscience. I felt it might kill me.

How much money was I willing to pay for change? All the water already over the dam, all the first $34,000 I had spent in my efforts to educate Ruffin to date.

What did I need not to give up? All the future costs of completing Ruffin's home CARD program. I could not sacrifice his chance at continuing development on the altar of advocacy — Ruffin and I needed a second $34,000.

After sitting down with the two of them and with their agreement, I was able to offer Donna's and Lisa's names up to become direct employees of the school authorities at $6 per hour, provided they also received family health insurance coverage and retirement benefits. Another CARD family's therapists were receiving these benefits in Brayton, in Heartland AEA. I drafted a little provision on how to choose and train replacements for Donna and Lisa, if necessary.

Then, I offered two options for summer services (EYSE): either at my home, with a loan of items from Ruffin's classroom, capping the cost at $10,000, or in a classroom where the Medicaid waiver program for children with disabilities did not meet, with the educators supplying their own certified staff.

I offered to contribute any Prudential insurance recovery beyond what was necessary to cover my own costs to date.

What was the state-wide change I hoped to buy for my first $34,000 of water over the dam? How would I have liked to have been served and supported as a parent with a newly diagnosed child with autism? What choices should public educators offer to new parents to consider, to reject or accept, for the education of their children?

All this was a Saturday morning romp, a trial lawyer's indulgence I needed to get off my chest and then abandon. I needed to leave what I envisioned in Curt's capable hands for him to reshape, tamp down, and mold toward a more reasonable individual settlement for Ruffin. Off went my morning's daydream of advocacy in the late afternoon Saturday mail. Together, Ruffin and I walked it down to the Post Office.

I turned to the planning of our summer nursery school that Sunday afternoon. I had Seamus look at my garage. With his power-washer could he blast out all the cobwebs and dirt? With his power-sprayer could he lay down a couple of thick layers of non-toxic latex white paint to lighten up the inside? Could he install some rudimentary lighting overhead? Could we round up some salvage carpet squares and the right adhesive to lay them in patches over the cold concrete floor?

I checked with Julie and Lisa about where to find good second-hand plastic playground equipment and called RoJene to see if she would like to bring Chance over every weekday this summer to teach.

Our plan was that when school let out in two months, Ruffin would be doing his hardest work, his CARD drills, in the morning while he was fresh, and playing all afternoon in our remodeled garage and backyard pre-school with five or more typically developing girls and Chance, under RoJene's supervision as my certified teacher.

Meg reported to me on Ruffin's progress over the last week or so toward his IEP goal of counting and making sets. Ruffin had been out of it with no concentration, looking off into space, spaced out, distracted, and playing with the objects and not concentrating all last week and again on Monday. By Tuesday, she had moved on to his IEP goal of Ruffin telling whether some school activity, such as gym, music, or speech occurred yesterday, or today, or would occur tomorrow, and had concluded that he seemed upset by these questions about time, was unable to respond, and was "not ready for this yet."

Inge, Emily, and Kim were scheduled by Bridgewater to present in late March at Sue Baker's Clear Lake meeting about Lovaas. I had been invited, too, but unfortunately, I had an evidentiary hearing and was unable to go. It would be easier to call Dr. Tristram Smith afterwards to get his account of how both the late March and the early

April meetings had gone. I focused on the meeting in Clear Lake where Inge, Emily, and Kim had presented, since Sue had been unable to videotape it.

Tris had found the audience of special educators friendly, until Kim approached him at lunch to ask if a child who had a diagnosis of PDD rather than classic autism, and who was a mild case, really needed an intensive Lovaas program. Tris explained to her, "Yes, but such a child might complete treatment sooner than two years." So, Bridgewater had been favored with an informed third opinion.

Tris had also been questioned about how much it would be possible to back off the hours of programming and still get the same results. He had been pressed to defend the measure of intensity — of 40 hours per week — supported by his and Dr. Lovaas's published research and by the latest reports of other researchers such as Dr. Sallows in Wisconsin.

He had also been asked, "What happens if you just put these children into ECSE classrooms?" Tris had pointed to the control groups in his and Dr. Lovaas's 1987 and 1993 studies who hadn't done very well in California special education programs. When given toys and group encouragement, they had not learned much.

Kim had protested from the floor, "That's not always clear."

Inge, Emily, and Kim's presentation that afternoon never mentioned Ruffin, his early delays, or his recent progress. Inge described and dismissed Evelyn's November workshop at my home as a mere reminder to her of well-known behavior management techniques and how to work on teaching abstract language. Tris thought she had damned Lovaas with faint praise.

Emily offered an account of her trip with Kim to Los Angeles. Oddly enough, Tris found her the most positive of the three, focusing in on the psychological aspects of the research, but discussing Dr. Lovaas's 1987 paper as dating back to 1967. Tris found that amusing — nearly a Freudian slip — since it had taken Dr. Lovaas from the early 1960s to the late 1980s to develop his methods and document their success by publication of his data in peer-reviewed scientific journals.

But it was Kim who had really ripped into our project. Tris thought she seemed overwhelmed by the Los Angeles conference, openly questioning whether Dr. Lovaas had included speech and language pathologists like herself on his UCLA research-group staff, or whether he collaborated with her cherished discipline. She claimed "discrete trial training" was passe. "It used to be done, but now we ought to teach more naturalistically." She questioned whether college students and laypeople, including parents, could do the professional work of qualified speech therapists.

Kim conceded that intensive treatment might be called for in cases of severe autism, but not for those who were more mildly affected. She trotted out a remark attributed to Dr. Norman that "pneumonia and the common cold might fall on the same spectrum of infection, but they didn't call for the same treatment." Tris found Dr. Norman's quoted remark shocking. As Ruffin's mother, I had always been more concerned that a little cold might develop into pneumonia.

Kim caviled too against the lack of developmental sequence or the full coverage of all developmental domains in Lovaas's early drills, claiming they might teach a child to rote-count, without being able to grasp number concepts in any functional way. She imagined that children so treated would grow up to be "little robots."

Of the four AEA presentations about their experiences with home Lovaas programming, Bridgewater's was the sole negative. Loess Hills, treating the little girl in Council Bluffs; Heartland, treating two boys working with Inge's counterpart there, Marion McQuaid; and a presentation by St. Ambrose College in Davenport, treating Chris Foster's son all gave positive and enthusiastic video presentations. The ironies didn't escape me. Every one of those programs, valued by all the other AEAs, could be traced to Sue referring a family to me for information and assistance from Dr. Granpeesheh and Evelyn — both of whom had trained with Dr. Lovaas and Tris at UCLA.

Finally, Tris said Sue had presented in a supportive manner, while confessing that she was unsure how to proceed statewide. Financing should not be a real issue because families would be able to rely on trained non-professionals. She did discuss funding alternatives and passed out her own and my written resource materials, including copies of Catherine Maurice's 1993 book, *Let Me Hear Your Voice,* in boxes — one for each AEA's regional special education library.

Meanwhile, Mr. Montague sent Inge's assignment back to her with his corrections. He had scribbled out Inge's final paragraph, which might have seemed to him — as it certainly did to me — to contain a legally damaging admission. "Because Ruffin has experienced such rapid growth during the 1994-1995 school year, the team recommends that his IEP be concluded in May of 1995." Mr. Montague let Inge know that he expected to see a final clean copy from her soon.

Sue Baker had invited our local support group to attend a long afternoon meeting about auditory integration training (AIT). We managed to arrange for six hours of babysitting so we could all drive down to her chosen venue.

Although Sue and I had been working together closely over the phone for the better part of a year, this visit of hers to our region would provide the first opportunity for us to meet in person. She seemed to be the large woman, with a broad face, a wide smile under a mop of wiry hair, bustling and fussing over the audio-visual equipment, trying to be a friendly presence, and still defer to her local autism resource team (ART) members, Ryan Duffy, a Bridgewater school psychologist, and Dot Gordon, both from Decorah.

I kept my greeting to a quick hello. I imagined Sue and I would have time to visit afterwards. Ryan and Dot were anxious that their meeting start and end on time. So were we, all the travelling parents.

For a couple of hours, Ryan and Dot droned on through their agenda about the history and current professional opinions concerning auditory integration training (AIT), passing out a list of resources and position papers, both positive and negative, but none of the primary materials — most of which we parents were already familiar with — since members of our group had reported back with books, papers, and videos after attending last fall's conference on AIT at Gundersen.

Transparency after transparency went up with, "Oh, sorry, no time for questions. We need to keep this moving."

Finally, we came to the real point of this meeting. Ryan and Dot wanted to be able to *study* our children's behavior both before and after the AIT treatment our group had arranged to take place in early June in the attic of my home. Bridgewater hoped each parent would complete four written behavioral surveys for Sue — one before treatment and three others after treatment, each month through next September.

The parents attending were more than a bit disgusted that we were not being offered anything for the privilege of being studied — no audiograms, and no financial participation by Bridgewater. After sitting captive for hours, no one held back very much at the end. The mood of the meeting changed to something approaching rump ugly.

Sue, Ryan, and Dot seemed bewildered and suddenly in a hurry to get on the road back to Iowa City and Decorah. I managed to catch Sue briefly at the door on our way out to ask if she would send me copies of all the primary materials from the list that had been handed out.

"I'd be happy to copy them at my office to circulate to the other parents," I offered.

Sue looked at me, nodded, and ducked out through the door to her car.

So, our AIT meeting broke up in disappointment and anger. None of the parents by then gathered as a knot in the parking lot cared much for the thoughtless exploitation of this exercise. We were not pleased. And we were more determined than ever to go forward as a group with our planned experiment with AIT in June.

CHAPTER TWENTY FOUR

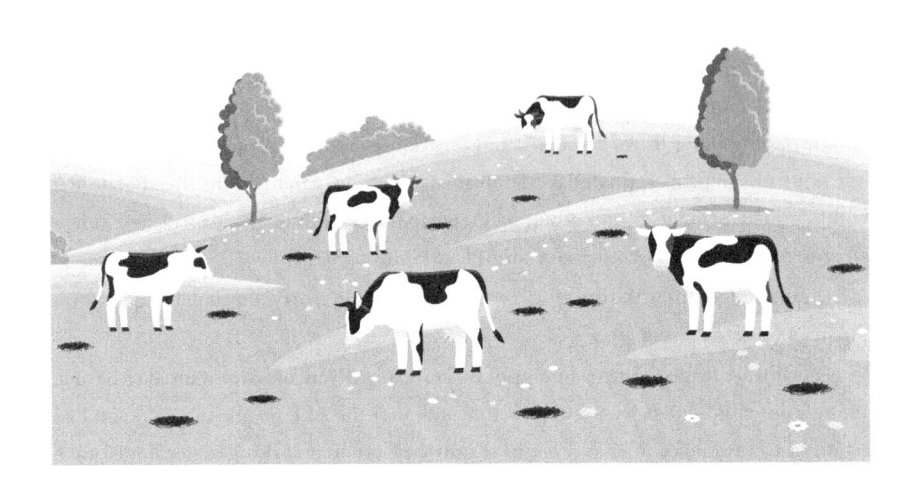

WET COW-PIES

There was a bomb sitting in my mailbox — from the school authorities. It came typed in large, bolded print on heavy laid and vanilla-creamy paper. I didn't need to sign for it, but all this heaviness seemed meant to intimidate. Mr. Montague had written to me and Curt submitting a proposed educational plan for Ruffin — from our local school district (ACSD) and Bridgewater. Everyone concerned was politely copied in.

I had to admire Curt's strategy as I read the document's *Preamble*. By simply reading this, Curt and I would be able to gather both valuable legal admissions and the functional equivalent of "discovery." What do those with whom you found yourself in disagreement think? Without knowing this, it would be more difficult to move effectively toward compromise.

Although there might be internal disagreements between, say, Mr. Montague, who might want to extend me a secret olive branch, and Miss Hobbs, who wanted to steadfastly defend her new special education program to her superintendent and school board, their two agencies were joined at the hip in their legal responsibility to Ruffin.

Because of Curt's gambit, the two agencies were forced to present a single face to me in mediation or litigation. As in any case of *joint* legal responsibility, each agency stood at risk of paying for the legal slipups of the other. The two school agencies acknowledged this as "a joint responsibility to provide special education services to Ruffin White. These obligations are set forth in existing IDEA Regulations and the current Iowa Rules of Special Education."

Curt and I both knew that was not the half of it. The governing laws of special education were found in federal statutes, the *Individuals with Disabilities Education Act* (IDEA), *Section 504 of the Rehabilitation Act*, and the *Americans with Disabilities Act*, all written and passed by Congress. The U.S. Department of Education then proposed and adopted rules binding on the states in the *Code of Federal Regulations*, with interpretative *Comments*. Written to conform to the *Code of Federal Regulations*, Iowa's laws of special education were passed by the Iowa Legislature, and the State Department of Education issued the *Iowa Rules of Special Education* which were published in the *Iowa Administrative Code*. The AEAs also issued thick, printed binders of procedures and rules that differed from region to region. Local school boards passed their own rules, too, that differed from time to time. So, special education law inhabited a shifting, messy five-story house — under constant reconstruction.

For Ruffin, time was moving quickly beneath him. He was now a swiftly moving target. His language development was running now at a pace twice that of a typically developing child. With our experience of Ruffin so quickly surpassing his original August 1994 IEP goals, there was no realistic way to plan in March of 1995 for the Ruffin he might be in the far-off August of 1996.

Dr. Granpeesheh and I had planned from the beginning of Ruffin's home program that Evelyn would visit us on a quarterly basis over his two years of treatment — to assure that our home program kept up with him, continued to challenge him, never bored him, or wasted any of his precious early developmental time. We were aiming for him to enter a mainstream classroom before his expected entry into kindergarten. This individualized aspect of Ruffin's potential was something his educators needed to become nimble enough to accommodate.

Far and away the best disclosure in this passage of the educators' most recent settlement offer was learning exactly who Curt and I needed to deal with as the real decision-makers: Mr. Lord for ACSD and Mr. Montague for Bridgewater — the two administrators at such high remove from Ruffin's small world as never to have taken the opportunity to visit us, or ever meet him, as far as I knew.

The 1995 EYSE Issue

1. Ruffin was evaluated for EYSE by the staffing team during December of 1994 to determine critical skills for EYSE. Ruffin does not qualify for EYSE under the existing Iowa Rule. However, the team does feel that Ruffin would benefit from some structured instructional and socialization activities during the summer months, and are therefore, recommending the following:

> A. To ensure that Ruffin's progress continues over the summer it will be important for him to continue to have group experiences. Specific options are being explored including Ruffin's possible participation in the summer experience program offered by the local group home for the disabled, or a play group set up by his mother.

That was a straightforward admission of one aspect of Ruffin's educational needs over the summer. His interaction with other children lay at the heart of every critical skill I had proposed we track over his Christmas holiday school break. But neither placement option had been nailed down yet. There was no firm offer to provide either group as a part of Ruffin's *free* appropriate public education, and no offer to *pay* for either group.

So, what *was* their offer?

> B. From Ruffin's IEP for 1995-96 critical skills must be identified that will be used in the fall of 1995 to evaluate Ruffin's qualification under (a) of Rule 41.17(8) of the Iowa Rules of Special Education. This rule will be the guideline to determine Ruffin's qualification for EYSE in the summer of 1996.

This legal-sounding gobbledygook seemed to be designed to kill two summers of Ruffin's EYSE entitlement with one stone — a single 15-month-long IEP that somehow encompassed both the summer of 1995 and of 1996. Under this proposed scheme, Ruffin's critical skills were not to be identified until *after* whatever he might receive as services for the first summer.

Then, to qualify under the specified part "a" of the carefully cited Iowa EYSE rule, Ruffin would need to show regression over the summer of 1995. This scheme was ripe for manipulation to foreclose any EYSE services for the summer of 1996.

It also sought to limit Ruffin's right to establish his need for EYSE under other parts of the rule, specifically part "b" regarding his uniqueness — as a child with autism on a rapid road to a mainstream classroom. Wickedly clever, I thought, but this failed to honor the spirit of the IDEA or the Congressional intentions in enacting it. Niggardly was the ugly word for it.

Then, a bit of a bomb went off.

C. As a pilot project for the summer of 1995 only, assigned to Ruffin White only, the AEA will hire an aide currently trained in "Lovaas" to work with Ruffin in structured group activities associated with the Medicaid Waiver/ACSD project, and/or a home program set up by Mary Jane White in the afternoon. The period of employment will not exceed 5 hours a day for 5 days a week. Terms of employment will be coordinated with the starting or ending of the above program.

This amounted to an offer to pay for 25 hours of educational services per week for the summer — to offer more services to Ruffin than had ever been offered to any child in our multi-county autism support group over any earlier summer. It looked like an offer to hire either Donna or Lisa to help Ruffin enter the mainstream.

It might be too much to ask Donna and Lisa to work with Ruffin in the morning on his one-to-one CARD drills, and then ask them to work all afternoon to help mainstream him into a 5- or 6-child playgroup. When I discussed this with Donna and Lisa, they each thought so, too. Their own one-to-one work was very demanding and required careful recordkeeping during Ruffin's brief trampoline breaks. It was physically and mentally exhausting, which was why Donna and Lisa ordinarily divided a day's work of CARD drills between them.

I had another concern. Was this crack in the façade something I ought to share with my autism support group? It presented me with a personal dilemma. While every detail of special education was supposed to be cloaked with *confidentiality* — a legal protection written into the IDEA with the best of intentions — to protect the privacy and dignity of the student with disabilities and his or her family — frequently *the observance of confidentiality* was a pavement straight to hell.

School authorities were able to keep news about what they might be willing to do for the child of a demanding parent from the parents of similarly situated children with similar disabilities. *Confidentiality's* shield became a convenient excuse used by school authorities not to share the availability of needed services. But I knew that everywhere in the law, *confidentiality* was subject to *waiver* — right along with the right to remain silent, or the right to a jury trial — rights of constitutional dimension that criminal defendants gave up routinely to acknowledge guilt when entering a guilty plea.

Could I look anyone in my support group — my newest friends — in the eye and keep this offer to Ruffin a secret? If I disclosed it, what did I really disclose to them about Ruffin? Every single one of them already knew Ruffin had an autism diagnosis. That was how we came to be friends.

No mention was made, nor any consideration given to Ruffin's continuing speech delay at the 20th percentile, or his general knowledge delay at the 30th percentile, or how, if at all, to address these accumulated developmental deficits so recently reported by Kim.

Any consideration of Ruffin's CARD drill program seemed to have been evaded. In this respect, Curt's gambit got us no further along than my earlier requests. By then, the death knell to my request for one-to-one CARD drills ever being incorporated into Ruffin's special education rang in as no surprise.

The remainder of Ruffin's ECSE programming should continue to occur in the ECSE classroom. In this setting Ruffin will have the opportunity to learn and have reinforced many skills that occur during regular programming. These skills and concepts are outlined below.

Time for some jujitsu thinking. How could I use this latest "no" to Ruffin's advantage? As I continued to read, I discovered what followed was a long description of exactly how Meg ran her ECSE classroom.

From Inge's early draft in Ruffin's educational file, I could see that she had been responsible for including it, and for taking the time to write it out in exquisite detail. Here was something I could share with RoJene as a template for our daily play group's routine in our garage classroom this summer and share with other parents in my effort to recruit a smaller group of typically developing girls — as recommended by Dr. Granpeesheh and Evelyn — to form the sort of summer mainstream group setting Ruffin needed to be driven to communicate.

Thank you, Inge, it was a structure.

When I showed it to RoJene it was all familiar to her as a teacher certified to teach Ruffin's age group. She was ready and willing to meet with Evelyn when she returned for Mother's Day in May to learn from her what more and what exactly she would need to do to support Ruffin's *integration* into a small, select group of friendly, chatty little girls and Chance.

The mail also brought a breath of fresh air now and then with the new season. A thank you note came from Clear Lake, from a speech and language pathologist on Northern Trails' autism resource team (ART) for my funding memo and the Maurice book. Northern Trails and the local school district responsible went on to provide and pay for a home drill program for another CARD family, agreeably, and without cavil.

There were always a few nice local people, too, reaching out to help, under the administrative radar, like Mrs. Wonderlich at the junior high school, to whom I owed a thank you note for sending me Sarah, Heather, and Tina. They had become cheerful and diligent workers on our project of providing research and related materials to families and professionals who contacted my office. "Enclosed is a gift certificate for pizza for them to enjoy." Since requests continued to pour in, I asked if she could send me a new team in the fall.

Despite these momentary uplifts, I was feeling deeply discouraged by our latest IEP meeting for Ruffin, and by what I had heard from Dr. Tristram Smith about Inge, Emily, and Kim at Sue's statewide meeting. Deflated, set back on my heels. I had to be tired. Donna and Lisa could use a break, too, to get over the flu, get healthy, and spend an uninterrupted spring break with their own children and families. I called Evelyn and she and I decided to call a halt and not have Ruffin work through spring break, as he had over Christmastime.

For two weeks then, Ruffin and I travelled back to North Carolina to visit my parents. I wanted them to see for themselves the good changes in Ruffin's behavior, his growth, and language development. I needed to know they would have my financial back for the upcoming summer. As a rule, the law business slowed down for the summer. Mounting a summer school experience for Ruffin while hosting ten days of auditory integration training (AIT) in my attic were going to be expensive and disruptive.

Ruffin handled the long two-day drive to North Carolina well enough. We were able to run between snowstorms and the sleet still sweeping the plains. Having outrun the one at our backs, we stopped for supper at The Red Hen in Mahomet, Illinois. I detached Ruffin and his car seat, as a single unit, and carried him in under one arm, under his blue blanket. That woke him up, but he wasn't free to run around, or run off, as I plopped him down on a red vinyl bench beneath a clouded window. I needed hot food, without a scene, and without having to make any explanation beyond asking for chocolate milk, please, for Ruffin's vitamin bottle.

We travelled down to our family's rented vacation spot at Myrtle Beach to celebrate Ruffin's fourth birthday there on April 9th. It was fine to watch Ruffin running down to the waterline, running back ahead of a breaking wave, turning to investigate small breathing holes in the wet margins. He wore himself out, running this pattern over and over, while my parents and I talked about money. Together, we worked up a budget for the 91 days of Ruffin's coming summer: $17,448.

Back in Iowa, the mail continued to pile up. Sue had written, responding to my earlier out-the-door request for copies of all the auditory integration training (AIT) resources in Ryan and Dot's handouts. She sent three recent articles, together with a parent-author's description of how to condition our children to wear headphones for the extended periods of time needed to administer the treatment.

Then Sue's letter took a measured turn — speaking as an advocate who had spent a long time in the trenches — to me, the newest, impatient autism parent on her horizon. "Your group has much energy to channel towards improving services you feel are appropriate for your children and your area. . . .. Your group might consider becoming a chapter, with an invitation to send a member to sit on the Board of Directors, as another option for sharing your concerns with the Society."

I needed to call Sue for contact information. I didn't imagine sharing this idea that we parents all pitch in *more* was going to fly with my beleaguered friends whose experience had been the Society had never been very helpful to any of them over the years since their older children had been diagnosed. When I paused to consider my own true feelings about this suggestion, I was more than a little miffed. Having to organize a summer nursery school that Ruffin needed, it wasn't like I had nothing better to do.

Sue's letter ended on a discouraging note. "The Bridgewater auditory integration training (AIT) study may take additional efforts to coordinate and sift out confounding treatment techniques which will be a focus for the months ahead. Attributing any results to the AIT procedure itself concerns me."

Several members of our parent group had been working hard to schedule our children's AIT treatments over ten days in early June — just after school let out. There was no way any of us were going to *focus for the months ahead.* Or wait for Ryan and Dot to morph into rigorous scientific investigators. Nor were we going to allow them to divide our children into treatment and control groups or require us to suspend *other confounding therapies.*

As always, Sue left the door open for me to call. So, I did. As it turned out, it would have been better had I waited. I opened her letter, after a long cross-country drive. My temper was short. After jotting down the contact information I needed, I unloaded, outlining, and ruminating over the details of the school authorities' most recent written offer for Ruffin, and passing along every negative remark from our local autism parent-group.

In high dungeon, I snapped our conversation to a wicked close. "Just *when* may I expect the courtesy of your written reply to my unanswered letter of a month ago?"

In late March, here came Sue's courteous, but clipped reply to my late February questions about her *Fact Sheet on Lovaas Behavioral Therapy*. It made clear she had no more information than had been published last fall in *The Advocate* interview. Sue had no more special access to knowledge than I did. She provided a published academic article by Schopler, Short, and Mesibov she had cited.

"This is belated, but we did discuss my busy schedule."

I had hurt Sue's feelings.

It was a poisonous thought to imagine myself as some sort of hero. Seamus had been right on that score. Advocacy was a pipe dream I needed to let go of to meet Ruffin's immediate needs this summer.

I needed to drive across a couple of counties to attend a brief court hearing. It occurred to me as I turned my gaze out over every newly green pasture along my route, that every one of them was sprinkled with wet cow-pies. It had always been a delicate matter for me to cross such a pasture — and manage to keep both of my feet clean.

CHAPTER TWENTY FIVE

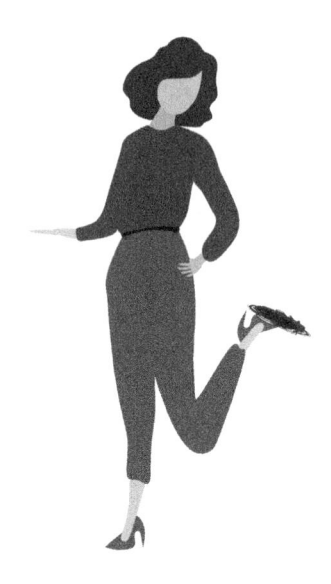

PUTTING MY FOOT IN IT

Another letter arrived from Dot Gordon, like as not prompted by Sue. "Some of the items on our list of auditory integration training (AIT) references are not available to me. I'm sure that you could get any of the books through inter-library loan." Well, Happy April Fools' Day! I slapped my knee and sent Dot's missive flying across my living-room office. This was our Bridgewater autism resource team (ART) — boldly citing sources they had lectured us about — but had obviously never read. I was still pacing around my dining room office, laughing, and choking in a fit of outrage when the phone rang.

It was Curt. I needed to get a hold of myself. He was barely over the flu, croaking in a low whisper. We needed to put together our overdue offer of settlement for Ruffin. I was the over-emotional client, ready to listen, to trust Curt, and be persuaded. The schools' most recent offer didn't meet the legal benchmark of "appropriateness." Curt agreed that to accept it for Ruffin would not materially advance our shared aim of making peaceful state-wide change in the education of young children with autism. We would work from *inside the state's mediation system* should the school authorities refuse our offer — now that Curt knew *who* to write — Mr. Montague and Mr. Lord — as the real decision-makers. He warned me this might take all summer. After talking about money with my parents, I was prepared for that.

Curt sounded hopeful he could settle the case in Mason City and wanted to do that first. I could appreciate that a high, early benchmark settlement might lead to our having a fair opportunity to settle with Bridgewater and my local district later. Curt could be aggressive, and planned to be, in his settlement demands there, he explained, because the child had moved out-of-state with his mother, eliminating the possibility of the schools retaliating against him and his family. The possibility of retaliation against a child and his family had never occurred to me. Curt explained it was frequent enough, as well as illegal under *Section 504 of the Rehabilitation Act.*

Dr. Hagen had assigned Dee Ann Wilson to mediate the Mason City case. Yes, the same person whom I had offended by writing to her as "Dianne." "Don't worry about that, Mary Jane," Curt assured me, "Dee Ann can get past that." I wasn't so sure, but then, I didn't know her; Curt did.

Curt's offer on Ruffin's behalf cracked me up when it arrived. It read just like Curt spoke, whether in court, on the phone, in a meeting, or over coffee. He began with the execution of a perfect pirouette — before falling on his own sword for me, his restless client.

"I was lately stricken with a pernicious and malicious flu, and, as a consequence, I have caused a delay in your settlement negotiations with Mary Jane White. I am truly sorry.

"I am pleased, however, that Mary Jane has put such a high premium on cooperation over confrontation, in the enclosed Offer of Settlement. While the settlement is not cheap, it is very reasonable, and I firmly believe that it would be in your best interests to accept it. The reasons are threefold.

"First as the cases in our booklet reveal, Mary Jane has a viable claim for the very substantial reimbursement items submitted to you at our last meeting. If this matter is forced to hearing, Mary Jane could easily recover sums two to three times larger than the costs of her proposed settlement.

"Second if this matter is forced to hearing, it is apt to be one of the most difficult and protracted in the history of special education in Iowa. As cases from other jurisdictions reveal, the proper prosecution of the issues requires substantial expert witness testimony, and I personally believe that the attorney fees on each side could run into the tens of thousands of dollars. If Mary Jane prevailed, as I personally believe she would, the school and the AEA would be liable for *her* attorney's fees as well as your own. The attorney fees alone could readily exceed the cost of her proposed settlement. At this juncture, the matter can be resolved amicably without paying any fees.

"Finally, our agency is working hard to find and promote proactive methods of securing financing for Lovaas-type training for young children with autism and developmental disorders. We believe that parents and schools, AEAs and advocates, must work together to make that financing viable — and that a decision *forcing* the financing of Lovaas would therefore be counter-productive in the long run. The State Department of Education has concurred in this reasoning, and I sincerely hope that you do as well."

I leaned back in my office chair, closed my eyes, and let an image run backward of all the money I was letting go rush over the dam. When I opened my eyes, I used the meaty parts of my palms to wipe away a few tears, picked up my fountain pen, signed our offer, and faxed it off to Curt, for him to deliver.

Then the wait began. Barring delay, we could hope to hear something back by early May — plenty of time to reconvene Ruffin's IEP meeting to consider again what Ruffin needed this summer, I imagined, as I consoled myself.

Two days after Curt's offer, Mr. Montague engaged Bridgewater's attorney, Mr. Allan J. Carew, a leading partner in what passed then for a large, partnership firm in Iowa. The firm dated back to 1854 and in the 1990s, consisted of five country-club, Catholic gentlemen, headquartered in Dubuque, an old, redbrick river town, long the seat of our Archdiocese, just a couple hours' south down the Mississippi for local gamblers bored with our smaller riverboat casino, and a bit beyond my own usual nine-county practice area.

I had run across Mr. Carew from time to time in our northeast Iowa courthouses, since his firm practiced widely, ranging into both Wisconsin and Illinois where its excellent reputation preceded him. Always, he entered our small, local chambers moving with his tall grey gravitas, ducking his head through the low doorways. He was a man fully at ease in his suit, tie, and the pair of flashing wingtips he crossed, using the long fingers of one hand to free up any fabric momentarily strained over his knee. I had never seen him carry more than a slender file in his other hand — just a few pages he might offer across the desk to our judge after waiting his turn and speaking his piece.

Mr. Montague and "Moe" would be visiting him together. They complained, "The focus of their proposal is the payment of money as opposed to our providing a program for Ruffin." I would have expected Mr. Carew to be able to offer Mr. Montague a more nuanced reading than this of Curt's and my offer, including my willingness to let

$34,000 go unreimbursed. But this was how our offer struck Mr. Montague, and how it pained him. "We feel we have acted properly in providing services to Ruffin. We feel we should proceed on to a due process hearing. However, prior to making a final decision, we feel we should discuss this matter with you in detail." They offered a document to give Mr. Carew all the background information to help him in advising them. That document compared Ruffin's diagnosis, evaluations, education, and CARD treatment to that of Bernard Smith in California.

Meanwhile, I was surprised by a call from a woman who re-introduced herself as one of the teachers for the private nursery school that Inge and I had visited earlier that spring. As a result of Miss Hobbs having asked their board of directors to admit him without regard to the usual lottery process, Ruffin would be welcome to attend next fall. However, to accept Ruffin's place, I needed to pay his registration fee and next school year's first month's tuition now. It seemed like a pittance. "I can run right down. See you in a minute." This was the best use I could make of my parents' birthday check for Ruffin and all the quarters from my change jar.

I was caught up enough on law office business by mid-April to let Curt know. "This is encouraging, but I've heard nothing directly from the school district, so I am concerned that the district may be getting me out of their hair by passing Ruffin on to be someone else's problem. Also, this is inconsistent with their pending late March offer to place Ruffin in their ECSE classroom for the foreseeable future.

"I did register Ruffin to attend the private nursery school in the fall on Monday, Wednesday, and Friday afternoons. Would it be possible for you to ask whether the public-school authorities plan to 1) pay the nursery school tuition, and 2) provide transportation to this private school placement that Miss Hobbs arranged, and that I have accepted for Ruffin? Can you also seek assurance that Ruffin will be able to attend ACSD on Tuesdays and Thursdays next fall?"

Meanwhile, Kim had re-tested Ruffin using the *Expressive One-Word Picture Vocabulary Test — Revised*, the same test Ms. Wilding at UIHC had been unable to score him on back in January because Ruffin had insisted on the word *clock* and would not be persuaded to produce the word *watch*. Kim's score sheet credited Ruffin with coming up with the right words for pictures of *bird, eyes, swing, train, apple, watch, bus, duck,* and *kite*, words most 2-year-olds can come up with; as well as *wagon, scissors, leaf, chickens, tiger, wheel, corn,* and *sofa,* with Ruffin offering *dolphin* for the picture of *a penguin* and *horses* for the picture of *a merry-go-round,* words most 3- to 3-and-a-half-year-olds can offer; *footprints, goat, suitcase, computer, animals, peanut,* and *computer* again for the picture of *a typewriter, fire come* for the picture of *a fireplace, cloth* for *clothing,* words most 3-and-a-half to 4-and-a-half-year-olds know to say, and *painting.* Donna painted.

Then as one might expect of a child with autism, Ruffin offered names he knew of concrete examples when presented with pictures meant to prompt a typically developing child of 5-and-a-half to 6-years-old to come up with group nouns: *apples* for *fruit, Jesus* for *statues, bee* for *bugs, girls and boys* for *children,* and *a building* for *walls.*

Using just this test of nouns, Kim was able to re-score Ruffin's developmental language age as the equivalent of 3 years, 7 months (a 5-month delay) placing him then at the 34th percentile rank of language development for his cohort of 4-year-old peers. It was another snapshot test, and I liked the trend — continuing rapid language development over the 8 months since August. By this same measure — Ruffin had managed to mitigate 11- to 13-months of his original 16- to 18-month language delay. Kim's assessment as a speech and language pathologist confirmed my untutored, personal impression, and my own mother's more experienced opinion as a trained classroom teacher expressed while she smiled from her beach chair.

As the sun came out in Iowa, while Curt and I were waiting out the time until early May, I succumbed to the sirens singing to me of state and nationwide advocacy. Since their Lovaas research and case law booklet's publication in early February, I let Joan know I had dozens of unfilled orders from all over the country. I needed a lot more copies.

Mr. Montague responded to the attorney Mr. Carew during the third week in April. "Enclosed you will find additional materials which I have assembled for you on Ruffin White. I have focused upon the early evaluation materials done by Bridgewater and other agencies and included the consultation materials from Dr. Sallows (pro- Lovaas), and the UIHC (pro-Bridgewater and ACSD?)."

Mr. Carew had assigned Mr. Montague and his right-hand man "Moe," some homework. Here they were turning it in. He must have let them know, as I always let my own clients know, that no lawyer could really help without having all the facts and the evidence. Turning a worrisome matter over to a lawyer didn't mean you didn't have to think about it anymore. Engaging a lawyer usually meant the client had just taken on a second job — rounding up, organizing, and handing in a coherent account of all the facts within reach.

That was not all Mr. Montague had sent. "You will also note a book of judicial and ALJ case interpretations which has been assembled by Curt Sytsma of Iowa Protection and Advocacy Services, Inc. and has been distributed widely in the state to parents and others interested in advocating for autism. It is not an encouraging piece of work if you are a public agency planning a case against Lovaas." This was exactly how Curt, Joan, and I had hoped their booklet would be used and read, and exactly how we hoped it would find its way into the offices of those members of the bar who advised school authorities.

"I have had time to reflect upon our conversation with you last week. I have also talked with Mr. Lord. We are still of the opinion that we have done what the law is asking us to do in this matter, and if we are to pay any dollars related to this case, we should be told to do so through the due process appeal procedures. (Reference: *Burlington School Committee v. Department of Education of Massachusetts*, U.S. Supreme Court, 105 S. Ct. 1996 (1985) (Enclosed)."

I couldn't imagine the Mr. Carew I had glimpsed slipping in and out of chambers was thrilled to receive a legal tutorial. Certainly not when *Burlington* was a case of considerably older vintage than the newer controlling case, *Shannon Carter*, also from the U.S. Supreme Court.

Mr. Montague had continued, dithering and whining, as an unsatisfied client pleading his case — just as I had — to his own counsel. "I keep asking myself: What did we do that was in error? Is the ACSD program an inferior program for Ruffin White just because it is not using the Lovaas method in the classroom as it is being used at home? Outside of the mother, who has gone on record as specifically recommending the Lovaas method for Ruffin White in the classroom? What are the pronged tests to be used to determine what constitutes an appropriate program? I always felt the standard set forth in *Rowley v. Board of Education*, U.S. Supreme Court, 458 U.S. 176, 182 S. Ct. 3834 (1982) provided that test. I believe we are meeting that standard in this case. You will recall we have prevailed in other cases using that standard to point out we have provided an appropriate program for students. How is this case different? If so, what is the new standard?"

Mr. Montague's last question was fair enough.

Shannon Carter set out the newer rule requiring the award of substantial reimbursement to parents who had provided uncertified but appropriate special education to their children when school authorities had failed to meet the legal mark of "appropriateness" — failing the children, their families, and the law as written by Congress.

Mr. Montague and Mr. Lord seemed hot to trot. "As for our coming up with a list of expert witnesses for our side, there are several possibilities whom we might consider in addition to our own people. They are: the people from UIHC who did Ruffin's most recent evaluation; Sue Baker, Iowa Autism Resource Task Force; Gerry Gritzmacher, Consultant, Bureau of Special Education; maybe Dr. Lyle Chastain, Minneapolis, Minnesota. Albeit, these are not as powerful as Ivar Lovaas, they are persons who are familiar with the program being provided for Ruffin White.

"What kind of a response are we going to make to their settlement offer, and when? This cannot be done until you and Mr. David Hunter, the attorney for ACSD, have talked with each other. Any thoughts on this? What is our next move?"

Meanwhile, Meg reported her last two weeks' work on Ruffin's IEP goal to answer three different "wh" questions for each picture she presented to him. By the end of two weeks, he had been able to offer brief answers to "who," "what," and "when" while still struggling with "where" and "why."

It was time to make up with Sue, to try to re-open the possibility of working together on auditory integration training (AIT) and keep her in the loop about developments in Ruffin's case. I let her know where I would be staying for the Society conference, hoping to meet up with her again there. I signed off, "Counting myself among the most impatient, your thoughts on avoiding problems would be appreciated."

But, at that juncture, I was so angry and resentful about our recent auditory integration training meeting and the upcoming summer, I wondered if I could ever bring myself to really mean it.

As wonderfully sympathetic and helpful as Curt had been, some of his passing remarks about Ruffin's appearance upset me too. I needed to let him know. "I've wanted to run down a medical book citation to share with you." Curt and I both knew that if a proper legal foundation were laid, such a medical treatise could be admitted as evidence in due process.

"Consider that until the stereotypies take over a child's behavior, until the 'light' of intelligence goes out of their faces, until mental retardation is fully acquired by a child with autism as a result of inappropriate education, many look very normal. In fact, there are many passing comments in the medical literature about the exceptional, even poignant beauty of these children's faces and the grace of their gestures. The comments are made against a background expectation, not at all counter-intuitive, that such a profound and until now intractable disability would carry some early outward manifestation by way of physical deformity.

"Why would this common expectation be wrong in the case of autism, particularly in cases of high-functioning autism or Asperger syndrome cases — like Ruffin? A good answer is suggested in the enclosed pages (303-305) from *The Biology of the Autistic Syndromes*. 'The face and body are fully formed during the first trimester. If the insult which causes autism attacks the fetus in the second trimester when brain development is crucially involved, then the face and body may be normal, intact, beautiful, and non-stigmatized, while the neurons of the brain migrating later in development may be badly and invisibly scrambled."

Ruffin had suffered many second trimester insults — premature labor, medications to halt it prescribed in high doses, a bacterial and viral infection triggering his premature birth near the end of the second trimester. "This point may be an important one to make in Ruffin's case to meet any naïve observations that 'Ruffin doesn't have autism,' or the argument that 'there is nothing much wrong with Ruffin' since he appears so unimpaired and attractive on the surface, and since he is now so very much better because of appropriate intervention."

CHAPTER TWENTY SIX

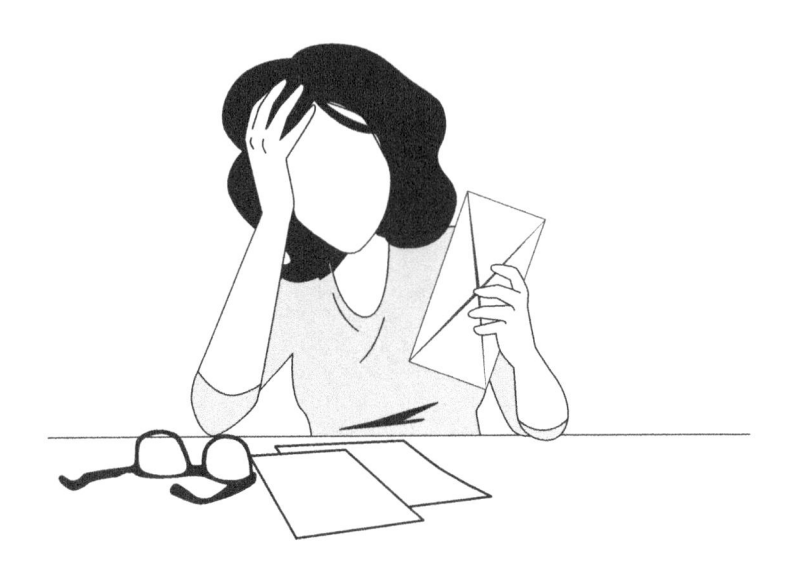

DO YOU HAVE A FAX?

Dr. Norman called Meg again at school in late April. He got more information out of her than I did.

"Ruffin is making good progress. He speaks in full sentences with much less echolalia and odd inflections. He exhibits some 'self-stimming' or self-stimulating behavior with facial grimaces — lots at home — only once at school. Meg thinks this behavior accompanies imaginary play and self-talk.

"Mom has still refused to sign Ruffin's IEP. She wanted to have the school district and herself submit proposals. Apparently, Mom is not happy with their proposal.

"Meg is now having Head Start kids into her classroom two days a week. Ruffin is getting along fine with them, especially in more structured activities. Ruffin is refusing by using 'No,' more often. He has developed a friendship with good play at the three-year-old level.

"Mom is trying to set up a play group for the summer. Also, Ruffin is set up to attend a Monday, Wednesday, Friday afternoon private nursery school with home Lovaas on the mornings of those days. Tuesday and Thursday all day ECSE with afternoon reverse integration. Friday morning some one-to-one with college students.

"Mom wants the school to pay for Lovaas drills this summer and next year and for the playgroup. School district does not want to pay for Lovaas or the summer playgroup but did offer to have Meg consult to the mother's summer program. Mom has Curt Sytsma, attorney for Iowa P&A on her case at this point."

That Dr. Norman could correctly spell Curt's difficult last name of Friesian-Dutch origin, suggested he was familiar with Curt's state-wide work as a child advocate. He offered Meg this advice, "Plan: I suggest the teacher, Meg, stay out of all the wrangling. Ruffin is doing well."

Meanwhile, Meg sent me her charting of Ruffin's IEP goal that he carry out a 2-part direction with each part having as many as 2 critical elements related to size, shape, and color, for example, "Get the big, red Lego and put it on the orange chair." This sort of "game" presented Ruffin with a good mental challenge — which he could manage by the end of the week.

Having gotten a couple more "we are in the process of reviewing your claims" letters from Ms. Crews in mid-March and mid-April, my other attorney, Scott Peters issued a blunt, final demand to Prudential. "You responded to my latest letter by stating that you are 'in the process of gathering additional information.' This matter has been before you since November of 1994, and the decisions of our Iowa Supreme Court clearly state that is an excessive amount of time and an unreasonable failure to pay these claims. Accordingly, unless our client has received your check within five (5) days of today's letter, we will file suit against Prudential for breach of contract and bad faith, including all consequential, punitive, cost, and attorney fee damages as provided by law." Scott's letter crossed in the mail with another "we are in the process of reviewing" letters from Ms. Crews.

Three days past Scott's deadline, Ms. Crews called me. She asked plaintively, "Do you have a fax?" It was highly inappropriate for her to contact me directly when counsel represented me. I wouldn't talk to her. I was busy, and I was cranky.

Mid-morning in early May, my fax machine spit out two pages on Prudential's letterhead. I had to credit Prudential as being nimbler than any of Ruffin's educators — from whom Curt and I had still heard nothing.

"After complete and thorough research on the information submitted regarding Ruffin's claims for Lovaas Therapy, our corporate office has determined that the services rendered by Autism Therapists of Northeast Iowa — my name for Donna, Lisa, and me as a small business — are equivalent to occupational therapy. Eligible charges will be processed for payment in accordance with policy provisions."

Prudential was going to pay Ruffin's claims. Eight days after Scott's firmest and final demand. Wow! I put my head down on the letter, on my desk, and started sobbing. When I could sit up, huffing, I wondered who to call first? Scott, of course, to thank him. Seamus, Donna, and Lisa, my parents, and Curt.

This would be good news for the school authorities, too.

Of course, Prudential's letter included some devilish details. "The invoices submitted for Lovaas drills by Lisa Murphy and Donna Schmidt cannot be considered as eligible charges without acceptable proof from the providers. We will need an itemized statement that has been signed by each of them."

That was just paperwork. One of my favorite things.

Also, coverage would be limited. "Charges for continued Lovaas Therapy will be referred to our medical department for review to determine the medical necessity of the additional treatment. All charges that are not medical expenses for Ruffin or are not listed as eligible expenses under the policy, will not be covered. These charges include airline tickets, hotel expenses, telephone, and food expenses, conference fees for Ms. White, Evelyn Kung's expenses to review videotape, phone conferences, and cost of her lodging, accompanying fees, books, computer programs, computer toys, drugs, medicines, and vitamins."

Berna Crews had signed this letter. May whatever gods they believed in and bowed down to finally bless Berna Crews, Dr. Northrup, Prudential's corporate office, and its medical department.

Curt was out of the office when I called to convey the good news. It was spring, the season of IEP meetings. Joan laughed, "He's running around like a chicken with his head cut off and will be every day until mid-June."

I promised her a letter that Curt could read later, explaining, "Prudential will pay something, but only after I pay a $1,000 deductible for each calendar year — a total of $3,000 for 1994, 1995, and 1996. My best estimate is that Prudential may pay as much as $6,000 for direct therapy services to Ruffin for the period covered by my statement of costs passed out at the mid-March IEP meeting."

Since the early May deadline to hear back from the school authorities had come and gone, we were working hard to get ready for Ruffin's summer play group. I arranged for liability insurance coverage and purchased art and other educational supplies. Seamus repaired my back-yard fence, installed playground equipment on a wood-shaving base, and converted my one-car garage into a shady play area with carpet, new interior paint, and shelving. I hired RoJene and a second experienced nursery school teacher, Elaine Mills, who would be Ruffin's teacher next year at the private nursery school, to lead his afternoon playgroup.

Meanwhile, Miss Hobbs thanked the president of the private nursery school "for considering saving us a spot each year for a potential student from our early childhood class." Not a breath about "special education." Those words might have been as scary to her as they were to me, at first, or off-putting.

"ACSD will pay Ruffin White's tuition for your nursery school program. We expect him to be successful. If he should require the services of a teacher associate, ACSD will provide those services for him."

None of these promises were copied to me, or to anyone else concerned. Even I would never have known of these arrangements for Ruffin, had I not been asked to pay for them, and had I not inspected Ruffin's educational files later that summer.

It was time to let the educators know about Prudential's agreement to extend coverage. When I let the cat out of the bag to Meg in our home school notebook, Emily called Mr. Montague immediately. None of this insurance information, nor Ruffin's private nursery school admission, was included in any of the ongoing negotiations between Ruffin's educators and me. Mr. Carew seemed to have passed on the assignment. Mr. David Hunter, ACSD's attorney, the newest man in the mix, working over in Waterloo — the farthest from Ruffin and the facts — had been tasked to respond to Curt's latest proposal.

Mr. Hunter sent his draft response to Mr. Montague and Mr. Lord in mid-May.

"Gentlemen, I am not thin-skinned. Please advise of any concerns or suggestions."

Right away, Mr. Montague replied, "David, my congratulations. You did an exemplary job on the Ruffin White letter. I have one minor, but important, suggested change. Insert the following, 'Enclosed is the preliminary IEP which was planned for presentation at the IEP meeting of mid-March. This IEP was formulated based upon many of the suggestions offered by Ms. White in her February 14th document titled: 'Mother's Draft IEP.'" Ah, yes, my unfunny Valentine. And then, in urgent caps: "COMPLETE AND SEND THE FINAL LETTER TODAY, IF AT ALL POSSIBLE."

The draft IEP enclosed was dated nearly a week after our actual March 16th meeting, on March 24th, as "amended" by Inge, but sloppily — which may have accounted for the lack of any reference to Ruffin's planned placement in the private nursery school or the recent availability of insurance resources.

Ruffin's case was quickly becoming one of too many cooks spoiling the broth — when Ruffin was just a little 4-year-old boy whose appropriate education required everyone's exquisite co-operation and co-ordination.

Mr. Hunter's first letter, echoing all Mr. Montague's suggestions, was duly faxed to all the principals and their attorneys, and then Joan faxed it on to me to read, as the legal gobbledygook it was — dressed up a bit to convey the message: We are very impressive people who have done all our homework. Was I supposed to be frightened by this peacock's display? Was I supposed to be afraid? I was not, not in the least, being familiar with working against big city law firms representing multiple opposing parties where the right hand rarely knew all the left hand was doing. The failure of such firms to communicate internally and among themselves was usually how, as one attorney, working solo, without so much as a legal assistant, it was possible to prevail against them.

Here came the bottom line on what I felt certain Ruffin needed — a summer with typically developing age-mates. "The ACSD rejects the offer of settlement presented with your letter of early April."

I called Joan to let her know I was perfectly willing to attend a pre-appeal mediation conference to try to resolve Ruffin's case whenever Curt felt it could be arranged, after the Mason City settlement, as he and I had discussed.

Meanwhile, Dr. Granpeesheh had offered me her written expert opinion, to present at mediation, or use in litigation.

"To whom it may concern: Ruffin White has been receiving supervision for his in home 'Lovaas' based behavior modification program from this clinic. An essential part of this program is based on the development of social skills and therefore necessitates the participation of the child in directed play groups or sessions. Therefore, Ruffin's participation in a play group that is supervised by trained teachers or therapists is an inherent part of his program and is necessary at this time."

Meg sent me her charting of Ruffin's IEP goal to make or count sets of objects up to 10. He seemed to have had an off day when he could get nothing right, followed by a better day the next when he was able to make sets of all the numbers up to 8. As other progress, she noted that Ruffin did an excellent job of batting a ball, and that when playing catch had managed to catch the ball 7 times straight.

On Mother's Day, Evelyn flew back to Iowa to spend Sunday with us — with Donna, Lisa, Seamus, Ruffin, and me — and assigned Ruffin a new, more challenging set of drills. RoJene and Chance came over for the afternoon so she and Evelyn could talk about how RoJene could best help Ruffin fully participate in our planned summer playgroup.

During one of the long calls I usually got from clients around suppertime, Ruffin slipped out of the corner of my eye, determined to show Rose, who was there to cook and eat with us, something in the driveway — our new Volvo station wagon. In his blind excitement he ran right through the glass of our front storm door, slashing one eyelid and his forehead. Suddenly, he was howling with surprise, and bleeding. Rose rushed into my dining room office to get me, her own face a frightened mask. I scooped Ruffin up to drive him to the emergency room, calling back to Rose to get Seamus, or call Donna — to have one of them meet us there.

I was devastated. How could I have let this happen? On Mother's Day? Our little, red hatchback had bitten the dust. How could I have ever imagined I could afford a safer car?

Ruffin had long since stopped howling. Donna arrived quickly, and she and I held his hair back and stroked his head as he fell asleep while the doctor on duty stitched him up. When I took him home and undressed him for bed, several other shards of glass were embedded in his torso — about which he had not complained — and which the emergency room examination had missed — what with all the fuss about his eyelid and forehead.

I didn't think I could manage a trip back to the hospital. I didn't want to report this embarrassing oversight. I didn't want to risk waking Ruffin. While he continued to sleep, I was able to tweeze out all the shards, clean Ruffin's wounds with peroxide and cotton, apply antibiotics and then a patchwork of little Band-Aids.

Mr. Montague issued a memo that next Monday on "the Ruffin White matter" to Jack Wallace, his mid-level subordinate, with instructions that he inform "all appropriate, subordinate Bridgewater staff."

"As you know, we have been meeting with attorneys representing the ACSD and our agency. Unfortunately, this has taken somewhat longer than we anticipated. I provide this general overview, with associated documents. This information must also be filed in Ruffin's folder, *less this memo*."

This amounted to a direct request for Jack to cull Ruffin's special education files, a violation of the federal law, *The Family Education Rights and Privacy Act* (FERPA), which governed the handling of a child's special education records. Perhaps Jack knew better than to violate federal law and left Mr. Montague's memo in Ruffin's file where I found it later. Maybe Jack just forgot.

Meanwhile, I was laboring over an Iowa Supreme Court brief defending a large wrongful termination jury verdict awarded to one of my clients who had been fired from his job as a long-haul trucker. He had told his employer to "stick your damn truck where the sun don't shine," *after* he had been told to keep driving regardless of however much his work-injured leg might pain him, and whatever his doctor's excuse said. It was due to be filed by the end of May.

School let out for the summer with Meg reporting again that Ruffin was "not really ready yet" to tackle his IEP goal to tell whether something occurred "yesterday" or "today."

I encouraged Jamie, Betsy, and Amy, three teenagers volunteering in Meg's classroom, who had also been volunteering all semester at my law office after school, "I could really use your help whenever you are ready to return. Mrs. Wonderlich and I expect to arrange for the three of you to get whatever credit we can toward your school or college, as you suggested. Thank you for all your help, and for the beautiful flowers. P.S. We are doing a research project for the University of Iowa with four children with autism during early June at my house. You three are welcome to come by and meet the treatment provider, and some of the children, if that would be interesting to you. It involves a new treatment to help the children listen more carefully and understand more of what they do hear."

Meanwhile, Mr. Montague had good news to share and issued another of his memos about a ruling in favor of a local district in Virginia involving the Lovaas method, a new opinion that had just issued in early January. "Recently, I received several documents related to current case law regarding special education cases from Dee Ann Wilson." Indeed, the same woman I had offended by mis-addressing her as "Dianne," whom Dr. Hagen had assigned to mediate the Mason City case for Curt and whom he had suggested we ask to mediate Ruffin's. Mr. Montague was encouraged by what Dee Ann had to offer him. "I noted this case with extreme interest, and then went to the *Individuals with Disabilities Education Law Reporter* (22 IDELR 88) for a detailed account."

The IDELR was a legal reporting service published by LRP Publications which summarized, collected, and published the full rulings of ALJs from every state and the written opinions of state and federal courts concerning special education law, including letters issued by the federal Office of Special Education Programs (OSEP) offering guidance and answering questions posed by the states. It was an expensive service to subscribe to. Most subscribers were larger law firms representing school districts. Curt's public agency couldn't afford to subscribe. He accessed this essential legal resource by going to the law school library maintained by Drake Law School in Des Moines, which was handy enough for him.

LRP also sponsored an annual training event to cover new developments in special education law. It could only be attended by ALJs and attorneys willing to certify that they had never represented parents in these disputes. In my experience later, the company was perfectly willing to take any attorney's money who approached politely, offering to purchase the written handouts of training materials prepared for the exclusive defense-networking meeting. This was an inexpensive means of eavesdropping on our adversaries, and it always tickled me to put my feet up with fresh highlighters to begin reading the enemy mail. Just as Mr. Hunter was not thin-skinned, I was not squeamish.

At the moment, it would be important for Curt and me to develop a legal argument to *distinguish* this newest Virginia case from Ruffin's. Mr. Montague remained hot to trot, crowing in his memo: "Inge and Meg have done an excellent job of comparing Ruffin's IEP objectives-vs-his generic classroom's curriculum skills, and the Lovaas drills. In Virginia's *Fairfax* case there were charts presented to the ALJ. These had an impact on the final decision since they were included in the case presentation in the IDELR document. This is the first case I have encountered where the schools have prevailed in a matter which is similar to ours, interesting reading to say the least."

Kim sent me an end-of-the-year handwritten note. "Ruffin has made very nice gains. I will be recommending that he be reevaluated in the fall to determine if additional speech services are needed at that time. Family members are encouraged to expect Ruffin to use his speech and language skills during the summer that have been worked on in speech this year." This was sealed with a silly, round sticker, "I heart speech" which, honestly, I didn't appreciate in the least. Nor the looming fight next fall that might be necessary to reestablish Ruffin's entitlement to continuing speech therapy.

As for what was stapled to her note, Kim reported that on the *Expressive One-Word Picture Vocabulary Test-Revised*, at 3 years, 9 months of age, Ruffin's score was the age equivalent of 3 years, 7 months (a 2-month delay), amounting to the 34th percentile. This particular test was one Ruffin would be expected to score strongest on — coming up with a word when shown a picture. It just tested for nouns, not sentence structures. On the *Boehm Test of Basic Concepts — Preschool* Ruffin's percentile rank dropped 14 points to the 20th percentile.

Yes, Ruffin had made some nice gains this year, but I hardly thought we were done yet. But it sure looked like Kim was ready to be done with him, or, more likely, I had to admit, with me.

I ran Ruffin over to Decorah the next day to Bridgewater's audiologist to have her perform a pre-AIT audiogram on Ruffin. "Your child has a hearing loss which may warrant medical attention. Please make an appointment with your doctor and take the audiogram and the Doctor's Report form with you to return to us." This audiogram showed that Ruffin's hearing loss was limited to higher frequencies between 4000 and 8000 Hertz, more in the left ear than in the right, "indicative of fluid" in both middle ears.

Ruffin and I went straight to see his pediatrician Dr. Olson for an antibiotic. I asked him whether Ruffin would be okay to begin auditory integration training by early June. "I don't know if it will help his autism, or his hearing," Dr. Olson opined, "but I can't see any way it would hurt him. Good luck. Let me know how it goes."

Then, he looked at me kindly, and said, "His autism seems much better. And, here, give me that," gesturing for the form Bridgewater wanted returned to them. "We can mail it back for you." He did, diagnosing Ruffin with "Serious otitis media, on medication with a good prognosis" and writing, as a specific comment on Ruffin's upcoming auditory integration training (AIT), "Sounds should cause no harm to him."

Ruffin's summer school began at home on Tuesday, May 31st. Every morning Donna and Lisa continued their one-to-one direct teaching using Ruffin's newest drill book written by Evelyn on Mother's Day, and that afternoon our playgroup began in my refurbished garage. Elaine Mills, who had agreed to teach for me, had suddenly backed out. Donna, who knew her as a friend, confided that Elaine needed to keep her job at the private nursery school. She had been warned not to involve herself in anything as unprofessional as we would be doing this summer. With that information, I simply let her go without a fuss.

RoJene was able to recruit Pine Wilson, a certified special education teacher from the Decorah school district to come and serve as my second teacher. RoJene and Pine agreed to teach on alternating days.

In early May, I had advertised in the newspaper to have local mothers volunteer their preschool girls and boys to attend our summer playgroup. At no charge, it looked like free babysitting, but in every admission interview, I explained to each mother exactly what we were up to, and why, and how we were doing this — for Ruffin.

RoJene taught the first day, with one of our new junior high school volunteers, Zoe, as her aide. The group included 2 boys and 4 girls, joined the next day by another boy. We offered a snack. At first, I kept daily notes, as did RoJene. Pine was not a writer, but she reported in daily.

Our first day, Ruffin had trouble sharing the balloon pump and his black pickup, a large riding toy, and needed a short time out with me. Later, he announced, "I'm happy, Mom," and went on to play well otherwise, attended well at story, and prompted the other children at "pick up" time. I was able to watch the group play *London Bridge is Falling Down.*

One little girl's mother sent me a note which I welcomed after the first day. "Our daughter seemed to enjoy herself on her first day at your house. I found it interesting, yet typical that she behaved better when I was not there. Kids, they're so unpredictable!"

RoJene made more detailed notes to share with me and with Pine.

Circle: The children gave their names and ages. I shared my pink rock and invited them to bring objects to share. I tried reading *Farmer in the Dell* by Mary Mabi Rae, but was unsuccessful. The three-year-olds needed to wander, but they were extremely interested in all the new toys and equipment.

Free Play: Everyone tried out everything. Chance initiated the ladder-rope up the wooden tower and ran over to me, yelling, 'I did it.' Then everyone followed his lead, and the ice was broken. We picked dandelions to swirl in the water.

Snack and Story (at the same time): *The Rainbow Fish*, Marcus Pfister. The children had good attention span for this story, and we talked about Ruffin sharing all his things with his new friends. Then we colored fish on paper to take home. Ruffin drew a whale.

PE: Running with large balloons in and out of the bushes.

Music: *The Mulberry Bush*. Ruffin never joined in but had fun watching.

Sharing for Ruffin was very difficult, however he improved greatly as the afternoon went on. He had one major tantrum. At the end of the day, Ruffin individually told his friends goodbye. Ruffin paid more attention to story time than any of the others.

As when I had engaged Donna and Lisa, I gave RoJene and Pine the opportunity of a week to get to know Ruffin and his behavioral challenges on their own.

We held our second day of playgroup with Pine teaching a group of half a dozen. I tried to help Pine as her aide. Pine read *Farmer in the Dell*. Art was sidewalk chalk. The focus of circle time was names, ages, and colors.

Mr. Montague issued a second memo about the location of additional records related to Ruffin's special education file maintained by Bridgewater. These file materials included his and my correspondence, research material I had sent him, and "Correspondence to attorneys representing Bridgewater, and ACSD," and letters Mr. Montague had written "to various persons and agencies as requested" by me. *"Please notify the Director of Special Education by phone if a request to release records is presented."*

His memo created a special segregated file — located in an office several counties distant from our home and local district — concerning Ruffin, which I, as his parent, had every right to inspect and photocopy under FERPA. Perhaps unadvisedly — his memo also operated as a clear, written waiver of the attorney-client privilege by Bridgewater with respect to all Mr. Montague's earlier letters to Mr. Carew and Mr. Hunter.

On Friday, playgroup was a small group with RoJene who brought baby chicks in from her farm. Ruffin wanted batteries for his train, not friends, or even chicks. He threw another tantrum. I needed to take him upstairs. Then, he had trouble sharing again — dinosaurs, an airplane, and his computer — and trouble attending to RoJene's reading group a book about chickens, but played well later — *Ring Around the Rosie*, *London Bridge* and helped make a "caterpillar" rope. He played a balloon-ball game of catch and pretended well with our new play food. Arranged on our new rope, the group walked to the library, where they played with puppets. As soon as the children were gone, Ruffin wanted his batteries, again, right away. The social difference between Ruffin and the others, especially the girls, was glaring.

I opened RoJene's notes to learn what she might have seen differently with her teacher training, and from her own perspective as an experienced mother of three. "Ruffin sat by Mary Jane more than joining in, but he was always interested and aware of everything the other children did."

Another day, I spent the first hour of playgroup picking up a little boy from his home out in the country, a beautiful summer day's drive into the foothills near the river. RoJene let me know Ruffin did better with the group when I was unavailable. After reading *The Very Busy Spider* by Eric Carle, all the children, including Ruffin, made construction paper spiders. RoJene and I hung them from the garage rafters.

By the end of the first week in June, Ruffin was able to manage playgroup without tantrums. The little boy who lived so far out in the country wanted Ruffin to visit. As I eavesdropped, the two of them chatted back and forth in the back seat of the Volvo. His older sister, in a wheelchair, had been in Amy's classroom across the hall from Ruffin. Ruffin recognized her. Her mom was staying home all summer to care for her.

Meanwhile, Tris, Dr. Tristram Smith, Lovaas's co-researcher wrote me to share his new address and phone number at Washington State University, and to let me know he expected "Ruffin will continue to progress rapidly." This arrived as a comfort. I was able to send a copy to my parents, and to show it to Seamus. And I held on to it as a talisman.

CHAPTER TWENTY SEVEN

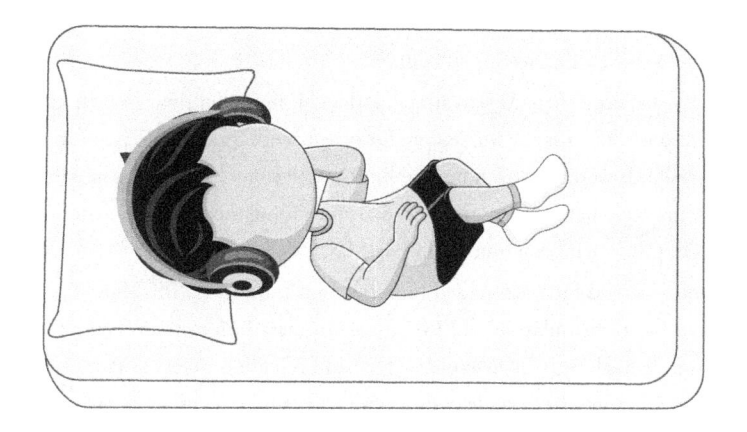

AUDITORY INTEGRATION TRAINING

Back in early November, the director of training for the Judevine Center for Autism in St. Louis, Missouri, had gotten back to our parent group about their recent experiences with auditory integration training (AIT). The parents of their clients were pleased afterward. This treatment of their children's ears seemed to have produced improvements in both language and behavior. She assured me, too, Judevine was "not aware of any negative results being reported when AIT is conducted following a proven format."

Our AIT experiment began in early June. Lisa Toalson drove in from Moline and was pleased to have our third-floor attic as a quiet space for treatment. After she assigned each child their daily treatment slots — one late in the morning and another late in the afternoon — Ruffin and I entertained the three other children and their parents who had travelled in from neighboring counties as guests downstairs throughout each day. That first day, it was non-stop pandemonium.

The visiting children became more accustomed to our home over the weekend, and somewhat more accustomed to being together. That Monday, I needed to travel to Des Moines for the *Ezzone* appeal arguments *en banc* before the entire Iowa Supreme Court. It was a command appearance for all counsel.

Tuesday, between their AIT treatments, the children, and their parents each travelled back and forth across the Mississippi for private audiograms in Wisconsin. Ruffin's hearing thresholds were all within normal limits, with some hearing loss in one ear. His tympanograms were flat, suggesting he needed continuing medical treatment for the ear infection Dr. Olson had seen him for in late May.

My forty-second birthday passed unnoticed on June 14th. This should have been Ruffin's own fourth birthday — had I been able to carry him to term. Happy Birthday to us! Seamus brought me the newspaper. He had been a bit unnerved that everyone in town had read a front-page article, continuing to a good part of an inside page, headlined, *"New treatment for autistic children is tried here."*

Robin Ouren, a young feature reporter who was attending Luther College had written the piece and came to be fascinated by autism. Her article was accompanied by her own photographs of Lisa Toalson and her equipment, seated with Renee and her mother Ruth, and one of Ruffin and me, with Ruffin lying down in his sleeping bag with a pillow cradling his head in a pair of huge earphones. After she graduated, Robin asked to join me as my legal assistant — where, among many other duties, she supervised our photocopying for parents and our junior high-school volunteers for several years.

By the next Sunday, Lisa Toalson had completed all our children's AIT sessions, packed up her equipment and hugged everyone goodbye.

Later, I sent a copy of Robin's article to Sue Baker. "We publicly credited the cooperation of Bridgewater, and your office. We tried to help the reporter explain the disability of autism to our community."

"Here are Ruffin's audiograms done before and during auditory integration training (AIT). An earlier audiogram of Ruffin done in the fall of the year is similar in its overall pattern to Ruffin's pre-AIT audiogram. The mid-treatment audiogram is quite different. Ruffin did take some Bactrim after the pre-AIT audiogram and during AIT. He experienced very little distress during AIT, probably the least distress of any of the children. Our worst experiences during AIT were trying to keep Ruffin awake. He kept falling asleep during even the loudest music, especially during the late night we had when both Lisa's earphone-sets bit the dust.

"Fortunately, we got Dr. Rimland and Dr. Steve Edelson on a conference call and learned that Lisa could purchase a set of replacement earphones at Walmart with the right specifications. Otherwise, with a gap of more than two days in the treatment sequence, we would all have had to start over again.

"Ruffin's principal home therapist has reported that Ruffin had several exceptionally good morning drill sessions during and since AIT. A task he is doing exceptionally well on, which she mentioned, is a drill during which she reads him a 5- to 6-sentence story without pictures, or any visual support, and then asks him as many 'wh' questions as she can imagine. Ruffin can listen to the story, process it, put the information into memory, discriminate the question, and provide answers on topic.

"He has also been doing better on 'giving things up,' not perseverating verbally or insisting on a demand, doing better with transitions, and accepting uncertain answers I offer him — 'maybe' and 'perhaps.'

"Our summer playgroup is going well. Ruffin was really on a roll from mid-June until just before the Fourth of July. I noticed a tremendous change in his speech inflection and the feeling expressed in his speech when he was talking to and responding to typically developing playmates. He got quite caught up in his friends, and for several days he would come into the house — for a drink or to go to the bathroom — and take no notice, or merely passing notice of me. This is a great improvement over his appealing to me over every issue of doing or not doing something or sharing something."

During AIT, Ruffin also had his second appointment with Dr. Funk, his special needs dentist at Gundersen. By then, Ruffin anticipated the visit as "fun." Unlike his first visit last December, no one was required to hold him down or steady him in the chair. He opened his mouth on request and tolerated the examination and cleaning without undue distress. No sweat! Dr. Funk observed, "Ruffin is a different child." And surely, he was.

Later, that summer, I continued to report back to Bridgewater, Sue Baker, and Lisa Toalson more about the results of AIT with Ruffin. "The areas of most improvement I see are Ruffin's greatly reduced resistance to change and parental direction. Very frequently now, if given a reason, he will transition without undue fuss. He will leave objects behind that he is attached to; if told, for example, that taking a plumber's friend into a restaurant will cause other people to laugh at him, he is satisfied to be reassured the object will be 'safe' at home.

"The last weekend in July, Ruffin and I got through Saturday and Sunday without any help from therapists, and he did very well at church, finding a friend from his playgroup to visit with during after-church coffee. We went shopping on Saturday, going in and out of several stores. Ruffin had a haircut for which he waited patiently as other customers had theirs first. I no longer feel a desperate sense of dread and anxiety when I need to run an errand with Ruffin. I mean, now I do go, rather than do without.

"The other area in which Ruffin continues to improve is his ability to put sentences together. Today, for example: 'Would you please move those papers, so I can lie down here?'

"His home therapists have commented that he has had several remarkably good therapy sessions involving sequencing card tasks, appropriate use of pronouns — I, me, she, he, him, her, and you — and use of complete sentences. For example, in conversation today: Therapist: 'Could we work at the park again?' Ruffin: 'That'd be okay. My mom won't mind.'

"He's able to settle down in distracting environments like the county fair and the Decorah swimming pool, enjoy himself appropriately, and keep up with the group." This was my perspective, of course. RoJene saw Ruffin as still having more of a problem in these challenging environments than other children of his age.

Much later in January of 1996, I was able to report back to Dr. Rimland, "Enclosed please find a pre-publication copy of an AIT study which was completed recently in Wisconsin. It is not supportive of AIT, and I understand from Dr. Palm, the audiologist involved, that he entered the study with the attitude expressed in the introduction. There seems to be little detail provided of the actual data gathered."

As promised, Dr. Palm had sent me the Gundersen AIT study, *A Double-Blind, Placebo Controlled Study of the Efficacy of Auditory Integration Training*. It had involved 30 multi-handicapped full-time residents of Chileda, age 7 to 24 years, 22 males, 8 females, 3 African Americans, 2 Latinx and 1 Asian American. There was no report of how many, if any, had a diagnosis of autism. The audiograms and AIT treatment described were both similar to what our autism support group had arranged for earlier in June, and the rating instrument for behavior change was the same ABC checklist we had used, before for a baseline, and afterward repeatedly for 9 months out.

The Gundersen researchers had concluded that "there was uniform improvement of all subjects, including the controls," which simply suggested to me that if caretakers paid close attention to the behavior of their wards, their behaviors might well improve — echoing Ruth's earlier common-sense speculations of last fall.

CHAPTER TWENTY EIGHT

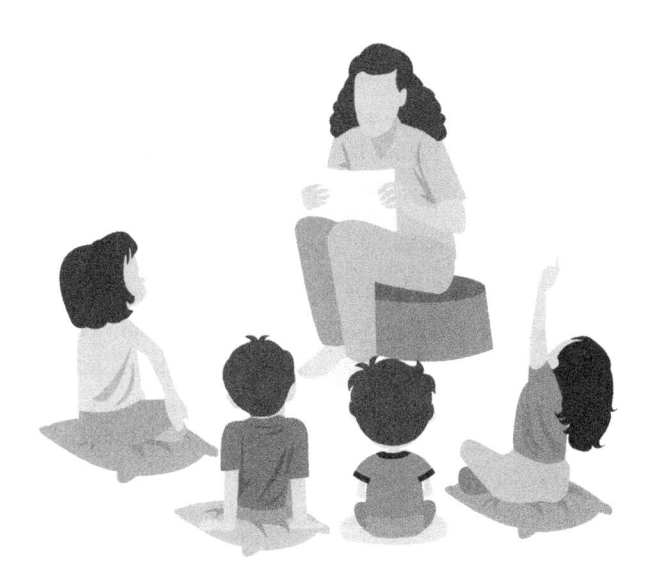

DEMANDING TO BE HEARD

Our playgroup resumed with Pine on the Monday after auditory integration training, but only one little girl and our faithful junior high school helper, Zoe, showed up to join Ruffin. I called all the parents to remind them our activity was still available.

By Tuesday, attendance was back up, but it was blazing hot, so RoJene and I took all the children back to the pool in the city park where they could play on swings, slides, and merry-go-rounds. All the children had extremely short attention spans in the heat.

After a two-week break, RoJene felt it was like starting the group all over. She and Pine were discouraged and wanted to consider shorter hours or fewer days per week. Ruffin wouldn't hold the pink shell at circle or speak out loud.

Otherwise, he did well, but some of his behavior disappointed me. He ignored his special education classmate at poolside while playing with our group. He ignored all my efforts to prompt him to greet this little boy who clearly recognized him. Later, on Sunday, Ruffin and I saw him and his mom again, and Ruffin waved and called out to him delightedly.

Donna's daughter Danielle and Ruffin burst in late one summer morning, after walking across town, with a little note from Donna. "I'm sending Ruffin home with Danielle because people are coming to pick my van up for repair and I would like to talk with them." It was a mark of Ruffin's behavioral progress that he could be entrusted to Danielle — a girl who was responsible well beyond her eleven years — and safely complete such a walk.

The playgroup that afternoon was with RoJene, and 5 children, headed back to the park. This proved to be an exceptionally good group day for Ruffin. "He showed much better behavior, joining in, and making conversation without Mom. Ruffin never actually played the same games as the other children in the pool, but he observed everything and knew all that was going on. He lay down and walked with his hands in the water for the first time — he was not ready to blow bubbles yet. Ruffin is a good serious color-er and *loves* story time. A remarkably successful day." Before she left for the day, RoJene and I talked about my fading out, especially at circle time.

I read RoJene's notes for this day with relief. This was going to work out. Maybe I would be able to fall back and even get some legal work done and make some money to help support all this effort.

With the pandemonium of auditory integration training behind us, and just as I imagined Ruffin's summer schedule was up and running again, Curt and I scheduled a long telephone consultation about responding to Mr. Hunter's letter of mid-May. Curt was pressed for time, working hard to try to settle the Mason City case and other matters. We decided that I would write back directly to Mr. Hunter, working from my notes of our agreed-upon strategy.

I had never run up against attorney David Hunter in any of my cases nor in any courtroom or chambers. Waterloo fell just beyond my northeast Iowa orbit. He practiced as part of a large firm, established in 1903 and housed by now in a reclaimed downtown brick building.

With Ruffin busy in good hands, I was ready. "Please accept my personal apologies for a tardy response. Throughout this time Mr. Sytsma and I have been hard-pressed to get a letter out to you. Yesterday, he suggested that I write to you directly.

"In this letter I will offer some explanation of our delay, a description of current developments, some of them positive, and describe our current negotiating position.

"As Ruffin's parent, and as a taxpayer, I am equally disappointed that your client has chosen to reject my early April offer of settlement. Nevertheless, I remain willing to attend a pre-appeal mediation conference to try to resolve these matters.

"The end of May and beginning of June were difficult times for Ruffin and me. First, it became clear that the group home's 'summer activity' program outlined in your late March offer was inappropriate for Ruffin and presented no opportunity for savings to any party.

"As I checked into that program with the director, it did not appear appropriate for Ruffin because no children who have enjoyed normal development would be attending, nor would there be any children attending who, although physically handicapped, could have modeled appropriate speech and social skills for Ruffin.

"The school district and Bridgewater seem to have been unaware that the group home intended to charge someone — either me or the public education authorities — $10 per hour, or $30 to $40 per day for Ruffin to attend that group because Ruffin does not have Medicaid funding for his disability or any other public or welfare money to support him. Ruffin's IQ is too high to qualify for a Medicaid Mental Retardation waiver.

"It became clear that I needed to put together an appropriate summer program for Ruffin here at home. Without structure, he still drifts back into self-stimulatory behavior. So, attending to Ruffin's actual education and occupation became my first priority."

In rejecting this part of the educators' offer, I wasn't just writing to their attorney. Again, I was writing over his head to any eventual due process decision maker, first an ALJ, and then either a state or federal judge on appeal. I was "making a record," to either introduce as evidence, or to use to refresh my own recollection should I need to testify in any later proceedings.

This was going to be a long letter. I described my own recent practice. "I am sure you can appreciate the demands of those legal tasks."

I described how we had started our playgroup. "It began a week after the end of school but was interrupted by auditory integration training sessions for four children with autism." I described that effort in detail, too. "It was convivial, but not a good environment in which to write this letter."

"Ruffin's present, regular summer program provided by me is: He works from early morning until noon with his home therapist Donna Schmidt. At noon he has lunch with me. Each afternoon for three hours he attends a playgroup with several children who have enjoyed normal development. I review the day, and problem-solve with the teacher. Then, Ruffin and I transport the other children home. In the late afternoon, for a couple of hours Ruffin works with his home therapist, Lisa Murphy. Then Ruffin has supper, bath, works on his computer, watches television or videos, and is read to by me until bedtime.

I documented RoJene and Pine's certifications to teach. "Mrs. Holub, Ruffin's special education classroom teacher, advises that Inge Nilsen, Ruffin's Bridgewater case manager, is acquainted with both teachers personally, and has expressed a high opinion of both of them to her."

"The parent of one child or a junior high school student offer their services as an aide on Mondays and Wednesdays. I also help, but we find Ruffin integrates more easily into playgroup when I am unavailable. It is a big challenge for him to share his whole backyard, most of his toys, his garage, his home, and his mother with a group of new friends, as it would be for anyone. The constant challenge to share everything in his personal world interferes with some of his best efforts at integration."

Would Ruffin's acknowledged special needs even meet with "good faith" on the part of his educators? I thought a later decision maker might be interested, so I offered them a cost-free opportunity.

"It would be a helpful gesture and would allow the school district to mitigate my damages, if the district would be willing to loan Ruffin's playgroup some of the books, puppets, and paint storage cups which I purchased for the district in the fall and which his playgroup teachers would like to use this summer. I would gladly return these items at the end of the summer and replace anything that might be consumed or missing. The playgroup could also use a music set — sticks, bells, drums, etc. on loan, and I would return and replace any missing items."

Although I remained willing to work within the mediation system, Curt and I had agreed we now needed to go for broke, so I let Mr. Hunter know, by dropping that bomb. "I trust that you will understand that in view of the very good possibility of Ruffin's entering a mainstream classroom by kindergarten, and his probable ability to pursue higher education, as well as the loss to me of substantially all opportunity to practice law over the last year, my position going forward must be to seek full reimbursement of all the expenses of Ruffin's special education to date. It is with the greatest reluctance and deep personal sadness in the face of near-overwhelming frustration that I withdraw my early April offer which Mr. Sytsma and I had crafted to be as generous as I could afford it to be.

"I am disappointed that the school district cannot see its way to providing what data-based research indicated would be appropriate for Ruffin in the fall of 1994, and what has proven to be very successful with him to the present day.

"I am also disappointed to see all the signs that your client ACSD is blindly following the very provincial lead of Bridgewater in making unsupported clinical judgments about Ruffin's programming. The beginnings of this 'thoughtless follower' role were evident in Mr. Lord's deferral to Mr. Montague and Bridgewater in our March IEP meeting. He, the school board, and you continue such blind deference at the taxpayers' peril. You need to think for yourselves. Continuing hand-in-hand with Bridgewater may leave you relatively isolated in the position you have chosen — perhaps by default — to defend.

"Many other AEAs in Iowa have been willing at least to fund a trial of Lovaas home programming. Thus, they join many other public education authorities across the country who have generally settled along the lines of my earlier proposal: school provides 30 hours per week of Lovaas programming; parents provide 10 hours per week.

"I feel the greatest personal sorrow and frustration to foresee how very much Ruffin's case could come to cost the public education agencies and their taxpayers in litigation and transaction costs. All the money you and the other lawyers, including me, may earn could be better spent on the education of children, including the provision of appropriate one-on-one intensive educational services to more preschool children with autism and other developmental delays, who also need them.

"The local group home 'summer activity' program is just one of a number of collateral issues which color my feelings about whether this school district and Bridgewater are prepared to meet their responsibilities straightforwardly and in good faith, or whether by their actions they unwittingly invite an 'attitude adjustment' by the only effective means — brutal litigation."

By using the brand-new cut and paste software feature on my computer, I found it easy to share a full list of other parents' grievances I had shared earlier with Sue Baker, and I added a couple more particular to our school district. "The school district was unwilling to transport the special education students to Luther College's superb facility for adaptive physical education on Fridays until the Association for Retarded Citizens (ARC) agreed to donate toward the cost." Local parents had been well-aware of the Luther College program because of the many earlier years their children had been bussed over to Decorah to attend special education classrooms there.

I recounted all the difficulties parents had encountered so far in trying to get ACSD to participate and contribute to raising funds to adapt their school playground to the physical education of children with disabilities. In my experience it never hurt to let opposing counsel know exactly what sort of people he or she might be working for — since he or she had a unique opportunity and responsibility to counsel his or her people confidentially and privately — to do the right thing and get credit whenever possible by doing it ahead of any court order.

As far as I could see from his own correspondence to Curt and me, Mr. Hunter remained totally in the dark about what Miss Hobbs had arranged for Ruffin so he could participate in the mainstream.

"A commendable development is the school district's response to my request that Ruffin be offered an appropriate *integration* or *mainstreaming* component by beginning the Head Start integration visits on Tuesday and Thursday afternoons to Ruffin's ECSE classroom during April and May after our mid-March IEP meeting. I am willing to have Ruffin placed for further integration and mainstreaming in your client's ECSE classroom next year on Tuesday and Thursday afternoons only, those being the afternoons that Head Start children will be present.

"I also appreciate the school district's response to my request that a place be secured for Ruffin in a private nursery school, the only available program for typically developing 4-year-olds in our community besides Head Start. I am willing to have Ruffin placed there in the fall for integration and mainstreaming on Monday, Wednesday, and Friday afternoons, providing that the following concerns are addressed:

1. "Elaine Mills, Ruffin's private nursery school teacher will be free to consult with Evelyn Kung of CARD as needed on integration issues. I'd like her to have the opportunity to consult with Ruffin's summer program teachers and therapists as well before he begins attending.

2. "Transportation is provided to and from and between all Ruffin's educational sites. Donna Schmidt and I would be willing to bring Ruffin to either the private nursery school or to your client's campus each morning after his home-based training if it would be cheaper to reimburse us than to run a school bus or car.

3. "Ruffin's tuition at the private nursery school is paid by the public education authorities out of his 'weighted' state funds.

4. "A fair division of Ruffin's remaining 'weighted' state funds between ACSD, and the private nursery school will be made to improve the nursery school environment as their board deems most appropriate. The private nursery school has no computers, and it looks like there are some things their board might like to buy or refurbish.

5. "The lack of outdoor physical education facilities at the private nursery school will be appropriately addressed. I would be willing to consider sending Ruffin to Luther College on Friday mornings, unless it works out that he is at your client's campus in time for daily recess.

6. "A home-school-school-therapist notebook will travel with Ruffin from site to site.

"On Monday, Tuesday, Wednesday, Thursday and possibly Friday mornings until noon or until lunchtime, Ruffin will be working with Donna Schmidt, his home therapist. He will also continue to work with Lisa Murphy, his other home therapist, at the accustomed two hours in the late afternoon after school."

Also, as far as I could tell, Mr. Hunter remained unaware of Prudential's willingness to provide some coverage. "This insurance coverage came about, just as I predicted and planned for in my earlier December letter to your client and Bridgewater. Unfortunately, the coverage only amounts to about 50% of the actual cost of the CARD program because Prudential is not yet accepting responsibility to pay for teaching materials, airfare, and the like. Also, I carry a high deductible of $1,000 per calendar year (amounting to a total of $3,000 over the applicable two-year CARD therapy period for Ruffin from November 1994 to November 1996).

"I have a letter from Dr. Granpeesheh of CARD opining that this summer's playgroup is necessary for Ruffin. I plan to use that opinion letter to gain as much insurance coverage as possible for Ruffin's playgroup, but I expect Prudential will begin to balk at paying for what more nearly approaches an educational effort. Prudential agreed to provide coverage for some of Ruffin's home programming because: 'After a complete and thorough research on the information submitted regarding Ruffin's claims for Lovaas Therapy, our corporate office has determined that those services rendered are equivalent to occupational therapy.'

"Perhaps we can work more easily toward settlement now that this additional funding stream is available, and in view of Bridgewater's sole responsibility to provide for 'support services' in the form of occupational therapy."

I was not above trying to drive a wedge between his client and Bridgewater. While visiting our special education classrooms, I had learned most of the children with physical disabilities received both physical therapy and occupational therapy and that those therapists, like Ruffin's speech and language therapist Kim, were Bridgewater employees.

"I doubt Bridgewater is in agreement that 'the compensation for any aide employed by Bridgewater for such a summer program would be governed by your client's collective bargaining agreement.' I am certainly not in agreement, since the option is available to both the school district and Bridgewater to contract outside the collective bargaining agreement for services with any private service provider.

"In my view, therapist and playgroup services were not provided to Ruffin in a timely manner, so I have done the best I could to put appropriate programs in place for him, and to hire appropriate staff. Many families on the east and west coasts are paying $30 to $40 per hour for these services. Occupational therapists would be more expensive for the school authorities and for Prudential, but would not be Lovaas-trained, nor specifically trained to work with Ruffin.

"Teacher's-aide wages are set at $5.50 per hour. I am paying my two certified teachers $10 per hour, the same as I pay Donna Schmidt and Lisa Murphy. Ten dollars per hour is comparable to what Medicaid pays our local group home for respite and recreational services. Ten dollars per hour is a most acceptable professional service rate to Prudential.

"As I think about the possibility of compromise, if the public education authorities paid $5.50 per hour and Prudential paid 50% of Ruffin's program (about $5.50 per hour), we'd be close to covering the cost of staff between us. Since staff for Lovaas therapy and the playgroup are the costliest items, the possibility exists that our sitting down to a hard-headed economically driven negotiation of the remaining costs could be fruitful."

Again, I reaffirmed my own willingness to mediate. "Speaking for myself and Ruffin, I hope you would find it worthwhile to meet for pre-appeal mediation now based on this letter. I'd prefer to meet in our town, since most of the principals are here, and because of the demands of running Ruffin's program."

As a potential mediator, Dee Ann Wilson was required to pass on information both widely and even-handedly — so she had also shared with Curt a copy of the *Fairfax* decision that had so delighted Mr. Montague earlier. I had heard about it too, through the grapevine over *The Me List*. Curt and I both had copies of it in front of us, as we had strategized.

"As a final matter, Mr. Sytsma and I caution you, the school district, and Bridgewater against placing an undue reliance upon the January 9, 1995, result in *Bequai v. Fairfax County Public Schools* as a case of 'dual programming.'

"Dual programming — my allowing Ruffin to return to an ECSE classroom without integration peers present — has ended. Toward the end of last school year, Ruffin began to notice and verbalize the difference between himself and other children with autism and other disabilities who do not talk. He has described his ECSE classroom as a place where 'kids don't talk.'

"My concern in this regard prompted me to visit the classroom toward the end of the school year to observe. I am confident that Ruffin's CARD programming and his response to it has been carefully documented. I have seen the school's documentation of its programming and Ruffin's response to it, and I am not terrified to see those writings surface as an exhibit in court.

"Unlike Mrs. Bequai, I will not be agreeing that 'there were no procedural objections to anything,' because that is not Ruffin's case. Before his first IEP meeting in August of 1994, I noticed and raised the issue of summer programming for Ruffin, but public education personnel at the meeting were unprepared and without authority to discuss that issue with me.

"Ruffin then quickly met the great majority of his original August 1994-1995 IEP goals for the year, leading to my request to reconvene his IEP team as early as November. An IEP meeting was held December 8th, 1994, but not completed because the public education personnel at that meeting were without authority to discuss the noticed issues of summer programming and reimbursement for CARD training. Effectively, Ruffin has been without an IEP since early November of 1994.

"The preliminary IEP for Ruffin for the 1995-1996 school year which you enclosed with your May 12th letter bears fax transmission dates of March 24th, being most oddly the exact date of the school district and AEA's first outline of a settlement offer to me. Thus, I am left with the puzzling inference that the school district's draft IEP was available to be sent to Bridgewater on March 24th, but for some strategic or tactical reason, after its transmission to Bridgewater, it was not available to be sent to me. Accordingly, I inquire what is the reason for this 47-day delay in your transmission of this important information to me?

"Now that I *have* seen it, in my estimation — and the estimation of Ruffin's summer teachers and therapists — the preliminary IEP of March 24th will no longer state unachieved goals, skills, and concepts by the end of this summer. Ruffin's skills which continue to emerge may result in his passing some, if not all, of those proposed goals.

"So, I request that Ruffin be assessed and evaluated at the end of this summer by either the Gundersen or the UIHC. It appears that the UIHC group charges less, and writes more detailed reports, so I would prefer the UIHC to do this work.

"Nor will I be agreeing as Mrs. Bequai did 'that experts would not be identified as experts but would simply be referred to by their qualifications.' As Mr. Sytsma advised during our mid-March IEP meeting, he and I will be challenging the autism expertise of all district and Bridgewater personnel, and it will be — his word — 'bloody.'

"If the new developments since our last meeting of mid-March as set forth in this letter do not seem to you and your clients to provide a good platform for fruitful settlement discussions, then to avoid litigation of the sort described by Mr. Sytsma, might we agree to the following? 1. We will await the results of the pending case concerning Lovaas home programming in Mason City before resuming our settlement discussions; 2. With the assistance of Prudential, I will front the on-going cost of Ruffin's programming while we await the Mason City case results, reserving my right to seek full reimbursement; 3. Co-operate in the provision of education for Ruffin in the fall along the lines outlined above in this letter.

"The advantage to your client and Bridgewater would be that Mason City's local district and its AEA would bear both the blood and the dollar litigation cost of coming to an answer with respect to whether special education programming currently on offer remains appropriate for a preschool child with a new diagnosis of autism or PDD-NOS.

"Curt and I will appreciate hearing from you soon."

Having left my draft to cool overnight, I ran it by Curt the next morning, saying, "This is a long, detailed, carrot and stick to divide ACSD from Bridgewater and *is what I want to communicate.* I want to send this *as is,* no changes. What do you think?"

"Go ahead, and send it — by fax, if you like. No, use snail mail. We need to buy more time." Curt explained he was still up to his armpits in alligators trying to settle the Mason City case.

My late June reply to Mr. Hunter quickly reached everyone else concerned. Bridgewater's assistant director "Moe's" copy showed neatly penned marginalia, indicating that my description of the local group home's program and my objections to it as a summer placement for Ruffin was "correct," and that as of our last IEP meeting in March, Bridgewater did "not know who was in this program."

The *Iowa Pilot Parents* summer newsletter printed a brief article about a telephone survey of parents, conducted to determine how many children with disabilities in Iowa were receiving summer services. It turned out only 2% of children with disabilities did statewide — a little over 500 children. In one of Iowa's AEAs, as many as 250 children with disabilities did; but just 10 children with disabilities did in Bridgewater. That disproportion made no sense. Why would disabilities be more severe in one geographical region in Iowa than in ours? This helped me to appreciate why Curt and his agency were focused upon the EYSE issue as an institutional priority.

The local paper that Seamus brought and left on our kitchen counter had become something I read now with greater interest. In tiny print, in the legally mandated *Public Notices* ACSD regularly set out all its expenditures. Mr. Hunter's law firm had been paid $330 for the month of June — which would have paid for 33 hours of Ruffin's special education, or 66 hours of it — by partnering with Prudential as I had proposed.

I was disgusted. When I explained this to my parents, they were disgusted.

CHAPTER TWENTY NINE

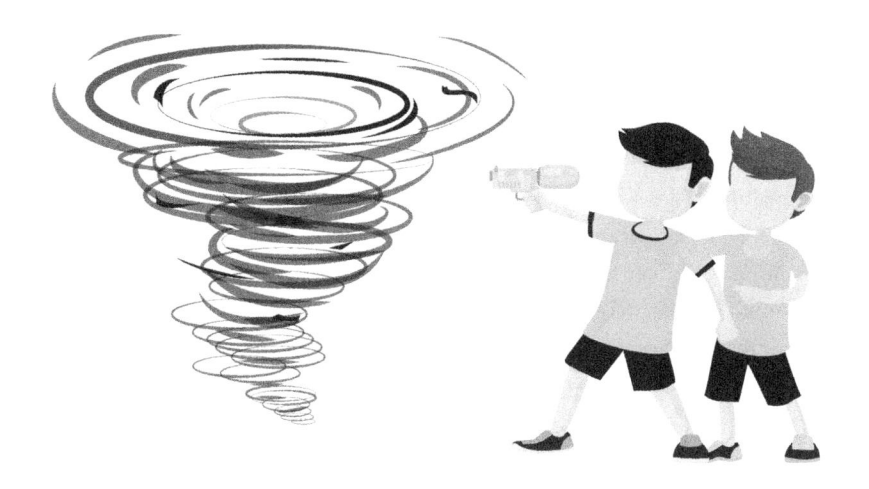

MIDSUMMER HEAT

Midsummer, I sat down with a *Flowchart of Key Programs* from Lovaas's own clinic at UCLA. His 1990 flowchart listed 11 developmental domains, from the earliest and easiest to teach, and for the child to master — to the last and most difficult and subtle developmental domains. Within each domain, scattered out across the page were the focused areas for treatment within each domain, from the earliest and easiest — to the last and most subtle.

With Ruffin having been in treatment for 7 months, having received about 30 hours per week of one-to-one instruction, and 30 hours per week of ECSE in public school through the end of May, and then 15 hours per week of our summer playgroup, while continuing all the one-to-one instruction, I wanted to assess for myself how far Ruffin seemed to have come by highlighting the domains and focused areas he seemed to have mastered. I needed to have some sense of how many remaining domains and focused areas Ruffin had yet to master. This would help me budget financially, too — to gauge how much farther and longer we needed to be able to go for him to complete his CARD program.

Over the internet, on *The Me List,* I learned about an Australian effort to replicate Lovaas's results published in an academic journal. I was able to track it down in a library at the University of Dubuque. The librarian there sent me a copy without charge. This small kindness had made me weep, uncontrollably. I had never wept like this before, that I could remember. I had to leave my office desk and retreat into an upstairs bathroom where no one, not Ruffin, not RoJene, not Pine, not Donna, not Lisa, and not Seamus, could ever hear me.

We all had a brief treatment team meeting every Friday night to adjust schedules, raise, and solve treatment issues, make a list of questions for Evelyn, pass out new drill materials, and share little episodes of success, for example, Ruffin's recent observation, "My Mommy loves paper!" And laugh. I needed to pull myself together to cheer everyone else along, to seem to be both confident of our success and happy despite the unrelenting stress.

Managing without an aide, for Friday's playgroup of 4 children, Pine grabbed juice and snacks, and fled the heat to the city pool and the park. She reported a particularly good group day, for the group, and for Ruffin. Circle time lasted half an hour with all the children attending and participating.

On one of the early crazy days of auditory integration training, Dr. Norman had called me, noting to himself everything I told him Ruffin was doing this summer, and everything I planned for him next fall. I made no secret of my legal aggression. "The mother is working with Curt Sytsma on a legal arbitration for Lovaas programming for a Mason City family which if they win or settle, she feels may bring Ruffin's school and others along."

Then, Dr. Norman asked me to sign releases of information if I wanted him to be able to talk to the private nursery school next fall. He let me know how frequently he had been talking with Meg, Kim, and Miss Hobbs's secretary since January, and that he had made notes of each conversation.

"I'd like to see those," I said in the calmest voice I could manage — because I was unhappily surprised.

"Sure," Dr. Norman responded. As Ruffin's parent, I was entitled to see his telephone contact notes. He knew I knew that I was entitled to see them.

Still, I continued to report to him openly. "Ruffin talks more and more all the time. He attempts much more elaborate narratives of past events. He has quite a bit more 'theory of mind' in the sense of offering to show me things he is looking at. Earlier he assumed I was all-seeing, all-knowing, and omniscient — especially about the location of missing objects — still a problem. He regularly proposes and imagines what he will be doing in the future, including when he is grown-up. He pretends best with his playmates using puppets, and dolls.

"He is verbalizing the differences between himself and non-verbal children with autism. 'Those big girls don't talk.' Ruffin made this comment again during our recent experience with auditory integration training. Also, late in the school year, Ruffin began to make comments about the odder behaviors of his classmates with disabilities. As a result of direct teaching of the concept, he is beginning to comment about or ask my opinion about whether certain behavior is 'silly' or 'will make people laugh at me.'

It was this last little account that prompted Dr. Norman to write me back. "To me this represents a big step forward in self-awareness, perspective taking, and some concept of social norms."

I responded later with what concerned me most, Ruffin's future development. "It is hard to know exactly how much Ruffin's use of the label 'silly' reflects a true step in self-awareness. We are teaching him this pejorative label by rote, and then explicitly connecting it to situations where his behavior is not appropriate, so that he will have feedback he can understand, and have a way of talking about these matters himself — an intellectual handle, a 'hack out strategy,' if you will.

"Many of Ruffin's remaining difficulties seem to relate to 'mind-and-feeling blindness.' We continue with a lot of direct teaching of his emotional vocabulary. We are trying to consistently label all his emotions which naturally occur, so this generalizes.

"It is encouraging that he is beginning to use the 'silly' label and routine to ask ahead of time before acting, and comment on his own behavior and the behavior of others, sometimes quite openly, and thus, tactlessly — perhaps a hopelessly inherited trait. He can also use and distinguish the use of 'silly' to describe okay kinds of silliness in the sense of okay fun."

In a follow-up phone call from Dr. Norman the next day I continued to update him on Ruffin's progress — as he made more notes. "Slow and steady — Mother continues to have concerns about language and language generalization to social situations. She is also concerned that the speech and language pathologist working with Ruffin is not supportive of her programming efforts outside school and may not give non-subjective evaluations." Yes, I was concerned about Kim, especially after what I had seen at Lovaas's January conference in Los Angeles, and after hearing Tris' accounts of Kim's open hostility at the state-wide meeting earlier last spring.

Monday's playgroup was 4 little girls and Ruffin, led by Pine. Ruffin was a "chatterbox" in circle, offering his account of an impressive tornado. "The clouds were heavy. It was dark. There was lightning. And thunder. I got a gun and banged the storm. I saved Chance Beard." He had been at RoJene's house with me when we had spotted the funnel.

Tuesday's playgroup, led by RoJene, was Ruffin, Chance, and 3 girls. It was cooler. Ruffin had no problem taking turns during a walk around the block, with each child taking a turn as the leader. The group stopped to discuss a roof project in detail. "Why would they need a new roof? What happens when it rains in? What are the tools?" They spotted new cherries in a tree and a big tractor and many other things on their simple short walk of three-quarters of an hour.

Wednesday's playgroup with Pine was small again, Ruffin and 3 little girls. I was able to work all afternoon since Ruffin ignored me.

Thursday's playgroup, rounding the end of June, was led by RoJene: Ruffin and his 3 girlfriends. Ruffin discussed his giraffe t-shirt and the giraffe's long neck. RoJene read *Mouse Paint* by Ellen Stoll Walsh. When she asked if colors could really mix to make new colors, only Ruffin agreed because of his prior knowledge gained at school. The group mixed purple, orange, and green using soft clay. They ended up at the library for books where Ruffin remembered the whale puppet he liked the best — but this time he agreed with RoJene that it belonged to the library rather than fussing to try to take it home with him.

That evening Ruffin had another accident. He fell and cut his chin while we were attending a jazz concert at Luther College. We took a quick trip to the emergency room in Decorah, where Ruffin had five stitches. I wasn't as devastated as before. The doctor on call seemed to take the whole matter in stride, as not terribly unusual. The next day, at circle, Ruffin told his friends, 'They sewed my chin.'"

The Monday before the Fourth, with no playgroup, Ruffin and I entertained a visit from a mother and her child with autism. This resulted in a *folie a deux* of two children with autism feeding off each other to engage in their individual worst behaviors. She and I had a difficult time visiting. I was moved that this mother had driven all the way from Cedar Rapids to pose her list of questions. She left with a load of papers and borrowed books.

To celebrate the Fourth, Ruffin and I took a trip across the river with Seamus to watch a tractor-cade under an array of fireworks. Ruffin was delighted with the tractors, even with the explosions, the lights, and all the noise.

By Wednesday, Pine was back with 2 little girls to join Ruffin.

After our 4-day holiday break, Ruffin had a tantrum transitioning to playgroup, but not to his CARD therapy, and a tantrum to try to escape picking up afterwards, because I was present for him to appeal to.

Pine reported that while I was absent, Ruffin had asked one of the little girls, a little inappropriately, if she loved him. She had said, 'Not really,' but played quite a lot with him as I watched from the steps — swinging together, playing house in his new tent which he shared readily, and taking turns pushing each other on the merry-go-round octopus.

The next Thursday, RoJene, 3 little girls, Ruffin, and I decided to go to the county fair, a noisy public event that would be a great challenge for Ruffin. At first, he was unwilling to keep up with the group, and extremely demanding. He could see the Midway rides and kept insisting we go there to play. We were *not* taking these kids into the Midway. The first greater part of an hour or so was rough with Ruffin not wanting to see the livestock. Then he settled in, and we listened to a couple of bands perform, watched the animal showings, and toured the 4-H displays. More tractors were the most fun. Toward the end of the afternoon, we picnicked on the lawn and the children played copy-cat games. Ruffin needed to be the leader. RoJene was not sure he would have copied the others.

Ruffin had his stitches out that day, too, at the hospital in Decorah, where he had been treated earlier. He had tantrums on the way home over his seat belt. The little girls helped, by counting one, two three, to encourage Ruffin to buckle up. I stopped the car twice along the way to resolve the seat belt issue safely.

On Friday, Seamus, 3 little girls, Ruffin, and I visited the trout hatchery. This was a quieter natural setting and seemed to work out better. We fed the trout, by sharing the feed out of a bucket, and picnicked outside in Ruffin's tent. Seamus taught the game of tag, and the concept of 'It.' The children competed, racing from tree to tree and playing beanbag toss. We saw a baby bird. Ruffin had another small tantrum over his seat belt.

That night, I contacted Tris, now at Washington State, trying to track down yet another academic journal article he might have better access to than our interlibrary loan service. "Ruffin continues to do well."

I wanted to wish Tris well. "I hope you and your family enjoy the Northwest. I loved being there as an undergraduate — at Reed College in Portland, Oregon. As I recall, there were many, many students there studying B. F. Skinner in the 1970s, and so intent on their experiments that when the war moratorium took over their lab in the basement of the administration building, they insisted on not interrupting the operant conditioning of their rats for even one day! And I thought they were nuts."

Later in the summer, there came an answer from Tris. "I am glad that Ruffin continues to do well and that you have finally succeeded in obtaining some insurance funding for his treatment. I enjoyed your story about the highly dedicated Skinnerians."

Ruffin played for a couple of hours on Sunday after church with the little girl who "didn't really" love him. He seemed to be very attached to her.

Our playgroup the next Monday was RoJene, Chance, Ruffin and 2 little girls. When RoJene called, "Put the toys down and come to circle," Ruffin did it readily and happily.

Each child shared a toy for the first time ever. It was hard to get Ruffin to listen to the others, but he shared his Etch-a-Sketch and talked about getting his stitches out, reporting that it hurt, and admitting that he cried.

When it was time for water-play, Ruffin found and put on his swimsuit "by myself" and was very proud. In the back yard, it was hot again.

RoJene organized a lost shoe hunt, hiding one of everyone's shoes for the children to find. Ruffin was dead set against joining in at all, but RoJene insisted. The second time they hunted, he had fun. As RoJene observed, "The first time for new things is awfully hard for Ruffin."

The group discussed the word "pairs." RoJene had pairs of socks, mittens, gloves, and children's shoes. Ruffin was the only one who knew the word "gloves."

The afternoon temperature by mid-July was over 100 degrees. Three new girls joined our group. RoJene brought them all inside where it was a few degrees cooler. She tried coloring, play dough, computer, blocks, and UNO as play stations. Nothing worked. Ruffin had a hard day, on the verge of a tantrum at all times. The little girl Ruffin "loved" cried all day. The new girls didn't talk or move until the last few minutes. It was ridiculous in the heat. The heat had us all down.

RoJene's considered opinion was, "Ruffin is losing out with this new group of 10 different children. I can't deal with all of them at the same time and do much for Ruffin whose 2- to 5-minute attention span is even shorter in the heat."

Maybe it would cool off, but likely not. I needed to take RoJene's view to heart. The heat was taking a real toll, and certainly, a larger group of children offered Ruffin more confusion than support.

Time to "tickle" Mr. Hunter since we had heard nothing from him. "May Mr. Sytsma and I have the courtesy of your reply to my June 21st letter?"

CHAPTER THIRTY

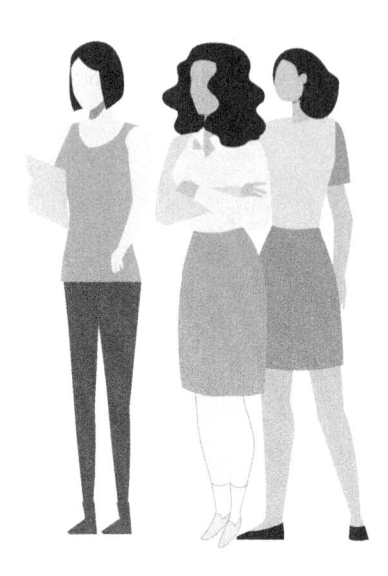

FIRST ANNIVERSARY

July 12th marked the first anniversary of Ruffin's diagnosis. Did I have time to reflect over the last year? Not much. But, as I discovered later when I inspected Ruffin's educational file, I *had* moved the school authorities to reflect on how to respond to Ruffin's needs and to my own unrelenting and annoying demands.

Mr. Montague was using a yellow highlighter to read my late-June letter. A large yellow question mark in the margin might have expressed his surprise as a trained audiologist, that Bridgewater, Sue Baker, and as many as four families were participating in a research project on auditory integration training (AIT) to determine the efficacy of this controversial treatment for children with autism.

Another large yellow question mark might have expressed his equal surprise that I had made substantial financial gifts to furnish Ruffin's classroom and playground last fall, yet none of those items were available to Ruffin this summer.

He noted Prudential's characterization of Lovaas therapy as "occupational therapy," and my assertion that if this were so, then Bridgewater was solely responsible to pay for it.

Finally, Mr. Montague highlighted my suggestion we wait for the results of the Mason City case, while I carried on for the summer with Prudential, reserving my rights to seek full reimbursement, so that Mason City and its AEA risk all the blood and dollar litigation cost of coming up with an answer to his problems with me.

Miss Hobbs's marginalia on her copy disputed my claim that Ruffin's classroom was unavailable to me, noting that I "didn't ask to use it; all that space can be rented." In her view, it was "not true" that the school district was unwilling to transport special education students to Luther College, crediting her own activism. "I went to ARC. They gave a donation, and our district paid the remainder."

Mr. Montague was talking to both the school attorneys, Mr. Hunter, and Mr. Carew, about Ruffin, and Mr. Hunter was supposed to be talking to mediator Dee Ann Wilson about scheduling a pre-appeal mediation conference. Together, Bridgewater and ACSD were taking the first steps to sue me in due process to obtain an ALJ ruling or court order on appeal that would require me to affix my signature to their late-May IEP prepared by themselves in my absence.

But Mr. Montague had responded more kindly to Renee's mother, Ruth, who had let him know that Bridgewater's autism resource team (ART) had been the only one in Sue Baker's statewide network not to apply for a $500 state-funded autism grant. "The team was planning to use the grant dollars to bring in some resources related to the TEACCH program to be shared with staff and parents. Unfortunately, when this project did not materialize, the team did not proceed on to another project." As the autism resource team (ART) leader last year, who had dropped the ball? We thought we could guess. And, as we knew, no project just "materializes."

"The new autism resource team (ART) leader Mary Carter has assured me that the team will be taking advantage of the grant this next school year. I am not sure you know that since the appointment of our ART, I have allocated a sum of $500 to the team to use as they have deemed appropriate. Therefore, the team has never been without fiscal resources. This is the same amount we have allocated to our Assistive Technology Team. Projects which exceed the above amount must have my approval prior to implementation."

Ruth, Jan Newmann, our county case manager, and I looked at each other. This all seemed rather pitiful. There was zero information about how the ART had chosen to spend their $500 pittance. We went on reading, Jan and I, by peering over Ruth's shoulder.

"To say" as Ruth had complained, "that members of the ART 'do not care about the needs of children with autism' is simply not correct. The members of the team have *volunteered* to serve because of their intense interest in learning more about autism and sharing that information with others about this unique disability. Their service on the team is above and beyond their regularly assigned duties."

I was grinning like a Cheshire cat at this point and explaining to Jan and Ruth that this letter contained significant written admissions that would be invaluable to Curt in executing our plans to *distinguish* the recent *Fairfax* Virginia loss.

Ruth offered without a moment's hesitation, "Go ahead, make a copy, if you need it."

The next time I visited with Sue, I ventured an observation that Mr. Montague's characterization of Bridgewater ART members as "volunteers" seemed contrary to our impression that our ART members were "drafted" and not nimble being given yet another hat to wear without further compensation.

"Nevertheless, they need to meet us, and our children, and get fascinated."

Ruffin's playgroup had a visit on Thursday from Emma Smith and her mother, Rebecca. Emma's father was Peter Smith, the principal of St. Patrick's School which rented space to Head Start and to the private nursery school. I hoped Rebecca would consider having Emma join us, but they never returned. Maybe they were just looking us over. Or, it could have been just the heat. The next afternoon's playgroup failed to meet because by that time the temperature in our garage classroom had risen to 106 degrees.

Instead, Ruffin and I went to meet RoJene and Chance at the larger Decorah pool. Like our trip to the fair, Ruffin was close to out-of-control for the better part of the first hour, yelling, hitting, fussing, whining, and always wanting something different. Later, he settled down.

RoJene thought the noise and confusion of these big, crowded places set Ruffin off. We talked about how she hoped he could be trained to tolerate these conditions by warning him what to expect, talking about his reactions, and repeating the crowded environment often. Age might make a difference. For me, our conversation provided a valuable view of Ruffin, seen through a teacher's trained eyes, and helped reinforce my choosing gradually more and more challenging environments for him then, and through the end of next summer.

Our playgroup had ballooned up again by mid-July to seven children — time for everyone to learn new names by passing the pink rock around the circle so each child could introduce him or herself before discussing rainbows and walking around the block to encounter a man cleaning fish.

Mr. Hunter finally got back to Curt. "Because of the approaching school year, we have been in touch with Dee Ann Wilson to schedule a pre-appeal mediation conference. My client and Bridgewater look forward to the assistance that mediation can provide." Maybe with this letter, Mr. Hunter felt he had moved Ruffin's file off his desk and back into the filing cabinet, but a letter of my own was crossing his in the mail.

Curt had advised me that the time was ripe now to exercise my rights under FERPA to inspect Ruffin's complete educational files to see what evidence might be there. I wrote to arrange that. So began a great paper chase that ran through the rest of the summer.

We had been faxing all our correspondence to Mr. Hunter, but he had not been faxing us back. This put him right back at the top of my "tickler" list. Time to prod him again.

"Settlement is not likely if we come to the table without your full responses to my inquiries delivered sufficiently in advance (within 10 days) of the pre-appeal mediation date for me to have given them thoughtful consideration with Mr. Sytsma."

This little tattle-tale letter was widely copied to everyone concerned, including our proposed mediator, Dee Ann Wilson.

Time to learn what more I could about Bridgewater's autism resource team (ART) and see what more information Mr. Montague might disclose about Bridgewater's expertise — or lack thereof — in autism. Time to provoke him openly. Any more information he might disclose could be relevant to Curt's theory for advancing Ruffin's case around the discouraging *Fairfax* decision from Virginia.

I sent him an aggressive letter which I also copied out widely.

Finally in mid-July, Mr. Hunter responded, but his message was disappointing. "ACSD and Bridgewater are well aware of your rights as Ruffin's parent to his records and as a citizen to their records under Chapter 21 and 22. We will be in touch with you to carry out the exercise of your rights."

What did I expect? I berated myself. It was summer.

Our playgroup continued to burgeon, with RoJene observing how it split into genders. "The group is quite different now with Sam and Chance, as two boys for Ruffin. The boys aren't interested in the same things as the girls."

Meanwhile, Bridgewater was scrambling to get its file on Ruffin in order before Dee Ann Wilson requested her copy to prepare herself to preside over mediation. Inge reported in to Mr. Montague offering a defensive chronology to meet my earlier assertion that Ruffin had been without an effective IEP since late last November.

"This is my best recollection of the events and chronology relating to Ruffin's IEP. I hope it offers some clarification of the issues."

It certainly did, as Curt and I came to read it just before our late summer mediation. It fully documented all our worst suspicions that Ruffin's educators had made a practice of flagrantly violating the IDEA's procedural protections requiring them to include Ruffin's parent — me — whenever making special education decisions affecting him, and before making any changes in his IEP.

At the tail end of the workweek, Mr. Hunter faxed me another letter — redolent of both panic and delay. "You and Mr. Sytsma have my assurance that the information necessary to respond fully to appropriate inquiries in your earlier letters is being gathered. I will be conferencing with Mr. Lord and Mr. Montague in late July and will advise you immediately of the time at which and the way you may expect the requested information."

For me, it was time to turn to the matter of scheduling re-evaluations of Ruffin in late September at Gundersen. I was eager to have Ruffin strut his new stuff there, too. Although I never seemed to get any concrete information out of Mr. Hunter or any of his kick-the-can-down-the-road letters, I disclosed all my latest plans — because it was important to Ruffin's future and to his success.

"I have made arrangements to schedule independent evaluations of Ruffin as follows: in late September at Gundersen, at an estimated cost of $2,000; and at the end of August at UIHC with Ms. Wilding for a comprehensive speech and language assessment, at an estimated cost likely to be minimal."

I planned to keep the Gundersen appointments should mediation fail.

"I am willing to consider that the appointment with Ms. Wilding may be all I need to help Ruffin should the establishment of his free, appropriate public education be along the lines I have previously requested."

"Also, Ruffin's Lovaas training consultant, Evelyn Kung of CARD will be returning on Saturday and Sunday, August 19th, and 20th to spend one of those days with Ruffin and his home therapists and to review Ruffin's summer playgroup experience with the teachers I employ. Ms. Kung will be spending her other day in town training a home therapy team organized and funded in part by Mental Retardation Medicaid Waiver for an older child with autism in ACSD." For Ruth's daughter, Renee.

"In her three to four years of working exclusively with children with autism, Ms. Kung has participated in the successful mainstreaming of numerous children like Ruffin into regular preschool classrooms of children who have enjoyed normal development. I want Mrs. Holub and Mrs. Mills both to conference with Evelyn Kung, RoJene Beard and Pine Wilson, my playgroup teachers, and with Donna Schmidt, my home therapist, for a couple of hours to help prepare Mrs. Mills to succeed in integrating Ruffin into her group of typically developing 4-year-olds.

"Donna Schmidt has indicated to me that she would be available to come to the private nursery school with Ruffin to help him there as a one-to-one aide, if necessary, to be faded as quickly as possible. I think this group and I ought to try to come to some consensus as to whether Donna's presence is necessary there, or whether we want to try integration without Donna at first, and to discuss with Mrs. Mills what behaviors, if any, would prompt her to seek Donna's assistance or further telephone consultation with Ms. Kung."

A handwritten note arrived from across the state, from a mother in Council Bluffs. "I wanted to send you a copy of our daughter's IEP and give my permission for you to distribute it if you feel it might be helpful — 30 hours a week of Lovaas paid by my AEA; 22 hours a week of Lovaas paid by Medicaid Mental Retardation Waiver for a total of 52 hours a week of Lovaas services. Can you believe it? I almost have more funds than I know what to do with and our daughter is doing great!"

I called her immediately and together we walked through her daughter's new IEP. Scott Peters had been the advocate for the family. I hoped this result would help pave the way for settlement of the Mason City case, and, of course, Ruffin's case, too. My fax whirred all this new information off to Curt.

By now, across Iowa there were a dozen children whose parents had organized and arranged funding for Lovaas home programming (ABA). Another dozen children were expected to begin programs in the fall of 1995.

CHAPTER THIRTY ONE

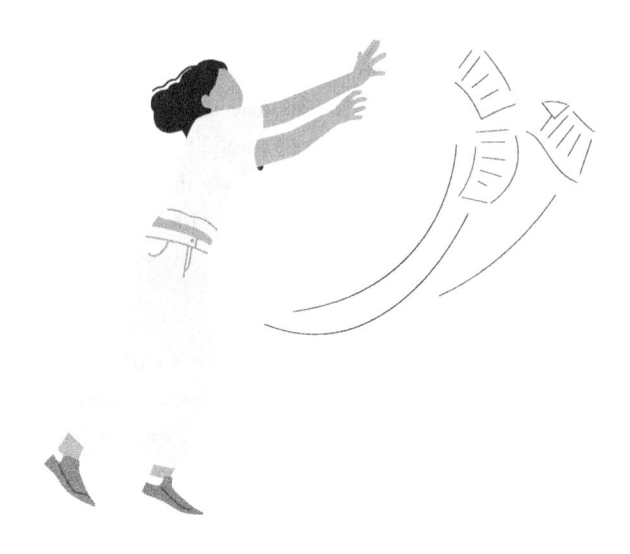

THE PAPER CHASE

The lawyer Mr. Hunter was scheduled to meet with Mr. Lord and Mr. Montague on a Monday in late July about gathering up Ruffin's educational files. Meg was called in from summer vacation to write a memo about all her phone conversations with Dr. Norman. By that time, she was unable to remember the dates or even who had called. She thought she had been asked about Ruffin's tantrums and "closure on the IEP." All she remembered was: "A head cold and pneumonia are also on the same continuum, but you would not treat them the same," the same remark Kim had offered to Tris back in March. Meg's memory — or reticence — offered a good illustration of why it was important to keep a running, written educational record. Otherwise, no one recalled dates, names, or even the substance of fairly important conversations about Ruffin.

Meanwhile, Mr. Montague, back from vacation, promised Mr. Hunter a memo from Kim. Her memo was brief. "Sometime in January prior to Ruffin's visit to Iowa City, I had one conversation with a gentleman there. The caller wanted to know about

Ruffin's behavior, for example, would it be difficult to test him formally. I responded that Ruffin should not be difficult to test. He was sitting well for me and was responding well to both verbal and visual stimuli."

During our earlier exchanges about Ruffin's use of the word "silly," Dr. Norman had fully disclosed the dates of every earlier contact between himself and the school authorities and their employees and promised to send his handwritten notes to me.

I had agreed, and let him know, "I will appreciate a copy of any records or notes you may have of our telephone contacts to help me refresh my own recollection." Dr. Norman responded now by faxing them all. The most important and damaging information he had noted was Meg's frank admission to him that the school authorities reached their decision to deny Ruffin Lovaas programming *before* meeting with Curt and me in mid-March — something which Meg had neglected, forgotten, or known better than to mention in her own memo written recently and long after the fact.

This came as no real surprise. It was surprising that there would be this undeniable documentary evidence of it.

Seamus came by to leave me the paper. I turned to the small print *Legal Notice* section. Our local school board had paid $1,942.37 to Mr. Hunter's law firm for the month of June. Making a rough back of the envelope calculation, I was dismayed to find that by partnering with Prudential, this money would have funded 388 hours of Ruffin's CARD program.

Meanwhile, RoJene had Ruffin and his 5 playmates dip their hands in paint and press them onto 50 benefit posters to raise money for the CARIN' group's effort to install adaptive playground equipment at school. After washing their hands under the garden hose, the children made their own peanut butter and jelly sandwiches. Only one of them had ever done this before. They had fun and ate them all up!

My deliberately provocative letter to Mr. Montague about Bridgewater's autism resource team (ART) failures finally drew a predictably touchy defense. But he had ended his letter with a significant admission. "You have expressed serious concern about the lack of parental input into this process. I agree that the autism resource team (ART) has not done as good a job of this as we might have. To ensure that you have a voice in this process I invite you to submit any suggestions you may have to Mary Carter."

Ruffin's playgroup celebrated Chance's birthday on July 27th. We had a thunderstorm that turned the sky black as night, so we retreated inside to eat cake and drink lemonade on the kitchen floor. Chance got a present from Ruffin who was very excited about giving it. Bubbles. A gallon of bubble solution and we made hundreds of bubbles, while the junior high school volunteers assembled large packages for the Society, and for Mary Carter, the new Bridgewater autism resource team (ART) leader.

As the party broke up, Renee's mother Ruth brought over a reply she had received from Mr. Montague full of interesting information about Bridgewater's ART. He had liked her newsletter, asking Ruth, "Please give me more details on how you wish Bridgewater to assist you" in its distribution. Ruth looked up at me, "Really, how hard is distribution for Bridgewater? We get all kinds of bookbag notes from them. Why not just throw this in, too?"

She continued reading aloud. Mr. Montague promised to inquire further "into how the schools might use sign language with Renee" since "Sue Baker has offered some technical assistance when my staff returns to work for the 1995-1996 school year."

I looked back at Ruth. "Sounds exactly like his response to my call a year ago when Ruffin was diagnosed. We're all going to just die here in the summer heat, waiting for the cavalry to arrive."

He had sent a copy of a recent letter from Sue. "It spells out in detail the circumstances related to our AEA's ART grant application."

"That's something," said Ruth, hopefully.

"Well, you got a letter," I replied.

And then we both laughed, a bit cynically.

Mr. Montague had also sent Ruth "several documents which are related to our ART which you may find of interest. One is a draft copy of the overall goals for the coming year." Ruth and I looked these over together, eagerly. "Awareness" began with "What we can and can't do." This was familiar territory to both Ruth and me, as were the "clarification meeting or phone call" that came whenever either of us had reached out for professional help.

Bridgewater's focus was clearly on staff development and indirect services, with "increased parental involvement and input" frankly characterized as "secondary." The most ominous "Staff Development" topic was "legal issues." The ART had an in-service presentation for local teams only, not parents, titled "Do's and Don'ts in Autism." They also saw themselves as having some function in the arena of "Assessment," where their lack of expertise was likely to be dangerous. There was some interest in exploring the topic of whether there might be unique features in the development of IEPs for children with autism.

But Mr. Montague had closed his letter to Ruth with an invitation. "You have expressed an interest in having some input into the ART process, and I invite you to submit any suggestion you might wish Bridgewater's ART to consider which would assist parents more effectively.

"This is the only way we will identify and resolve problems. It has been my experience that when parents and service providers disagree on issues it does not mean that one group is *against* the other. It simply means we disagree on a particular issue and such issues need to be resolved through discussion, compromise, and better understanding of each other's position."

By that time, with Ruth reading out the end of Mr. Montague's letter, I was rolling on my dining room carpet with laughter, and as Ruth finished, she asked me if I didn't have a cold beer in my refrigerator.

"Yes," I choked, "Why don't you take one of Seamus's?"

Time to tickle Mr. Hunter again. "May Mr. Sytsma and I have the courtesy of substantive replies — something beyond polite acknowledgments — to my three earlier letters?

"We face a final practical deadline of about August 29th, being the approximate date school resumes. It appears to me that we are unacceptably close to running out of time without any firm arrangements for Ruffin's education being made, much less agreed to, before school starts."

Because he and I had had a good visit after his little daughter visited Ruffin's playgroup, I felt comfortable reaching out to Peter Smith, the principal of St. Patrick's Catholic School to lend him the 1987 Lovaas documentary and ask him to pass it on to Elaine Mills, who would be Ruffin's teacher in the fall at the private nursery school. I was concerned because Elaine whom I had recruited to be a playgroup teacher had backed out at the last minute. After playgroup finished for the summer, I would let Donna pass the notebook of materials Pine returned to us on to Elaine who took it, then, readily enough, directly from Donna, her friend.

Mr. Montague faxed Kim's latest memo to Mr. Hunter late in the day on the last day of July. He included it in a longer fax to me of two separate letters. He assured everyone concerned that Meg's and Kim's memos had been added to Ruffin's educational file and that "a survey of their respective staffs by Mr. Lord and Mr. Montague discloses no other contacts with the medical team at the UIHC during the time period indicated by you." Now, I had them to compare with Dr. Norman's much more detailed handwritten notes of the same conversations which he had jotted down at the time.

But no one was going to make it easy for me to inspect the rest of Ruffin's files. "Both the ACSD and Bridgewater maintain required files regarding Ruffin's education. We are not aware of any requirement that these files be gathered at any one place. Please contact Mr. Lord and Mr. Montague directly, and they will make reasonable arrangements for your examinations and copying." I was scolded, "Your comment advising our client and the AEA not to cull items from Ruffin's file was unnecessary, as ACSD and Bridgewater are both well aware of legal requirements and professional standards on this subject."

As for Mr. Hunter, "I had hoped to provide you with a comprehensive answer to the many points in your lengthy letter of June 21st. However, I find that summer schedules have made this difficult. We will begin providing you with responses to portions of that letter as each is completed and hope to have these to you in the very near future in sufficient time for your review prior to our pre-appeal mediation session."

Mr. Hunter's other letter was an apology addressed directly to our mediator, Dee Ann Wilson. "I had talked to you by telephone in mid-July regarding a pre-appeal mediation conference and believed that the formal processing of that conference had been accomplished. The suggested date of August 18th was cleared with everyone from ACSD and Bridgewater, Mr. Carew's office, and my office.

"When I spoke with you this morning by telephone and received Mary Jane White's latest letter, I realized that you were waiting for formal written request for the conference and that you had had no communication with her regarding that date. For my part in that misunderstanding, I do apologize."

It seemed to me Mr. Hunter might not know what he was supposed to be doing to handle this legal matter for our local district. That concerned me. It was always more difficult to work with — and against — an adversary who didn't have a clue. As an officer of the court, bound by the rules of legal ethics, working against a clueless adversary meant you had to do their work *and* your own work *and* bend over backwards to be fair to help the court, the decision maker, or the mediator to reach a fair and just result. It was always just a huge pain in the ass.

And what would have happened had I not written my latest tickling letter? Nothing. Nothing. Nothing for Ruffin.

I needed to get up early on the first day of August to answer Mr. Hunter, when my mind would be fresh, and when, hopefully, I had left any anger and frustration on my pillow. I was able to fax my reply to him out to the world before Ruth arrived with her daughter Renee. Donna was there, ready to watch Ruffin and Renee until this afternoon's playgroup.

By the crack of dawn, Ruth and I had begun our three-hour drive south to Cedar Rapids where the Society, the Woodward State Hospital School and a group home partnership were putting on an all-day Structured Teaching Methods workshop. The TEACCH presenter, Ruth Hurst — whom Bridgewater's autism resource team (ART) had failed to connect with for their overdue grant proposal — was going to be presenting, along with several other TEACCH-certified speakers.

Since I had read all the published TEACCH volumes, I was curious to see how this methodology differed from Lovaas, and Ruth wanted to see whether TEACCH might have something appropriate to offer her older, non-verbal daughter Renee.

Ms. Hurst worked at the Woodward State Hospital School, a locked residential placement for children with autism who were unable to live at home due to their difficult behaviors. She reported the incidence of autism then at approximately 15 in every 10,000 people, with perhaps 26 in 10,000 when Asperger's syndrome was included — which sounded like a small percentage of the population, unless, like Ruth and me, you had such a child at home, in which case you had autism 100% — in your family.

Ms. Hurst assured us that 70-80% of people on the autism spectrum were also mentally retarded, with IQs below 70. However, she offered the names of Temple Grandin, Donna Williams, and Thomas McKean as examples of three people with autism without mental retardation.

Then she ran down the overlap of autism with Tourette's, pica (the eating of inedible substances), anxiety, anorexia, bulimia, obsessive compulsive disorder, Down syndrome, Prader-Willie syndrome, fragile X, tuberous sclerosis, and general seizure disorders. As treatments, she mentioned megavitamins and facilitated communication.

And then, she turned to her treatment of choice, Structured Teaching or TEACCH. Her talk was full of anecdotes of horrors, resolved by structuring the child or adult's environment around unbroken routine.

The next speaker offered several tips for structuring a child's environment by establishing physical boundaries, with partitions, shades over the windows and mirrors, or using tape on the floor to mark off leisure space from workspace, minimizing distractions by structuring a barren environment, and the use of noise-cancelling headphones to avoid the child picking up extraneous speech.

The facilities for teaching at Woodward were described as very highly structured in this way, with children set to work in cubicles. In the living quarters, round tablecloths marked the tables for eating, with a change to square tablecloths signaling the tables could be used for leisure. Visual and object schedules were assembled for each child's highly structured day.

Children in cubicles proceeded from bin to bin of tasks, left to right, top to bottom, with transition objects such as clothespins, and rewards of popcorn and soda. Most of the children's work amounted to "make-work" which the staff then took apart. Obviously, everyone stayed busy. The staff ratio at Woodward was characterized as "rich" — at 1 adult to every 4 children with autism.

To me, this seemed a bizarre and isolated life.

Dee Ann Wilson issued her notice to all parties concerned and to her colleague Gerry Gritzmacher, that she would be our mediator at a pre-appeal review conference to be held on Ruffin's behalf on Mr. Hunter's August 18th date at 9:00 A.M. in the library at the high school in our town, giving us all her phone number to call "if you should be unable to attend."

Curt needed to clear his busy schedule and I needed to file numerous motions in all my Tuesday morning motion hearings in a distant county on behalf of my clients there to ask the state courts and all opposing counsel to please reschedule all those other matters to later dates.

Mr. Lord was required to complete a special education pre-appeal review checklist and return it to Dee Ann, with a copy of Ruffin's most recent staffing report or evaluation, and Ruffin's most recently developed IEP. Since Ruffin had long since mastered all his August 1994 IEP goals and had submitted to two "independent" outside evaluations as well, the material Dee Ann had requested was likely to leave her in the darkness of ancient history as far as Ruffin was concerned.

RoJene reported in about playgroup. "It was an interesting boys-only day. The boys drove cars on the road-mat for 30 minutes at first. After reading *The Very Hungry Caterpillar*, we colored pre-cut butterflies and hung them up in the garage with our spiders. Ruffin shared nicely today of his own accord without being prompted."

It was the end of the day. Mr. Montague had yet to return my call about when and where he would share Ruffin's Bridgewater files with me.

CHAPTER THIRTY TWO

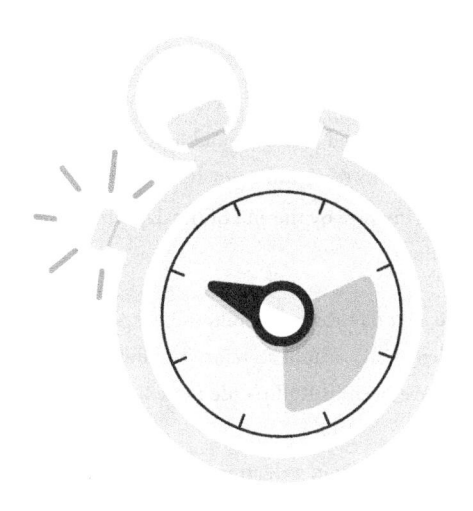

DOWN TO THE WIRE

Mr. Montague called finally, well after the close of business. I could see Ruffin's Bridgewater files on August 15th at 9:00 A.M. at the local field office — what he called the two co-joined trailers across the blacktopped playground from our junior high. A scant three days before our scheduled mediation. He and "Moe" would bring all Ruffin's files over from Elkader, except Inge's and Jack's which were in Decorah, locked up because neither would be back from vacation until late August. He promised not to charge me for the first 100 copies. After that, the copy charge would be twenty cents per page.

I listened without arguing and sat right down to write Mr. Hunter a smoking fax.

"Mr. Montague advised me today that it will not be possible for me to inspect the files Inge Nilsen and Jack Wallace kept on Ruffin until late August, *after* our pre-appeal mediation, when they both return from summer vacation. Surely someone has a key to the Decorah field office and can retrieve their two files so I may inspect them."

My phone rang early the next morning. The woman calling introduced herself as Caron Angelos, one of Mr. Hunter's law partners. He was on vacation. She was monitoring his cases and had my most recent fax.

Caron agreed that my asking to see Inge and Jack's files "seemed to be a reasonable request," and that people being on vacation "was no excuse" for my being unable to exercise my rights as a parent under FERPA.

Everybody, it seemed, was on vacation, except Caron and me. Who needed a vacation anyway? I was so hopping mad that if I could have disappeared on vacation myself, I would never have been able to relax and enjoy it.

Fine, I was in a towering rage by the end of the day when Seamus ventured to stick his head in my kitchen door.

I spent most of the next day at the schoolhouse, inspecting and copying what Miss Hobbs had given the elementary school secretary to offer me. Many items that I knew existed — that should have been in Ruffin's file there — were missing. I simply took a copy of all I was offered.

Caron called again that evening, well after suppertime, to assure me Mr. Montague had just committed to producing "all files" for me on August 15th. "Good," I thought, and filed her name, Caron, under the word — Good — where I would keep her in mind.

First thing in the morning, I called Miss Hobbs to ask, "Where are all my letters to school? They were not in Ruffin's file yesterday."

"They are in my file and Mr. Lord's file, which are *personal* files, *not* available to you."

I tried to talk to Curt. He was in Mason City with Dee Ann Wilson, working on trying to mediate the case there. I didn't want to disturb them, but I did want to talk with someone knowledgeable and experienced in FERPA law and practice — the norms of educational file-keeping, if you will — and about what I thought smelled fishy.

So, I called Gerry Gritzmacher. We had spoken before, at Dr. Norman's suggestion.

Gerry told me he did a lot of pre-appeal mediations in autism and behavior disorder cases. That made me wonder why he wasn't in Mason City, but he didn't say, and I didn't ask. He told me that he and Dee Ann usually worked together on them, as the neutral parties in mediation, as a resource to both sides, particularly if there were questions about the administrative rules of special education. He and Dee Ann shared an expertise on the rules, and on methods and best practices in behavior management in special education. They tried to stay neutral without advocating any particular method.

I began to ask as many dumb questions as I could think of to continue to engage him. It seemed to be a good time for him. Summers must be slow even in Des Moines.

Gerry explained what would happen at our upcoming mediation.

He pulled up the state mediation file on Ruffin at my request and confirmed it would be Dee Ann who would be handling it. She had already written to request Ruffin's special education file, but nothing had arrived there yet in Des Moines from either ACSD or Bridgewater.

I explained that Ruffin's educational files seemed to have been "culled" by ACSD and might not even include the files kept by the most important people working with Ruffin at Bridgewater. Gerry agreed this would present a serious obstacle to mediation and to Dee Ann as the mediator.

We talked over the sort of letter I might write to remedy this problem for Dee Ann.

That afternoon, using Gerry's suggestions, I faxed out another letter about Ruffin's educational records. "I had the opportunity to review some of ACSD's records on Ruffin yesterday morning. I very much appreciated Miss Hobbs's willingness to provide the copies I made yesterday at no cost. However, I could not help but notice as I inspected Ruffin's school records, that very few of my many letters to school authorities, teachers, speech therapists and the like were in the file." Then, I recounted my unavailing call to Miss Hobbs.

During playgroup, RoJene reported Chance's cousin, Sam, got stung by a bee and Ruffin was extremely sympathetic.

Miss Hobbs called. I could re-inspect and "amend" Ruffin's file there on August 14th in the early afternoon.

With Ruffin sound asleep, I prepared an updated accounting that Curt needed for mediation, documenting my costs of Ruffin's special education to date of over $60,000. This was a net figure — less the claims Prudential had already paid.

My home treatment team videotaped the day's activities that Monday, CARD drills in the morning and playgroup in the afternoon as an exhibit for mediation or due process, showing Ruffin learning new things, and right in the thick of it all afternoon.

Taking my own binders of chronological files with me, I drove back to the vacant schoolhouse to re-inspect Ruffin's ACSD files. Someone had already returned most of my letters and videotapes to Ruffin's file. Nevertheless, I sat for several hours under the watchful eye of Miss Hobbs's secretary, as I paged through the school's file and my own binders, page by page, checking carefully so that the result by the afternoon's end was that each file became a complete duplicate of the other.

I discovered that Kim had written another memo indicating that she would be keeping back in her "personal" file all Ruffin's test protocols. "I have nothing else that is not already a part of the file. I like to hang on to the protocols so that I can track changes easily." Well, as Ruffin's cranky mother, I thought, I would like to see his protocols, too, and assess his developmental changes for myself.

First thing in the morning, I drove over to Bridgewater's cobbled together trailers and lugged my set of Ruffin's binders up the metal stairs, looked around and found Mr. Montague and "Moe" waiting for me, drinking coffee, and eating pastry. I said hello, nodding, and shaking each of their hands, indicating that I was ready to get to work. They asked that I sign a written request form to inspect Bridgewater's files first.

Then several piles — one for each Bridgewater employee concerned — were set out on a desk they invited me to sit at and use, while they watched. As with the day before, this was a matter of hours, with poor "Moe" needing to use a tailbone donut to sit on a molded plastic chair.

I began to leaf through each sliding pile, while Mr. Montague and "Moe" fell to chatting with each other first about agency matters and then about their personal lives, hobbies, and families. Eventually, they simply ignored me.

After all, Mr. Montague's secretary, Joy, was there to make copies of anything I needed. Most of the piles were so poorly organized it seemed easier to me for Joy to just copy each pile. I would be able to sort them out later at home, by working all night.

The way it went was I looked through a given pile, identified whose file it seemed to be, and then handed it over to Joy for copying. A half hour later, Joy would bring me back my photocopy. I would set the original pile by my photocopies, and compare every photocopy with every original, checking to be sure no page had slipped by in the copier's feeder. Joy and I both knew it happened. She was patient and professional. I'm sure the air conditioning helped.

The piles Bridgewater offered me included Mr. Montague's own sequestered file from Elkader with all his correspondence with the two law firms — even the evidence of Mr. Carew's earliest advice to the school authorities to grant my requests for Ruffin without cavil. Joy copied it all right under Mr. Montague's and "Moe's" noses as they continued chatting idly with each other.

"Thanks so much," I said, with genuine cheerfulness at the end of our long day. "See you at mediation."

In response to Dee Ann's request that ACSD attach a copy of Ruffin's most recent staffing report and a copy of his most recently developed IEP, the only documents attached were the original August 1st, 1994 Bridgewater evaluation team report, suggesting that Ruffin was moderately mentally retarded with an IQ of 50, the August 25th, 1994 IEP, the December 8th, 1994 draft IEP, and the most recent January, 1995 evaluation report from UIHC. None of the fall 1994 Gundersen Clinic autism evaluation material had been included.

All this would help Curt and I know what our mediator, Dee Ann, had seen about Ruffin beforehand — and what she had yet to see — that Curt and I would need to share, or point out to her. For example, that Ruffin's most recent IQ score was 97.

Mr. Hunter had written me, too. By then, he was back from vacation and seemed confident he had run out the clock. "In response to your letter of June 21st, we would like to provide you with a limited response to some of your inquiries. You discuss the fact that Ruffin's IQ is too high to qualify him for a Mental Retardation waiver. You also discuss the summer activity run by the group home as not having an appropriate student body to provide Ruffin with appropriate speech and language models. We agree with your statements.

"We also believe that there are many areas of agreement concerning Ruffin's IEP and look forward to the opportunity to review this information during the mediation process on Friday."

With his limited response to my long-ago midsummer inquiries, Mr. Hunter had discarded a few losing cards from his client's hand — the possibility of cost-shifting Ruffin's special education to Medicaid — and any contention that the school's EYSE offer before this summer began was in any way defensible as "appropriate."

The great paper chase, such as it was, was at an end.

It was still early in California, so I could visit with Evelyn on the phone. She needed a fresh written report of exactly how Ruffin was doing to review before she arrived just after mediation. Curt was due to arrive Thursday night before Friday's mediation. I had two days to kill two birds with one stone. My written report for Evelyn could easily double as a draft present level of educational performance (PLEP), in case we were able to write an appropriate IEP for Ruffin, either at, or after mediation.

I gathered around me all Donna and Lisa's daily CARD drill therapy notes and RoJene's daily playgroup notes and began compiling and writing. Clean copies of this document were helpful to circulate back to Donna, Lisa, RoJene, Pine, Evelyn, and Dr. Granpeesheh, and to sit and discuss with Seamus, or to have a phone call with my parents about, and to pass on to later evaluators.

Someone at school later, Meg, or Inge, or the two of them working together, circled, and carefully underlined this document of mine — noting all the progress Ruffin had made over the summer.

Then, I turned to the school authorities' late-March plan to gauge Ruffin's progress toward those proposed annual goals and objectives. No one from school had even seen Ruffin since late May. Over the summer Ruffin had already achieved many of the year-long goals and objectives planned for him by the schools for next year. I faxed this, together with my PLEP, to Evelyn in California for her to review with Dr. Granpeesheh and to mark up on the plane as she flew to see us in Iowa.

Rose had answered the door, and in walked Curt, who greeted Ruffin, squatting down to meet his little client for the first time, peering into his face, and waiting for eye contact, before saying, "Hello there, little fellow," holding out his hand for Ruffin to shake. Ruffin took it and smiled, but quickly broke away, his own curiosity about the doorbell satisfied, to return to his Legos.

Then, Curt turned to say hello and goodbye to Donna on her way out the door. Rose was cooking, so we would have dinner. Lisa was expected to arrive before long to work with Ruffin afterward.

"Come in, come in," I invited him, handing him a copy of all I had prepared, which he flipped through briefly.

"Good, can I take this back to my motel? It should be useful if we manage to get to a settlement tomorrow."

Curt and I swapped good news.

Curt went first. "We've just settled the Mason City case. Of course, the child's not coming back to school anywhere in Iowa, but the district agreed to pay the doctor and his family a reimbursement." The amount struck me as right in the ballpark of all the earlier settlements in other states.

"Congratulations," I grinned. "Maybe that will be helpful to share with everyone else tomorrow."

"I think so."

"And, I have good news from Evelyn, too. Grant Wood AEA in Cedar Rapids is going to pay CARD for a two-day training workshop for a child there this fall."

"Excellent, more good information we can let drop tomorrow in negotiations."

Curt and I sat down after dinner to work through our understanding of the most recent results of the great paper chase, paging quickly through Ruffin's chronological file, hitting my yellow highlights, each one of which I had tabbed with a colored paperclip.

Our two legal heads were better than one. While my own great skill as a litigator was the skill of "the second chair," the person on the litigation team who knew all the details and "owned" every scrap of the evidence by having it organized and readily indexed and tabbed so any member of the team could have it to hand in a moment, Curt's great skill as a litigator and appellate brief-writer was the skill of "the first chair," the team member who could view the whole case from 30,000 feet up, who could summarize Ruffin's case to simple clarity for our mediators.

Curt was able to shape Ruffin's case to a persuasive and winning three-pronged set of legal themes designed to undermine the objections of our adversaries, the school authorities — very politely — in a way they need never feel the sharpness of the blade we hoped would dispose of them, so they would give up and give in — nearly thankfully.

By midnight, Curt and I were both ready to print and collapse. I laughed, "Best preparation for trial is a good night's sleep."

"Yes," Curt agreed, as he loaded up his briefcase and headed out into the soft, summer dark.

CHAPTER THIRTY THREE

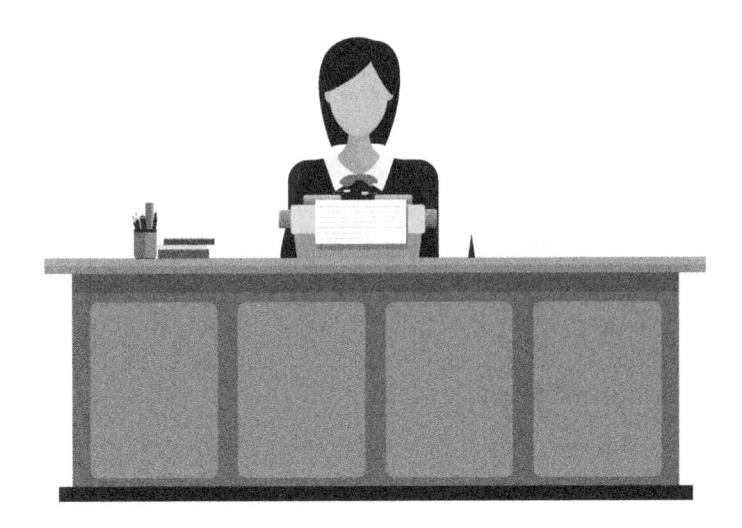

MEDIATION

On the appointed Friday in mid-August, while Donna put Ruffin through his paces, Curt and I walked into the high school library together. He greeted Dee Ann, introduced her to me, and me to her. Gerry Gritzmacher was there, too. "Hello," I said, "Nice to put a face to your voice." I recognized Bridgewater's attorney Mr. Carew, of course, and said my hello.

Mr. Hunter's absence was explained by Caron the Good who was here from his firm to represent ACSD. Curt knew Caron well. He was pleased to be working with her, and quietly let me know.

I agreed, "Yes, Caron has been good, helpful, much more so than Mr. Hunter, on the FERPA issues — getting all the paper rounded up."

Jan from county case management walked in to join us, at my invitation. She gave me a hug. She was there, purely for support. Then, Shirley K. Paradis arrived, the private court reporter, whom I had engaged to come and make a permanent record of the proceedings. As they each arrived, I introduced them to everyone.

With the group gathered, we got down to the business at hand — not Ruffin, necessarily — but procedure. Everyone was uncomfortable with the presence of Shirley, my court reporter. I thought to myself, what a bunch of scaredy-cats. Were we all likely to keep complete and identical notes of these proceedings? Not a chance. Not while everyone was thinking, talking, and planning to talk — like lawyers.

Finally, in a failing effort to lighten the mood in the room, Dee Ann offered, "I will just use first names unless anyone has any problems with that. I will try to keep this as informal as possible."

Dee Ann called on "Gus," and Mr. Montague responded, with great formality. "I have been asked to make an opening statement on behalf of ACSD and Bridgewater." Woah, I thought, were I in Caron's shoes, I would feel more than a little wobbly about this. It crossed my mind, then, that Caron was a woman here, bearing no resemblance to a Roman emperor. No waving of the olive branch though, no proposal of any "marriage."

Curt then spoke for me at length and with passion about our mid-winter IEP meeting. "I find this flabbergasting. It's bad enough we had a meeting of the school members of Ruffin's IEP team in advance of the real IEP meeting with his mother, it's bad enough the meeting before the meeting made important decisions in her absence, but afterwards, at the *real* IEP meeting the school members of the IEP team told her that they were prohibited from discussing two subjects: her proposed methodology for the education of Ruffin, and summer programming for him — in other words, the IEP team couldn't address anything that was important.

"That is so blatantly illegal — procedurally — that I find it appalling. Evidence of all this is readily available in Ruffin's educational records. You will be able to find it, because — as is her wont — and it is a good practice — Ruffin's mother has kept good records of all these proceedings."

After that, Dee Ann and Gerry separated our group into two caucuses. Negotiating went smoothly and steadily on for three hours that morning and four more hours that afternoon.

Mr. Montague rallied the educator group to wave his olive branch, and we all managed to contract a shotgun marriage of Ruffin's school and home programming along the lines I had suggested in my late June letter.

I provided the dowry by backing down on my money claim, as I had planned to do, being careful to secure the educators' agreement to pay the target amount I knew I would need to finish with Ruffin's CARD program, whatever else might happen.

The reimbursement to be paid me by ACSD was later published in the school board minutes as $20,000. The unpublished reimbursement to me from Bridgewater raised the "confidential" total settlement amount above the Mason City case settlement, the one Dee Ann and Curt had just mediated there.

As it turned out, without my court reporter, Shirley, we would have had no accurate record made of the agreements we reached, nothing to rely upon during the coming months as the agreement needed to be reduced to written settlement documents, signed, and carried forward.

We agreed that an IEP meeting would be held early that evening when a goal would be written to address Ruffin's social skills. To meet that goal for the next school year, Ruffin would attend the private nursery school Monday, Wednesday, and Friday afternoons, with tuition paid and transportation provided by ACSD who would also pay Evelyn for 10 hours of consultation with Meg and Mrs. Mills, the private nursery school teacher. The IEP team would discuss having a computer available there.

For more integration, Ruffin would attend ACSD on Tuesday and Thursday afternoons when Head Start visited.

At ACSD, on Monday, Tuesday, Wednesday, and Thursday mornings, either Donna or Lisa would attend school with Ruffin as my employee to carry out Ruffin's CARD program there. ACSD would reimburse me a flat $5 per hour for that work.

Ruffin would continue to attend the adaptive physical education activities provided at Luther College on Fridays.

An independent educational evaluation paid for by Prudential would be obtained from UIHC as soon as possible. There would also be a follow-up evaluation by the UIHC in the spring, and Bridgewater would pay for that. Afterwards, we would reevaluate Ruffin's IEP.

It had been a long, productive day of negotiations. Dee Ann finished up just before suppertime, and left with Gerry for Des Moines, a five-hour drive, west and south, on the available two-lane rural roads — which brook no diagonals, leaving them no choice but to drive Etch-a-Sketch fashion, first straight into the sunset, and then with the sun setting to their right.

Curt and I had a couple of hours to eat, breathe, and regroup, before reconvening with some of the educators early that evening to write an IEP to implement our settlement.

As we decompressed, I congratulated Curt on the result of his hard work for Ruffin and for me. But I told him it grieved me to know that Ruffin's education should not have cost a cooperating group of people any more than what I scribbled for him on the back of a napkin:

$14,550.54 for Ruffin's CARD home program for the school year and summer months

$ 500.00 for Ruffin's participation in a summer Playgroup

$15,050.54 for Ruffin's TOTAL 12-month free, appropriate public education (FAPE)

Less $-6,382.79 contribution from Prudential

$ 8,667.75 Net Joint Cost to ACSD and Bridgewater

That was several hundred dollars *less* than what ACSD and Bridgewater would receive in 1994-1995 state funding by "weighting" Ruffin as a 2.4 special education student — approximately $9,140. Except that Curt and I had agreed at the educators' request to "weight" Ruffin as a 3.6 "severe and profoundly disabled child," so they could collect $13,680 on his enrollment for 1995-1996.

Meg came to Ruffin's IEP meeting that evening with handwritten goals and objectives and a typewritten PLEP which we needed to revise together.

Since Kim was not in attendance, there was not much we could do to elevate her speech and language goals for Ruffin. She was planning to cut services to Ruffin anyway. Meg reported the results of Kim's two February formal testing sessions of Ruffin on the *Preschool Language Scale — 3* and *Boehm Test of Basic Concepts — Preschool Version*. Those results indicated an approximate 6-month delay in overall language skills, representing much improvement over previous testing.

Emily, the school psychologist, was also conspicuous by her absence.

Miss Hobbs sat in silently.

Working together, Meg, Inge, and I made short work of re-writing Ruffin's annual goals and measurable short-term objectives to bring Ruffin's language skills into the normal range as measured by formal testing by August of next year.

Ruffin's CARD drills were explicitly acknowledged to be part of his IEP, as part of his free, appropriate public education (FAPE). This was the concession I was willing to buy for Ruffin — and hopefully for Renee and others in Bridgewater — by compromising on my claim for past reimbursement.

Other *Annual Goals* included: "(1) Ruffin will be mainstreamed with language developmentally appropriate children, in order to develop social interaction skills appropriate to the setting; (2) Ruffin will increase his social interactions with peers and other adults including the initiation of interactions." There were appropriate math goals and the promise of a "kindergarten transition plan."

Meg and Inge quickly filled out the rest of the federally mandated state form.

But the cover page still included a statement that "EYSE issues are not yet resolved." The truth was we were all dead tired after a long day of negotiation, and more of the truth was — as Curt had argued earlier in the day — the Iowa EYSE rule for summer services was ridiculously illegal.

Curt and Dr. Hagen would be working on revising it over the winter. So, for the moment, then, we all punted again on the 1996 summer services issue.

We quit.

When I got home late that evening, hoping to cuddle with Ruffin, he was already asleep. Rose was asleep too, but stirred as I came in the door, and gathered her things to go home, asking softly, "How did it go?"

"Well enough," I smiled through my weariness.

"I'm glad then. See you tomorrow."

While I had been unable to see Ruffin all day, his schedule had run like clockwork in my absence, thanks to Seamus, Rose, Donna, Lisa, RoJene, Pine, and our junior high school volunteers. Did I need to wake Ruffin? I wanted to hug him, to have a hug *from* him. Instead, I stroked his hair, watched him sleep on a while, before heading back downstairs to call Seamus and my parents.

Finally, stepping out on the porch in the dark to retrieve the day's ungathered mail — I was delighted to find a New Jersey educational materials supplier had sent a new set of "I Feel" cards for little exercises Evelyn and Dr. Granpeesheh had suggested we try using to introduce Ruffin to the trickiest thickets of human nature by arming him with a robust working "theory of mind."

CHAPTER THIRTY FOUR

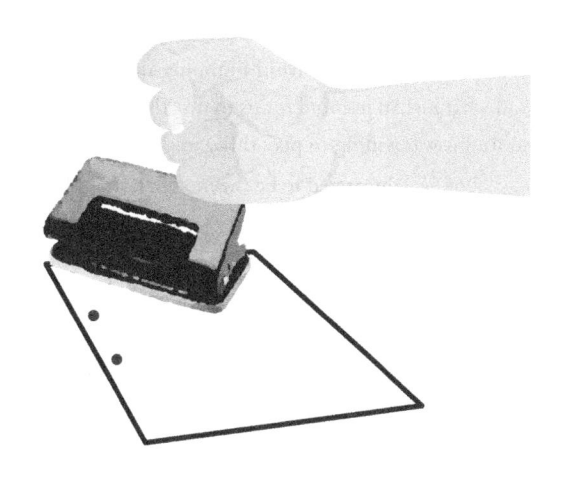

BLOWBACK

Evelyn arrived from California, that first weekend after our long day of mediation, familiar enough with Iowa by then to be driving a tiny, red rental through the high corn and bright green soybean fields away from the farm of the Smith family near Brayton deep in central Iowa to our home in the far northeast corner close to the Mississippi. She was eager to watch us put Ruffin through his paces, first with Donna and Lisa, and then with Seamus and me.

Afterwards, she set right to work at my kitchen counter, perched on a wooden stool, writing out a new set of drills for us to use with Ruffin over the next semester, focused on further elaborations of his early childhood pre-academic skills. They included a new introductory set of higher-level "theory of mind" exercises that Dr. Granpeesheh had been developing during and since her graduate studies with Lovaas at UCLA.

Evelyn explained them all, while we tried them out. One exercise included my wearing a blindfold while Ruffin talked me through a tour of our home, room by room, prompted by my brief, repeated question whenever he fell silent, "What next?" This disarmingly simple exercise was meant to offer Ruffin a concrete demonstration of what I could not see, of what I could not possibly know. The blindfold literally blinded my mind, so Ruffin could see the necessity of telling me everything that was around me, everything I needed to avoid bumping into, given where he had in mind for us to go and what he had in mind for us to do. This played well into his strong desire for control, so Ruffin was willing to play this game over and over, with everyone.

Donna volunteered to be the member of our home treatment group to attend school with Ruffin every morning in Meg's classroom. Lisa made it clear she preferred to continue to work with Ruffin after school in my home or hers. An after-school session would dovetail well for her with the hours of her second job at TASC, a workshop for disabled adults where the strong behavioral training she had received from Evelyn was valued.

After our staffing broke up, after Evelyn headed over to her bed and breakfast to lie down and nap, after Seamus bowed out, after everyone else had gone, Donna was still there, lingering, wanting to talk. She was concerned about being able to dress professionally. Her usual sweatpants and slippers, topped by an embroidered seasonally themed sweatshirt were unlikely to pass muster, or meet our local school district's dress code, however informal. This hadn't crossed my mind, but I heard her out, as Donna recalled how she herself and her brothers and sisters had been treated as students in our district, each of whom had been counseled in turn that he or she would never be "college material." As I reflected over last year's IEP meetings and Ms. Wilding's comments in the January evaluations down at UIHC, I shared Donna's concern she might not be treated professionally at school or might not be recognized the way Lisa was by then at TASC.

Both she and Lisa were due to be rewarded for their success in treating Ruffin. I decided to pay each of them — equally, to avoid favoritism or dissention — a bonus for the year. We had all worked hard. We had reason to celebrate, didn't we? Evelyn had been pleased with Ruffin's progress. I certainly was. We were succeeding, weren't we? It was past time to thank Donna and tell her to take a day to drive up to LaCrosse to go shopping at the nearest Macy's or wherever she and Danielle might enjoy going. It was the season for back-to-school shopping.

Evelyn trained a TASC respite care team on Sunday for Renee, Ruth's daughter. Renee's program differed from Ruffin's early intervention program. It was individually tailored to Renee's own special needs at home — with her Medicaid respite care workers, her parents and her siblings all being trained how to help her there. It incorporated some of the computer programs Renee had tried and seemed to enjoy. For Ruth to continue to work and go to college to study accounting, for her husband, Al, to continue his farm and factory work, and for the two of them to have any time to devote to Renee's siblings, Renee needed to learn some meaningful activities to keep her occupied — even for a few minutes — on her own. Renee needed to be taught how to communicate "yes," and "no," to avoid her repeated but effective resort to difficult and time-consuming tantrums. Both Ruth and Al hoped Evelyn's training of a home care team and a structured program of activities at home would make living with Renee much easier — day by day — and over the long run.

By Monday, our summer playgroup was beginning to wind down, with just one little girl coming over to visit with Ruffin. Ruth dropped by, waving a copy of an agency-wide Bridgewater memo Mr. Montague had just issued approving the circulation of our autism support group's newsletter.

Curt called to suggest that we let Caron handle getting the necessary approval of all the financial terms of our mediation. He and I didn't know whether ACSD's school board had any inkling our day-long mediation had even occurred, or that it had been resolved at the district's considerable expense. It was possible that Mr. Lord and Caron would be selling our school board an unpleasant surprise. Since I had learned during mediation that the school board could back out of our "agreement" for any reason, or no reason at all, I thought, why give them any reason? Or any occasion?

My plan for going forward was to keep my head down and try to make this shotgun marriage work with the help of Meg and Inge working below the administrative radar as quietly as we could so the IEP — which *was* legally binding — could be implemented smoothly. Goodwill and continuing success with Ruffin were obviously the best way to seal the deal.

While I waited for the school board's approval and for their promised reimbursement check to arrive, I needed more money than I had on hand. My parents had already helped so much over the summer. No one in town needed to know exactly how hard-pressed I was now. A couple of local bankers had family ties to members of the school board.

So, with my *Ezzone* jury verdict in hand and my court reporter's transcript of our recent mediation agreement I drove past every bank in Iowa and down off the high prairie across the Mississippi and walked into the first bank I saw in Wisconsin. There

I explained how much I thought I needed to borrow and offered what evidence I had of my expectations.

The middle-aged man behind the loan desk wanted to know why I needed the money and why I didn't seem to be working.

I laid it all out for him, and waited, on the verge of tears. "I need to save my son's life."

"We could offer you a personal signatory loan."

"On what terms? On what security?" I swallowed.

"Reasonable enough terms, with a second mortgage on your home. You sound to me like someone worth betting on. I imagine we'll make our money on you. You look like another gambler to me."

I signed his thick sheaf of papers, opened a new account there with the loan proceeds, and he and I shook hands. I waltzed out the heavy glass door feeling fortunate that so much of the Wild West ethic had survived into the late twentieth century in a small, sleepy Mississippi river town.

That night I attended a brief half-hour private nursery school orientation for parents and nursery schoolers for the Monday, Wednesday, and Friday afternoon class. Elaine Mills, who would be Ruffin's teacher, passed out her daily schedule, a list of the names of Ruffin's fourteen classmates, and introduced her aide. I sat well back in the room, kept my mouth shut, smiled, keeping a watchful eye on Ruffin's behavior as he wriggled in his seat beside me. Ruffin would need to manage this experience — Elaine's classroom — on his own. I was determined to stay out of it.

Our playgroup of Ruffin and his little girlfriends finally petered out that Wednesday with hugs, goodbyes, and promises, "See you in the park." "See you at the library." "See you in church."

Our house descended into happy chaos over the next week at the end of August. My parents and my sister's younger son, Ruffin's year-older cousin, Robert, arrived for a visit before school started.

By noon, the first day, life had unpacked and re-ordered itself around three sit-down meals a day — run along the lines of my mother's weekend custom — clean up and dishwashing afterwards — with Ruffin and Robert in constant motion underfoot, in and out the back door into the backyard garage of paints and scissors, books and blocks of Ruffin's disbanded summer playgroup. Donna and Lisa, RoJene and Pine, even Rose stopped in at various times to stay in touch with Ruffin, visit, share a meal, and meet my parents. Seamus visited to join in and pick up gossip. None of us worked on Ruffin's home program. Evelyn's recent visit insured that we would all be hard at work again soon enough.

Late that first afternoon, I slipped away from the commotion for a moment to check the mail. Even at the tail end of the slowest legal month of the year, it remained dangerous to neglect the mail for so much as a single day.

A one-page, unsigned typewritten note had arrived in an envelope. "As you may know, there is a fine line between genius and insanity. We believe you may be precariously balanced on this line. It is never apparent to the person in this situation. 'Those who think they are insane never are.' Strange behavior is seen by others as strange, but never by oneself. We could point out the problem areas, but to you, that would not be apparent. It is up to you to start looking at things in a rational way. That may only be successful through therapy. A decision to seek professional help can only be made by the individual. For the sake of those around you, specifically your child, please help yourself. Our intent is not to be malicious; we are only concerned for the welfare of your son."

Out on the porch by myself, I turned the envelope over, this way and that. It offered no return address but had been post-marked in town — as it turned out, on the day after a Bridgewater meeting during which Mr. Montague had disclosed to all his staff — including Emily and Kim, who had both been conspicuously absent at mediation — what must have come as the surprising result of our agreement and the terms of Ruffin's newest IEP.

I looked off into the warm, sunny day, into the depth of a perfectly blue sky, took a shallow breath, folded the single page back into its bed of three sharp creases, and slipped it into the envelope I knew I would keep. But this was nothing I cared to share with anyone now. Nothing I wanted to share with anyone here visiting. I was far too angry. I was suddenly truly angry. I fumed, quietly to myself. Who writes such a thing? Who types such a thing up, carefully, and deliberately? Who doesn't tear such a thing up, having read it over, or slept on it? Who creases such a thing, and mails such a thing to anyone?

Wasn't it enough that I had my own doubts about my sanity without some anonymous "we" calling me out on it? An anonymous "we" whom I realized, I had just "agreed" to entrust Ruffin to, to whom I had "married" the better part of our highly-effective home program — Ruffin, Donna, and me. What had I been thinking? And were they really going to succeed in driving me crazy?

I walked the envelope into my living room office and laid it carefully face down on my desk. I returned to our celebrations, to dinner, to dessert and the dishes, to watching the national news with my father, to settling Ruffin and Robert in on the computer, so I could visit with my mother and hear the latest news of my brother and sisters.

But, of course, the letter continued to rankle, to burn on the horizon of my brain, to worry me like a sore, until after everyone else in the house was asleep, I crept back downstairs, reopened and re-read it.

Finally, I did what I could to dismiss it, what I did to any upsetting paperwork that arrived once I had given it the thought it deserved. I stapled the envelope to it. With a sharp whack, I applied my two-hole punch to it, and secured it on the prongs of the latest volume of Ruffin's chronological file. There, it was. *Filed*.

I imagined I had dealt with it. I was never going to talk about it, never going to complain about it. Whatever I felt about it, I was going to have to work with whoever wrote it — for Ruffin's benefit.

The private nursery school sent me a check refunding my summer deposit made toward Ruffin's tuition. It came with a stern note declining the offer of "a computer for the education of your son" due to "limited time and space," and because "it would greatly alter the educational structure" of the program "whose teachers collectively have 29 years of teaching experience." These were early days for personal computers. There had to be some accounting for the fear of something so new-fangled in a small town without so much as a McDonald's or a Walmart.

Within the next day or so, finally, some mail arrived worth handing over to my mother to read. Professor of law, parent-advocate, Jay E. Grenig of the Marquette University Law School in Milwaukee sent a brief thank you for his copy of Curt and Joan's booklet and promised to mention its availability in the next issue of his Wisconsin newsletter.

Then on the verge of the new school year, my running conversation with my parents, my attention to Ruffin and Robert, to meals, to dishwashing and housework was interrupted by longer calls from new parents who had been offered my phone number by Sue Baker. When I had listened, when I had spoken and whomever had called was calmer, I referred each one on to Dr. Granpeesheh of CARD, or Dr. Sallows in Madison, or to Keli Larsen in Des Moines, who had worked a brief stint in Lovaas's UCLA clinic as a front-line therapist. As I hung up the phone, and it rang again, repeatedly, I could tell my mother was puzzled.

The significance of all this distracting activity escaped her. She and my father were happily focused on how much better Ruffin seemed to be — playing with Robert and talking. Why wasn't I? The sirens of advocacy called to me. Ruffin's improvements no longer struck me as encouraging, unusual, or remarkable. I was used to them arriving now, more and more quickly. I expected them and expected them to continue.

Ruffin's second year in preschool special education began in late August. I alerted Meg, "Ruffin was up early to say goodbye to his grandparents and little cousin this morning, so he could be tired.

"Ruffin won't be in school tomorrow. He and I will be taking a trip together.

"Ruffin asked a very unusual question this morning. 'What is 'double duty'?' about dialogue he overheard on a video. His cousin Robert modeled this type of question to Ruffin all weekend, and Ruffin is now copying his behavior."

I wrote to the school nurse, separately. "The vitamin and DMG doses are both the same as last year. Do you need a prescription from Ruffin's doctor? If so, just let me know. You have one from Dr. Olson from last year. Thanks."

As it turned out, school recessed two hours early due to extreme heat. Ruffin handed me Meg's quick mimeographed note. "What a great first day! All the kids got right off the bus and started playing. We had get-acquainted time, then went to music and recess. After recess, it was time for lunch and then we rested for a while. By then, it was time to get ready for the bus."

Ruffin's book bag was stuffed with school bus rules, a community mobility consent, a photo release form, a Luther College consent for adapted physical education, reminders to send toothbrushes and blankets, diapers and clothing changes, and a strong suggestion to those of us who didn't qualify for free or reduced lunch to please buy breakfast tickets so our children wouldn't feel left out. New home-school notebooks were promised to be ready for us all soon.

Meg's first lesson plan was announced as: "Who Am I?" There would be new special needs children in Meg's classroom this year. Ruffin made Meg's now a class of nine.

Jack Wallace sent over all the Bridgewater paperwork I would need to fill out for Ruffin's full re-evaluation at the UIHC in the spring and let me know that Mr. Montague and "Moe" might pay for Ms. Wilding's speech and language assessment there — the occasion for Ruffin's missing school to take a trip.

Inge filled out Ruffin's Bridgewater information sheet — keeping Ruffin's disability as "non-categorical," without changing it to "autism." This failed to comply with Congress's 1990 amendments to the IDEA, which had added "autism" as a specific disability category, and with the September 29, 1992, *Rules and Regulations* published by the U.S. Department of Education in the *Federal Register*: "'Autism' means a developmental disability significantly affecting verbal and nonverbal communication and social interaction, generally evident before age three that adversely affects a child's educational performance. Other characteristics often associated with autism are engagement in repetitive activities and stereotyped movements, resistance to environmental change or change in daily routines, and unusual responses to sensory experiences." *Comments* to this passage, also published in the *Federal Register*, clarified that children with Ruffin's exact diagnosis — PDD-NOS — also fell within this official federal, educational definition of "autism."

Inge also completed all the new paperwork to raise Ruffin's financial weighting from last year's 2.4 to this year's 3.6 — the highest available special education funding. Mr. Montague signed off on this increased state funding in early December, as Ruffin's paperwork churned through the system.

From Iowa Pilot Parents, on the far western border of the state, I began to borrow and review a series of videotaped lectures by special needs attorney Reed Martin, an author-attorney Curt and Joan had recommended. He had written about the 1990 IDEA amendments with respect to autism. "Autism was added to the IDEA as an eligibility category. 'Autistic condition' had always been served as 'other health impaired' but Congress recognized that some children with autism 'continue to face difficulty in receiving a free appropriate public education.' Congress emphasized that autism is a disability in its own right and not some form of mental illness or other health problem. This poses implications for: 1. The credentials of evaluators and opens the door for independent educational evaluations; 2. The qualifications of personnel at the IEP meeting who have 'expertise' in the disability; 3. The credentials of teachers who teach children with autism; and 4. Questions about placement of children with autism in 'generic' classes with students with mental illness, mental retardation, behavior disorders, or communication disorders. Has your state developed new standards for each of these?"

Meanwhile, Dot Gordon who had served on Bridgewater's autism resource team (ART) last year had engaged Gerald L. Hammond, staff counsel for the Iowa State Education Association to write me "about a letter you authored this summer to August Montague, at Bridgewater" which "was also copied to approximately twenty-three persons including Ms. Gordon." Indeed, I had written directly to her director and to everybody in my wide circle of advocacy and had copied it to Dot herself. Now Dot was accusing me of "libel *per se* under Iowa law."

Indeed, and since Mr. Hammond and I both went to law school, he and I knew: Truth is a complete defense to libel. I considered that this seemed to have arrived in a letter, not a lawsuit. Dot had been removed from the autism resource team (ART) leadership by Sue Baker and Mr. Montague, after Ruth's letters about Dot's failure to meet Sue's grant application deadlines.

By the time I had written Mr. Montague so aggressively later that summer, Mary Carter had already succeeded Dot. So, I applied the two-hole punch to Mr. Hammond's missive and consigned it to Ruffin's chronological file. I had written and reviewed enough of these letters in fifteen years of trial practice to know Dot's whining was going nowhere but into Mr. Hammond's own file, too.

My suspicion was confirmed by a letter Mr. Hammond left Dot to write on her own the next day — to Ruth and her husband — which Ruth brought over to share. No attorney planning an actual lawsuit for libel would have permitted his client to pen such a letter, much less mail it.

Dot complained about me and claimed great expertise in autism and a record of being helpful to "many parents, teachers, and colleagues with questions of diagnosis and treatment for their children with autism" over the last two and a half decades. "I do understand that as parents of a child with autism, you wish to have the best possible service for your child. However, when parents take the adversarial position of damning the professionals, the child is the one who suffers." Ruth was not pleased, and not intimidated, either.

Obviously, Dot had no idea what Ruth had written earlier to Mr. Montague about the autism resource team (ART) and no recollection of Ruth's years of requests for help with Renee and having run into nothing but dead ends with Dot.

Neither Ruth nor I had any willingness or reason to discuss anything further with Dot. Since last summer we had counted her as irrelevant to any planning for our children. We imagined that because of our joint efforts, writing and registering our separate complaints, that she had been safely sidelined.

CHAPTER THIRTY FIVE

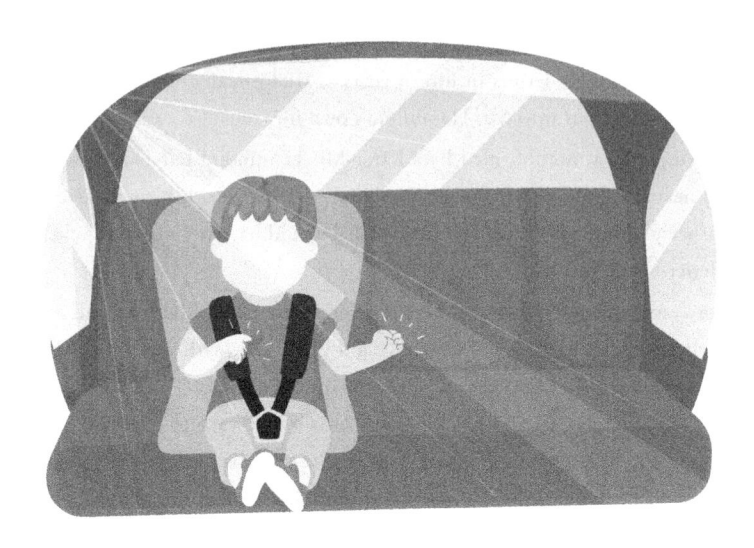

PROOF OF OUR SUMMER'S PUDDING

Ruffin and I had an early morning appointment with Ms. Wilding in Iowa City. In his car seat, with little to entertain him over a three-hour ride, in my rear-view mirror, I could see Ruffin engaging in self-stimulatory behavior for the first time in a long while, babbling nonsense syllables and flicking his fingers in front of his face to manipulate the strong, low light of sunrise entering his back seat window. Music on the radio which I hoped might capture his attention was unwelcome. I worried that all this was not a particularly good prelude to what I expected to be another long day of testing.

The drive was what it was, over narrow two-lane roads before navigating a dozen bothersome stoplights at the tail end of Iowa City's morning rush hour. There was no way to get there any faster. I struggled to make it to the clinic — with just enough time to find a parking place on the roof level of the oversubscribed parking structure.

Our visit resulted in Ms. Wilding writing a ten-page, single-spaced highly detailed report of her evaluation of Ruffin's recent speech and language development. After she walked me through her results briefly, as she and I agreed, she sent it directly to me. After last spring and summer's paper chase, after all I had learned through that long process, I wanted to review Ruffin's medical records first to have an opportunity to arrange for the correction of any errors, and to address any quarrels or concerns I might have with Ms. Wilding before agreeing to release her report to his educators.

Thankfully, for this latest report, there was no such need.

"Ruffin White is a 4-year, 4-month-old male.

"Background Information: Ruffin was last seen by this speech and language pathologist during his evaluation at UIHC on January 23rd. His mother requested this special evaluation near the beginning of the new school year to look at the progress Ruffin has made in the elapsed time since his last evaluation and to look specifically for concepts which may need further intervention.

"Speech: Informal observation of Ruffin's articulation revealed that there remain developmental articulation errors which do not impact on the intelligibility of Ruffin's speech.

"His voice continues to be high pitched, although not as high as we recall from the recent past. He only occasionally used a loud volume which he used quite frequently during the last evaluation. He also tended to use appropriate prosody whereas during the last evaluation he was using patterned inflection and tending to sing some of his responses." Yes, I thought. We had nailed *that*, Donna, Lisa, Evelyn, and I, in part by using Meg's trick of lowering the pitch of all our women's voices.

"Language: During today's evaluation, Ruffin was successful at providing some of his personal information, including the town where he lives, his address, and his phone number. He was able to tell the name of his teacher and where his school was located." Ms. Wilding's earlier January complaints about Ruffin's rote echolalia had vanished.

"Ruffin was compliant to directions primarily for taking breaks and coming back to the working area. He did follow 'listen and look' type directions also. Ruffin's student behaviors such as sitting, looking, staying in his own space, and being task-oriented were all appropriate. He tended to look at this examiner as I talked to him and presented information to him, and he also looked at this examiner when he was presenting information to me. We noticed a little twinkle in his eye, and he seemed to orient to the face." This last observation of Ms. Wilding's particularly pleased me, of course.

"There were occasions as we were passing in the hallway and using some terminal greetings that Ruffin needed to be cued to look at the examiner by his mother, but during the time when we were in an organized situation, he had the conversational eye gaze well under his control." I felt a wave of relief flood through me. Ms. Wilding made it sound like Ruffin would be unlikely to have any problems navigating the private nursery school on his own.

"Sentence length was variable for Ruffin today. The longest sentence that we recorded was a novel sentence of nine words, 'I got a big one that doesn't make stars.' We were talking about flashlights, and he was using my flashlight that made stars. As one looks at his sentence, Ruffin makes a statement and then modifies the information. When I asked him if he had a flashlight, he remarked, 'Yes,' and then made the modification statement. This indicates maintenance of an initial topic which is brought up by another.

"Ruffin is using the pronoun 'I' to refer to himself appropriately. We noted that he is using *is* verbing occasionally although he isn't using it all the time. He is contrasting the *is* verb especially when he's asking questions. We did have several 'wh'-type questions today except for 'why' questions. 'How' questions are difficult for him in terms of response on the formal measures and this is supported also in conversation with his mother. He is negating appropriately in the sentence format with statements such as 'I don't want that,' or 'It's too loud.'" Ms. Wilding was listening to Ruffin, and listening to me, with greater respect than earlier. I admit, I liked that.

"Sentence formulation skills are appropriate with some inconsistent type errors. Ruffin is still working on his formulation skills, and this is evidenced by the fact that he does have occasional false starts in his sentences where he re-evaluates what he is organizing and then changes the way that he is starting the sentence. This however indicates that his language system is a functional language system, and he is attempting to meet the demands that he feels he needs to present and also meet the demands of his communication partner." Dr. Granpeesheh and Evelyn would be sure to appreciate this observation. This is what we had been aiming for in guiding Ruffin's development over the summer.

"Pragmatically, he is making comments, calling attention, requesting, requesting information, requesting permission, using socially appropriate words such as thank you and please. We noticed occasional echolalia as information became too difficult. We noticed less echolalia of verbal reinforcement that we offered. What we noticed was that at times when we used verbal praise, he tended to look at us and smile as opposed to recreating that information verbally. We noticed he occasionally talked about numbers when he was uncertain about issues he should be bringing up." Ruffin's resort to bringing up numbers in conversation sounded remarkably true to my own recent experiences with him, and indicative of some continuing residua of his autism. We still had work to do, but we also had a full year before Ruffin entered kindergarten.

"During his breaks, Ruffin did select various toys from the toy shelf, and he tended to bring those toys to the table where I was seated to play with them. Occasionally, he called my attention to a particular toy with a 'Look, you have a ____' type strategy and then would complete that with, 'Can I see it?' as a question.

"He was interested in how things worked and did not use toys in a particularly repetitive fashion. He used toys carefully and appropriately. He picked up all the toys when I said it was time for us to leave. He was noted to line up small cars and to spend some time observing toys that moved around in a circle very quickly." Only the final observation of this paragraph suggested, again, some faint continuing residua of autism.

"He did attempt imitation of several things that I presented to him such as whistling and winking. He thought this was fun and enjoyed these silly little interludes. Ruffin was having a good time here and seemed fairly settled in a strange place. He did ask for his mother initially, wondering, 'Where's Mom?' and then seemed settled knowing that she was in the waiting room."

Would I have preferred to have observed all Ms. Wilding's interactions with Ruffin myself from a respectful distance, or from behind a one-way mirror? Of course, but I felt our home team had much to be pleased with in her detailed written record of Ruffin's ability to interact alone and without support during her evaluation.

DIAGNOSTIC MEASUREMENT:
Expressive One-Word Picture Vocabulary Test — Revised
Raw Score: 39 (up from 25 on 04/12/95 by Kim)
Age Equivalency: 5.0 years (up from 3.7 years on 04/12/95 by Kim)
Percentile Rank: 73 (up from 34 on 04/12/95 by Kim)
Standard Score: 109 (up from 94 on 04/12/95 by Kim)
Stanine: 6 (up from 4 on 04/12/95 by Kim)

Kim's report that I used as a baseline for Ms. Wilding's newest report had arrived in late May, reporting her own mid-April testing. Bringing Kim's earlier testing to bear offered me some formal measure of Ruffin's language development over the past summer. With his early morning drills, and afternoon playgroup with typically developing girls and boys — Ruffin's speech seemed to have developed nearly 18 months over his last month or so of school and the most recent three months of the summer.

Ms. Wilding explained, "Single word naming is a strength for Ruffin. On this measurement he scored at a higher level than he scored on some of the others. He enjoyed this task and had a good deal of success. He was also able to practice 'I don't know that' and 'I need help' strategies several times on this diagnostic test.

"It did seem as if Ruffin had difficulty with group nouns such as fruit, vegetables, furniture, musical instruments, and categories of that sort. He tended to call these by other group names such as food, things, sitting, and so on, naming them by function, and he seems to be learning in this way.

"We always want things to be functional for Ruffin. A grocery store activity, looking at the various fruits and other items, might be appropriate." Going to the grocery store as a learning experience would be possible now since Ruffin's public behavior was so much improved with his tantrums now fewer and farther between.

"Today Ruffin had difficulty with ostrich, octopus, leopard, raccoon, and so on. Granted these are fairly obscure animals, but for a child as bright as Ruffin and one who has a variety of interests, these are things that he would enjoy.

"His last administration of the *Expressive One-Word Picture Vocabulary Test-Revised* in January could not be scored because Ruffin did not attain a basal level on that measure. If we go back and assume a basal level on that, then we would realize an approximate 2-year gain in the approximate 7 months since his last evaluation."

"In summary then, Ruffin is experiencing good growth in the language area. He has made progress in all the areas that we looked at today. He has made growth in his social communication interactions and in his pragmatic language skills. He did not particularly initiate any topics for discussion today, but he tended to call my attention to things with a look at what you have kind of approach. But calling my attention always related to something immediately in this room. He did not initiate about any topics which were not in this room and about which we could not share visual regard."

This last observation of Ms. Wilding's reinforced the continuing need for a home-school-school notebook to circulate with Ruffin as he moved through each instructional day. Otherwise, there would be no way to prompt conversations with him about either his past or his future experience.

But I could hardly wait to show this conclusion of Ms. Wilding's report to Seamus, Donna, Lisa, RoJene, Pine, Meg, Inge, Sue Baker, Evelyn, and Dr. Granpeesheh, and to call my parents. I would give Donna an extra copy to pass to Elaine at the private nursery school.Ruffin slept most of the way back. I woke him in Elkader where we stopped to eat an evening meal. We had some trouble in the restaurant. Ruffin was unfamiliar with the available "salad bar" routine. He expected and insisted the waitress should bring his food to him.

After several days of unstructured family activity, Ruffin had been up the last couple of days very early and had gone through many transitions — saying goodbye to his playgroup, to his grandparents and cousin Robert, had gone back to school and then down to Iowa City. Upon reflection, I thought he was coping well with a lot of schedule changes after the breakup of his summer routine. Even with this morning's self-stimulation and this little balking at supper, I was elated we had taken the time and the trip.

CHAPTER THIRTY SIX

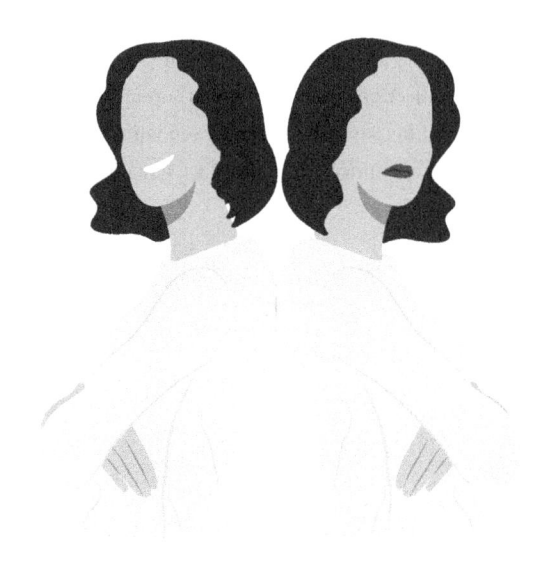

TERROR AND JOY IN EQUAL MEASURE

I offered a summary to Meg of what I had learned from Ms. Wilding, hoping that Elaine at the private nursery school would read it, too. "Yesterday, Ruffin saw the same speech and language pathologist who evaluated him last January. His *Expressive One-Word Picture Vocabulary Test-R* score, measuring his knowledge of nouns, was the age-equivalent of 5 years, that is, 8 months above his chronological age.

"She also administered the *Sequenced Inventory of Communication Development* and found Ruffin was able to test beyond its parameters, to the age equivalent of 3 years, so she used a new test developed in 1991 designed to cover more complex grammar and concepts. Ruffin's age-equivalent on this newest test was 3 years, 9 months, that is, a 7-month delay.

"Her overall impression was that Ruffin is developing a good vocabulary but continues to have problems putting the words he knows together, especially in the absence of his knowledge of basic concepts of time, space, causation, and relationship which have usually been picked up by other children his age.

"Her written report will follow in about a week, with details as to which concepts Ruffin seemed unfamiliar with, with her."

"The name tag enclosed is for Ruffin to wear to the nursery school's first day, at their request." Ruffin's teacher there, Elaine, had shared her daily schedule. As I looked it over, it would be a good replacement for Ruffin's summer playgroup. I was delighted when a photo arrived of Ruffin at his first day of nursery school wearing his name tag, and pleased to hand this to Seamus, who also knew most of the families of Ruffin's new classmates.

While Ruffin was in school, I filled out all the paperwork "Moe" wanted for Ruffin's full re-evaluation in the spring, adding a note. "I appreciate Bridgewater's willingness to pay for Ms. Wilding's speech assessment of yesterday. I didn't want to miss that appointment because it is so difficult to schedule with UIHC without having to wait months for an appointment. Bridgewater's willingness to pay for that assessment, and the tone of your recent calls is very welcome and reassuring to me as a parent."

At Ruth's request, I disclosed to Curt the full controversy surrounding Bridgewater's autism resource team (ART) and Dot Gordon, asking him to attend an early September IEP meeting for Renee, "age seven, so she may have a CARD program at school, too."

Renee's classroom teacher, Amy, had indicated a willingness to be trained, "but it is hard to say what may really happen." Then, I ran down our difficulties with Dot in detail with a little summer timeline, referencing some thirteen items of correspondence, adding, "The state autism specialist Sue Baker is aghast that her autism resource teams (ARTs) presume to diagnose autism, or not. She indicated to me since we reached our mediated settlement on Ruffin's case, that ART teams are not qualified to diagnose autism, much less question the diagnoses made by qualified medical professionals at Gundersen or UIHC. The executive director of the Society, who was copied on my allegedly libelous letter, and who lives in Bridgewater, has written to Mr. Montague about her own concerns about the same ART team problems, too."

The phone rang. It was Meg. Ruffin couldn't manage in the severe heat of her public-school classroom. "Could you come get him? I'm sorry he got so sick."

Ruffin's school nurse was satisfied with last year's vitamin and DMG prescription from Dr. Olson, but I needed to fill out a form to formally request that Ruffin get his prescribed medication at school.

Ruffin's new school year was beginning with a widespread sense of distrust in every quarter after our hard-won mediated settlement in mid-August. I was as distrustful as anyone, and all the careful jockeying left me feeling deeply sad. I had wanted to mediate to meet Ruffin's special needs, and for peace, but found myself uneasy in the shotgun marriage I had arranged.

On a happier note, Mr. Montague issued a memo to all special and general education personnel serving children with autism in Bridgewater, circulating the parent support newsletter Ruth and I had mailed out so widely. "In 1990, then President George Bush signed into law the *IDEA*. This law included two new disabilities: autism and traumatic brain injury. Following the addition of these new disabilities, parent support groups were formed across our nation and state to make other parents and members of the professional community more aware of all aspects of these disabilities."

Sadly, Mr. Montague had his history backwards. Without parent support groups, the original *Education of the Handicapped* federal laws — creating his publicly-funded special education profession as an audiologist — would never have passed Congress. This early special education legislation was the outgrowth of parent support group litigation against the public schools for disability discrimination.

"Bridgewater is asking your assistance in forwarding *The Northeast Iowa Support Group Newsletter* to as many parents and professionals serving children with autism at your school or field offices as possible."

As parents, Ruth and I were mildly surprised, and pleased.

My Thursday morning note to Donna and Meg ran, "Hopefully, Ruffin will do better today in the cooler weather. Donna, Meg and I discussed you working with Ruffin at home in our air-conditioned upstairs bedroom tomorrow if the heat returns, so he can stay in good shape and not miss Elaine's private nursery school class that afternoon."

"Meg, has anyone at school visited with Elaine about her participation in the full UIHC re-valuation 'Moe' and Mr. Montague want? She could probably use some information about this aspect of 'special education,' and a copy of Ruffin's IEP." I remained wary about communicating directly with the private nursery school. Thankfully, Donna and Elaine were longtime friends. I had that back channel available, but, if Ruffin were to have issues that led to problems in Elaine's classroom, they would become legal problems under special education law.

Meg's end-of-the-day note came back. "Ruffin seemed *great* today. Ate well. I am enclosing a release of information form for the private nursery school so we can meet about Ruffin's IEP. Also, we need Ruffin's enrollment form as soon as possible."

By now, the simplest request for any release raised the level of my concern. I found this one disquieting. But Meg called, and I was able to talk to her and tell her how I would be conditioning my release. Having gained access over the summer to records of Meg's spring conversations with Dr. Norman, I felt I could trust Meg to keep Ruffin *safe*, but I knew I could *not* trust Meg to advocate for Ruffin. That was my responsibility.

I didn't want to upset the implementation of Ruffin's newest IEP by sharing anything yet about the anonymous note that had arrived between our mediation and the start of school. But I needed to proceed with caution and document every concern I had about Ruffin somewhere in his educational record. The readiest, the least confrontational but effective level was to write in Ruffin's home-school notebook. I needed to be clear there, among the quotidian. "I came by to see Rose, the school secretary after you called, to enroll Ruffin. She just took his lunch and breakfast money. I don't have an enrollment form."

Meg sent her aide Ella to the private nursery school with Ruffin. She offered the first report back that Meg and I had of Ruffin's day there. "Nursery school went well. Ruffin did a nice job listening and following directions. He talked to the other children and seemed to really enjoy playing with a train with the other boys. He also played on the slides and in the kitchen area."

But here was joy and terror in equal measure. Ruffin's book bag also carried the private nursery school's written reminder that Elaine needed the completed paperwork for Ruffin's medical physical back to her by next Wednesday since they "could be inspected at any time and need this form on record in order to comply with state regulations."

This was the first I had heard of any need for a physical. And, firmly stapled to Elaine's note was a *Discharge Policy*, new that year, with this explanation offered. "According to our licensing survey, we are required to have a discharge policy. The following is our policy: Your child will be discharged if his or her behavior is disruptive to the staff, other children, or beyond that which we are adequately capable of handling. Unless circumstances determine otherwise, a two week notice of termination will be given except when your child shows behavior causing injury to self or others. A parent-teacher conference will be held during this time to determine other possible options."

From what I had heard, the cream of our town's healthiest social crop of families attended this private nursery school. With Ruffin's history of autism and spectacular meltdowns, I was terrified for him.

I took Ruffin straight in that very afternoon to Dr. Olson for a physical. Although we came on short notice, he was accommodating as always, willing to see Ruffin immediately whenever and whatever our need might be. I was grateful that his was one office where I never ran into any trouble, where I could count on getting nimble help and good support.

He remarked at the end of our appointment with some amazement, "This is a different child." He even scribbled "speaks well" on his examination sheet for the private nursery school. He was pleased, too, that despite Ruffin's prematurity, his being born at only 31 weeks, his weight and height now fell into the 90th percentile.

Ruffin was getting to be a big boy. Seamus would enjoy seeing this report, and those numbers.

With the school week and our medical errand behind us, with the long Labor Day weekend ahead of us, Ruffin and I changed into jeans, boots, and our warmest plaid shirts. We were heading out to meet up with RoJene and Chance at their farm. From there, we would follow RoJene's small truck out to our first rodeo.

Her red taillights turned off the gravel into a larger pasture that was filling up with pick-up trucks and livestock trailers, the small, closed ones for a single bronc, the long, open aluminum ones for the rough stock, the calves raised to be roped, the bulls raised to be ridden. I tried to park my teal-green Volvo station wagon in a spot I could get out of easily enough if this didn't happen to work out as an adventure Ruffin could handle.

As I bent to unbuckle Ruffin from his car seat, the sharp smell of urine rose from the grass into the sweeter aromas of manure and hay. The heat of the ground still held these smells, and the smells of clover and alfalfa. The air above began to cool finally as the sun went down. I handed Ruffin his quilted jacket and grabbed my own.

The sky was clear, full of stars with the waning crescent of a fingernail moon above the farthest tree line. We were somewhere out in the country. It was dark. The pasture was rough underfoot. I took Ruffin's hand, so we could manage if either of us stumbled. Moving ahead of us, RoJene was carrying Chance on one hip and waving us in the direction of lights strung through the trees, and then around a circle of low poles that lit the rodeo arena, the judges' stand and a small set of bleachers.

The voice of the announcer opened the event, warming up the loudspeaker overhead by ribbing one of the contestants, "Give that cowboy, a hand. He had a lot of try." He continued joshing his way through a jumble of nicknames, reporting out the averages of the earlier slack competitions, the warm-ups before the public event.

The four of us climbed to be able to sit high up over a scattering of ordinary daytime feed caps, and a few more ostentatious cowboy hats. RoJene pointed out the bucking chute and the roping chute at opposite ends of the arena, where the rough stock would be held in position before each new contest began. Ruffin was transfixed by the scene, following RoJene's finger with his gaze. He was wriggling in his seat, and pulling my hand, wanting to go back down and explore.

"No," I warned him. "We can't go near them. These are not horses and calves for petting, like Seamus's."

And, yes, Ruffin understood, from what Seamus had taught him, bulls were dangerous wherever they were, whenever you saw them.

With sticky homemade bars in hand, and small drinks from the concession stand, Ruffin and Chance settled in, content to watch the clowns and barrel men gather in small knots in the ring, making their plans, working out their assignments. Flags fluttered in the stiff, fall breeze. RoJene explained how each might drop to signal the timers to start the clock and pointed out the flags stuffed in the back pockets of each judge that would be thrown into the dirt to signal the timers to press their stopwatches.

The first bareback rider exploded out a gate. His hat flew off, as his body flopped forward and back like a rag doll, laid out across the horse's back as it bucked. Eight seconds and he was done. Then the gate opened on another, and another. It was a small, private rodeo, and we were on to steer wrestling, a matter of three seconds, if that, as the hazer on his lighter horse channeled the steer breaking from the gate straight into the arms of the cowboy dropping from his larger mount. The show clamored on to team roping, with two horses, two ropes, and the head-roped, heel-roped calf strung out in the middle between the noses of the horses and the cowboys raising their hats. This event could have been designed as a favorite for Ruffin.

Then on to tie-down roping, calves turned unceremoniously on their backs with their hooves in the air, as the cowboy signaled his tie was complete by raising both arms high in the classic, "Look, Ma, no hands!" Then the saddle bronc riders, three in quick succession, one losing his hat, one losing his seat, and the third managing a full eight seconds before turning himself loose and leaping deliberately away.

Then came a bit of a break with some music, Tim McGraw's *I Like It, I Love it*, for the barrel men to roll out the barrels to mark off a cloverleaf pattern to be ridden in something between fifteen and sixteen seconds. Ruffin found the quick repetition exciting. He seemed to shut out the noise and the glare, turning to Chance to be sure he missed nothing, saying, "Look, another one coming!"

Bull riding as another bareback event, and our rodeo was over.

With Chance, Ruffin was disappointed it was over. They liked it; they loved it; they wanted more of it, like any young boys at their first rodeo. I had been foolish to worry Ruffin wouldn't be able to manage the noise of the loudspeaker and the crowd, the glare of the lights or the excitement. For the first time I felt certain life could come at him, and engulf him, and he could embrace it on its own terms. And this is what I wanted for him. It was.

After Labor Day, the stubby bus came to pick Ruffin up. I was settled at my desk to work when there was a hard knock at my front door. I opened it to find Deputy Rosendahl, a large red-headed barrel of a man, whom I also knew to be unfailingly kind. He looked uncomfortable as he handed me the papers that were the occasion of his errand.

He apologized. "Sorry, you've been sued. Now, you've been served. Sorry."

My stomach flipped over for a moment as I struggled to keep my hands steady. All these papers were likely to amplify any motion of my own. I didn't dare move. Or show any weakness, even to a kind man.

I managed to say, evenly enough, "It's your job to serve, and mine to get sued. No need to be sorry. So, let's see what it is, then, shall we?"

He was curious, too. Running my eyes down the first page and flipping to the bottom of the final page I could see I had indeed been sued, along with my trial partner, Mark Soldat, for a quarter of a million dollars — as the fair amount to replenish the defense fund for the school district Mark and I were suing out in his western reaches of the state.

We represented the district's superintendent of over thirty years, together with those parents who had supported his efforts to guide the consolidation of four rural school districts. It was a difficult political task to have undertaken and had resulted in his being fired — wrongly — in his and in our clients' views.

The district's defense lawyers had exhausted all the available insurance funds to continue paying their fees. At hundreds of dollars an hour, it hadn't taken all that many days of trial. Our adversaries knew as well as Mark and I did that we still had many days ahead of us to prove up our client's multiple claims that the school board had violated Iowa's open meetings law through a long series of controversial public meetings.

Yes, Mark and I were being sued for a quarter of a million dollars to replenish the defense fund. I was shocked, but this was laughable. The big lawyers' self-interested lawsuit failed to account for the distinct possibility that Mark and I might *win* the underlying case for our clients, as we were working hard to do and feeling hopeful that we would.

We needed to win, or we'd never be paid.

Mark and I were that sort of lawyers. We were working on contingency and in reliance upon the strength of a fee-shifting statute. As with many civil rights statutes, this fee-shifting provision meant that if the district were found to have violated this sunshine law, the shade that would fall on the losing district would be full responsibility to pay not only for their losing defense, but to pay all Mark's and my fees as well. This fee-shifting provision had been passed by our state legislature to encourage and support private litigation for enforcement of the open meetings and public records laws — just as Congress had written the IDEA to encourage and support parent litigation to enforce the laws of special education.

I didn't imagine our Judge Carroll would think much of this tactic, and as I expected, he would make quick work of dismissing this suit, and ordering the defense lawyers to continue to appear before him even if they were to go uncompensated.

For the moment I fought the urge to get back to my desk to get Mark on the phone to give him a heads-up in case he had yet to be served. Yes, he and I would need to talk, and get something on file before Judge Carroll to join the issue for him. As I began to think quickly through Mark's and my next moves, I *chuckled* to myself.

I looked up to find Deputy Rosendahl still loitering and more obviously curious.

I took a deep breath and then ran down the whole foreseeable scenario, as if he were a client of mine.

He nodded his understanding, wished me luck, and finally turned to leave, headed back to his patrol car, parked there, in front of my house on Main Street. My explanation offered him a new role, as my messenger, if he wanted it.

Absent any explanation, this sort of visit could tempt him with a knee-slapping story to tell back at the county jail, or over cards at night, or over the local café's morning coffee table. As long as his patrol car had been parked outside my house on Main Street, I could see he was going to be asked about it and would have to tell anyway.

Ruffin came home very cranky from the heat. It was 90 degrees, probably hotter in the small metal bus. Strangely, it was also windy enough that his hair was snarled and needed combing. He seemed to collapse and fell asleep on the sofa, under the ministrations of the comb. It was clear he was tuckered out, completely. I gave in to letting him rest and called Lisa to let her know he needed a break this afternoon.

Mrs. Wonderlich had sent a note in Ruffin's bookbag that her latest group of junior high school students were willing to donate their time and talents to help. So, I called her with my thanks, to let her know last year's students had volunteered all summer, and, yes, I would be delighted to train another group this fall.

Meg sent a welcome note, describing her ECSE class this year. With four children and Ruffin returning from last year, and four new children joining it, Miss Hobbs had assigned Meg a second classroom aide. My employee, Donna, assigned solely to Ruffin, went unmentioned.

"Two special programs we are planning on continuing this year are the Head Start dual programming (they come to our room two afternoons a week) and the Luther adaptive P.E. program on Friday mornings." I was alert to the Head Start reference, of course, since it was a principal term of our mediation, but was especially pleased that Meg had also written, "Ruffin told us about the horses at night with RoJene — very excited." Meg reminded me Ruffin still needed his blanket and a toothbrush at school. Yes — O, dear, bad Mommy — I had left his blanket in the dryer. I rustled up a fresh toothbrush. Stuffed both in his backpack, so they wouldn't slip my mind again in the morning.

When Ruffin came home on the bus the next day he seemed better, ready for a little snack and eager to work with Lisa who said, "Ruffin, I missed you!" Ruffin took her hand to lead her up the stairs. On the landing below them, I reached into his backpack to fish out Meg's latest note. "Ruffin had a great time outside with hoops. Boy, can he run! He worked well with Donna — he sure must enjoy her as he *never* resists going to work. Head Start's first full day is today, so it will probably be a couple of weeks for them to settle in before they begin to visit us."

I felt uneasy about this delay, unimpressed by the reason for it, and the minimization of what amounted to a violation of Ruffin's written IEP, but the ringing phone broke the worrisome thread of my thinking. It was Sue Baker calling to ask how Ms. Wilding's most recent speech evaluation of Ruffin had gone. I was able to run down all our good news and Sue seemed as genuinely delighted as I knew I was.

"Really! Could you fax me a copy?"

I owed Sue a heads-up about Dot Gordon's threats to sue for libel because Sue had written letters about Dot too, to both Mr. Montague and Ruth. Then Ruth herself burst in through my front door during our gingerly discussion of this sore subject, with news. "Renee's going to have a CARD program at school! Miss Hobbs told me it was Mr. Lord's decision."

I handed the phone to Ruth and got on an extension so she could join our conversation and tell her story directly to Sue. "Mr. Lord decided. Before he even got my letter asking for CARD!"

To me, she said, in a shared aside, "We won't need to have Curt come to tomorrow's IEP meeting after all."

That would be doubly good news for Curt. He could avoid wasting a workday on the road. I had to wonder how Miss Hobbs might have felt about all this, but why bring that up now and throw a damper on Ruth's excitement. Here was an unexpected occasion for unmitigated joy, so the three of us just hashed it over and savored it as the breakthrough it seemed to be.

I caught up with Curt late that afternoon to free up the next day for him and ask him to give some cool thought at a distance to how Sue, Ruth, and I might speak to Dot's feeling we might have libeled her. Even with the law and the truth on our side, I hoped we would have the benefit of his counsel on some form of diplomatic clean-up.

Ruth, Sue, and I had *all* written to complain about Dot to Mr. Montague. Curt suggested some language for Ruth and I to use, to share with Sue, and with Mr. Montague, if need be. "Do we as parents not have the freedom and privilege to seriously question professional judgment with respect to our children? Should a questioned professional sue the questioning parents for libel and threaten harm to our children?" We would address the libel issue with questions, should it resurface. That should head off any need for Curt to file counterclaims for retaliation against us as special education advocates on my or Ruth's behalf under *Section 504 of the Rehabilitation Act*. I didn't imagine Deputy Rosendahl was likely to show up at my door to serve a libel suit — but better if he never did.

Nevertheless, later I sat down to puzzle through the results of Ruth's own FERPA inspection of Renee's files as a part of our efforts to unravel the workings of Bridgewater's autism resource team (ART). I worked up a more fine-grained timeline for Curt's back pocket in case Ruth or I, or even Sue was ever sued. But, neither Ruth nor I, nor Sue ever were.

Early that evening, Ruth and I walked across Main Street to our first, fall autism support group meeting at the local pizza parlor, now Ruffin's and my go-to place for quick, hot food, including salad and lasagna. Our group was pleased that Mary Carter from Dubuque, school psychologist Lanny Strasser from New Hampton and Gay Doyle from Elkader all attended, participated, really listened, and made concrete offers to help parents get the help they needed: good medical evaluations, assistive technology, and encouragement to ask for services in which they were already interested.

Ruth announced her news that her daughter Renee would have a CARD program at school. At least two other families were there from other school districts and freely expressed some of their concerns and frustrations about the failures of their older children to develop speech. Ruth seemed much empowered by recent developments — hopeful and realistically reserved — in a very good place.

Meanwhile, Mr. Montague was writing to the UIHC group to arrange for Ruffin's future full re-evaluation there. "This evaluation should be considered by your clinic as an *Independent Evaluation,* allowed under Section 300.503 of the *Individuals with Disabilities Education Act* (IDEA). As such, it shall be at no cost to this parent.

"This is the second evaluation of Ruffin by your clinic, and his mother has requested specific attention be paid to 'social skills and curriculum suggestions related to his educational program.' Bridgewater AEA and ACSD are also requesting that you address these concerns. We further ask that you consider inviting Sue Baker, M.S. Autism Services Consultant, Child Health Specialty Clinic-Hospital Schools to participate in the post-evaluation staffing, as she may be able to help us related to Ruffin's educational program.

"This evaluation is the result of a pre-appeal mediation conference held in August. We are, therefore, very anxious to have this evaluation scheduled at the earliest possible opportunity, in order that all parties might implement the most appropriate educational program for Ruffin as soon as possible."

What a change from last spring this represented at the upper reaches of Bridgewater. Nevertheless, Mr. Montague dinged my reimbursement claim for $1.50 for the parking ramp charge during Ruffin's visit to see Ms. Wilding, demanding that I produce a receipt.

Petty? I wrote to Mr. Montague, "I do not have a receipt for the parking ramp on the enclosed claim because I was unaware that I needed to ask for one. I will understand if the power of your discretion as director does not include persuading your business office to waive the provision of a receipt in the amount of $1.50 for parking for an appointment at the UIHC which required two-and-a-half hours of medical service. Kindly process the claim in accord with the powers of your discretion. Thank you."

I tried to catch up on more overdue correspondence. I asked Chris Foster down the Mississippi in Davenport to send drill cards that her Noah had already mastered for Renee. Ruth was working a factory shift and going back to school for her accounting degree. She had no time to cut up catalogs and paste pictures on notecards as I had done so many nights last fall when Ruffin's home-based program began.

Chris was someone whom I could always turn to, someone well out of my own neighborhood, with whom I could safely share my troubles and frustrations. "Besides the 'hate mail' I got just after our settlement, I now have one member of Ruffin's autism resource team threatening, through an ISEA attorney, to sue me for libel!

"Dr. Glen Sallows will be coming to Iowa to speak at the October Society conference in Des Moines. All his families' home Lovaas programs are funded by EPSDT Medicaid funding. Should be a good talk." In a P.S. I shared the latest good news about Ruffin from Ms. Wilding.

To another couple out in Elkhorn, Nebraska, I sent information they had requested over the phone. "It is wonderful to hear that you folks have had your CARD workshops out there already — just since your June diagnosis. Good luck in all your endeavors. I know you will find them extremely rewarding, not only for your own child, but also for others, and personally for yourselves. It's up and down. Pace yourself, and call when you need help or want to share good news."

This was just one of dozens of letters I wrote, trying to pay it forward. It was a matter of superstition as much as anything. I thought of every letter to each new parent, interested teacher or school superintendent as a penny thrown in the wishing well with my hope Ruffin would enjoy a full recovery, a full life of joy and human sorrow.

CHAPTER THIRTY SEVEN

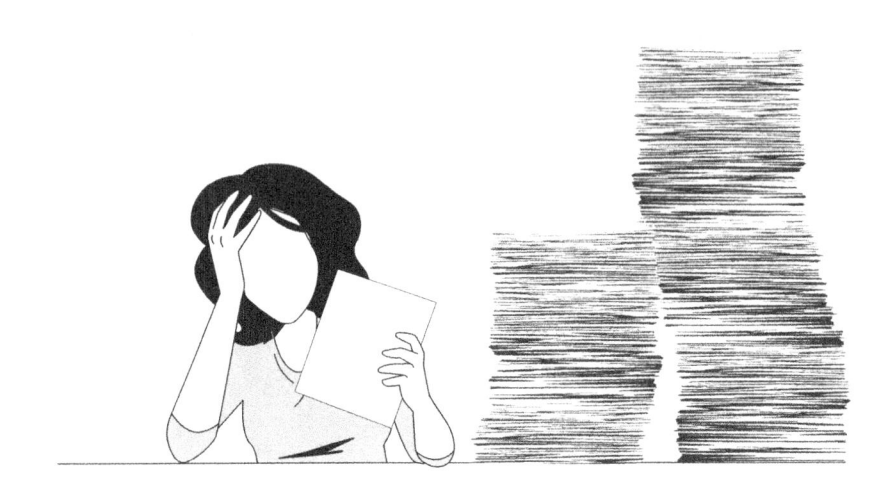

WHO TO TRUST?

Ruffin had a swollen upper lip. He denied being stung — he was playing with his flashlight and batteries when he began complaining — maybe this was battery acid? But no leaky battery. As an older sister, as a babysitter, I had never seen anything like this. By morning Ruffin *denied* it hurt, but it must. Finally, he told me, "I put my lip on the battery" — so it was an electrical burn.

Based on Ms. Wilding's latest report, Donna, Lisa, Seamus, and I decided to re-visit categories with Ruffin. Under our mediation agreement, I could no longer just order whatever instructional materials Ruffin might need. So, I had to prompt Meg to provide materials Donna needed to use at school — attribute blocks Donna hoped would keep Ruffin interested — available through Bridgewater's media library. It all amounted to more work for Meg. Ruffin had mastered and become bored with his "feeling" materials. Donna needed fresh materials for this subject, too.

We took photographs to reflect the sequence of his new daily and weekly schedule for a drill, "Then what?"

We passed around the newest songs he needed to learn for Elaine's class at the private nursery school and planned what to do for Halloween.

We brainstormed how to keep Ruffin listening and giving his various teachers the eye contact they expected.

All the changes were hard on Ruffin. Meg reported a couple of toileting accidents at school. "He may have waited too long to tell me."

But she also handed me Ruffin's art project. He had added curly hair, eyes, nose, and a smiling mouth to a pre-drawn gingerbread-shaped figure onto which he had also carefully pasted pre-cut clothing: a blue shirt, green pants, and two black shoes. This went up on our refrigerator. I looked at it with some amazement, thinking, this seemed normal.

With Ruffin settled upstairs working with Lisa, I went back to school with Ruth to attend Renee's IEP meeting with her, at her invitation, to provide support. This was a hard meeting, hard for Renee's teacher, Amy, who sat quietly with tears collecting on the bottom of her eyelids, threatening to, but never quite spilling over.

Ruth was firm: Renee hadn't made much progress in school ever, or last year. Change would be hard. A change of educational methodology would be particularly hard.

But, with the outcome assured by Mr. Lord's offer, it wasn't a very long meeting. Ruth and I were able to leave in time to pick Ruffin up after Lisa's drill session. We walked over to the local pizza parlor with Ruffin to eat dinner and stay for an early evening meeting of the CARIN' group.

A father from Dallas, Texas had shared all the diagnostic and progress evaluations for his son, who resembled Renee more than Ruffin did. He shared what seemed to have worked for his son and shared his son's drill book developed over the first six months of treatment. With his permission, I passed all this material on to Ruth, for Renee, who, like his son, had little echolalia and was highly distractible.

For the first time at the end of the school day, Elaine added a note. "At nursery school, Ruffin was a little wound up, but still very manageable. He enjoys all we do."

I decided to skip an evening meeting of the Cedar Rapids chapter of the Society, where there was going to be a discussion of auditory integration training. I felt the need to pace myself and concentrate on Ruffin. When I put him to bed, he stayed awake, whispering, sometimes explosively, to himself in a residual 'babbling' episode — the first he had experienced in a long while.

But that Monday morning Ruffin came downstairs fully dressed. This was the first time he had ever done this on his own. He announced, "I beat you, Mom."

Meg wanted to know, "What day can you meet with Elaine, her aide, and me?" She had also mentioned something about Head Start. "I am enclosing a snack calendar. It will change when we start integration with Head Start, because snacks for Tuesdays and Thursdays will then be provided." School had started in August. It was mid-September, but Head Start integration had yet to begin.

Elaine had written something, too, fairly encouraging. "At nursery school, Ruffin enjoys airplanes during playtime, is very attentive during circle. He participates in everything. At snack today, it was Ruffin's turn to pass out napkins to his table — he needed help with this. He was coughing at different times today. He needed to be reminded how to hold a crayon while coloring. A good day."

Elaine also sent home Ruffin's tracing of his name with glue and green glitter on red construction paper, and the pre-kindergarten edition of *The Weekly Reader*, which I remembered as an old chestnut from my own childhood, along with the lyrics to the little nursery school song *Wheels on the Bus*, so Donna, Lisa, Seamus, and I could rehearse it with Ruffin. Through Elaine's class, Ruffin was invited to buy his own books through Scholastic. This was one of the first times that Ruffin's childhood began to echo my own.

Lisa was working hard upstairs with Ruffin, but he needed some cough syrup. He took it without balking. He even held the spoon *himself*. Last year, I would have been *covered* in syrup, and so would have been half the kitchen. Under the influence of cough syrup, he went down for the count early.

I called "Moe" to let him know December would be the earliest that UIHC could see Ruffin for a full re-evaluation. I also had appointments scheduled at Gundersen for late September. I offered Bridgewater the choice of appointments, since I didn't know whether Mr. Montague would prefer a report from Gundersen as soon as possible or a later report from UIHC. "Moe" promised me a decision.

When "Moe" called back he repeated what we had agreed at mediation. "We get better reports from UIHC, better follow-up and better outreach." He asked if there were specific problems in either of Ruffin's classrooms that would preclude waiting for UIHC. I agreed Ruffin could go later, provided Evelyn could visit Ruffin in both of his classrooms in early October and offer us any advice needed on integration issues.

This led to a longer conversation with "Moe" about pretending, and social stories. I mentioned Francesca Happe's recent book from Harvard, research studies on pretending, and particularly those showing that attempts to teach adolescents social skills seemed to have failed. Most typically developing 4-year-olds have some theory of mind skills. "Moe" was curious and much easier to work things out with than Mr. Montague, but he didn't have anything to do with Head Start and couldn't answer my questions about that.

Meg reminded me, "School pictures tomorrow. Ruffin finger-painted and loved it." My first thought was, tactile defensiveness, much improved. I asked, "Could the photographer try to get Ruffin's 'good side' by turning his eyelid-scar to the background?"

Elaine sent some homework for Ruffin and me to "see how many circles you and your child can find at home tonight." A pleasant task at the end of this day. Also, Ruffin had traced his left hand, and colored each finger a different and beautiful color, each of which he could name. Ruffin's first show and tell would begin next Monday. "Our purpose is speaking in front of a group and to listen when others talk."

Seamus brought the newspaper. In *Public Notices*, I found the late August school board minutes. "The Board entered Closed Session as per Chapter 21.5(c): To discuss strategy with counsel in matters that are presently in litigation . . .. The Board entered Open Session at 8:16 PM" — after beginning the meeting at 7:30 PM — so, about 45 minutes. "No action was taken." Curt and I had no way of knowing what went on with our school board unless Caron might confide in Curt for some reason.

Although Ruffin had always been reluctant to wash his hair, by the middle of September he *changed his mind*. It helped to remark *benignly*, 'It was a good idea for you to *change your mind*. Thank you.' He proudly held his head back and got no soap in his eyes.

In Ruffin's home-school notebook I began to share with Meg everything "Moe" had been curious about. As much trouble as I was having puzzling out the special education system Ruffin and I were now enmeshed in, I doubted I was the right person to teach him how to avoid being hurt by deception, lying, or trickery — or how and when it might ever be appropriate to practice those dark arts.

Ruffin was invoking school rules at home. He told me, "Don't talk with your mouth full." And "That's a rule." I asked him who said that, and he replied, "Mrs. Holub." It was adorable.

Bridgewater's audiologist evaluated Ruffin's hearing for the first time this year after our summer experiment with auditory integration training (AIT). "Both ears: Normal hearing; within normal limits." It was Ruffin's best hearing test ever.

Meg had good news, too. "I administered *The Brigance* today which is a checklist, not a test, but there are some age equivalent measures.

"Syntax: Ruffin has all the skills through 3 years, 6 months. The only remaining item is 'Asks definitions of words,' listed at the 5-year-old level. I haven't heard him do this at school, so I didn't mark it.

"Sentence Length: Still measuring. I know he has some long ones — they want an average.

"Personal Data: Ruffin has scattered skills up to age 7 years. A little confused about his birthday. Almost had mastery of his phone number and complete address.

"Social Speech: Ruffin has all the skills through age 4. Others are emerging: 2-part oral message, answers the phone and summons a person, participates in conversation without monopolizing, says 'excuse me' to interrupt. (This is listed as a 4-year, 6-month-old skill, but I know 10-year-olds who don't!).

"Verbal Direction: Ruffin has all the skills through the 5-year, 0-month level (as high as this checklist goes).

"Naming Pictures: The checklist only goes up to 4 years, 0-month level. Ruffin got them all except a 'nail,' and he understood that receptively.

"Articulation: Ruffin did very well, able to articulate some sounds through the 7-year level. My scoring is not a very specific check. Kim would have better information on this.

"Repeats Numbers: Sequence of 3. Ruffin did one set of 4; has all the skills (goes up to 4-year level).

"Sentence Memory: 6 syllables imitated (3 years, 0 month). Ruffin did not do 7 or 8 syllables (3 years, 6 months). I would like to re-check this.

"Singing: Ruffin has all the skills through the 4-year-old level, which is as high as this checklist goes.

I replied to Meg. "I remember *The Brigance*." Both she and I had completed this checklist on Ruffin back in late November of last year, so we had those early measures to compare against these later ones to gauge his developmental growth. I offered Meg what I was seeing at home.

"Syntax: Ruffin is asking the definitions of words here at home — so, maybe that skill is emerging? He asked, 'What does it mean?' of a word this morning as we were reading.

"Personal data: Here at home, he gave his address and phone number yesterday afternoon to me and to Lisa, but he needs to *generalize* this skill.

"Sentence Memory: I'm not surprised that this is a weakness. Any auditory sequence is still hard for Ruffin to listen to and copy. This did get better early last summer, *after auditory integration training* (AIT), and he continues to improve. Remember, late last spring, Ruffin was still speaking telegraphically — especially away from home?

"Yesterday Evelyn said she has a tried-and-true social skills curriculum she uses with children once their speech comes in fairly well. She'll bring it when she comes in early October. Thanks for all your information from *The Brigance*. I'll pass it on to her."

"The neighborhood grandchildren came over to play with Ruffin and stayed for an hour in our backyard this afternoon, mostly throwing a ball back and forth over our volleyball net and using the playgroup equipment. Ruffin had a great time. These are the children who teased him and deliberately broke his toys last year so he would get mad for their amusement."

I brought Evelyn and Dr. Granpeesheh up to date by sending them a mid-August video of Ruffin with his summer playgroup, all RoJene's summer notes, Ms. Wilding's late-August report and Meg's latest *Brigance*. "We are getting no complaints and some compliments on Ruffin's participation in a private nursery school group of 15 typically developing 4-year-olds."

The next Saturday, while Donna and Lisa drilled Ruffin, I tried to help Gay Doyle, Bridgewater's parent-educator who was struggling with insurance coverage for her older daughter with autism, by sending her a half-dozen items I had on hand.

Then, since she had Mr. Montague's ear, I pointed out, "Even children with 'PDD' and 'autistic-like tendencies' are supposed to be categorized under the IDEA as 'Autistic' (AT — on the Bridgewater computer form).

"This issue was hashed-out before Congress in the 1990 IDEA amendments. Under the IDEA "Autism" is a very broadly defined disability. Here are a couple of pages from attorney Reed Martin, one of the foremost practitioners of special education law who represents families and students. He poses four hard questions about the implications of the 1990 special designation of autism as a separate disability category. Iowa has yet to address any of these four questions — not in the five years since the 1990 IDEA amendments.

"I hope the items you asked me to gather will be helpful to you, and to other parents."

Ruffin had a great weekend. Saturday, he did well eating out and shopping, and a good job helping with house-cleaning and washing our new Volvo. He caught a frog, drawn out of the lawn by all the water from the hose.

Sunday, he played in the park, where he spoke at length about catching and caring for his frog — not present for mutual "visual regard" — with another child and his mother. I sat back, eavesdropping on their conversation. Ruffin told them how he caught a frog, what the frog ate, that it was only one frog, that he kept it in a jar, and that it jumped.

Miss Hobbs called later in the day. Some educators from the North Fayette school district wanted to attend Evelyn's training for Renee. She volunteered to take care of bringing in or ordering all the food. North Fayette would be contributing money to the cost of the training, all very cordial.

As soon as this surprising phone call ended, I thought of two families in our support group who lived in North Fayette — both with older non-verbal children. I called one of the mothers to let her know, and she told me that after our last support group meeting, she and the other mother had gone in together to their administrators to ask for new programs for their three children with autism. Such good news, I called Ruth at the community college to leave her a message.

Meg crowed, "Ruffin had a great day, very relaxed and content today. He talked a lot to us and to the other children. He told me all about his frog!"

Elaine added, "Nursery school: Show and tell went well — Ruffin showed how his puppets work. Great time during playtime, interacting with many. He was very social today. We talked about feelings today; Ruffin responded appropriately. He continues to be very attentive during all listening times."

Everything was running like butter, except that I needed to make banana bread. Since tomorrow was a Tuesday, Meg needed a snack. Wait, that meant Ruffin and the rest of her class had yet to host a visit from Head Start.

It had been over a month since our hard-won mediation, and there had been no money in the mail either. I called Curt to ask, "What's up?" He reached out to our mediator Dee Ann. Her assistant issued a memo to everyone concerned. "My sincere apologies. I thought this agreement for Ruffin White had been mailed out the first week of September. Therefore, should there be any changes we will need them by the end of September, and if changes are made, an updated version will be mailed out in October."

As a result of what I thought was an agreement, taken down by a court reporter, in mid-August, I had materially changed my position for Ruffin and entered into a written IEP. Now anybody who wanted to could make changes? It was "an informal process," but where was my reimbursement? I needed to fly-speck Dee Ann's text of the agreement against my court reporter's transcript. I called Curt, to okay Dee Ann's text from my end, and hoped there wouldn't be any changes proposed by the schools.

The intake coordinator for UIHC issued a letter covering a myriad of forms for me to complete for the re-evaluation of Ruffin there at Bridgewater's expense. I decided to tackle all those later. I just couldn't face anymore paperwork.

Ruffin told me that his "old Mom" lived a long time ago in a log house — "You remember? We passed it?" We *had* recently driven by it. I showed him videos of himself and me there and pointed out that *I* was his "old Mom." He was reluctant to believe this. We had moved out of my log house when Ruffin was 15 months old — then he spent a month with my parents before we moved to our Victorian in town. It was amazing to hear Ruffin talk now about our old log house — which he did seem to remember — now that he could talk. He recognized himself easily as the baby in the log-house videos but was insistent that I was just his "new Mom." How strange.

In the morning, I saw Meg had written, "Ruffin had some resistance (not overt) to Donna's call to come work today, but it was probably due to his being at the macaroni tables — it is a favorite activity. And Donna does great, using his resistance to discuss and explore his feelings."

I explained, "Sorry, yesterday Ruffin got only about one-fourth of his morning vitamin and DMG dose. He was much better with Lisa by the afternoon. I visited with Donna about what happened."

According to Donna, what had happened was a big tantrum.

It was past time to tackle the pile of UIHC paperwork. The first form's bottom line was "What kind of help would you like us to give you and your child? (Specific requests or questions to be answered)." I replied, "1. Support his CARD program as appropriate; 2. Curriculum to teach social skills and theory of mind 3. Systems advocacy from your institution to begin meeting the medical 'standard of care' by recommending more appropriate programs for PDD-NOS and autism in preschool (i.e., Lovaas)."

I filled out the pages of a mother's questionnaire, a new addition since last spring, marked *Confidential* about my own health and mood over the last three months of July, August, and September — covering the time we had been running a home drill program and summer playgroup, preparing for and holding mediation — with tens of thousands of reimbursement money still hanging fire.

"Do you feel miserable or depressed?" I marked most or all the time. And yes, my appetite was poor sometimes, and yes, I had a hard time falling asleep, was tired, had difficulty concentrating a good part of the time, resorting to a daily written list of "things to do." I found myself easily upset or irritated. No, that didn't touch my extreme fury, my volcanic anger. "Have you lost interest in your work, your friends, or your appearance?" I reported I was unable to practice law as before.

But, although I continued to worry a lot, I didn't feel like a failure, or cry a lot, or contemplate suicide. Of course, I *had* thought of suicide last year when Dr. Caldwell had first delivered Ruffin's diagnosis, but I had not given it any thought since. The frustrations and successes of advocacy seemed to have kept that at bay.

I didn't have backaches, or bad headaches, nor a fast or irregular heartbeat, but I had "vomited violently three times while reading Ruffin's school file this summer." Yes, I was tense and nervous sometimes, but I wasn't afraid to be alone, or go out and meet people. I wasn't scared or anxious for no good reason. Did I feel that everyone was against me? No, I wasn't paranoid, but I reported having received vicious hate mail and written threats about my efforts on Ruffin's behalf from school people or people privy to school information.

No, I didn't take medication for my nerves, or feel I might have a nervous breakdown. Finally, I offered this comment: "It has been very encouraging to get word that more than a dozen Iowa children are partially funded for CARD training, three in Bridgewater now, besides Ruffin. Several school officials are coming around, but without apology."

Clearly, I was in rough shape and had been over the last year since Ruffin's diagnosis. Even with the help of my parents, Seamus, Donna, Lisa, Rose, Evelyn, and Dr. Granpeesheh, Dr. Rimland in San Diego, Curt and Joan, RoJene and Pine, my new legal assistant Robin Ouren, and a clerical staff of teenage volunteers, the last three summer months had been difficult. Inspecting Ruffin's full educational file just before mediation had undermined my trust in Meg and Inge, and even Sue Baker. The state mediation system seemed riddled with error and uncertainty, distant and weak.

Who would I have seen for *more* help? When would I have had the time? There was not a licensed psychiatrist within a hundred miles of our town, and not a mental health counselor within a hundred miles with whom I did not work professionally. Who would I feel comfortable confiding in, or trust to keep his or her mouth shut? I didn't have two hours to drive back and forth somewhere to spend luxuriating at length on some couch.

That was the way I saw it: getting Ruffin what he needed was much more important to me now and would be for the foreseeable future.

CHAPTER THIRTY EIGHT

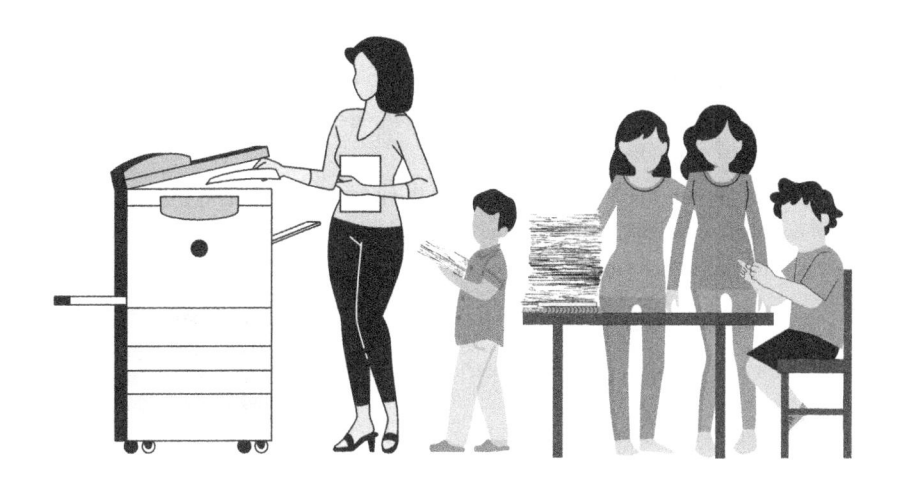

BACK TO GUNDERSEN

Ruffin and I were due to be seen at Gundersen soon, but our mid-August mediation agreement was still hanging fire. The newspaper Seamus had left on the kitchen counter reported that the next school board meeting would be Monday, *after* Ruffin's Gundersen clinic appointments. I called the school. There was no time left to notice a special meeting. The school board could not meet legally any earlier. I understood that. I called Gundersen to explain our dilemma. They were not sympathetic. The clinic expected to be paid.

I tried to reach Curt without success. Then, I took an hour to visit the gym and think. Finally, I called "Moe" and explained. "Moe" said Bridgewater's board was waiting on my school board's approval before it could issue me their portion of the agreed-upon reimbursement. But "Moe" agreed to pay for Gundersen. I would need to sign and return some forms. Not a problem. He and I both had faxes.

Again, "Moe" seemed very cordial and to have all the time in the world. So, without mentioning anyone's names — as a mutual bow to the sacred confidentiality of special education matters — "Moe" and I had a good hair-down discussion about the three families and their new CARD programs he expected Bridgewater and their local districts to cooperate in providing that year.

Meanwhile, Miss Hobbs issued a memo to all interested parties about Evelyn's upcoming early October visit. The group Evelyn would train had expanded to include two dozen people from two school districts, Bridgewater and TASC. Costs would be split between the two districts and Bridgewater.

A relief, as this, too, arrived by fax. Everything promised to go off without a hitch. More goodwill prevailed. Mr. Montague fully reimbursed my travel expenses and parking for Ruffin's and my earlier trip to see Ms. Wilding.

Ruffin was back, off the bus, at the door, for a hug and little snack before heading upstairs for his afternoon drills with Lisa.

Now our weather had turned suddenly windy, cold, and rainy. Meg reminded everyone to dress their children warmly, with hats, and, yes, mittens.

Elaine had written, too, with some concern. "In the bathroom, Ruffin became fascinated with the mirror and didn't want to wash his hands and get back in line. Then, he became fascinated with pulling the sleeves of his shirt over his hands and waving his arms in the mirror. I went in and gently touched his arm and physically directed him back in line — no problem.

"It was his turn today to pass out napkins at snack time. He doesn't understand the task of giving napkins to each person at his table. I physically directed this. He had started to go to another table." Meg had a different routine for passing out napkins in her classroom. That was bound to be confusing for Ruffin.

Ruffin came home sick with Donna the next morning before lunch. Thank goodness for Donna. I had too much work to do to get ready to take him back to Gundersen on Friday to manage him. The junior high school volunteers would be copying and filing overtime by the afternoon.

I tackled Gundersen's *Child Behavior Checklist for Ages Four to Eighteen* for their full re-evaluation. The first question was about what sports Ruffin liked: Swimming, batting and catch. Then, what hobbies and activities: Computer (educational software), 'reading' books, feeding animals. Next, what organizations or clubs: I listed our summer playgroup, noting that Ruffin had attended every day of the summer. Next, Ruffin's jobs or chores: Ruffin did like to help around the house as a go-fer, and cleaning and washing the car. How many close friends? Thinking of Chance and the little girl who "didn't really love" him, I checked the box for two.

As for questions about how well Ruffin managed to get along with others and behave, I offered my observation that Ruffin was "mind blind" still but improving with language and training. Describing his school placement, I recounted the complicated two-campus placement reached in mediation, and Lisa's continuing therapy in the afternoons with Ruffin. All weekends were free time to spend with Seamus and me.

I gave his medical diagnosis as: PDD-NOS.

What concerned me most about my child? 1. Finding a curriculum for "theory of mind" and social skills training; 2. That an "appropriate placement" would be with a small group of 4- to 5-year-old typically developing classmates for 30 to 35 hours per week, but this was *not* available in the schools' continuum of services; 3. Fear that continuing exposure to ECSE classmates may provide poor language and behavior models; 4. Fear that an unstructured, upcoming summer would lead to language and behavioral deterioration; 5. Concern that Ruffin was currently mis-classified as having a "non-categorical" disability when he was entitled to the benefit of an "AT" autism classification under the 1990 amendments to the IDEA.

Please describe the best things about my child? He was talking. He was getting to be much easier to care for regarding his behavior. He was very affectionate. He was eating, sleeping, bathing, dressing better and more independently.

Then followed a lengthy list of 113 disordered behaviors for me to rate Ruffin as having or not, and comment upon.

Using Lovaas's *Flowchart of Key Programs* again, I updated Ruffin's progress over Lovaas's usual 2-year curriculum. Ruffin had mastered all the early work of the first 4 domains, and in the remaining domains he had mastered a great many focus areas. With my yellow highlighter, I circled those areas I thought he had emerging skills in, or were part of his current drill book from Evelyn that Donna, Lisa, Seamus, and I were working on: speech volume and inflection, the abstract concepts of categories and emotions, listening to and telling stories, describing past experiences and future tense, reading, writing, observational learning, conversations, getting and giving information, pretend play, one-to-one playmates, group play with age-mates, dressing, placement in a nursery school, and skills for community safety.

Out on the farthest fringes at the end of Lovaas's curriculum were areas I trusted Evelyn and Dr. Granpeesheh would get to when the time for Ruffin might be right: describing topics, worksheets, problem-solving, joining a pre-existing conversation, interviewing, board games, play talk, scripted play, asserting himself, playing teacher, helping others at school and with household chores and errands.

I sent this chart to Gundersen, so Ruffin's team, and Dr. Caldwell, especially — who had written Ruffin's CARD prescription — could see how far along Lovaas's own *Flowchart* Ruffin had come since last year.

Then Mrs. Wonderlich's volunteers and I assembled fourteen indexed tabs of information for Gundersen, as background for this, their second full evaluation of Ruffin. Those documents fully described all our efforts with Ruffin since last fall.

Without Mrs. Wonderlich's teenaged volunteers, without a filing system they had learned to pull from to make copies, without their busy hands and interested questions, their checking back, "Is this the right one? This the right tab for it?" I would never have been able to assemble Ruffin's case in any meaningful way for Gundersen.

As the copier whined in a fume of hot toner and warm paper, Donna walked downstairs carrying Ruffin, who had been sleeping all afternoon, slowly improving, and getting better. Ready, I imagined, to be up all night. I took him in my arms and looked forward to reading to him. I could go upstairs and lie down to do it, because Rose was there, reliably, to cook dinner.

When Ruffin had fallen deeply asleep, I took that final midnight opportunity to carefully check the volunteers' work and read back through the documents we had assembled. After the busy summer and settlement negotiations I considered how far Ruffin had come, thought about where he needed to go next, and how far he would need to go before he could join a class of typically developing boys and girls.

I typed out a brief agenda for the interpretive staffing at Gundersen. 1. Medically necessary prescription for CARD services to August 1996; 2. Strong support for educational diagnosis of "Autism" under federal and state IDEA special education regulations and *Section 504 of the Rehabilitation Act*, signed by all; 3. Detailed assessment and testing, to identify missed concepts and language elements; 4. Social skills and theory of mind curriculum; 5. Anemia; 6. Ear Tubes — risk of yeast infection with repeated antibiotics; 7. A buddy in preschool integration.

Gundersen's report issued after our Friday and Monday visits: "Ruffin is a 4-year, 5-month-old child who was originally seen here in 1994.

"Staffing Summary: Following Ruffin's evaluation, present at the staffing were Dr. Ladd, child and adolescent psychiatrist; Dr. Caldwell, pediatric neurologist; Dr. Kondrick, neuropsychologist; and Mila Sokolov, speech and language pathologist. Absent was Dr. Palm, the audiologist." I was pleased with the reappearance of all the big guns on Ruffin's earlier team.

"Dr. Caldwell, Pediatric Neurologist: Ruffin presented for follow-up of his PDD-NOS. As before, he continues to make good progress. Part of this is attributable to his LOVAAS program, part to the intensive interventions he has received, and part to general maturity. His mother has him on megavitamin therapy with B6 and magnesium and a substance called Dimethylglycine. I am not sure what impact the B6, magnesium and Dimethylglycine have had.

"Impression: PDD-NOS. A letter was sent renewing his Lovaas CARD program through August of 1996."

Check, then, the first item on my personal agenda. I needed this to get Prudential to help me keep my end of the bargain — the mediation agreement obligation I had undertaken to help pay Donna to attend school and do her therapy with Ruffin there.

"Mila Sokolov, Speech and Language Pathologist: Ruffin returned for a speech and language evaluation. Growth was documented in all language skills, especially social communication interactions and pragmatic language skills.

"Ruffin was reevaluated using the *Reynell Developmental Language Scale*. Ruffin evidenced more than a year's gain in a year's time. He continued to have trouble with longer directives involving a variety of concepts. Attention was variable and waned when directions became more complex.

"Impression: This young boy continues to present with deficits in language comprehension and expression of less than one year with some scales being at age level. Continuous and progressive improvement has been noted from previous evaluations. Deficits continue to be influenced by the nature of PDD-NOS.

"Dr. Palm, Audiologist: Ruffin was seen for a repeat evaluation today. I saw him on October 5th, 1994, at which time he had grossly normal hearing. Again today, his audiogram confirmed grossly normal hearing levels bilaterally with flat tympanic membranes in both ears.

"Dr. Kondrick, Neuropsychologist: Ruffin was seen for intellectual assessment. Ruffin gave good cooperation and effort during today's test administration such that obtained scores are judged a fair estimate of his current abilities. He entered the test environment taking mom by the hand. He was reticent to let her leave the room, and she sat behind and observed testing.

"On the Wechsler Preschool and Primary Scale of Intelligence-Revised, Ruffin earned a verbal IQ of 92, a Performance IQ of 134, and a Full-Scale IQ of 112."

Since Ruffin had last been seen at Gundersen about a year ago, before his CARD programming began, his Verbal IQ on this same measure had risen from 74 to 92 (an 18-point gain), and his Performance IQ had risen from 86 to 134 (a 48-point gain).

Dr. Kondrick pointed out though, "His Performance IQ is believed to be inflated secondary to the fact that Ruffin is well practiced at tasks such as block design, figure copying, and construction. Ruffin's performance for verbal subtests is also particularly of note. He performs in an age-appropriate manner when the tasks require single word expression or understanding. He also performs in an age-appropriate manner when he is allowed to point to answers. He has a good understanding of the concept of 'same.'

"When these oral reasoning subtests require that he demonstrate understanding of the semantic structure of language, use conceptual reasoning or reasoning via categories or word relationships, his performance falls off relative to the typical peer. There are times when Ruffin simply does not understand a question he is asked.

"The most pronounced difficulties were seen on the Similarities subtest. This subtest requires an understanding of similarities, differences, and category membership. Responses, however, require more than just a mere understanding of category membership and require reasoning or explanation for why things belong together. Ruffin has difficulty with such elaborate use of language."

How did I feel about this IQ? It still exhibited an "autistic profile," a large imbalance between verbal and non-verbal IQ, but I was deeply comforted by the near-normal measure of Ruffin's verbal IQ. He certainly had the potential to learn whatever he might need to through language and otherwise, and to learn to communicate his own discoveries.

With this IQ measure, Ruffin entered the educational arena of the "twice exceptional," populated by those children with difficult disabilities in the presence of other exceptional strengths and abilities — easy to tease or bully — who required thoughtful teachers willing to suspend a belief that weakness in one academic or behavioral domain was a clear proxy for a student's potential in other academic or behavioral domains. Unevenness of potential remained something to be aware of, to work with, and to work around.

But, after this IQ measure, Ruffin could never be described as "retarded," nor could I be dismissed as a mother whose furious advocacy was the result of some personal failure to face that she needed to cope with a child who simply needed care, love, and comfort. I could not be dismissed as the mother of a child for whom the schools should abandon all ambition. I need not fold, with grace, to the unchangeable, or kneel with thanks to Providence who had sent this child to instruct and humble me to be grateful. I could just *be* humble, and grateful.

"Dr. Ladd, Child Psychiatrist: Ruffin is now 4 years, 5 months old. He has made some significant gains since last year, most notably in language, but continues to have problems in language and socialization.

"For example, in the office, he spent very little time interacting with me. At home, when children come over to play, he will often stand only a few minutes with them, and then wants to come in.

"He continues to meet the criteria for PDD-NOS. From a medical point of view, the diagnosis is probably Asperger's, a subtype of PDD-NOS. As I look through the educational material, he continues to meet the criteria for autism as defined educationally. It should be remembered that the current law was written prior to the medical diagnosis of Asperger's being accepted. That only occurred this year."

Of course, I was incredibly pleased with these paragraphs since they addressed the complex interaction between medical and educational definitions of autism spectrum disorders in a more nuanced manner than he had offered last year.

His report continued, "Ruffin should continue in a highly structured program such as the one that he is currently involved in, based on models from southern California. I would like to see him integrated with average children as soon as that is practically possible, since social skills are probably the most important aspect of his ongoing educational program."

"Debbie Olufs, Learning Disabilities Section: I saw Ruffin for the educational portion of his exam. In general, he did a lot of smiling and fidgeting during the assessment process. We began with a measure which is highly nonverbal in presentation, and which utilizes a lot of manipulatives. This was obviously an area of comfort for Ruffin, and he engaged quite readily, enjoying the work.

"When this measure was done, we did begin a test that was more verbally directed. Ruffin did not like this measure, and more inappropriate behavior was noted. He was much less engaged in the task, somewhat avoidant, and quite likely to say 'I don't know' for questions, simply to get out of the task at hand.

"This indicates that environments which are laden with oral directives are going to be quite challenging for him. It will be important for his teachers to realize that when these types of behaviors occur, it may be due to the contextual environment of the classroom, and not simply because of misbehavior on Ruffin's part. Classrooms which are highly verbal will impact more directly on his disability and may prove to be much more disconcerting for him.

"Academically, Ruffin has made some impressive gains in the past year. Although his profile remains quite similar to his previous profile, gains of nearly a year in a 1-year period were frequently noted. This gives support to the quality of educational support he has received in the past year.

"At this point, Ruffin appears, in many ways, to be academically ready for kindergarten. He knows basic colors, at both recognition and recall levels. He knows basic shapes in the same way, except for triangle, which he relatively consistently confused with rectangle. He knows some concepts such as big, little, and small, but is not very flexible with the use of synonyms in these concepts. He can read the numbers 1 through 10 and has one-to-one correspondence well above that. We measured it to 20, but it is probably even higher. In general, he knows his letters fairly well, and can both recognize and read lower- and upper-case letters. He is beginning to show the ability to write numbers from a model.

"Two behaviors were noted which were pleasing. He was asked to build a tall tower when given some blocks. He turned the jar over that had held the blocks and stacked them on top of the jar to make them even higher. Another time he was asked to engage in imaginative play with puppets. Through this, he showed good initiative of conversation and good expression. In addition, he displayed consideration towards a puppy puppet which he was not holding.

"In general, he did best with tasks which required imitative modeling. On these, he was fairly compliant. He is somewhat concerned when he does not feel he does a job at the level he expects, and frequent erasures and retrials were noted. Some academic behaviors on the PDD-Autism Spectrum were noted.

"For example, he showed an affinity for numbers, completing some basic addition and subtraction facts with no concrete reinforcers. In contrast, when he was shown a picture of a fireman and asked what this gentleman did, he initially said, 'saves people' and then he said, 'puts water on fire,' but no matter how many times he was asked, he could not come up with the fact that the fireman is supposed to 'put out the fire.' I would guess, therefore, that there will be times in the classroom where his inconsistency will be puzzling, not only to his teachers but to his peers."

Dr. Kondrick had this to offer: "This 4 year, 5-month-old boy is seen for Intellectual assessment, as a part of a comprehensive workup relative to developmental delays and oddities in emotional and social relatedness.

"According to his mom, Ruffin has received 30 hours a week structured activity in the home via the LOVAAS method of behavioral management. Three adult providers provide this. Additionally, he is now enrolled in an early childhood classroom, 35 hours a week. Therefore, he is in structured programming from 55 to 60 hours a week.

"His mom says that he is well practiced at block design drills. She elaborates that this requires him to take a two-dimensional picture and construct a three-dimensional structure of blocks from the image. He is also well practiced at figure copying in art at school and on the computer. At home he practices cutting and pasting and the use of scissors.

"Ruffin carries a previous diagnosis for PDD-NOS. Hypotheses include possible Autism and possible Asperger's."

Then, Dr. Kondrick described how Ruffin entered the room and how I remained with him to watch. "He was content to proceed in this manner. He only turned around a few times to look at his mother, and this did not interfere significantly with standardized test administration. Ruffin is quite wiggly in his seat. He did become tired toward the end of testing."

Dr. Kondrick set out Ruffin's new, much higher IQ scores and commented upon what she judged they meant and offered a bit more detail. "For example, when he is asked to name three animals, he has great difficulty in understanding this request. Ruffin can name and point to animals but has a difficult time in complying with the oral direction to name three in a spontaneous manner. He did eventually say 'cows, sheep, and dolphin,' earning credit. He has similar difficulty when asked to name a vegetable. He offers fruit. When the question was repeated, he offered 'salad.' His most pronounced difficulties were seen on the Similarities subtest."

Mila Sokolov, the speech and language pathologist, reported: "Ruffin was seen approximately 1 year ago. At that time, he was demonstrating deficits in both language comprehension and expression of more than 1-year.

"Since that time, he has received intensive speech and language therapy with emphasis placed on improving language relative to structure and formulation as well as the pragmatics of language.

"A very comprehensive evaluation was conducted recently in late August at the UIHC. Developmental articulation errors were noted with an accompanying 'mild high pitch.' Growth was documented in all language skills — especially social communication interactions and pragmatic language skills.

"Since Ruffin had undergone some very extensive testing, it was decided that re-evaluation using the *Reynell Developmental Language Scale* would be utilized for comparative purposes. On the Verbal Comprehensive portion of the *Reynell Developmental Language Scale,* Ruffin achieved a raw score of 53 with a corresponding age equivalence of 3 years, 7 months and showing more than a year's gain in a year's time.

"He continues to have difficulty with longer directives involving a variety of concepts. Even though he clearly understands these concepts individually and in shorter directives, he cannot maintain the integrity of the message as it increases. For example, when told to 'put the 3 short pencils in the box,' he responded by putting only 2 of them in the box and forgetting a third one even though he clearly understands the concept of 'short' and the number concept of '3.' Attending was variable and waned as directions became more complex.

"The *Test of Auditory Comprehension of Language-Revised* which assesses knowledge of vocabulary, morphology, and more complex sentence structures, was administered. Ruffin achieved a total raw score of 59, and a Standard Score of 101, with a corresponding age equivalency range of 4 years, 4 months to 4 years, 6 months.

"He scanned his choices carefully while making a selection. It was noteworthy, however, that several of his errors involved misinterpretation of concepts on his part. For example, when asked to show me a 'large blue ball,' he pointed to a smaller blue ball. Later, since this was surprising that Ruffin had missed this, I went back to these items and asked Ruffin to name each of the pictures. He correctly named 'a small green ball, a big blue ball, and a large little ball.' It is unclear whether he confuses 'large' and 'little' or if this was only an isolated incident.

"In talking with the mother, there are instances where Ruffin will misunderstand words and these merely need to be taught at the time the error occurs and then he should be given an opportunity to practice that concept or misunderstood language item several times in a variety of contexts.

"Language Expression: The Expressive Language portion of the *Reynell Developmental Language Scale* which assesses language structure, vocabulary, and content yielded a raw score of 45 with a corresponding age equivalence of 3 years, 6 months which, again, demonstrated more than a year's gain in a year's time.

"He was able to talk about pictures although his verbalizations, today, were somewhat limited. He was battling a cold which also limited the amount of conversation that was gathered. However, he was heard to speak in a variety of contexts that have also been noted by those speech pathologists working with Ruffin including commenting, requesting information, and answering questions. There do seem to be, however, some limited memory strategies which might be something that could be worked on in a practical manner.

"Impressions: This young boy continues to present with deficits in language comprehension and expression of less than 1 year with some skills being at age level. Continuous and progressive improvement has been noted from his previous evaluation. Deficits continue to be influenced by the nature of pervasive developmental disorders.

"Recommendations: It is recommended that Ruffin continue to receive speech and language therapy with emphasis placed on continued improvement relative to following directions involving a variety of concepts, improving comprehension and formulation of question types, recognizing any 'gaps' in language concepts (i.e., The concept of 'large') and working with them on an ongoing basis, and continuing to work on interactive communications.

"One area that may need to be addressed in an organized, yet practical manner might include working on short- and long-term memory tasks and understanding the learning style of children with PDD.

"Ruffin has had excellent intervention for the past year with good follow-up by the speech pathologist at UIHC. There is no further need to see Ruffin for language follow-up at Gundersen."

Sadly, Ruffin missed his picture being taken at the private nursery school, individually and with his classmates. Donna, Lisa, and I needed a picture to be able to teach him their names. We were able to get one from Elaine, cut it up, and have Seamus identify each child for us.

CHAPTER THIRTY NINE

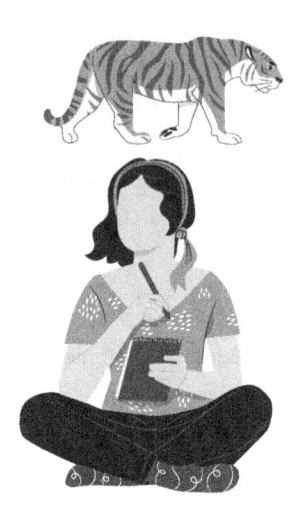

PACING LIKE A TIGER

When I asked Ruffin over breakfast at our downtown café, he said his little girlfriends from summer playgroup had never come to visit him at school. It was late September. I would need to ask Meg. Their mothers had both been delighted when their daughters had been admitted to Head Start. This needed attention. I had spent too much time enjoying the O. J. Simpson trial. I needed to get my head out of that.

Meg was cheerful enough. "Ruffin took a note to the office *all by himself!* His interactive play outside was great. He answered more readily in group than he has so far, all year."

But at nursery school, Elaine seemed concerned. "We noticed that Ruffin needed to be reminded about our routine today, probably because of his missing two days. We cut out colored circles for a stop and go light. He had trouble following directions for this project, especially using a glue stick on brown paper. Not as good a listener today."

Seamus brought the paper that afternoon. The school board had paid $626.10 more for legal fees. I had yet to see a dime of the tens of thousands of reimbursement promised me at mediation.

"They're not going to pay you. What makes you think they ever will?"

Then I was furious with Seamus.

Ruffin was up all night — very hyper. It was the first time in a long time and was *so scary*.

I suggested to Meg and Elaine, "If he needs to sleep or rest today, I think that's okay. I wonder why Ruffin is having trouble with directions in nursery school. He's usually so compliant. What are the directions? How long and cluttered (linguistically) are they? I'm thinking about what we learned from Ms. Wilding's late August report."

The doorbell rang. It was a mother who had driven a long distance to visit and gather copies of whatever autism resources we had. The teenaged volunteers picked a full set of helpful materials from their carefully filed, labeled, and pre-copied caches of documents. She headed out the door after an hour with an armful of reading, and a box of a dozen yellow highlighters, with our best wishes.

Ruffin arrived home on the bus for hugs all around, and a snack, before heading up the stairs for his last session of the day with Lisa.

Elaine had sent a general announcement that her class had 16 children now, 10 boys and 6 girls, with a nicely detailed summary of her curriculum, including a full list of books she would be using, and Ruffin's cut and paste project of an autumn tree with leaves in the branches and on the ground around its roots.

Meg had included an October snack calendar.

A small wispy cloud passed briefly through the sunniness of this productive day. Wasn't Head Start supposed to take over providing snacks on the days of their visits? No Head Start appeared on Meg's snack calendar for any day in October.

Ruffin was still full of energy after his afternoon session with Lisa and wanted to play outside until after dark. He cried broken heartedly when the neighbor children went home to go to bed, "I want my friends." Then, he ate well, bathed, and dressed himself in his pajamas, picked a book to read, and had a good, sound uninterrupted night's sleep. We were back on track.

I assured Meg and Elaine that Friday, "He should have a good day. Ruffin went swimming a lot this summer. He doesn't put his face in the water yet to blow bubbles but might copy someone after one or two refusals." Meg replied that afternoon, "Ruffin's new Luther friend is a young man. Ruffin was not too happy in the water but didn't fight it. He cried at first — okay after that." This regression surprised me.

Elaine had added, "Good day, here." She was agreeable to meet Monday after school in Meg's classroom with the two of us about Ruffin.

We enjoyed our weekend — shopping, eating out, going to the gym, As I worked out, Ruffin played patiently for twenty minutes with his blue glitter ball. At Sunday school, he volunteered answers when called upon. He went out to Seamus's farm, where the two of them worked at wood splitting and hauling, fed animals, burned trash, harvested the garden, and hammered nails. He and I went to the park for several hours. It was Ruffin on the go all the time.

We were half-way through the first semester. Meg and Amy were sending home their fall harvest, mid-term reports. Meg reminded me, "Ruffin's snack day is tomorrow." Some sort of subtle clue? Still no Head Start?

Monday afternoon's meeting with Meg and Elaine went well enough, until Elaine bowed out. As soon as Meg and I were alone, it was another ambush reminiscent of last year's mid-winter IEP.

After I stormed out, I wrote to Meg, in a large, slashing hand, heedless that Elaine would see it, too. Too bad. "When did you first learn Head Start was not going to show up?

"It is clear what Ruffin's needs — what his *unique* needs are. The problem here is one of administrative inconvenience. Frankly, *that* is Miss Hobbs's problem to resolve, not mine, but I will be as clear as I can be about what *various options might meet Ruffin's unique needs in my view.*"

I could not have been more furious. At Miss Hobbs for making Meg the messenger again — just like last year. And at Meg for caving into this craven role. Hadn't I learned last summer I could not trust her to advocate for Ruffin? None of this was good for Ruffin. And this matter could not have surfaced at a more delicate time with Evelyn due in a few days to set up Renee's program and train so many people in Bridgewater. Copies of my letter to Miss Hobbs went out widely to everyone even remotely concerned. I wrote in a white heat.

"The agreed-upon IEP program reduced the number of hours of integration with typical age-appropriate classmates from 3 hours per day to 2 hours and 20 minutes per day, at most — that is, from 15 hours per week to 11 hours and 40 minutes per week. But, since the Head Start Tuesday and Thursday integration has never materialized, Ruffin's integration time has fallen to 7 hours per week — less than half of last summer's program.

"The agreed-upon IEP program also reduced the number of hours of intensive one-to-one CARD drills by Donna from 4 hours a day 5 days a week (total 20 hours per week) to 3 hours a day 4 days a week (12 hours per week). This reduced amount of time with Donna is further diluted by Ruffin's participation with ECSE and severe and profoundly disabled classmates in music, physical education, and library, all of which take place during the Monday through Thursday morning hours."

I set out dates and details from our home-school notebook: the early promise that Head Start would be there in "a couple of weeks;" Ruffin missing his summer girlfriends; Meg's most recent ambush when "she proposed we draft and sign an IEP amendment" to eliminate Head Start because "Ruffin had already met several of the stated objectives." It seemed that this year's IEP, like all others before it, had set the bar too low for Ruffin and endangered him.

"There is some evidence from the reemergence of self-stimulatory behaviors, toileting accidents, night-waking, and breakthrough babbling, that the transition from last summer's program to the two school programs has been somewhat difficult because Ruffin's educational plan is insufficiently rigorous.

"At the recent meeting with Mrs. Holub and Mrs. Mills, I advised them of Gundersen's most-recent IQ testing results of 112. However, the averaging of IQ into a single figure obscures the effect of Ruffin's autism on his various skills. Ruffin's verbal IQ remains at 92, or about ½ a standard deviation below the mean of 100. Thus, Ruffin presents a range of IQ from 92 to 134 which spans 3 standard deviations from the mean.

"It would seem most appropriate to concentrate on remediating Ruffin's nearly 1-year delay in syntax, pragmatic use of language, and shallow general knowledge base by putting him in the company of typical children doing typical pre-school activities every afternoon for as long as possible, in hopes of narrowing the very wide gap between his verbal and non-verbal IQs which make him a difficult child to teach.

"In order for Miss Hobbs to do the administrative groundwork to prepare a continuum of options for placement for Ruffin's Tuesday and Thursday afternoons, from which we might choose as a team," I indicated several placement options to explore: 1. Further integration into the private nursery school; 2. Reverse integration from private nursery-schoolers; or 3. Integration up into kindergarten.

"I hope this offers some insight into the continuum of placements I would like to have us consider as a team. I do want the people necessary to make an appropriate decision to meet quickly so we can replace the missing component of Ruffin's agreed-upon IEP." In other words, I didn't want Miss Hobbs to notice me into another mid-winter IEP meeting like last year's.

The next day, Meg answered my most direct question — whether she remained worthy of my trust. "I only knew last week. I waited to tell you during our meeting as it was already scheduled." She filled out the daily note form of our home-school notebook but offered no anecdotal comments about Ruffin. She knew I loved those, that I relished them. In this silence, I could sense that I had hurt her feelings. She was drawing back from any semblance of partnership. What a coward she was. In a worthless allegiance with another coward — Miss Hobbs. What did it take to be my working partner? Courage. Like Donna's bold and brassy, or even quiet, distant courage, like Lisa's.

Neither Meg nor Miss Hobbs was, or ever could be, my partners. I would never win them over. And, certainly, I had no control over either of them. Neither of them was Ruffin's mother. Why was I expecting them to take a motherly interest in Ruffin? That was expecting too much of them, as working professionals. Even a reliable working partnership was too much to expect of either Meg or Miss Hobbs, but I felt like a manipulated fool to have decided to try to partner with either of them — to Ruffin's detriment. I was flooded with regret. By depending upon them to keep their word at mediation, by depending on them to carry out the IEP plan, I had placed Ruffin and his development at risk. Or slowed it, at the very least.

It would be difficult, and monumentally inconvenient to withdraw Ruffin from public school now and reconvene his summer playgroup somewhere in a heated room for the winter. None of Ruffin's summer playmates were even available — most of them were enrolled in Head Start.

Time for more firmness with myself, to take myself in hand and work myself back up into some transparently fake cheerfulness. To Meg and Elaine, I sent the best I could manage. "I love his school pictures. So will the rest of his family."

Once the stubby bus picked Ruffin up, as always, my legal work, and our autism advocacy helped me push away worry. Helping and talking to other parents and connecting them to each other helped me to feel better about myself and to erect a façade that looked like the patience I really could not muster. The work of somehow paying it forward helped and appealed to my deepest superstitions — that unless I did this, there was some awful chance Ruffin would suffer, and unaccountably regress.

Advocacy and the usual fall run of divorces to file before my new clients would be facing the holidays — the Thanksgiving and Christmas family dinner tables — the drunk drivers, the teenage burglars, the petty drug dealers, domestic abusers, and parents in juvenile court seeking reunification with their children begin to stream again through my office to drown my own sorrows.

Meg continued to remain very cool, writing little more than was needed to fill out her daily note form. It was time for more on my part. "Hooray, Ruffin's understanding of occupations is taking hold. Donna showed me the *ABCs of Emotions*. I think that's just what we were looking for as fresh drill material. Ruffin is using 'disappointed' now. He told me he painted apples, leaves, and a stem in nursery school. Tonight, he was exceptionally talkative and sweet.

"All the plans for Evelyn's visit came together beautifully today — she will spend Saturday in West Union with the North Fayette district people and their parents. Donna, Lisa, and I will meet with Evelyn on Sunday at my home in the early afternoon. Please come and join us. Elaine is welcome, too."

As to our unresolved inclusion issue, I suggested, "Please send Ruffin to kindergarten and first grade library and recesses on Thursday and Tuesday afternoons until Miss Hobbs can get back to me about the other options."

Seamus arrived with the paper. "You made the paper. I've been hearing about it all week. The school board had a special meeting just about you, last Monday." This devolved into some ugliness about his not having any control over me.

"How embarrassing," I said, "for you." Acidly. And then shook open the paper to the *Public Notices*. "This is the first I've heard of it."

In the tiny print, it appeared the school board had met for an hour and a half long special closed session with "visitor Caron Angelos, attorney," about "the determination of a course of action the district will follow on a financial settlement requested by a patron."

Here I had thought, silly me, we had all *agreed*, not that I had "requested," not that I had begged.

"I compromised." I told Seamus, and then explained how little Ruffin was getting this year compared to last summer. "I offered them a bargain. What is this? 'A motion was made and seconded that no action be taken until additional information is received from legal counsel.'"

Seamus had no answer. Not so much as a whisper off the grapevine.

"What did you expect?" he asked, and then left in a huff of his own frustration.

Curt promised to call Caron and find out what was happening with the school board. I could well imagine what was happening.

Curt and I knew we could sue to enforce our mediated agreement, since I had detrimentally relied upon its terms and sent Ruffin back to school, legally "sealing the deal." Or we could back out and sue in due process for the amount needed to reimburse me in full. Curt counseled we should bend over backwards for the moment and give Caron the professional courtesy of another chance to persuade the board to pay up without a fight.

I agreed, "Fine."

Then Curt and I walked through the inclusion failure problem of no Head Start and brainstormed what we could do about that. Curt was concerned that our whole mediation effort and agreement was going to unravel. I was so furious I didn't care whether that happened or not.

But Curt agreed — the IEP was legally binding.

I was whining about being ambushed again by a beloved teacher who had been pressed to sweet-talk me into signing away Ruffin's established entitlements. Fortunately, Curt had a little legal ace up his sleeve to show me, to direct my anger in a productive direction.

Chris Foster had sent me a truly cheerful note. I was happy to have her card with a hummingbird sipping at a row of Dutchmen's breeches. Why not pretend it was spring, if it lifted my spirits as we headed into winter? Even a little, even if only for a moment?

Meg responded at length finally, but defensively, falling on what was Miss Hobbs's sword to fall on, again. "Regarding the delay with Head Start, I was the one informed. The administrators of both programs gave permission for the integration program to occur — it was up to the teachers to work on details and schedules. I apologize for the delays, but I was trying to be as organized as possible with alternatives."

I wrote Meg back, utterly unmollified, and then struggled again to get back on a cheerful mommy track with her, using the product of my brainstorming with Curt.

"I enclose a letter about an interim IEP for 30 days' time at most. It should allow Ruffin to go to kindergarten and first grade library and recess *by next Tuesday* until we can find something appropriate. Miss Hobbs needs to call me ASAP."

I had written Miss Hobbs again, too, as the special education director for our district, in the most fruitless effort to be informative, businesslike, and conciliatory. This letter discussed the applicability of two particular *Iowa Rules of Special Education* to Ruffin's situation.

"First, Section 41.70(6) *Amending IEPs* clearly provides: 'An IEP cannot be amended without conducting an IEP meeting and following all requirements pertaining to an IEP meeting.' Thus, the recent Monday afternoon meeting with Mrs. Holub was not an appropriate occasion for proposing or signing an IEP amendment, nor was the IEP amendment issue noticed to me in advance as required by the IDEA.

"Second, Section 41.70(4) *Performance contract* provides that while the IEP carries no outcome guarantee, still 'the agency *must* provide special education and related services in accord with the IEP . . .' That is, the IEP doesn't guarantee, for example, that a given speech pathologist will succeed in teaching the child to speak, but the IEP *does* guarantee that speech pathology services will be provided in the amounts agreed upon, even if the speech pathologist is pregnant and ordered to bedrest or, Heaven forbid, is hit by a Mack truck, either of which circumstance would generate the administrative problem of quickly engaging a substitute, and then hiring a replacement.

"Ruffin's agreed-upon and signed IEP provides under the heading *Extent of Participation in Regular Education* . . . Dual programming with Head Start will be 180 minutes per week. Since school began six weeks ago, 18 hours of this agreed-upon regular education service has not been provided. Ruffin has lost something we all agreed he needed. Spending 18 hours in ECSE is not *Regular Education*, nor does it meet Ruffin's agreed-upon need for participation in *Regular Education*.

"I wrote to Mrs. Holub in the home-school notebook earlier, giving my permission as follows: 'Please send Ruffin to kindergarten and first grade library and recess on Thursday and Tuesday afternoons until Miss Hobbs can get back to me about the other options.' With my permission to do these things, it is incumbent upon the school to do them without further delay to avoid damaging Ruffin by confining him in a more restrictive environment than we have all agreed he needs.

"Certainly, we may agree to do so under Section 41.70(6) *Interim IEP*. While an IEP must ordinarily be in effect before special education can be provided, "this does not preclude the development of an *interim* IEP . . . when the IEP team determines that it is necessary to temporarily provide special education . . . as part of the evaluation process, before the IEP is finalized, to aid in determining the appropriate services for the individual.' A minimum IEP team for this interim integration issue is me and Ruffin's teacher, and she and I agree.

"So, Miss Hobbs, please do call me today with an update — whether you have good news or bad, best to get it delivered quickly — and get me directly involved in whatever you and anyone else may be working on."

Meg replied, "No time to write. Ruffin had a great time at Luther. Ran hard, played with balls and ropes. Have a great weekend." Elaine had dropped out of writing in our notebook. This latest dispute was just the sort of thing to scare the bejesus out of her.

Late in the afternoon, as Ruffin was working with Lisa, I got a call from Miss Hobbs, who asked if we could have an IEP meeting for Ruffin. Well, of course. We agreed on a day in October, after school. If I got there and all we had were tiny, wooden preschool chairs, I would not be sitting. I would be pacing around like a tiger.

CHAPTER FORTY

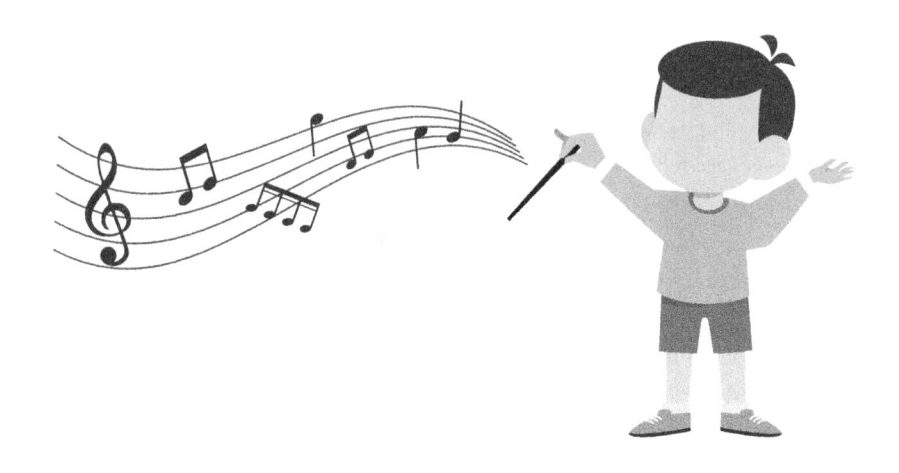

THE INCLUSION KERFUFFLE

My latest letter drew a response from the president of the private nursery school — addressed to Miss Hobbs but pointedly copied to me. "After our phone conversation on Friday, concerning your request for Ruffin White's further integration into our school, I wish to clarify some fallacies in Ms. White's letter."

At least her response provided some concrete information. And I needed to cut this mother with children in our local district some slack. It was not her fault that Miss Hobbs needed her little nursery school to fill in for the missing group from Head Start.

"Miss Hobbs, I'm sure you understand that we cannot, in good conscience, admit Ruffin to *another* preschool class, should an opening occur, without first offering that position to those that are currently on our waiting list. We feel that every child is special and unique, and our priority lies in meeting the needs of those who have been waiting patiently for any type of placement within our program.

"Ms. White assumes that our school would be 'unwilling' to accept Ruffin in other preschool classes and that 'by sharing information . . . about Ruffin's unique needs or sharing information about special education law' would make a difference in enrolling him in further of our classes. This is not true. Our enrollment is regulated by the state of Iowa based on the square footage of our facility — so many square feet per child depending upon the age of the child. We cannot deviate from our enrollment limits, or we will lose our license to operate.

"Also, Elaine Mills is rightly concerned that some of her comments about Ruffin's behavior have been misconstrued. In Ms. White's letter to you, she states that 'Mrs. Mills reported that Ruffin is a very attentive academic student . . . He responds spontaneously to topic, out of his acquired general knowledge (which, however, remains relatively shallow).' The phrase in parentheses is Ms. White's assessment, not Mrs. Mills'. Mrs. Mills has stated that Ruffin is ahead of the other children in the class in this area." Yes, I had written *with parentheses*, so it would be read exactly this way, as my own assessment based on the recent Gundersen reports — but maybe I had met my match here as a pettifogger. Now, I was not only a bad mommy, but also an unreliable reporter at best — a liar.

"Mrs. Mills also states that Ruffin's 'self-stimulatory' behavior of pulling his sleeves down over his hands causing 'hand-flapping' occurred only once. Although he did pull his sleeves down over his hands twice while waiting in line, it was noted by Mrs. Mills and her aide that other students of this age behave this way, too. The sentence, 'The danger is that this behavior can become habitual and can be noticed as "dumb" and "weird" by others,' is Ms. White's perception and not one noted by Mrs. Mills.

"The private nursery school board supports the qualifications and abilities of our teachers and aides. If asked by Mrs. Mills, I will be present at future meetings among Mrs. Holub, Mrs. Mills, and Ms. White so that any comments made by a teacher of our faculty will not be misinterpreted in future communications." Well, of course Mrs. Mills and the private nursery school administration should have been included in the IEP meeting for Ruffin back in August — if Miss Hobbs, as the local district's director of special education were offering their services to meet the district's legal obligations.

"In regard to Ms. White's desire for any reverse integration from our preschoolers, our school will not endorse this program. At the beginning of the school year, a class enrollment list went home with each student. If Ms. White wishes to contact these parents on her own, she may do so; but we ask that our school's name not be used."

All in all, I was grateful to have this letter as an educational record. Under FERPA, Miss Hobbs should have been fully documenting her phone calls with the private nursery school, but when I re-inspected Ruffin's file this letter was all the evidence there was of what, if anything, might have transpired.

In pressing a private nursery school for more special education services, Curt and I knew that we didn't have a legal leg to stand on. But Miss Hobbs was another matter entirely. And it didn't look like the private nursery school was going to step up and rescue her. As the hot potato he was, Ruffin had landed right back in Miss Hobbs's lap. A situation I had foreseen in August, during mediation negotiations, was staring us all in the face now. Where were we going to find all the *mainstream* placement Ruffin needed — and that had been promised him?

I took Ruffin to Sunday school where he listened attentively and colored his worksheet nearly within the lines. He also drew his own self-portrait with eyes, nose, mouth, hair, and body, arms with fingers and legs with toes.

That afternoon Evelyn met with Donna, Lisa, Meg, and me. Meg reported to Miss Hobbs. "The meeting was held at Ms. White's home to discuss Ruffin's progress and to make changes to his program as needed. I attended the part of the meeting which discussed how much direct drill time vs. shadow time for integration was needed for Ruffin.

"It is my view that Ruffin needs to interact as much as possible with other children to learn social skills and strategies. His program is set up to provide these opportunities. I stated that I felt he could benefit from having his therapist Donna do less direct drill and more integration shadowing to prompt attention and social learning. Evelyn Kung stated that Ruffin should have no more than 4 hours of drill a day and any other time should be integration shadowing. I left the meeting feeling that he would spend more time learning group dynamics than he had been. They then proceeded to discuss some specific drills they would implement and as I was not needed, I left." I appreciated that Meg took the time to attend a Sunday afternoon meeting and hoped Miss Hobbs paid her overtime.

Evelyn let the rest of us know Ruffin was ready for coloring books, activity books, including dot-to-dot, number-to-number work with crayons and markers. She suggested a guess-who game, and pretend play with airplanes, farm sets, and construction sets of more elaborate design, including micro-machines with motors and moving parts, K-Nex and anything else that might hold Ruffin's interest to help us elaborate his imaginative play.

CARD's bill for services to Ruffin for this visit was $108, which Miss Hobbs didn't or couldn't pay because the school board had so far failed to approve our mid-August mediation settlement. I needed to remind her, again, in mid-January to get this paid, when Dr. Granpeesheh's billing office dunned me.

Evelyn visited the private nursery school on Monday to observe Ruffin in Elaine's class of 16 students. It happened to be fire prevention week. As a careful and knowledgeable observer, Evelyn provided the first real report to me, and to Ruffin's IEP team, about how Ruffin — as a child still with some residual autism — was functioning there in an unaccommodated mainstream.

"1:30 PM to 2:45 PM: Free Play: Ruffin was playing with a couple of other children using a wooden toy airplane pretending that it was flying. I was delighted to see that he was initiating this play and displaying creativity as he had the toy plane land onto the back of a wooden flatbed toy truck.

"One of the children that Ruffin was playing with noticed that I had entered and came over to me. Ruffin saw me and appropriately responded with a 'Hi!' and walked over. He stood behind the other child and watched as the child asked my name and told me about his new hat on the shelf.

"The teacher then called out for all the children to clean up. Ruffin cleaned up all the toys that he was playing with and helped some of the other children.

"After this, he came over to me and immediately asked me what my name was using the phrase, 'What's your name?' This was an obvious imitation of what the other child had inquired of me. Ruffin's mom and therapists had told me that he did not ask other people their names spontaneously. I told him that he knew my name and he then laughed and told me my name.

"The teacher then called the children over to the carpet.

"Carpet Time: The teacher talked about what children should do if there were a fire at home using a reader with which they were familiar. She talked to them about what they should do if their clothes caught fire, pointing out that they should 'stop, drop, and roll.' It was very obvious that Ruffin did not understand these phrases as his attention was turned elsewhere.

"The teacher then told the class to get up and show what they were supposed to do. Ruffin was in the front of the line, and when the teacher told him to stop, drop and roll, he just stood there and looked at her with a blank face. Another child behind him immediately ran in front of him and performed these actions. As soon as Ruffin saw this other child, Ruffin imitated him.

"With Ruffin sitting on the carpet with his back to the teacher, she told the children that they should then go and seek a grown-up for help. As Ruffin turned around to face her, the teacher asked what they were supposed to do after they had stopped the fire on their clothing. The other children responded appropriately but Ruffin did not, as he had not heard the teacher when she had given the directions. His mother later also told me that she was not sure if Ruffin had understood the meaning of the word 'grown-up.'

"Ruffin then stood to the side and watched as the other children repeated the earlier stop, drop, and roll actions. After this, the children were directed to snack.

"Snack Time: Places for each of the children were set at a table. Ruffin went to the table; however he needed directions to find his name at the correct place.

"The teacher then showed the children the cereal that they would be receiving for snack. As she poured some into Ruffin's napkin, he pushed it away, while the other children began to eat. At this point I intervened, telling Ruffin that he only had to try it, and if he didn't like it, he didn't have to eat it. After some persuasion, Ruffin tried some, decided he liked it, and even asked for more after he had finished his portion.

"There were only a couple of other children at the table with him as the others were out sick for that day. I did not see either of these children interact with Ruffin at the table, however they did sit nicely at their places. The teacher later informed me that those other children did not speak very often. At the end of the snack, all the children were asked to throw their things away in the garbage can and return to the carpet to watch a video about fire safety.

"Fire Safety Video: Ruffin sat down in front of the other children and was very attentive to the video. Afterward, the children went back to their places at the table.

"Work in Readers: Ruffin opened his reader and was very interested in all the pictures that involved fire safety. The teacher began to tell the children what pages to look at, but Ruffin continued to look on his own. The teacher pointed out where she was in the book, and Ruffin turned to the appropriate page. He seemed to follow along well until they reached the part regarding what one was supposed to do if their clothing were to catch on fire. I then asked Ruffin what he was supposed to do, and he did not know, and looked at me. I then told Ruffin what to do. In three parts, as there were three actions, I explained to Ruffin and asked him questions to make sure that he understood. During this time, the other children were responding to the teacher's questions regarding this series of actions."

Miss Hobbs's written notice of Ruffin's upcoming IEP meeting arrived with its legally required list of prospective attendees: Miss Hobbs, Inge, Meg, Kim. And me. No one from the private nursery school was invited. And no one from Head Start either. So, the handwriting was on the chalkboard — maybe Miss Hobbs was going to offer some *mainstream inclusion* solution for Ruffin by working in-house on her own campus.

Meg reported that Tuesday, "Ruffin's play outside included thinking of new ways to play with the swings." That sounded ominously like Ruffin's earliest, concerning behaviors in the local park, when he had worked to set all the swings in motion so he could observe their relative and intersecting arcs, while ignoring all the other children around who wanted to swing together with him.

Meg warned me, too. "Mrs. Mills says there will be no early private nursery school dismissal on Wednesday, as we will have. You will need to pick Ruffin up then as our drivers will be all done by then. See you tomorrow later in the afternoon for our meeting."

With minor irritation, I noted that sluffing the transportation off onto me was another flagrant violation of Ruffin's IEP. Special education transportation was the responsibility of the school district. Hands down. What if I were scheduled into court? Or suddenly called in by a judge, as I often was, when he or she had a new criminal case to assign to me? Or had a regular 9:00 to 5:00 job, like most parents? This had been *why* Congress provided that schools had this responsibility.

Whatever, I thought. It wasn't worth bothering Curt. In the grand scheme of Ruffin's special education, it was a small matter, likely to recur all through the school year. As it did.

I sat down to sketch out some notes for the afternoon's IEP, about Ruffin's unique needs for language development: syntax, pragmatics, deeper development of his general knowledge, pretend play, and socialization.

Could we review all Meg's charting on Ruffin's IEP goals?

I wanted to raise the idea of Ruffin having a first-grade buddy and a kindergarten buddy for library and recess, to have Kim increase his speech therapy with children above his own speech developmental level, and to caution Kim not to interfere with Donna's time at school. If Kim couldn't manage to schedule around Donna, then Bridgewater could assign someone else to Ruffin's case.

We needed to tackle the EYSE issue for the summer of 1996, which had been left unaddressed in August. The IEP we agreed to in August had become, in my view, no longer reasonably calculated to work since Ruffin had lost so many weeks of Head Start integration, but I thought we could easily make that up this summer.

Having just learned Ruffin had an above-average IQ and was not mentally retarded, I wanted Ruffin removed as much as possible from the unnecessary "restrictiveness" of Meg's ECSE classroom and his exposure there to poor language and behavioral models.

Finally, I made copies of the August "hate mail" I had received. I was prepared to announce that I was not the least bit interested in getting any more of it.

Given my preparations, I was pleasantly surprised at how well the actual meeting went. Kim was a no show, as usual. Emily had not been invited and was not expected. Inge's face was an unreadable mask as I passed out the August "hate mail," and said my little set-piece.

We agreed to use the earlier August present levels of educational performance (PLEP) as still appropriate, but no one was prepared or willing to discuss summer programming (EYSE) or compensatory education for the many weeks of time with typically developing classmates that Ruffin had lost. I promised myself and Ruffin, silently, okay, later then.

Miss Hobbs's involvement in the process and her unexplained waving of some magic wand had somehow caused the Head Start group to reappear. I would never be offered an explanation for why they had refused to come earlier, or for why or how they chose to come back. I would like to have known how and why, but I didn't need to. I was prepared to focus on Ruffin's future.

Kindergarten shared reading, library, and the confusion of kindergarten lunch and recess with new, older classmates would present Ruffin with new challenges, but I imagined he might be ready for them, based on Evelyn's assessment of the sort of kindergarten academic activities she thought he was ready to tackle. And I knew Donna would be there to intervene quietly, if he needed help, or needed to have his attention redirected.

Now that we had at least an interim IEP for Ruffin's *integration* with typically developing boys and girls, Meg returned to writing freely in our home-school notebook. "Ruffin is playing fireman outside."

By the end of fire prevention week, Ruffin was doing a much better job of coloring within the lines on his fireman worksheet, focusing more on the hydrant in the drawing, and the hose in the fireman's hands, applying color to those objects with some care, while ignoring the human figure of the fireman. I might have been the only one who noticed.

Ruffin stayed home with a bad cough on Tuesday. On Wednesday, as Ruffin's cough improved, Donna and Lisa stepped in to babysit him while I drove up to Gundersen to review their written reports of Ruffin's most recent re-evaluation, and to have lunch with Dr. Porter who now led that group — to lobby him.

The documents I reviewed were dated October 4th. The first was addressed "To whom it may concern," and read: "The question has arisen whether or not Ruffin White's disability can be classified within the autistic spectrum. We feel that it can. His developmental disability significantly affects his verbal and nonverbal communication, as well as his social interaction. He is also characterized by some stereotyped movements, definite resistance to environmental change, and an inconsistent IQ profile. These problems are not due to an emotional disturbance on his part. Whether he is found to have Asperger's Syndrome or PDD, these all fall under the educational diagnosis of autism, and he deserves consideration for this disability as defined by the federal government." Every principal member of Ruffin's autism clinic team signed this prefatory statement: Debbie J. Olufs, M.A., Learning Disabilities Section; Irwin J. Ladd, M.D., Child and Adolescent Psychiatry; James Caldwell, M.D., Pediatric Neurology; Patricia A. Kondrick, Ph.D., Neuropsychology, and Mila Sokolov, M.S., Speech Pathology. Debbie Olufs had drafted this statement and gathered all the signatures.

I was pleased and planned to use this to ensure that Ruffin would be educationally categorized "AT" for Autism on all his special education census and financial-weighting paperwork. No more autism resource team (ART) member Dot Gordon or school psychologist Emily Knight or principal Miss Hobbs "un-diagnosing" Ruffin medically — or educationally.

Ruffin's IEP team met again in late October about how his interim IEP had been going. With the new Gundersen autism clinic endorsement that Ruffin was ready for kindergarten and integration, Miss Hobbs agreed to continue all the interim arrangements as a permanent amendment to Ruffin's IEP. Everyone initialed it, happily. Meg took me off the snack calendar since Ruffin would be snacking now with Head Start.

Of the 2,100 total minutes Ruffin was in school each week, he lost 2 hours per week of instructional time to transportation to get to the private nursery school on Monday, Wednesday, and Friday afternoons, leaving 1,980 minutes. Of those, he spent 1,140 minutes in various integration settings with typically developing boys and girls: nursery school, shared kindergarten reading, lunch, kindergarten library and recess, and Head Start, leaving only 840 minutes per week in Meg's ECSE classroom, where he worked with Donna 4 mornings a week on drills. On Friday he went to Luther College to swim or play in the gym with the multi-school group of disabled students.

At our meeting we were also able to discuss the high points of Ruffin's new Gundersen autism clinic evaluation. I asked Inge to have Bridgewater change Ruffin's disability category from NC (non-categorical) to AT (autism).

I reaffirmed my mid-August mediation agreement to change Ruffin's disability-severity weighting from 2.4 to 3.6 to raise the money available to the local district from $9,120 it had received last school year to $13,680 for this school year (a total of $22,800), so that, eventually, the $20,000 the school board needed to approve to reimburse me would net them $2,800 toward the fees the district had paid their attorneys.

I thought this came close to a win-win on the money, and my own advocacy goal of introducing Lovaas's methodology into the schools, but, of course, the matter of bruised feelings was another unaccountable matter entirely.

Ruffin was an absolute pistol that night. He pulled down his *Snow White* and *Little Mermaid* books and "read" each page to Rose and me, and then asked us to sing it back to him while he directed us with a Tinker toy stick. I was surprised at how much he remembered of the stories. He also *bragged* to Rose about going to kindergarten with "the big kids." He seemed very proud and eager to tell her all about it.

CHAPTER FORTY ONE

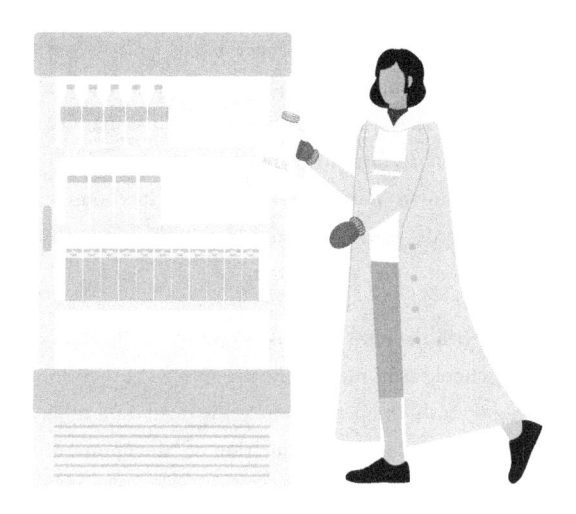

MY OWN WORST ENEMY

Ruffin was "afraid," he claimed, to go upstairs because of "monsters." When I asked what they looked like, he told me they had hair like spaghetti with all sorts of foods as body parts.

There are no monsters up there,
Except ones that you can eat
With hair that's like spaghetti
And meatballs for their feet!

He and I made that up to march him to bed by. Later, Meg sent me a song her class had been singing, one verse of which was:

And his hair was made of spaghetti,
Spaghetti, spaghetti,
And his hair was made of spaghetti.
And his name was Aiken Jones.

So, I let Meg know about our marching to bed at home, and this, too. "Ruffin said Mrs. Mills was there to talk to you. He can tell me quite a bit more about his school day now."

I was quietly pleased to find that Elaine Mills was passing out printed worksheets to color at nursery school and giving instructions on exactly how to color them, and that Ruffin had followed them. In his bookbag there gathered a veritable litter of other worksheets from kindergarten where Ruffin went with Donna. On these, he had traced broken lines learning how to form his printed letters correctly, circled pictures whose names began with a common, initial letter, and underlined simple sentences of mostly three-letter rhyming words, "cat," "sat," and "mat." The kindergarten teacher came to adore having Donna as an "aide" to her group.

Seamus arrived with the newspaper as always. At my kitchen counter, he read out the minutes of the school board meeting finally approving their mid-August mediation with me. On October 16th, in open session at the regular monthly meeting it had taken a scant three minutes to handle the question of "the approval of an agreement for student program cost."

All ayes, with no attorney present, the matter of Ruffin had been raised and resolved "authorizing the payment of $20,000 to the parent of a special education student for reimbursement of program expenses associated with providing a free public education, provided that the school district obtains from the parent all Lovaas reference materials, and home Lovaas program materials. We recognize the parent's contribution of materials to be used in the special education program."

Here in the smallest possible print, I had achieved my personal, advocacy goal. I had introduced Lovaas therapy into our local school. Now, the school wanted my entire autism library.

I chuckled to Seamus, "Yes, they want it out of my hands."

"I'm surprised," Seamus admitted. "This was not what I was expecting."

"Me, either" I said, and threw up my hands with mixed feelings of celebration and exasperation. I explained to Seamus that the condition that I turn over all my Lovaas materials to the district had not been part of our original mid-August deal, but that it suited me. I would just have the teenaged volunteers make me copies of all the materials that might be worth keeping for myself or might be worth sharing with others.

"Taking that much money from them is worse than you donating all that money last fall."

"Everything this year was supposed to remain confidential."

"People downtown are already talking. There and at the hay sale. I'm getting a lot of questions."

"Well, now you have some answers. It can't go on much longer. Ruffin is getting better. Every day . . . something new."

Whatever was new with Ruffin offered us a happier subject. When Ruffin arrived home on the bus, I offered Seamus our notebook. Meg had written, "Last week I checked Ruffin on a 12-piece puzzle, and he had a lot of trouble, so I had that as this week's IEP objective — but he fooled me! He will be working on a 100 piece one now as he does so well on 12 pieces.

"Mrs. Mills just stopped in yesterday to tell me the nursery school schedule this week. I passed her a copy of the Gundersen full evaluation report so I wouldn't have to send it over in Ruffin's backpack. I'm glad you have arrangements made to pick Ruffin up this week since Mrs. Mills said she loves having him and hoped he could stay the whole time for her class."

As I read over Seamus's shoulder, I thought to myself, subtle and unsubtle messages received. Meg and Seamus, both. Maybe. Who could ever be certain? I had learned to stay alert and remain doubtful.

Just as Ruffin and Lisa arrived from school the next day, so did the teenaged volunteers ready to hug Ruffin and chat with him for a few minutes before settling into their tasks. I dug Ruffin's book bag out from under their coats to find Meg had sent along a notice that our parent-teacher conference for Ruffin was scheduled for November 7th, right after school — when I'd promised Ray DeNeve I would be with his group in North Fayette. He had called earlier to introduce himself and asked me to attend an IEP meeting for one of the students whose teachers had trained with Evelyn. I assured him that I would.

But I had also decided I had paid about as much forward as I could afford to by working as an unpaid volunteer on these autism issues. It was no longer fair to Ruffin, or to me, to have our bank account threatened with being overdrawn while we waited months on end for reimbursement. Over the next week at the request of four different families I began to work as a legal advocate for their children. And it was time to put my efforts to advocate on a more businesslike footing. I was tired of being the only professional at the IEP table who was not being paid. If I were successful in improving programming, I told my clients, we would ask the schools to pay my fees.

Upstairs, Ruffin and I played a long, long game of pretend with a family of snakes represented by rubber belts from his Gear polis, a toy Evelyn had suggested he might enjoy. We broke the belts into a boy, a mother, a father, grandparents, sister, and brother and invented many activities and stories. Ruffin called this game "a story" and wanted to return to it "to finish the story." Usually, I played the boy, and had him play the mother. Whenever I was negative, resistant, and perseverative, Ruffin proved to be surprisingly resourceful in suggesting compromises, changes of mind, using a lot of techniques of persuasion, and re-direction, that he must have picked up from Donna, Lisa, Meg, Elaine, Seamus and me. I was delighted.

I let everyone know about this. "He is watching us all very closely. He cited a lot of 'rules' in his role as the mother: 'Kids obey grown-ups; grown-ups don't have to obey kids.' 'You have to eat if you want to grow big and strong.' He also offered up some original and sensible proposals of his own as I acted up. Our scenarios included eating, being sick, going to the haunted house (which we really did Saturday night — he wasn't scared a bit), discovering a fire, calling an ambulance, and getting ready to go visiting and shopping."

Honoring my earlier commitment to Ray, I added, "Meg, I need to see you for parent-teacher conference on some other day. I need to be out of town."

Ruffin worked with Donna using the school's computer and printer to make me a printed Halloween card, a house with jack-o-lanterns, a scarecrow, and a flight of bats, one crossing the moon, and inside, in orange crayon, Ruffin's drawing of himself, with a printed message, "Happy Halloween, from your little spook," signed across a background of tiny ghostly ghosts, "Ruffin," in his own handwriting.

The private nursery school class walked across town to parade through the kindergarten to show off their costumes and stay the afternoon to play games, and gorge on treats.

"He's come quite a way since last Halloween," I observed to Donna. She had chosen to stay the afternoon for the celebrations, and after Ruffin had thrown up, to bring him home. She thought it had been too much candy. At home, Ruffin threw up again, but didn't seem to have a fever, or want any rest. Donna and I laughed about the horror of last year, so long gone, as finally, she came out with the whole story of her first terrible trip to Walmart with Ruffin.

Meg had written, too, "Ruffin carried a verbal message to another classroom."

Over the first weekend in November, I marked the one-year anniversary of Ruffin's CARD program. How far we had come. His IQ gains were impressive and very much in line with what the academic peer-reviewed research showed could be expected as a good response to Lovaas programming. Ruffin's original Bayley Scale IQ in August 1994 had been 50. On the WPPSI-R:

Before CARD October 5th, 1994	After CARD September 25th, 1995	Change
Verbal 74	92	+18
Nonverbal 86	134	+48
IQ 78	112	+34

These IQ gains, and Ruffin's accompanying rapid acquisition of meaningful language were like those described by Catherine Lord and Andre Venter in *"Outcome and Follow-Up Studies of High-Functioning Autistic Individuals"* in the TEACCH volume, *High Functioning Individuals with Autism*, edited by Eric Schopler and Gary Mesibov (Plenum 1992), citing Lovaas's 1987 study, the first, brief mention I had noticed last summer of Lovaas.

How much help I had needed to reach out for and received. How grateful I was. And, how insistent I had needed to become.

And, what if? Those black thoughts, too, passed through my heart as well. Sadly, as observed by Lord and Venter, it did appear that "even the maintenance of relatively high preschool IQ depends heavily on the acquisition of language before age 6, otherwise IQ may fall into the mentally handicapped range in later childhood." I thought it was past time that educators seriously consider whether young children with autism were at risk for acquiring mental retardation if they were not given an intensive enough early intervention effective to help them securely acquire language or some equivalent form of common human communication.

What if I had trusted to the expertise of Bridgewater and its autism resource team (ART), or Ruffin's IEP team? What if I were not a rabid reader and researcher? What if I were not a writer? Or too timid to ever write what I learned, what I knew, what I thought, and what I was witnessing?

What if I were not a lawyer? What if I had represented myself? And Ruffin? What would have become of Ruffin? Or of other children of his generation like him? And of me, had I folded? I swore to myself, I would never fold until every child and family facing a new diagnosis had the information and access to the resources to step out and move loose in the universe if they chose, and if they dared.

Ruffin and I walked downtown to the barber shop Saturday afternoon. All the men who had been talking fell silent as we came through the door. No one asked what I was doing in the barber shop. No one dared ask what I was planning to do with $20,000 of good taxpayers' money. Let that struggle like a swallowed canary in everyone's throat,

I thought. I sat down and thumbed through an old swimsuit issue of *Sports Illustrated* while Ruffin had a haircut. I wanted him to look nice for the evening. Seamus and I were planning to take him out to a cavernous barn of a restaurant nearby, for a celebratory dinner. Before dessert, Seamus taught Ruffin how to play bar darts.

At Sunday school, Ruffin sat as still as a little angel, coloring like the devil, and teasing his favorite summer girlfriend. That afternoon he lay in my lap on the couch while we watched a nature show on monkeys. When it was over, he sat up suddenly, and confided by whispering in my ear that he really wanted a big ball with feet, like the one at the Luther College gym, for Christmas.

Seamus came back over to romp with Ruffin on the carpet. They were having so much fun Ruffin didn't get to bed until late that night. I didn't care. Who needed sleep then?

It was still the weekend. Our weekend.

Ruffin colored a cornucopia with foods pasted in it in nursery school and told me, "That's a cornucopia," and spun out a long story about a little girl with a nosebleed there who bled on the rug and whom Mrs. Mills had helped. It was okay, the little girl was able to stay in school.

This was the first week since school began that I was seeing the language and behavioral progress at the rate I had become accustomed to see last summer. The fall transition had been rough. Maybe things were finally swinging along. Then, due to parent-teacher conferences, school let out first one and then two hours early, and by Friday there was no school at all.

More of the paper began to shuffle to implement our mid-August mediation agreement as Thanksgiving vacation approached, over a month after the school board had voted its approval. Mr. Lord sent an early childhood placement agreement over to the private nursery school for Ruffin to continue to attend — where he had been attending since late August. Fortunately, Ruffin never experienced, nor caused any serious problems in Elaine's class under this special education agreement — not seen by me until my next FERPA inspection of Ruffin's files on Valentine's Day — after most of Elaine's class lay well behind us.

Caron wanted my signed release of any further liability on the part of Ruffin's educators. I spent time reading and flyspecking Caron's draft, found it good, signed it and walked a copy over to Mr. Lord, who was friendly and eager to have it in hand. He let me know he was acquainted with my client, the former superintendent out in western Iowa and the open meetings, public records, and contract termination litigation in which Mark Soldat and I represented him.

He expressed sympathy for our client and his predicament. "It was an impossible task for him to try to manage grade-sharing among four school districts. Consolidation is inevitable for the smaller, rural districts."

I acknowledged this. "Inevitability seems particularly hard to bend to for the one district populated by fairly hard-headed Century farmers, all those grandsons of German immigrants."

That got a chuckle out of him, then, as I handed over my sealed envelope.

Donna let me know she was uncomfortable at school. Meg and Miss Hobbs had invited her out socially, for drinks. Since she had turned down these invitations repeatedly, now she was feeling pressured. My appearances at IEP meetings as an advocate for other families wasn't making her work at school any easier either. Donna wanted me to know how she felt. "How so many women can be so unhappy and catty when Ruffin is making great progress really beats me!"

But now Meg had confided, "Ruffin had library and two recesses with kindergarten. Yesterday, one of the teachers was sick, so he stayed here — Donna used that time for extra drills." No problem. I thought we were finally rocking and rolling in good faith on giving Ruffin what he needed as his special education according to his IEP.

Then, there were little red flags and irritations. They irritated me anyway. In December Bridgewater scheduled a meeting about autism without inviting any parents, so Ruth and I agreed to crash it.

Ruth and I drove south into the next county. We met up in person with parent-educator Gay Doyle, and Ray DeNeve from Bridgewater. Although we had crashed his party, Ray turned out to be a peach of a guy, and this meeting was a positive experience which left Ruth and me feeling hopeful. He had invited all the local district superintendents and principals from his southern sector. The Lovaas topic was addressed by two experienced preschool teachers, Gay, and a psychology student at Mt. Mercy College who had been trained by Dr. Tristram Smith.

Our home-school-school notebook had lapsed into disuse. I was writing to myself. I wanted to see some daily individual report about Ruffin at nursery school. "I hear *nothing* in this notebook from Elaine. Meg, can you follow-up on this for me please?" At least I had Donna with eyes-on Ruffin, and Ruffin himself now to talk to.

Finally, I was able to spend an hour at the gym on weekends. There, Ruffin busied himself without requiring my close attention. He introduced himself to another, older child, and invited her to play with a ball he had asked the adult attendant to get for him out of a locked closet. Then, at his new, shy friend's whispered request, he approached the adult attendant again — to ask for and get a second ball.

By mid-December, Meg's lesson plan was Christmas, without any more community objection to that religious theme than there would have been in the 1950s of my own southern childhood. Ruffin ran late getting dressed. I realized we had missed the bus and drove him into school where he was marked "Tardy."

Then, I scurried off to court so as not to be late myself.

We lost another school day to teacher in-service. Donna and Lisa worked with Ruffin at home. Ray ran the paperwork to reimburse my late October mileage picking up Evelyn and ferrying her around his North Fayette district and eventually down to Moline, where there was a small airport. Being Evelyn's driver gave me a welcome opportunity to pick her brain.

No school, again, for the same reason. Donna and Lisa were working overtime while I went over to the courthouse for a day of juvenile court appearances. From Des Moines, Curt prompted Caron. "Please have your clients make out the settlement check to Mary Jane White and Iowa Protection & Advocacy Services, Inc."

Meg resumed writing in Ruffin's notebook. "Ruffin played great outside with kindergarten to second grade recess, and Head Start was here. Donna said he had a great lunch. Elaine says the kids ask for Ruffin when he isn't there yet." Ruffin was always a little late to Elaine's class after eating lunch with kindergarten and catching his bus to ride the few blocks across town.

School bus transportation remained very inflexible and unable to respond to the differing schedules of Ruffin's public and private preschools. With so many recent schedule upsets Lisa was having some problems with Ruffin settling into his afternoon drill sessions. When he did, he was learning well.

The next day, I needed to write to Meg. "We have a safety problem with the bus. Ruffin has grown and in his winter boots when he sits on the seat, his feet stick out and his legs don't bend at the knees. The seat is too deep. His feet are jammed against the seat back ahead of him. A quick stop of the bus would break his ankles or legs. Please observe Ruffin in his bus seat and ask Miss Hobbs to have the bus garage provide a safe way for Ruffin to get to school." Meg sent me a student transportation form to be completed for all special education students, upon which I could convey my concerns. Until we got this matter attended to, Lisa picked Ruffin up from school.

Ruffin developed a bad cold and was too sick to send to school the last couple of days before Christmas break. Donna and Lisa kept him busy at home with CARD drills, and Seamus and I were able to spend time with him together until early January of the New Year, 1996.

Elaine sent a postcard to Ruffin over Christmas. He found it exciting, as the first mail that had come to him from someone other than family. I was always getting lots of mail, and he had yet to have *any*. "Read it to me, Mom." So, I squatted down beside him, and read, moving my finger along each line. "Thank you. The jack straws were delicious! I hope you had a nice Christmas. See you in January! Mrs. Mills."

The matter of Ruffin's safety on the school bus had yet to be resolved, but here was another form from Meg that might do the trick, so I filled it out and sent it in. Next Monday, the bus driver tried a kangaroo seat for Ruffin — his own idea.

When I said that didn't look very safe either, he threw his hands up and confessed he had told Joe, the head of transportation, earlier, that the seating for Ruffin was too big — not the right size. Joe had told him, "One size fits all."

The driver still hoped to persuade me to accept the kangaroo seat, and argued, "Besides, I never go more than twenty-five miles per hour in town."

I'm afraid I replied, sharply, with what I thought was obvious, "*Someone else* could hit you, you know, going fifty miles per hour."

Then, I called Joe, in high dungeon.

By mid-morning Ruffin had been switched to a new bus with several more inches of leg room.

As school moved back into the swing of things, Elaine offered a suggestion to foster recall and discussion with Ruffin. "*Charlotte's Web* is a chapter book. Ruffin may be ready for this — read a chapter a night. He will need to discuss and remember what has gone before to be ready for the next chapter." While Lisa worked upstairs with Ruffin, I was out the door and around the corner to the public library to check out E.B. White's wonderful book so we could begin reading it that night.

We were due to have another visit from Evelyn in mid-January.

Curt called. A $20,000 check from the district had arrived, but he didn't have a check yet from Bridgewater. Caron was busy working on a brief, but he would have her call Mr. Carew to get their money moving our direction.

Elaine had written to explain, "I cannot meet with Evelyn on Sunday — I'm taking my daughter to college where she will start as a freshman at Iowa." I understood. This was once in a lifetime for Elaine — and something I still hoped to be able to do one day with Ruffin.

I alerted Miss Hobbs to Elaine's conflict, suggesting a solution. "If Elaine is not available during Evelyn's visit, I'd be willing to accept a one-hour telephone conference consultation time with Evelyn, Elaine, Meg, Donna, and me as an acceptable alternative way of completing the quarterly consultation we agreed to at mediation."

Time to begin looking at kindergarten class sizes. The ones at St. Pat's were 14 to 15 students. The ones on Miss Hobbs's campus were a third or a half again as large. I wanted to observe individual kindergarten teachers this spring, at or before the early February kindergarten round-up.

Principal Peter Smith at St. Pat's and I visited about his two kindergarten classes. Based on what he had seen of Ruffin on his campus at nursery school, he assured me Ruffin would be welcome to attend St. Pat's kindergarten next year.

I called Miss Hobbs to follow-up about getting Elaine and Evelyn together. I shared what I had learned about St Pat's. She didn't seem pleased, seemed really upset and let me know she expected to have four kindergarten classes next year, each with 18 to 26 students, depending on enrollment. Her preschool classes were designed to be smaller. This year, her smallest kindergarten class had 22 students. It failed to cross my mind that by sending Ruffin to St. Pat's for kindergarten I might be robbing her public school of Ruffin's $13,680 of state dollars of special education funding — not that Miss Hobbs brought it up, but it could have been a specter in the background.

Blind to Miss Hobbs's problems, and blissfully, I reported to Curt and Joan, "These are just a small sample of the letters which have poured in recently concerning *Judicial and ALJ Interpretations of the FAPE Requirement for Preschool Children with Autism* since I last reported to Joan in late October. As you can see, many parent-attorneys are requesting your booklet from Arkansas, several from New York, Michigan, Massachusetts, and Wisconsin. It is also encouraging to see that organizations, libraries, universities, school districts, state departments of education, and HMOs are also requesting your information as a resource.

"In addition to the one settlement from Arkansas, I am also aware of the following settlements and decisions: Michigan: $27,000 reimbursement settlement for one year's Lovaas; Washington: $60,000 reimbursement from ALJ due process proceedings for one year's Lovaas for a set of twins; New York: $10,000 reimbursement; New York: family in the middle of due process; California: Ralph and Sherrie Lewis (both parents are attorneys) reached a confidential settlement for full reimbursement in mid-hearing at due process; California: another family is in the middle of due process.

"Many of the parents have made incidental comments in their letters about how well their children are doing with Lovaas programs, and about the difficulties they have experienced with their school districts. I hope this information will be helpful to you in preparing your annual report."

Ruffin's play continued to improve at home. Our weekend's puppet play became much richer, more elaborate than our earliest play with kangaroos. That Christmas, Ruffin had gotten small, stuffed Pooh, Piglet, Eeyore, and Tigger from his Aunt Susan. He knew these characters from books and videos and applied their names properly, identifying them rightly as the animals they were.

There had been a period when he played with animal figures but refused to give them individual names. Now he named all sorts of figures and the names given were remembered, and old scenarios developed into new ones — he was not bound to routine. He and I played up to three-quarters of an hour in long multi-episode pretend play with the new Pooh group — using their correct emotional attributes — Pooh was kind; Eeyore was gloomy and spoke slowly, with a low pitch and sadly; Piglet was squeaky and afraid, and Tigger bounced around with the greatest hyperactivity.

Ruffin played out entire scenarios of stories we had read, with flexible elaborations. As an example, Tigger was included in Eeyore's birthday and needed to bring a second balloon. We didn't have a Rabbit figure, but Ruffin picked up a nearby dinosaur and speaking in an aside from our scenario informed me the dinosaur would be Rabbit, but "just pretend."

Ruffin was also reading words in Dr. Seuss books and on our *Scrabble* board, and from television — the *Nickelodeon* logo and *Snick/Snack*. While watching a show on *Nickelodeon* with exaggerated plot deceptions — a girl bitten by a chameleon was turned into one secretly from her other family members — Ruffin turned to ask me for this confirmation, "They don't know she's the chameleon really?" I thought this was terrific theory of mind stuff.

The temperature was beginning to plummet the second week in January from a noon high below freezing toward a predicted low in the near single digits. Everyone was hurrying to get home by the time school let out. Ruffin was home on his new bus, ready for a hug, a snack and to work with Lisa. Lisa had just finished her session with Ruffin when I huffed my way in the door from the Post Office and spoke briefly to her in passing.

Once Lisa had left, Ruffin was usually ready to tell me all sorts of little stories about what had happened at school. But that day he didn't really seem to want to talk much. Suddenly he just seemed very tired after a long day of resuming his full school and therapy schedule. He fell into a sound sleep in the late afternoon after a brief tantrum, the first in a long while.

Then, as I opened the refrigerator I saw we were out of milk. I would need milk for his vitamin dose in the morning. How could I have let myself run out of milk? I woke Ruffin to dress him as warmly as would be necessary to drag him back out into the cold. The wind I had come in from wouldn't do his ears any favors. He'd already missed several days of school just before Christmas, and again after Christmas with snow days and in-services.

Ruffin didn't want to get up. He didn't want to go anywhere. He didn't want to get dressed. He didn't want to go back out. So, I made the worst mistake, the most consequential mistake, I had made so far as Ruffin's mother, a single mother's classic mistake. I tried to call Seamus, who was out with his animals, and did not answer. I didn't want to bother Donna, who was home at dinner with her family. Rose was still visiting extended family in North Dakota. I asked Ruffin if he would be okay, alone. He said, "Yes," but wouldn't look at me. Now, he was concentrated on building something with his Legos.

I slipped down the street to pick up a gallon of milk. Usually, grocery shopping represented a blissful errand for me to be savored alone, wandering the aisles, buying on impulse. I felt the tug of that oblivion briefly, walking through the grocery to where the milk stood like solid bricks of snow in a case against the far back wall. I hooked one with my mitten and headed directly back to check out.

Waiting in line, I overheard a terrible story told by the woman ahead of me about a 5-year-old who had fallen asleep on the school bus that morning. The child had spent the long school day locked on the bus, parked in the unheated bus barn, wetting himself with no access to a bathroom. When he was discovered at the end of the day, he had been simply returned to his home in that condition with no explanation.

As I arrived home with the milk, Ruffin was still playing quietly on the carpet with his Legos. He looked up to tell me, "The phone rang. I talked." But he couldn't tell me who he had talked to, or whether there was any message he had been given. I looked down at him and smiled. I praised him. At the moment, I was pleased he had been able to answer the telephone and talk to a person he had no way of seeing.

The next day, I thanked Meg, "Ruffin *loves* his new bus with two friends and Renee — it seems much safer." Then Gay Doyle called from Bridgewater. She had talked to Ruffin on the phone the day before, just before she was leaving work. "He was delightful. Did he tell you?"

"Yes," I said, "but not exactly what I can do for you?" as I thought to myself, mystery solved.

Later, that afternoon, I told Donna and Lisa the terrible story I had overheard waiting in line at the grocery, and about Ruffin answering the phone, and thought nothing more of it than I had passed along something else Ruffin had learned to do. We had been trying to teach him how to dial 911, how to call a fireman, or the doctor. It had seemed the next thing we needed to do.

That night, I picked up Catherine's book again, as I often did. She had written something about her daughter I thought I remembered. I found the right page, and re-read the sweet passage, "On August 30th, 1988, Anne-Marie invited me into a game with her. She picked up a toy phone, walked across the room, extended the receiver toward me, and said: 'Here. You. Me.'"

The next day, although the temperature had climbed above freezing, Ruffin came down with yet another cold and was absent from school the rest of the week. He slept in and busied himself on the computer until Donna arrived each morning and Lisa then each afternoon.

CHAPTER FORTY TWO

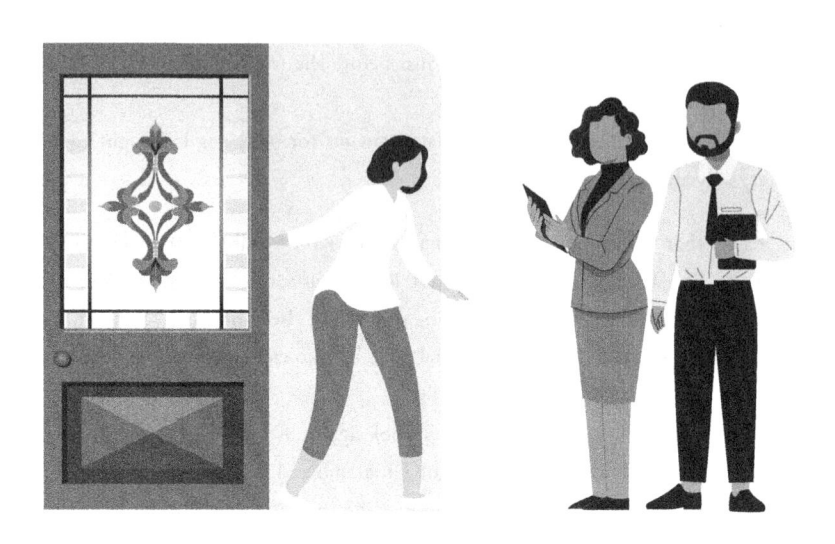

THE LESSONS OF EAVESDROPPING

Evelyn returned to update Ruffin's drill book that Sunday. Our home team planned for Donna to observe Ruffin at the private nursery school. We discussed whether Ruffin should attend kindergarten at St. Pat's or stay in public school with the kindergarten teacher there, who was familiar with him, in a special 15-child class where she would have the help of an aide. Evelyn thought this was the size class Ruffin would need, and Donna agreed it would be ideal. I was sure Miss Hobbs would not be willing to adjust her kindergarten class sizes. I had broached the idea with her, and she had already said to me, "I won't adjust class sizes."

The check for my reimbursement was still sitting on Caron's desk somewhere in Waterloo. I didn't have it yet. Evelyn said the district had not paid CARD yet, either, handing me another copy of their overdue bill. I promised her I would see to it.

Meg arrived, and then, as we turned to Evelyn's latest ideas for Ruffin, my doorbell rang again. Miss Hobbs and an older man were there, stomping snow off their boots and smiling. "Come on in," I uttered in surprise, as I took the man's extended hand, offered with his self-introduction, "Charlie Johnson, superintendent, Turkey Valley," and shook it.

"I can't stay long, but I'd like to sit in for a little bit."

Evelyn explained to our now-larger group it would be easiest for Ruffin to learn to take directions addressed to a group in a *physical* setting, playing soccer or T-ball. These activities would help him learn to listen to the teacher and copy the responses of the other children before generalizing this skill to listening to group directions in a classroom to perform academic tasks while seated. We could try using a token system to reward Ruffin's attention by letting him earn ten stars to trade for a treat. At her house, Lisa had been offering Ruffin stickers to eat more and different foods, and he had worked very hard to earn a clean plate "bear."

An especially good idea Evelyn offered was to use a *remnant book* to address Ruffin's difficulty in recalling past events. We would save physical souvenirs of events outside Ruffin's ordinary routine to help remind him of those events so he could answer questions about them or recount those events to those of us who had not been present. She explained this practice well for us in her written report to Ruffin's educators because they would need to help us in this effort.

Evelyn thought Meg was right on target by having Ruffin carry messages between classrooms and to the school office. That would be an appropriate memory exercise for him at this time.

Superintendent Johnson needed to leave, and as he was stepping out the door, here came the president of the private nursery school board, waltzing up the steps to my porch. I introduced the two of them, who nodded to each other, as the president told me she would be sitting in today for Elaine.

Once we were settled again, in our musical chairs, I said I was concerned Ruffin seemed to know only 4 of the names of his 16 nursery school classmates. Evelyn suggested inviting those classmates whom Ruffin could name over on the weekends. They were the most likely to be or to become his friends. She suggested Ruffin was ready to begin planning a party for the enjoyment of others — considering what types of games this or that friend of his might like to play. We should have him plan what to say to each person and think through how each person he invited might have a good time. We would need to formalize Ruffin's social approaches to others using memorization of some statements about his feelings, using mental sentences of rehearsal, and giving Ruffin direct permission and encouragement to express social feelings.

We would also need to begin asking Ruffin to describe to us what he heard. We needed to teach and encourage eavesdropping. It would be important to try to get him to ask more 'Wh' questions. And to teach him the meaning of a feeling and the word for it: "confused." And then hold back a bit on our help and let him use "I'm confused" to approach his classmates and others for information.

My raising the issue again of adjusting Ruffin's kindergarten class size resulted in Miss Hobbs producing a tape recorder, and sufficient interpersonal tension to put a quick end to our meeting.

Meg's later notes to Ruffin's file showed she had read and carefully marked Evelyn's report. Ruffin still had trouble following directions addressed to him individually. Meg agreed that he needed more memory drills. As a new behavior, she noted that Ruffin would share on request and sometimes offered gifts. His language ability had increased, including his ability to answer questions, to talk to others, both classmates and adults. There were lots of requests about his own needs and wants.

This last observation of Meg's was interesting to me when I came across it. In my earliest reading about autism, I had found several academic studies about children with autism who had developed speech. Those researchers had carefully counted and characterized the types and frequencies of these children's utterances and consistently reported a greater instance of "requests about their own needs and wants" and a paucity of those utterances designed for the social sharing of information, of remarks directing the joint attention of one's conversational partner to something interesting or amusing.

Being continually on the receiving end of lots of requests could be tiring, more than a bit wearing on any relationship. Had I recalled it at the time, I might have made a note to myself. Just as I imagined that most of my requests on Ruffin's behalf were welcome, and were being met, our shotgun marriage — between Ruffin's educators and myself — was about to hit the rocks — largely because of my own unforgivable error, my earlier lapse in judgment to have left Ruffin home alone while I ran to the store for milk.

No school next Monday to allow for a day-long meeting for teacher in-service. The private nursery school didn't hold class either. Since Monday was my busy legal morning, the only day we had a judge available in town to hear motions and pass sentences, Donna came over to work with Ruffin. He didn't need any more interruptions to his schedule.

After court, I decided to walk Evelyn's bill into school, and bring it to Miss Hobbs's personal attention. Rita, the office secretary, told me Miss Hobbs was still busy, meeting with all her teachers. I left Evelyn's bill with her and asked that she pass it to Miss Hobbs to see that it got paid.

"Please," I said, as I passed it over the little shelf that protected her from distracting eye contact from everyone passing in and out of the office to pick up mail and flyers from a wall of small, stuffed wooden slots.

"I don't know anything about it," said Rita.

"I know. It's about Ruffin and Renee's special education," I explained, smiling. "Just pass it along to Miss Hobbs. She knows all about it."

"I can do that."

"Thank you. I appreciate it,' I said, smiling again, thinking to myself, reinforcement, reinforcement, everyone in the world needs reinforcement.

And, of course, everyone who is fully human feels the need to share. I had shared with Donna and Lisa all about Ruffin having answered the phone in my absence. Donna had shared that with Meg. Now, a week later, sometime during this morning's in-service, Meg shared it with Miss Hobbs: I had left Ruffin home alone recently. Had Donna also shared that I knew all about that terrible story about the 5-year-old who had been locked in the bus?

By that afternoon, Miss Hobbs was on the phone to Donna, asking a lot of pointed questions and explaining it was Donna's duty as a person working at her school to make a child abuse report. Miss Hobbs explained the ins-and-outs of Donna being a mandatory child abuse reporter. "Why, they had been training on that very subject this morning. I don't expect you to know, but . . ."

Donna knew all about the ins-and-outs of reporting child abuse. Donna and I had passed once earlier in our lives, like ships in the night — years before we ever met and became friends.

It was my own first year of law practice, more than a decade and a half earlier. I had been invited by one of the most experienced of our trial court judges to attend an upcoming first-degree murder trial, a rarity in our thinly populated rural jurisdiction. Judge Keefe thought I might find it instructive. He would approach both the specially assigned prosecutor travelling in from Des Moines and the local defense team whom I knew. If they all agreed, I would watch the entire trial, beginning to end, and circulate freely between both camps as they discussed trial strategies, prepared their witnesses, and responded to unexpected setbacks. This would offer me a unique insight into whatever might happen next, before him and the jury in open court. I would need to respect confidentiality — strictly — here he raised an admonitory finger — and not share with anyone whatever I might overhear.

"Do you understand? No passing any information. And I don't want to hear any of it."

"I understand," I said, amazed and grateful for this rare opportunity.

"When nothing else is going on, you come sit back here in chambers, with me. I'll talk to you about what I am seeing and thinking, and why I will be making any rulings on the evidence and on any of the motions that have been argued to me at the bench. I can't let you approach the bench with counsel for those arguments. It might cause undue curiosity in the jury and bring on complications."

"I understand."

"But you won't miss much," he chuckled. "And if you do, I'll catch you up on it back here in chambers."

The trial I had watched then so intimately had involved the murder of a toddler by her mother's boyfriend. Donna had been the little girl's regular babysitter. As a young mother herself, just out of her teens, she had reported her suspicions of child abuse repeatedly. Although the mother, boyfriend, and little girl had been placed under a social worker's regular supervision, Donna had been persistent and insistent in reporting the child's newest bruising and injuries.

I was drawn into Donna's testimony, as she spoke clearly of her concerns and to everyone's failure to protect this child she had cared for a great deal. She was unshakable on cross-examination and obviously furious with the whole system.

Years later, as our paths crossed again, Donna and I discovered we had both participated in this notorious trial — which had resulted in the conviction of the boyfriend — and we frequently returned to discussion of it since I had been able to attend the whole trial, something that Donna, as a trial witness, had not been permitted to do.

Donna continued to harbor strong feelings about the matter. She felt the child's mother, her friend, should also have been prosecuted — for something. The point was: Donna didn't need any great instruction from Miss Hobbs on how to pick up the phone and report child abuse. As a young mother, she had done it when she had seen it as necessary to try to protect a child she cared about. She didn't need to be a mandatory child abuse reporter to do it.

Miss Hobbs insisted Donna report Ruffin's home alone incident immediately. As Ruffin's principal. Of Ruffin's school. Where Donna worked under her supervision.

Then, the local head of the Department of Human Services reinforced the same obligation to Donna over the phone.

Donna called me right away that afternoon while Lisa and Ruffin were working upstairs, to give me a heads-up. She didn't have any choice but to report. And she was furious with me.

"What were you thinking? Leaving him alone for a single minute?"

"It was wrong," I admitted.

"Anything could have happened," Donna said.

"And I would never have forgiven myself." It was true. I couldn't deny it. Not to Donna. And not to whomever came to the door to investigate.

"It was wrong," Donna agreed. "I know you love him, and I know you are anxious he never skip his vitamins, but, really, anything could have happened. Thank goodness, nothing did."

"I know, but it's not a matter of no harm, no foul."

"No," said Donna. "This is about being a mother. And you tell me, why can't Seamus bring you milk, as often as he visits? He should be doing that, but he'll never do anything for you and Ruffin unless you stand up to him and insist on it." She was righteously furious with me, and with Seamus, and what she said cut to the quick.

Donna was furious, too, to have been caught up in Miss Hobbs's and my mutual ill-will. Our prickly relationship was not good for Ruffin in any way.

"She's not all that hard to get along with. You could do it for Ruffin. It's not like she's pestering *you* to come have a drink at the country club."

"Is she still doing that? I'm sorry. I'm sorry this is happening to you. I know you need to do what you need to do. You do, too. And don't worry about it. It will be whatever it is. I'll need to admit it, and just deal with whatever the consequences are. You know I would jump in front of a moving train for Ruffin. Best to just get it done, without waiting."

"Yeah, well, I've already done it. Miss Hobbs had Meg report it, too. I just thought it was only fair to let you know someone will be coming to your door."

"You did the right thing. I know, like you did before," thinking back to that terrible child murder trial. "Thank you."

I couldn't imagine Meg had enjoyed her day off teaching, having a nice relaxing day of in-service. I didn't even imagine Miss Hobbs found leaning on Meg or making her phone call to Donna had been pleasant matters to attend to, not with everything else that was going on at school.

That winter the school board, staff, and community were beginning to hold a series of contentious public meetings to consider moving from a Jr. High concept to a modern middle school concept. This would move the sixth grade out of Miss Hobbs's elementary school building, and then the matter of who might serve as the middle school principal would be up for discussion.

With the district's exceptionally strong financial position relative to our neighboring districts, with an arbitrator's recent order to raise every single teacher's salary, the paper was abuzz with letters to the editor concerning our town's crumbling public school infrastructure. Why had it not been maintained? There were extended technical discussions by outraged farmers about the foundation of the Jr. High building, cracked and mis-repaired after a fire that had burned the old, adjacent high school to the ground a decade ago. The foundation had been rumored to be irreparable, but now Mr. Lord had an expensive engineering report he was standing up and slapping in his hand at meetings, confirming the whole building was dangerously unstable.

County property taxpayers could see it coming and didn't much like it. The district would be calling for the passage of a bond issue. It was just a matter of time. Seamus, for one, was following all these developments with a certain relish, predicting the farmers out in the country — even with the latest property tax relief on their agricultural land — were not going to be happy about voting to build a new school. Not when they all knew well enough how to hold their own buildings and machinery together through good times and bad with duct tape and baling wire.

With that behind us, finally, I was able to tell Seamus what I thought was coming — a DHS investigator within a day or so — to my door.

"Just keep me out of it. You always think you are so smart, so, you'll need to think of some way out of it. You'd be a whole lot smarter if you read the paper."

"And you could bring milk. With Ruffin, there is never enough milk."

That led to a fruitless argument that left me feeling abandoned and stupid. I had known when I moved into this town to be nearer Seamus, that in the 1990s it was mostly a throw-back to the 1950s. Most grandchildren lived within a stone's throw of both their grandmothers and within a tight circle of dozens of aunts, uncles, and cousins. Everybody in town ate home-cooked food, at home. I hadn't chosen to live in a diverse neighborhood with take-out or, even a sit-down restaurant beyond our take-out pizza and meeting room across the street. I had retreated to this place, without so much as a McDonalds for hot, fast food. Or morning milk delivery. What was I thinking? I wasn't thinking.

In our hilly river county, none of the men carried a cell phone yet in a little tooled-leather holster for someone at home to be able to call and ask, or remind them, to stop on the way home and pick up some milk or whatever. This was all my fault, all of it — the whole sorry situation, with Seamus, and I needed to think of something by myself and soon before the next day and the child abuse investigator came knocking.

So, I began to clean the house. Thoroughly and furiously.

I kept Ruffin home from school on Tuesday in our beautifully clean house. He was still sick that morning. I made myself some strong coffee and took Seamus's stupid advice and read the paper he had left behind as he had stormed out.

I turned straight to the letters to the editor page to put my finger on the pulse of the community. The paper had printed a long letter about the boy left on the bus submitted by his aunt who lived safely out of state. "This could have been a very tragic day."

Ruffin seemed better by the middle of the afternoon, so I took him over to Lisa's where she wanted to work with him. She would drop him back home when they were finished. I went home to wait for someone to come to the door.

I had just missed the investigator who had made an "unannounced home visit but found no one home." He called a bit later and found my line busy. Yes, I was trying to work. My phone rang immediately as I put it down late in the afternoon. It was the investigator. I recognized his voice as someone I knew, Charlie Coffey. I had worked with him often in juvenile court. We made immediate arrangements for him to come for a home visit.

Charlie walked in and told me that mid-afternoon last Monday "an informant" had called his supervisor, the head of the regional office. I knew her and had often worked with her too. According to Charlie, the informant alleged I had left my 4-year-old son alone without adequate supervision, that Ruffin had autism and was not capable of self-supervision while I went to the store to get milk. He was here to investigate that allegation as a "denial of critical care."

I understood and told him the allegation was true.

He had checked for my name in the central registry and there were "no prior founded or undetermined reports on record."

I understood that was a good result. As an admitted offender, at least I was no more than a "first offender."

Charlie asked if Ruffin was home.

I explained, "Ruffin is in therapy. I expect him home soon."

Charlie asked me why I had thought it was safe to leave Ruffin home unsupervised.

I admitted, "It was wrong. I wouldn't do it again. I think Ruffin knows 911. We are teaching him. Or he would know to go to a neighbor if there were a problem." But I wasn't sure.

As I spoke, I was thinking of a recent incident when Ruffin's bus had dropped him off at Lisa's after school had closed early due to a blizzard. This was where he usually went for his afternoon therapy right after nursery school. Lisa hadn't been home, but her door, like most household doors in our town, had been unlocked when Ruffin tried it, and walked in out of the blowing snow. Fortunately, Lisa's children had walked home from school and in the door within a few minutes of Ruffin's arrival.

I explained to Charlie how Ruffin received megavitamin treatment along with his therapy. The vitamin mixture was bitter, and Ruffin would not take it unless it was mixed with chocolate milk. I needed milk to mix with Ruffin's vitamins so he would take them. I described his behaviors when he missed a dose.

I must not have been communicating clearly, because Charlie didn't fully understand what I was talking about. He got the mistaken impression that Ruffin's medication was something to prevent seizures, since that's what he said in his report.

I told him I made a phone call to try to get someone to stay with Ruffin, but I couldn't reach that person. I remembered the weather was awful at the time and told Charlie I didn't want to take Ruffin outside into it, but I didn't want him to miss his medication either.

"What I chose to do was wrong. I asked Ruffin, before I left, if he would be all right if I went to get some milk. He said, 'Yes,' and I imagined he would be fine. I was gone for all of five minutes. I went up Main Street and came right back with the milk we needed."

Charlie asked to see Ruffin's medication, so I got up and brought it in to him. He examined it closely and described it in his report. "The supplement contained approximately the same type and amount of a normal supplement except for a large increase in the amount of B6 present. The supplement was a powder and was, according to Ms. White, recommended by the leading authority on autism. She advised Ruffin's program of therapy was now duplicated by about 20 children in Iowa."

I told Charlie I thought Ruffin knew 911. It was part of what we were trying to teach him at the time. "But this is my fault, for not making more calls before leaving. This occurred one time. It won't happen again, believe me."

I was fairly sure Charlie believed that much, anyway. He went on to ask me if there were any other problems with Ruffin, or whether I thought I had any need for services that might be provided through the Department.

I knew what he was talking about, and told him, "No, I don't think so."

Then he asked me who Ruffin's father was.

I told him, "No one is listed on Ruffin's birth certificate," which was true then, and handed it to him.

"Do you need a copy?"

"No, that takes care of it."

I was relieved we had gotten past that, since Seamus had already made it clear he was not eager to be dragged into court, nor willing to take Ruffin into temporary protective custody as a relative.

I was able to relax a little and began to talk with Charlie about the progress Ruffin had made with the megavitamin supplement and through therapy. I pulled out Ruffin's paperwork that showed his IQ had gone up from 50 to 112 between the testing dates of August 1994 and September 1995. I explained that Bridgewater had done the first test, while Gundersen had done the latest one. I explained how there remained a large difference between his verbal and non-verbal IQ scores. Charlie was familiar with some of these tests himself. He understood what I was talking about when I mentioned "three standard deviations."

Charlie seemed to relax a bit, too, and remarked, "We haven't seen that much of you in court, recently."

"No," I agreed. "I haven't been able to work as much the last year. I have had to dedicate most of my time to all this stuff," here I waved at a shelf full of Ruffin's various files, "to try to help Ruffin, you know, with his autism, if possible."

Charlie pulled out a little desk calendar and together we tried to puzzle out the day I had left Ruffin home alone. At the time, all I could tell him was I thought school had just come back into session after Christmas. It must have been well over a week ago, maybe as long as ten days. I told him I had told everyone working with Ruffin at the time, because while I was out, Ruffin had handled a phone call from someone.

And, I remembered, as I had told him earlier, "It was cold, and the weather was really bad."

Ruffin wasn't back from Lisa's, so Charlie asked if it would be okay if he came back about an hour later when I was sure he would be able to meet with Ruffin.

"Sure, I can give you a call as soon as he gets home, then."

When Ruffin returned and Charlie came back, Charlie asked about the scars on Ruffin's left eyelid and forehead where he had run through the glass of our front door last Mother's Day.

I had to explain that.

Charlie included his impressions about Ruffin. "I was introduced to Ruffin by his mother. Ruffin interacted well with his mother and was verbal. He was active and appeared healthy and well nourished. He appeared to be his stated age. I played a game with him and his mother and he would talk with me. He was appropriate in his interaction during the game but would not answer questions unless he felt like it. This is not atypical in children who have not reached school age and have not been trained to answer questions.

"Ruffin knew where the phone was and how to turn it on. He could dial 911 if you told him the numbers. He did not appear to know what 911 was or why you would call that number despite his mother saying she had worked with him on this. I did not believe he was capable of self-supervision, based upon my observation and interaction."

Although his would be a "founded" report of child abuse for which I was responsible, a case of "denial of critical care," Charlie looked at me over his reading glasses and said, "Promise me, you'll never do this again?"

"Never," I said, and hoped he believed it.

"Fine, well, Ruffin doesn't seem to be in any real danger here with you now, so I'm going to leave him with you. It seems to me you are trying to take good care of him," and here he looked around, opened my refrigerator and several of my kitchen cabinets, "and the house is nice and clean. I don't think we have a foster home that could handle a child with autism, anyway. Okay, thank you."

Ruffin hadn't misbehaved in any way with him, but I wondered if Charlie were not remembering what I was. Shortly before Ruffin had been diagnosed, my arrangements three-deep for sitters all collapsed and I brought Ruffin with me to a brief juvenile court "review hearing." For the five minutes it took to manage that in the courtroom, Ruffin had roamed around the edge of the room uncontrollably, babbling explosively. Charlie had been there, too. Ruffin must have seemed frightening and strange.

CHAPTER FORTY THREE

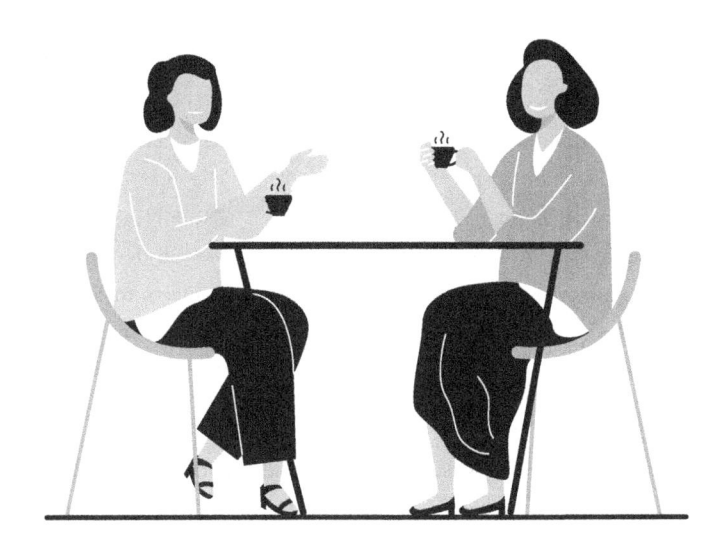

WHY CAN'T WE?

There was no school. The teachers and administrators were busy meeting with each other for another in-service. Ruffin was home for two days, working with Donna, and then Lisa. Evelyn checked in by phone, but I couldn't tell her much about how Ruffin's educators were following through on her suggestions. Our recent Sunday work session with her had been so odd and contentious, I needed to write to school to memorialize it.

While I typed fitfully, Ruffin played dot to dot on his computer. He enjoyed opening *Mario Teaches Typing* and *Math Blaster*, his newest computer programs. He was also asking when the clock would look like the time for the bus to arrive.

"Evelyn has left Donna a very full set of drills addressing 'theory of mind' tasks. These are Donna's highest priority, since Ruffin shows some small signs of noting and remarking on the mental states and emotions of others. Donna will direct her attention back to the storytelling, 'wh' question drills and prediction drills that she warned me in December were suffering from the burden added to her of pre-teaching all the kindergarten reading material.

"Theory of mind is an important deficit — perhaps the unique deficit of autism, present in the most high-functioning and high IQ sufferers — and it is important to address with Ruffin now, aggressively, before kindergarten, when he will fully integrate with his age-mates. I have loaned Francesca Happe's *AUTISM, an introduction to psychological theory* to Donna for her to read. This is the researcher Evelyn, and I were discussing in Sunday's meeting.

"Decoding written language is something we know Ruffin can learn — because he is sounding out and sight-reading more and more words all the time off the computer, the television, and in books at home. He is likely to learn to read regardless of his autism. But without theory of mind skills, this 'reading' may amount to little more than *hyperlexia* without comprehension, or any pragmatic or functional appreciation of complex human feeling."

Later on, as examples of Ruffin's theory of mind remarks, I was able to share these with Meg and Elaine. "'Danielle *knows* where the bakery is,' offered by Ruffin as he and I were on the way to the bakery and talking about how to get there. Reverse psychology was beginning to work with Ruffin. My teasing him, 'You can't have one!' succeeded in getting Ruffin to eat a popsicle. As we were looking for his cowboy costume, Ruffin remarked, 'I don't *know* what's in that box. *You never showed it to me.'* Ruffin remarked, 'I did that *on purpose*, sorry.' About squirting shaving cream in the bathrooms. He can answer appropriately if an accident occurs. He also uses, 'I made *a mistake,* or 'You made a *mistake*' — but still as a relatively concrete description or label of events observed behaviorally, not necessarily very psychologically."

But, to Miss Hobbs, I wrote explicitly to set the record straight about my feelings, "Every effort you can make to support and show respect for Donna's work will be appreciated. The 'anti-Lovaas' vibes Donna feels on the ACSD campus, and which she described to Meg before our Sunday meeting — are not okay. It was hard to hear Donna talk about how she knows her treatment of Ruffin is viewed by some there as 'cruel.'

"I felt embarrassed to have superintendent Charlie Johnson and the private nursery school president show up at our work session with Evelyn. It was impossibly awkward to ask them to leave in the face of their efforts to come on a Sunday morning." Meg had seemed as surprised as I was. Miss Hobbs's early January memo to all interested persons was hardly a general cross-invitation for all those persons copied on the memo to attend any meeting with Evelyn, regardless of their connection to a particular child, or the strictures of special education confidentiality.

"The private nursery school's willingness to adjust Mrs. Mills' class size to fit Ruffin's special needs, and the school's sacrifice of all the tuition from children left on their waiting list was a warm surprise. This generosity certainly was a contrast to Miss Hobbs's expressed unwillingness to consider adjusting ACSD kindergarten class size and her ready jump to bring out a tape-recorder at that moment. To fully mainstream Ruffin, small class size was the only, crucial accommodation Evelyn stressed earlier in the meeting.

"I did visit St. Pat's kindergarten recently for about two hours to observe. There were 14 and 15 children per class, an appropriate size for Ruffin, according to Evelyn. St. Pat's expects to have a similar or lesser enrollment for next year but will know more after their February round-up." At principal Peter's Smith's invitation, I had sat quietly in the back of a couple of kindergarten classrooms. I liked what I saw — small groups of well-behaved children focused on kind and interesting teachers.

"Why can't we just celebrate Ruffin's gains and arrange, or find an appropriately sized class to support him next year? Surely, with weighted funds at 3.6 for Ruffin, paying St. Pat's $710 annual out-of-parish tuition to put him into a small class would be a solution where everyone benefits — Ruffin's needs would be met, and Miss Hobbs could keep ACSD's kindergarten as large and evenly-sized as she likes.

"Please provide me with a copy of Sunday's audiotape for my files."

Miss Hobbs seemed stung hard by all this. She replied quickly with some heat. "In the past I have received letters from you which I felt contained inaccurate information. As you are aware, I chose not to respond. However, I now believe it is time to clarify inaccuracies as they are presented and will continue to do so should future letters contain inaccurate information.

"Donna Schmidt did not say anything at the meeting about 'anti-Lovaas' vibes at ACSD. She has never expressed these concerns to me or any staff members and said no such thing at the meeting. She did tell superintendent Charlie Johnson that it is sometimes hard for people to see the harsh way of talking to children using Lovaas so he would have some understanding of it.

"Charlie Johnson called me about attending the meeting and I referred him to you. He said he would call you and attend with your permission. The private nursery school president attended in Mrs. Mills' absence. As she stated in her letter of early October, she came so that comments made by a teacher of her facility would not be misinterpreted.

"Evelyn Kung made no recommendation for kindergarten class size. She did state that Ruffin was making good progress and that she had no concerns about him being ready for kindergarten. She also stated that he would not need a classroom aide. Ms. White, this is the very reason I asked to tape record that discussion. As in the past, you invariably inaccurately restate what was discussed.

"As I told you at our Sunday meeting, it is up to each parent to decide to send his or her child to public school or private school. I also stated that we won't know what our projected class sizes will be until after kindergarten registration in early February, and even then, the numbers continue to change until school opens in August. Should you choose to send Ruffin to ACSD, I will be making classroom assignments in May, with changes possible through the first two weeks of school.

"I have a copy of the audiotape you requested. I shall send it to you as soon as I received the copy of your videotape I requested in mid-November." The latter referred to a videotape Ruth had made of her most recent IEP for Renee.

I couldn't let Miss Hobbs's letter questioning my credibility as a fact reporter sit unanswered on the educational record to be read by a mediator, ALJ, federal district court judge, or heaven forbid, a juvenile court judge considering whether to put my parenting under juvenile court and DHS supervision, so, whether I wanted to nor not, I needed to write Miss Hobbs right back.

"The time to clarify perceived inaccuracies is immediately.

"My letter recounts Donna's expressions of concern about anti-Lovaas vibes *before* our Sunday morning meeting.

"*Before* our Sunday morning meeting Charlie Johnson never referred himself to me to ask my permission to attend.

"The private nursery school president arrived Sunday morning about the time Charlie Johnson left. She brought no report, oral or written, from her school. She brought blank paper. She had never attended Ruffin's meetings before.

"'Demanding' and 'picky' are two words Evelyn used Sunday to describe how other parents have appeared to school administrators as they sought to have their children who have completed CARD programs mainstream unaided into small-sized kindergarten classes. Accommodation by finding or creating a small-sized class into which to mainstream such a child avoids social stigma and more restrictive placement with a classroom aide.

"Please advise me soonest in writing of ACSD's projected class size after your February kindergarten roundup. I understand those projections are not firm.

"It is inappropriate to condition delivery of the Sunday meeting audiotape, a part of Ruffin's educational record, upon my producing to you the videotape of a meeting concerning another special education student."

And, of course, it was a bald violation of FERPA.

But Meg and even Elaine continued to communicate and follow up more helpfully. Meg added a note to Ruffin's educational file. "The attached integration worksheet reflects the addition of two kindergarten PE classes. These sessions were added as part of a drill to increase Ruffin's ability to listen and follow group directions as well as other group skills as suggested by the CARD consultant."

Meg also created a 'remnant book,' adopting Evelyn's suggestion. "Since I couldn't find a hot dog — we cut this shape out of a bologna sandwich — hope it works. Also, Legos — will get better as we collect more pictures and 'remnants.' Ruffin told us Grandma and Papa visited last summer, and with prompts we got, 'I called *them.*'" She prepared an integration notebook for Elaine, and Elaine began offering more structured and frequent written comments about Ruffin's daily behavior.

OBJECTIVES FOR INTEGRATION

1. Scripted narrative play
2. Conversation
3. Verbally plan activities with peers
4. Share skills
5. Follow peer suggestions
6. Abide by group decisions

With two columns below for Activity and Comments, Elaine could briefly note activities so I could ask Ruffin about what he might have done at nursery school. Her first comments offered that Ruffin had shown his pictures and talked about them at show and tell, played with blocks in a group, had no problems and no extra help on the daily worksheet, and that he had been very attentive to today's story.

This looked like it was going to work. Definitely an improvement, I thought.

Seamus arrived with the newspaper headline: *School may ask voters to approve high school addition.* He was pleased with himself to have seen it coming. I wondered, couldn't Meg and Elaine, Donna and Lisa, Seamus and I just get on with Ruffin's education quietly, since Miss Hobbs and Mr. Lord had much bigger fish to fry.

That same week the school board adopted a resolution in support of adequate funding for special education to be sent to all our area legislators. The resolution included an ominous sounding introductory clause: "WHEREAS it is grossly inequitable to pass along 100 percent of the excess costs of special education to property taxpayers, or to absorb the excess costs from the regular education budget . . ." After Seamus's kitchen counter tutoring, I was able to translate this with some crudeness and fair accuracy. Why should farmers and businessmen have to pay for other families' *retards*?

Donna called later in the week to warn me the school seemed to be trying to build a stronger child abuse case against me. Meg had noticed blood on Ruffin's lip and sent him to the office to be examined by the school nurse. Thankfully, the kindergarten teacher told Donna she had seen Ruffin fall on his face in her room, explaining the blood on his lip.

Later in the day a Bridgewater occupational or physical therapist came into Meg's room, concerned about Ruffin's facial scarring. Given the available explanation of the day's injuries, Meg sent the Bridgewater therapist packing and wouldn't allow her to test Ruffin's reflexes without having a signed release from me.

Later, Meg wanted me to sign a release to refer Ruffin for evaluation by a physical therapist because he had had some accidents this past year. She recalled that I had expressed concern earlier about Ruffin's protective reflexes. I considered whether I would consent, on condition I be present for the examination, but Donna warned me that Miss Hobbs seemed to be looking for evidence of injury attributable to child abuse. So, I remained wary. I listened to Donna, and simply set the referral paperwork aside. No one could examine Ruffin without my signature. I kept that paperwork on my "toad pile" — of bothersome paperwork I would get to sometime when I felt like it.

Donna was concerned that matters with Miss Hobbs were heading overboard again and would put her in a greater bind at school. Donna thought Meg was concerned, too. I asked about the effect of my latest letters-for-the-record. Donna told me Meg had taken the fact that I had written another couple of letters well, without being angry or upset, but then she didn't think Meg had had time to read all of them yet.

Meg had admitted to Donna as she was leaving that day, "I'm not really anti-Lovaas. It's just not for me."

Donna was also concerned that the kindergarten teacher was having a hard time controlling her large and unruly group. Donna had seen Ruffin working hard to copy another child's paper. When she pulled him back so he couldn't see it, Ruffin had wanted Donna's help. He had been rolling his pencil when he was supposed to be listening.

Donna also planned to go observe Elaine's class to see how well Ruffin was listening there. Since she and Elaine remained friends, Donna thought Elaine would just let her in.

As for Ruffin himself, he had dressed up in his cowboy outfit and pretended to talk on the telephone about a problem with his cousin. He had a good lunch talking with a little kindergarten girl. Ruffin had offered, "You're aut-y" to Donna when she had put her hands over her ears. And "You're stimming" to Donna, again, when she had objected to a smell. He had responded to Donna's brief hypothetical, "If you burned your finger," with his reply of completion, "You would feel pain."

Elaine sent us a little "report card," which was very welcome.

I have spent this month evaluating your child, checking readiness skills in preparation for kindergarten roundup in February. In most educational circles there are four kinds of readiness: academic, social, emotional, and physical. Each type of development can proceed at a different rate; no kindergarten-age child will be completely 'ready' in all four areas. Your child doesn't have to have it all mastered to be ready, willing, and able to benefit — and enjoy — kindergarten.

Personal: Ruffin knows his full name, birthday, parents' names, and his age.

Social Development: Ruffin plays cooperatively with friends, obeys rules, shares toys, communicates his feelings and ideas, waits for his turn, accepts routine but needs to be reminded to stop playing, and shows self-confidence, being very proud of his accomplishments.

Emotional Development: Ruffin says goodbye to parents and switches focus to a task, forms friendships with peers, and they enjoy Ruffin, too; is flexible when confronted with new situations or frustrations, shares his ideas, tries new activities, and is able to relax.

Academic Readiness: Ruffin can identify common shapes: circle, triangle, square, rectangle, can say the alphabet in sequence, understands counting order, counts to 20, recognizes numerals 1 to 10, can draw a person with many recognizable features, recognizes the primary colors, shows good listening skills most of the time and has a good attention span, but if he is distracted it's easy to bring him back to task.

Physical Development: Ruffin speaks clearly so that others can understand, dresses himself, zips and buttons, has good large muscle coordination, good small muscle coordination when painting, coloring, cutting with scissors, and putting puzzles together.

Ruffin is ready for kindergarten in the fall. He fits very well in our class, is well-liked by all. He has a very pleasing personality. We really enjoy him.

At the same time, Meg filled out a *Listening Self-Assessment* checklist, by adapting it to assess Ruffin's listening skills from her perspective. Listening skills that she judged Ruffin was good at were: listening to his own feelings, listening for another person's feelings, paraphrasing, expressing his feelings, helping other persons hear themselves, making eye contact, observing body language, taking note with retention, and establishing trust.

Listening skills that she judged Ruffin was doing all right on but needed to develop were: listening for facts, asking open-ended questions that require more than 'yes' or 'no' answers, being non-judgmental and open-minded, being willing to confront conflict, remembering information, letting other persons solve their own problems, being comfortable with silence, being other person focused, and encouraging feedback.

Listening skills that she judged Ruffin was having difficulty with were: not interrupting, not completing other people's sentences, not giving advice, not getting defensive, not evaluating, and not thinking of what he is going to say next instead of listening.

None of the current local nonsense and real troubles dampened my enthusiasm for advocacy. It helped to keep me from considering myself a hopeless idiot. Dr. Jack Scott from Florida Atlantic University and his group were going to hold a conference for two days at the Ft. Lauderdale Airport Hilton. I read his brochure in the middle of our Iowa winter and wondered if I shouldn't be considering a move to Florida. In my dreams. It would be too disruptive of all our lives. I needed to bloom — and advocate — where I had planted myself. There was a great deal more to do in Iowa, if I had any energy not already focused on Ruffin — always, always, I promised myself — my first priority.

Later, Dr. Scott scrawled a handwritten note thanking us for the information about Ruffin's home program therapists which he and his colleagues had used in a published article on therapist competencies, *Essential Content for Training Behavior Analysis Practitioners* in *The Behavior Analyst,* No. 1. (Spring 1995), 18: 83-91, and went on to include in Catherine Maurice's manual designed to help parents in running home-based programs. To our nationwide list of other parents, the junior high school volunteers distributed Dr. Scott's survey focused on the necessary support and requirements for being a successful home therapist.

On *The Me-List*, a parent from Michigan began keeping a partial list of school districts across the nation willing to pay for in-home Lovaas programs, including districts in Michigan, Maryland, California, and New Jersey. It felt good to log on to *The Me-List* and not feel so alone, and to have a list of districts to suggest to families of newly diagnosed children — where they might consider moving to access a real free appropriate public education.

Meanwhile, Ray, who was always the easiest person to work with in Bridgewater, was educating me about Iowa's special education "weighting" system for funding, and returning our Lovaas tapes, and our tapes of Ruffin after copying them with enthusiasm and thanks.

And here was my love. Ruffin brought home his nursery school worksheet and handed it over to me proudly. He had printed his own name at the top, and traced and colored the snowman, his green hat, his orange carrot nose, his red bowtie, his three purple buttons, and his brown-handled and yellow-straw broom.

Meg had noted, "Ruffin drinks his chocolate milk at breakfast right down, no problem. Ruffin did two PE classes back-to-back today. Since the purpose of having Ruffin attend PE is to follow group directions, maybe we don't really want him practicing in our ECSE session first, so we will just stick with the two kindergarten sessions unless you don't agree. Let me know if this is not acceptable to you." I was pleased. This sounded more like the Meg I knew and could work with easily enough if Miss Hobbs kept her nose out of it.

Elaine reported that Ruffin had followed his classmate's suggestions in playing with blocks and tractors and had abided by group decisions to read and act out a play in which his own part was the snail. This gave me subjects to bring up with Ruffin in our after-school conversations.

Donna told me about a "who has the button game" Ruffin's group had played in kindergarten music. Ruffin had been prompted to look at everyone's faces to try to use his "theory of mind skills" to be able to guess who might be hiding the button. Donna had been working with Ruffin in one-to-one drills, too, by being tricky herself, and helping him use his new skills of persuasion. Meg had complimented her, after watching, "That's where that one-to-one helps."

Donna had gone to both kindergarten PE classes with Ruffin, and it had been the same lesson, a good repeat for Ruffin. The kindergarten teacher had directed the PE teacher not to give Ruffin any special directions.

And Donna was trying to ask Ruffin more questions that required him to make inferences, questions like, "How does Donna know you washed your hands?"

I recounted to Meg, Elaine, and Donna in late January, "Ruffin saw a possum at Lisa's yesterday and told me it was 'pretending' to be dead after they turned it out of the trashcan. Also, Ruffin offered a long conversation about Renee and how he likes her except when she tears his paper. He said, 'She *wants* me to teach her.' He reported she doesn't tear his paper anymore.

"The remnant items in Ruffin's book are 'blind' to him — I don't let him know what I've put in. He is using 'proud' and 'excited' appropriately to describe my feelings and his and the feelings his friends would have if they could see his 'house-tent.' He says he 'misses' his summer friends — mentioning two of them by name.

"Everything in the purple picture represents a named object of some kind — he can tell you."

School dismissed early another morning due to heavy snow, while Charlie Coffey continued his investigation of the events of January 9th, when I had left Ruffin home alone. "CHILD ABUSE INVESTIGATION: On January 25th, 1996, this investigator spoke with Donna Schmidt by phone. Donna Schmidt indicated she provides Ruffin with intense behavioral modification. She indicated Ruffin doesn't have a concept of what an emergency is and said Ruffin does not have the ability to provide self-supervision." When I read his report later, I knew Donna was right. Ruffin did not yet have what our home team considered "mastery" of what to do in a variety of emergencies.

Heavy snow continued on Friday. I decided to keep Ruffin home from school. Donna came over to work with him, and by late that morning, school had been dismissed again due to the weather.

Ray DeNeve called me to give me the dates, times, and places to attend three IEP meetings for students with autism in his Bridgewater sector and apologized for superintendent Charlie Johnson not having contacted me in advance before attending Ruffin's Sunday meeting with Evelyn. I assured him we were all good.

At home, Ruffin did a lovely job of completely coloring his winter hibernation worksheet — his trees were green, the frozen water was blue, the furred bear, beaver, and squirrel were brown, and his sleeping turtle was whimsically purple. The word I used to tell him how I felt was "proud."

On Sunday during Catholic Schools Week, Ruffin and I toured St. Patrick's to check it out again. Seamus suggested that I carefully read the newspaper supplement describing the small parochial school. Based on Iowa norms for the *Iowa Test of Basic Skills,* the average achievement for each grade there was above grade level in growth as compared to the public schools.

Seamus and I discussed the smaller class sizes at St. Pat's, and I read all the published personal endorsements of community leaders whom we both knew. We talked over the experiences of the children whose families we both knew who had attended St. Pat's.

The supplement promised an active parent volunteer group, a schedule of field trips, and a regular latch-key afterschool program — so whenever bad weather called for an early release, I would never need to worry about where Ruffin might be dropped off, or whether anyone would be home from work to meet him.

There seemed to be a surprisingly large staff. Seamus took me through all their pictures, their little biographies in the paper, and gave me the benefit of all the gossip he had gathered back through to the first pioneer generations of each of their family reputations. Although Seamus had attended a one-room country schoolhouse through fifth grade, he attended public school only three years before he went back to attend high school at St. Pat's.

On Monday, there was still no school due to the weather. Donna and Lisa came over, morning and afternoon, at their accustomed times, to keep Ruffin on some sort of regular schedule.

A parent with a child with a new diagnosis called in from Coralville. The address went right to the teenaged volunteers — here at my home-office while there was no school — who quickly assembled a box of videos from Lovaas, my presentation at Western Hills, and a fat Bindertek of research and resources.

On Tuesday, I assured Meg, "Ruffin kept nicely busy at home for the two-school snow-days with his computer, books, and educational television. He is enjoying 'hiding' things and 'fooling' or being fooled in his theory of mind exercises."

Meg replied, "Ruffin told me you made the sharks out of paper, and that you and he made up stories about them and made a paper house on your couch for them. I showed him how he could tape the shark to a pencil to make it a stick puppet. 'Take it off' was the only comment I got. Lots of high voice talking today."

Preschool conference preparation day on Wednesday meant Meg's class didn't meet, but Elaine's class met in the afternoon to make up for a snow day. Early that morning Donna called to ask whether Ruffin had any school for the day, and then came over to visit. She and Seamus had discussed the child abuse complaint — Seamus had been very angry with Donna. I assured Donna, I hadn't asked him to be. I knew I had done what I had done. She and I were good. Donna told me she had unloaded on Seamus. "I told him he should be bringing you and Ruffin milk every time he visits here."

"When you were a child growing up here, was there ever morning milk delivery, you know, by a milkman?" I asked.

"I remember that." Donna said. "It used to happen when most women at home didn't have cars."

"What woman could live here now without a car of her own?" I asked.

"A woman with a milkman!" I looked at Donna, and she looked at me, and we both doubled over, snorting coffee out our noses.

When Donna caught her breath, she said, "Ruffin is still having some eating problems. He was not eating at school yesterday. He doesn't like being asked about it, either. I think we need to get all the food pictures out of his remnant book."

"I'll let Meg and Elaine know. I need to let you all know anyway I will be starting Ruffin on some iron for his anemia."

Then Donna and I descended into gossip. Donna told me how she had joined a hallway knot of elementary school teachers discussing the January boy-on-the-bus incident — they had blamed everyone but the school — the kindergarten child for falling asleep, the child's second grade brother for not being responsible for him. Only one teacher mentioned the "sweeping the bus rule" the bus driver had failed to follow with the possible tragic outcome and had walked away. Meg's classroom was in a truly angry mood — Donna found it the prevailing mood in her classroom.

So, the next time I wrote Meg, I wrote hoping to buck her up and still manage to get Donna's latest message across. "Ruffin was right on target with you about our shark play. He is having no problems putting the right number of jellybeans on cookies in *Millie's Math House*. He is also using his hands now to indicate his ideas of time — long or short — and of distance. Let's try something other than food remnants. Ruffin doesn't like being 'grilled' on what he ate."

CHAPTER FORTY FOUR

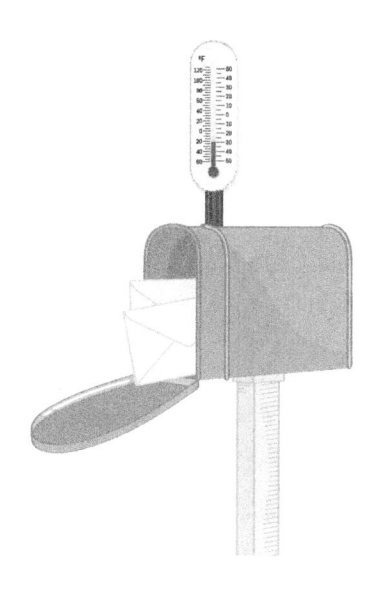

PLEASE BRING YOUR PARENTS

The National Weather Service: *From February 1st through 4th, 1996, artic temperatures overspread the Upper Mississippi River Valley. The culprit was a frigid airmass which moved into the region in late January. With clear skies at night, temperatures plummeted into the 30s below zero over much of the area. This blast of artic air set all-time record low temperatures for Iowa, Minnesota, and Wisconsin: Elkader, Iowa (tied the record at 47 degrees below zero).*

But, on February 1st, Ruffin had school. I was due to pick him up mid-morning to visit St. Pat's. He was marked absent from public school without excuse. In the car he told me that a classmate wouldn't share the tractor, and that another got into trouble for giving a razzberry to a grown-up and had to sit in a chair for being naughty. In a sort of chant, he was using the word 'plus' to string numbers together, using numbers like '30' and '45.'

Ruffin had received this invitation by mail. "We heard the good news that you are going to be in kindergarten this fall. We are excited about meeting you. Please bring your parents along. We have some important papers to give them that day. See you soon! Your friends at St. Pat's School."

Our visit was as welcoming and friendly as their written invitation. Ruffin was paired with a kindergarten child who would be a first grader next year and remain Ruffin's "buddy" throughout all next year. He was the son of St. Pat's Title I reading teacher. Ruffin seemed to know his way around the building and was comfortable to have his "buddy" guide him into one of the kindergarten rooms where I was welcome to follow them and stand with a group of parents as we watched a late-morning lesson. With his "buddy," Ruffin was more than willing to cross the street to try going through the lunch line and eat at a table with him and his friends in the church basement.

I tried to reach Curt and Joan that afternoon to have one of them call Caron to leave a message that somehow, we needed to discuss my choice of kindergarten for Ruffin.

That evening, Donna and Lisa ventured out into the bitterest cold so we could hold our weekly meeting on how Ruffin was responding to Evelyn's latest drills and integration suggestions. Donna suggested a capped cup for administering Ruffin's vitamins and DMG. It might appear more ordinary than a bottle to his various classmates, and still assure he was likely to take his full dose. She and I were also working on a home-school calendar for remnants. We were still trying to run down photos of all the groups of children Ruffin schooled with so he could learn all their names: Meg's class, Elaine's class, the group of Head Start visitors, and the various groups of kindergarteners in PE, library, and shared reading. They amounted to a formidable list of names to learn — even for the two of us with Seamus's help.

Word went out on local radio: no school Friday. It was too dangerous to be running the buses out into the rural parts of the county where it was always colder with the unbroken wind travelling over the prairie. Meg and Amy's plan to go bowling and have pizza for lunch in town was a casualty of the weather. These field trips always involved a lot of planning. I knew everyone would be disappointed. Ruffin certainly was.

Monday, as the cold broke, Elaine let me know Ruffin had pretended with her group that he was a groundhog and made a Valentine mobile. He had also done a great job on his matching shapes worksheet, drawing connecting lines from circle to circle, square to square, rectangle to rectangle, triangle to triangle, and heart to heart with a purple crayon with which he had also printed his name.

Meg sent some news about her class which had suffered so many short weeks with cold and snow, including the postponements of field trips and all Luther PE until mid-February. Her class would no longer be watching *Sesame Street* daily at nap time, after lunch.

Ruffin opened a second, mailed invitation that Tuesday. "At last, you are old enough to attend school. You and your parents are invited to come to kindergarten registration. Plan to stay an hour and a half. We will be visiting with you in one of the kindergarten rooms, while your parents meet with other school personnel. Someone will visit with them about things which will need to be done before school begins in the fall. Now that you will soon be coming to school you should be able to put on your coat and zip or button it, begin to tie your shoes, go to the bathroom by yourself, and leave mother for a few hours during the day."

Since a large group of parents and prospective students was expected, there would be no current kindergartners in attendance, and no kindergarten classes or teaching for any of us to observe. After the full crowd gathered, I got up and walked over to look at the completed sign-in roster. There were 63 students — which I calculated would produce 16-child classrooms if Miss Hobbs were to hire 4 kindergarten teachers again next year, as she had this year.

But, of course, not everyone was able to attend this mid-day work-day event — which was why each of Miss Hobbs's four classes were likely to be much larger than the 15-child upper limit Dr. Granpeesheh and Evelyn were recommending for Ruffin. Maybe I was being too negative now that I had St. Pat's for comparison.

If Ruffin were entitled to a free, appropriate public education here, I needed to gather my mask of attentive cheerfulness, take a seat in the back of the room, and listen. This was *information*. Information, for decision-making.

Miss Hobbs stepped up to lecture us on health records, cumulative folders, immunizations, school physicals, written consent to medicate our child at school, flogged the third-party, private insurance policy to cover our child's injuries at school, handed out yellow dental cards, explained how vision and hearing screenings and Bridgewater developmental screenings would be available to the disabled, explained when to keep our child home from school if he or she were sick, mentioned — here with a nod to the annoyed — that weather, the heat earlier and the cold at the moment, had really been hard on attendance this year, reviewed the need to call in by mid-morning if our children were going to be absent, and stated, possibly in response to the most recent letter to the editor, "If you have your child on the bus and we don't have your child here at school, we will be calling you to ask why they are not here."

We were instructed exactly how to write a note excusing an absence, and informed: "As your child's principal, I can request you to take your child to the doctor for an excuse."

Then the school nurse told us, "We don't have the money to screen all our students for hearing or developmental delays anymore — we used to."

Lists of supplies to purchase were handed out. The milk, breakfast and lunch program rules were passed around, as Miss Hobbs resumed the floor. "Put your child on the bus the first day, please. We really discourage visits to school by parents for the first six weeks, to encourage separation and make it easier for your child. After the first six weeks, you are free to visit here at any time.

"Remember, our playground near the edge of town is colder by 5 degrees usually."

We could expect a schedule of parent information meetings, and individual parent-teacher conferences. Miss Hobbs would be making a class list in May, for the four teachers. "You can't pick your child's teacher, but I will avoid a teacher for you, if she happens to be a neighbor or relative or you have some specific, legitimate concern. Special needs boys and girls will be balanced in each classroom. We will split up cousins or preschool friends on request, but be reasonable, people. These lists are a drag to make." There was some sympathetic, or nervous laughter. Ours was a small town in a thinly populated rural county.

"If you think you have a problem, phone the teacher first, before me, then call me, then call the superintendent, then a school board member."

"At home, cut your television off when you can. Here at school, we know television hinders developmental growth. Read to your kids. Remember, school is a lot of reading."

Here, again, the laughter was of the nervous variety. Just how many of these parents, most of whom appeared much younger than I was, might have attended kindergarten earlier in this same 1960s vintage, low, red-brick building?

"Here at school, we offer your child art, music, physical education, and one computer per classroom. Our kindergarteners are placed in shared reading time for 30 minutes a day in four different ability groups. Science is offered in mixed-grade smaller classes of 15 to 17 students. From kindergarten through second grade, your child will keep a writing portfolio. If you want to get involved here on campus, volunteer for our partners in education program. Those meetings are held here, in the library, at night.

"Remember, your children don't want to see you after fourth grade. Not at school, anyway."

I wondered if Miss Hobbs wasn't joking again, since I could see some of the other parents, those with older, additional children, were laughing.

We were all invited to come to an evening of open house, to tour the facilities, during carnival, and briefly introduced to the guidance counselor. Finally, at the door, Miss Hobbs had the counselor hand each of us a 4-page kindergarten checklist to fill out in September to help judge whether our children were really kindergarten-ready. I put this on my "toad pile."

Was I really being open-minded about this option? Honestly, my answer to myself, in the lingo of the moment, was: Not!

I went to get Ruffin from Meg's class to take him over to Elaine's, and glimpsed Ruffin's notebook where Meg had written, "The reason Donna has been putting food in Ruffin's remnant book is that is one of the few things that changes daily. However, if he doesn't like to talk about food at home, we will quit. It will limit us to what we can put in the remnant book. Daily routine such as drills doesn't change much. Any ideas for the remnant book? If you leave the pictures in the remnant book, he can use it for his yesterday and today drills. No kindergarten shared reading group today due to kindergarten roundup, so he got to go outside. He loved it! Big hills of snow. He really watched *Sesame Street* closely today." So much for cutting off the television, I thought to myself, a bit acidly.

Fay Hill, the nurse consultant at Gundersen assigned to Ruffin by his PICU team followed up on his development, asking that I complete a questionnaire about how Ruffin was doing medically, developmentally, nutritionally, and with his social status. I responded as fully as my teenaged volunteers were able, with an indexed booklet of all Ruffin's medical records and evaluations to date.

I reported that health insurance was not adequate to meet Ruffin's medical needs but nothing more could be done about it. Prudential had stopped paying for Donna now that she was working at school — the treatment she delivered was deemed "educational" and thus coverage was excluded under the express terms of my individual policy. Even Scott, as powerful an attorney as he was, could no longer budge them.

But, sealing the envelope to Fay, I had to reflect on how many ways Ruffin was a lot better than he was in July of 1994 when he was diagnosed.

Ray DeNeve called with an idea to share. He was toying with the idea of making a proposal to hire a Bridgewater employee to train teachers and aides in discrete trial training methods. It didn't cross my mind he was thinking of hiring Donna away from Ruffin's team. I referred him to Dr. Lovaas, Dr. Sallows, and Dr. Granpeesheh for help to arrange for training someone and offered him specific suggestions, volunteering to speak to any of these experts about any appropriate Iowa candidate.

Seamus and I made a tentative decision that evening to register Ruffin for kindergarten at St. Pat's. The school needed to hire a new maintenance man. Seamus agreed to apply. If he were hired, he would be able to keep an eye on Ruffin, during and after school there. On Ruffin's application, I fully disclosed his handicap as "PDD-NOS or Asperger's Syndrome, a form of autism," and hoped for the best — for his admission.

I needed to provide Ruffin's vaccination records for oral polio vaccine, diphtheria, tetanus, pertussis, and HibTiter, all given over his first and second years. On June 20th, 1992, he had received a single dose of measles, mumps, and rubella (MMR) — before the FDA required manufacturers to remove the thimerosal mercury preservative from multi-dose vials — the sort of vial Ruffin's dose was drawn from as I had held him, trusting him to the ministrations of the county nurse. In view of the live controversy then as to whether the MMR vaccine or the thimerosal might trigger symptoms of autism, Ruffin's family doctor, Dr. Olson, provided a written waiver for Ruffin from the state law requirement that he receive another MMR dose before entering kindergarten.

Wednesday began in our ordinary way. I scribbled to Meg, "Ruffin told me all about the big hills of snow — five minutes at least — in the car after kindergarten roundup without any remnant book reminder. He also recognized, greeted, and pointed out to me two of his nursery school classmates there. Television in school? Why not read, as suggested to parents at the public-school roundup?" I should have kept that last thought to myself. With so many demanding special needs boys in Ruffin's class, Meg probably needed television to complete her paperwork, just as I did at times. "What's the word on a pocket calendar for Donna? Cost is $35 in Decorah for a pocket and fillers — could save some if we just bought the pocket. Let me know."

When the mail arrived, I had a notice from my bank. I was twenty dollars overdrawn. But Joan had also written to me. "It is a pleasure to forward your reimbursement to you today. It was a long time coming." Talk about an arrival in the nick of time.

And Miss Hobbs had sent me a copy of the audiotape she made of part of our Sunday meeting with Evelyn. Maybe she had called Caron, and Caron had told her she had to — to comply with FERPA.

In the final envelope of the day was a $156,000 check, my portion of that part of the *Ezzone* verdict that my trial partner Mark Soldat and I had collected so far. I checked to be certain I had time to drive across the river into Wisconsin, to pay off my second mortgage, the one I had negotiated late last summer well out of town.

On the way back, I stopped into the local bank where I was overdrawn, and paid off my first mortgage, too. Then, I went home, and wrote out a stack of checks to pay every debt I owed, every credit card against which I had taken the maximum cash advance in this long, uncertain gamble. There was still plenty of money left over. Ruffin and I were home free. We were both going to be able to run loose in the universe again.

I called Lisa to give her the day off. I stuffed photocopies of all these transactions in my briefcase and called Seamus to come out to meet us in the park as I went out again to pick up Ruffin from Elaine's class.

"Look," I said, as the three of us sat on the swings in the suddenly balmy promise of spring weather. The snow at our feet was melting into running sheets of water. I handed over all my wrinkled photocopies to Seamus, and grinned, as he admitted he'd never seen that much money in one place.

"Me, neither," I admitted, and then dug into Ruffin's book bag as he splashed around at our feet. Meg had written to me, "Great about the conversations. Have fun with the puppet show. Great job for him to have earned it so fast." And Elaine had written for her part, "We will have school on Monday (public schools *do not* have class that day). We are making up a snow day." In our integration notebook she let me know Ruffin had watched St. Pat's second grade act out *Three Little Pigs*, and played puppets with a group of boys, and made a heart puppet. I dug around a little more and came up with it, twirled it between my fingers, winked, and handed it over to Seamus.

"You don't want to forget Valentine's Day, do you?"

No school again Thursday. Donna and I took the opportunity to confer. Ruffin had a hard time telling *her* about kindergarten roundup. But Meg had gotten Donna a pocket calendar and a collection of reward-stickers for Ruffin.

In shared reading, Ruffin filled in all the blanks on his worksheets and was learning to do upper- and lower-case letters. Without Donna to step in and direct Ruffin's attention, he was still missing any verbal directions addressed to the class. Donna was working with the kindergarten teacher to learn in advance what skills Donna could pre-teach Ruffin a day or two ahead of time to allow him to follow along with greater success.

Yesterday, Ruffin had recognized the teacher's *verbal* directions — he was listening, but not always beginning to end, but working to *listen*.

Donna had taken Ruffin's watch away yesterday, so he would not fiddle with it while listening. Later, he asked Meg where his watch was. She reminded him Donna had taken it. At that point, Donna *lied* — to set Ruffin up to stand up for himself. Ruffin held his own and got the other kids to back him up. Donna admitted she had lied and explained what "a lie" was. Then she and Ruffin discussed explicitly what lies were, as a theory of mind exercise.

As I was talking special education funding with Ray DeNeve again, he let slip that Mr. Montague would be retiring the end of the school year and repeated his earlier confidence. *"I'm hoping to propose hiring a Lovaas consultant to whomever takes his spot."*

Friday, I wanted Meg and Elaine to know, "Theory of Mind: I've heard Ruffin use, 'I believe . . .' Also, appropriate use of 'jealous.'" Meg shared, "Ruffin had a bloody nose at bowling — we couldn't rinse it out since we were at the alley. He liked bowling and pizza." Elaine let me know Ruffin met all his objectives for integration in group play with puppet shark games, and outside play on the newest snow hill. That weekend Ruffin made a popgun, like Pooh's — out of a balloon pump, stopper, and string, and it worked very well.

By the next Monday, Tuesday, and Wednesday, Ruffin was home with a heavy cold and went to the doctor for a chest X-ray, "which was clear, and some blood tests — all normal, including his white blood count and hemoglobin. Tonsils were normal as well." By Thursday afternoon, Ruffin seemed well enough to attend nursery school where Elaine let me know Ruffin played shark again with a couple of his classmates, rode bikes, hunted for hearts with the group, and opened Valentines in a sharing ritual.

I went into school to collect Ruffin's records and learned that a ninth child had joined Meg's classroom during the ninth week of school. I found several other disturbing things that I addressed later in an early March letter.

Then, I was on the phone most of the remainder of the day, calling other parents, calling St. Pat's principal Peter Smith about trying to get Ruffin's special education funding shared with St. Pat's, calling Evelyn about my choice of kindergarten class for Ruffin, reaffirming the maximum class size she recommended and what type of teacher, calling Ray, and calling Donna. Ruffin's new bus driver asked that I call him at the bus barn in the morning if Ruffin would not be attending. It was a reasonable request. Backing out of my driveway onto busy Main Street *was* dangerous.

I had been writing a longer letter to Mr. Terry Voy in Des Moines about ACSD transportation safety. All the parents concerned dropped by to sign it. Back in January, Betty, Ruth, and I working together had learned that he was responsible to handle bus transportation issues involving child safety. This year, Betty's daughter Bonnie had been delivered home late by an uninformed substitute bus driver. Renee and Ruffin had both been dropped off alone in a blizzard, too. Voy had urged me and any other concerned parents to please write him a detailed who, when, what, where, and why account of any incidents of transportation concern, and promised to refer them to the consultant who accredited our local school district to have any problems resolved. We were pleasantly surprised.

On a happier note, Meg reassured me, "Ruffin came in alert and seemed happy to be back. Played very well. Made and ate a 'Rainbow in a Cloud,' Ask him." And there was a little yearbook: Meg's class, Miss Meyer, Mrs. Weber, and their nine students, and Amy's class, Mrs. Muller, Mrs. Fischer and their five students. I thought we could use that, and went to find the scissors, to cut it up for flashcards so we could teach Ruffin all their names.

From Elaine's class Ruffin brought home his handprints in purple and yellow paint. No more tactile defensiveness, I thought. Then I laid my own hands down over these prints and was surprised to find that Ruffin's hands at nearly 5-years-old were easily the size of my own.

I needed to alert Meg, Elaine, Donna, and Lisa on Monday. "Donna reported that Ruffin had a nosebleed at school after blowing his nose. Lisa reported he had one at her house." Ruffin didn't seem to experience any pain with these nosebleeds, but I found them terrifying. There was always just a lot of blood, and it was hard to stop.

Seamus had walked in during one later Saturday afternoon. The floor at my feet was littered with reddened tissues and Ruffin was squirming to get down and get on with something more interesting to him than this battle to stop his bleeding.

"This looks like what used to happen to me when I was a kid," he announced.

"Thanks a lot," I huffed. "For your genetic contribution, then."

As always, he had advice to offer. "It's too dry in this house. If you go down to the auto body shop, they can make you some folded metal radiator humidifiers."

"What?" I asked, pulling another tissue out of the box teetering on the arm of the love seat.

"You slide them into each radiator, and then fill the little wells at the far end. Every day. With water."

Oh, I thought, that might work, and asked, "How much do they cost?"

"Twenty bucks a piece, I think. You could afford it."

Well, okay, it was true now. I could.

Ruffin had stopped bleeding, and while we ate, I was able to fill Seamus in on what else I would be letting everyone else know. "Ruffin began seeing a one-to-one friend at Lisa's yesterday. He's been asking for spring and summer to come and for me to call all his summer friends."

Ruffin piped up, "My bear is watching me play with the computer," and set his bear up in a position to see. He commented quite freely now about what was being seen by himself and others and what was consequently known or unknown to him or to them. And, he had whispered to me recently, "I'm lonely. I miss you. Do you miss me?"

Seamus was pleased to hear all this but stopped listening when I began to complain that except with Ray at Bridgewater, I seemed to be getting nowhere with my advocacy.

CHAPTER FORTY FIVE

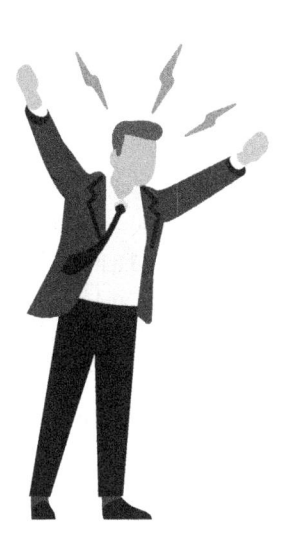

ARE WE IN DISAGREEMENT YET?

School had been called back into session over the radio — as a snow makeup day — even though it was President's Day. The nursery school planned to meet, too. I had hoped to be able to attend a two-day annual Parent-Educator Conference at the Hotel Fort Des Moines, sponsored by Iowa's AEAs, but it was clear from my latest FERPA inspection of Ruffin's educational records that every absence of Ruffin's was being marked whether he attended school part of the day, or not, for whatever reason. I remained acutely aware the child abuse investigation was still hanging fire and decided this was no time to be traipsing off to Des Moines, with or without Ruffin.

Not going would save $130 of childcare at the conference, enough to buy what I really needed now. I was able to let everyone know, "Since we've been filling our radiator humidifiers here, we've had no more nosebleeds at home."

I was surprised to find Mrs. Weber writing back in our notebook. "Mrs. Holub has gone to a conference today and tomorrow." It failed to dawn on me that Miss Hobbs must have sent Meg straight to the Hotel Fort Des Moines.

In Elaine's class, Ruffin had completed an eleven-dot drawing of George Washington's hatchet, colored well with crayons, including red on the four accompanying cherries. Seamus was pleased. He collected presidential memorabilia.

Ruffin himself was able to recount show and tell, telling me what was shown, who forgot to bring anything and what others had brought. He was doing a fair amount of spontaneous recall of past events by bringing them to bear logically and in argument on more immediate subjects.

The teacher from kindergarten shared reading sent home Ruffin's worksheet with a star, and the comment "followed directions," with Ruffin having to listen to words and mark whether a series of pictures matched or not a series of spoken words. Ruffin had also printed his name at the top of his paper.

Far away in Des Moines, after lengthy discussions and negotiations with Curt, Dr. Hagen had issued a memo to all AEA directors of special education to govern this year's cases of EYSE, or special needs summer school.

What would be the EYSE plan for Ruffin? His IEP team was well behind schedule in addressing this issue. We had no excuse now with Dr. Hagen's most recent memo having issued. On four days in late February and seven days throughout March, I requested information concerning EYSE. His educators were aware of these requests, but no one responded to them.

I continued to share our good news. "At Lisa's, Ruffin did a beautiful job of eavesdropping on adult conversation, making a nice interruption. I was telling her that according to the doctor, Ruffin had grown an inch and a half since his last visit. Ruffin broke in with his comment that when he stretches himself out, he can touch both arms of the small sofa, our love seat at home. He told Lisa he is taller now than he was as a baby."

By now, Ruffin offered a good recall of his whole school day for me. His conversation was well-peppered with comments about relevant past events. Donna had sent home Ruffin's latest shared reading paper — yellowish lined paper to guide the printing of capital and lower-case letters — on which Ruffin had written carefully, "Meg is a cat. Meg is yellow and fat." And he had printed his name, with backward turning 'f's and an 'n.' He told Lisa about hanging it on our refrigerator. When I thanked him for this at bedtime, he had a *very* emotional reaction — he cried, as when someone is too openly kind.

It looked like the little girl Lisa had chosen for him would be a good playmate. Her verbal skills were very high — and she seemed calm. Ruffin helped her with a puzzle. She was very pretty, and Ruffin complimented her on her clothes — a little boldly.

Ruffin was also getting fairly free with his advice to grown-ups on the rules. He scolded me that I hadn't worn my seatbelt — that it had been dangerous — I should put it on today. He advised Lisa not to go outside in her sock feet to put out the garbage — she could get sick — she should wear shoes. This seemed to be a mark of his intimacy with people whom he felt close to and comfortable with. Was he advising adults at school, or was he keeping a more appropriate distance?

Meg's report for the day struck me as more than a bit disturbing. "Donna noticed toe-walking today. I tried to stretch Ruffin's heel cords — can't tell if they're tight or not. I'm sending home a referral so a physical therapist can test Ruffin's reflexes and have her check his heel cords."

Yes, I thought. That made two of them, and I put this latest referral I would never sign on the top of my "toad pile."

"Inge is coming today — we will try to set a date to consider Ruffin's eligibility for EYSE."

I wrote pointedly to Meg. "I need to see any EYSE paperwork and Ruffin's IEP charting for the year, please. I noted Ruffin's toe-walking in my original August 1994 notes for the preparation of his first IEP. It is a neurological 'soft sign,' and is diagnostic of autism.

"In any case, I will need to be present for any exam to monitor it, participate, and inquire, and the physical therapist should be comfortable with that and prepared to answer questions about movement disorders in autism."

As I was coming to expect, Meg offered nothing by way of information about the school's physical therapy concerns. "Physical therapy is through Bridgewater."

Donna sent home some of Ruffin's free-form marker artwork — his drawing of himself and a classmate on the floor of Meg's classroom, napping.

A letter arrived from Charlie Coffey, finally, covering his report. It would remain on record and not be expunged for ten years, not until January of 2006. It was the answer I was prepared for and had expected. "Recommendation for Services and Juvenile Court Action: Although this is a founded report for denial of critical care, Ruffin appeared well cared for in other respects and I see no reason to take further action based upon this one incident which the mother has said will not happen again. There is no recommendation for services or court action."

From Des Moines, Terry Voy had responded with shocking indifference — a predictable effect of the power of local control in the matter of education — to the Palmers', Lembkes', and my joint letter of bus transportation concerns, by simply forwarding it to our superintendent, and an accreditation consultant for the state of Iowa. "If we can help, let me know." No magic wand from Des Moines was going to wave in our direction. I was afraid this might be disappointing to share with Ruth and Al, and Dave and Betty, but it turned out it wasn't. Nobody was ready to give up.

We moved on quickly to plan our next steps based on what we had learned from Mr. Voy's letters. David and Betty asked for an IEP meeting for their daughter, Bonnie. It was body-stacked with nearly four dozen Bridgewater and ACSD employees — all gathered in a wide circle in the cavernous, metal-sided city council room.

Mr. Lord stood up within five minutes of Bonnie's meeting being called to order and asked, "Are we in disagreement yet?" Which would have meant our meeting was over, and he could stop paying overtime to everyone there in attendance, and Dave and Betty would have had to have me file an appeal to Des Moines and litigate the matter out.

That was not our plan.

"No," I said, speaking as their attorney. "We're not in disagreement yet. We are here to discuss this matter. You haven't even heard from Bonnie's parents. Just have a seat. At times, it pays to take the time to listen."

Then David and Betty got up and made their strong, common-sense case that every long-haul truck driver they knew sat in an air-ride seat, and a lot of cargo in semi-tractor trailers travelled on air-ride suspension systems. They just thought their little daughter in a wheelchair deserved the same smooth, cushioned ride as a washing machine or a refrigerator.

And most air suspensions were more dependable, easier to maintain, and cheaper.

I could see Joe, the transportation manager, had begun nodding. That was contagious. Nearly everyone around this rural agricultural circle understood semi-tractor trailer truck transportation and began nodding.

Mr. Lord could see that giving Dave and Betty's suggestion some consideration made more sense for him — and Bonnie — than any of us chasing after a court order.

Seamus brought me a copy of Saturday's *Des Moines Register* front page headline article, *Fewer names on abuse registry* about the adoption of new rules designed to eliminate minor incidents of endangering children resulting in their parents' names being placed on the child-abuse registry — and being banned from jobs working with children for at least a decade. The new rules provided for expanded appeal procedures to consider appropriate past cases.

Seamus slapped it down on my kitchen counter.

"It's worth a try, don't you think?"

"Well, I didn't imagine I would get through the special education wars here without getting a ding in my armor, but you may be right."

"If you think about it," Seamus said, still standing, looking down at me, with his face reflected in my morning coffee, "I'm always right."

"You were right about folded metal radiator humidifiers," was as much as I was ready to concede, but I was grateful. I stood up and hugged him. To celebrate we took Ruffin out to the horse sale, and then out to dinner.

When the new law went into effect later that year, Iowa opened a path for parents who had been found to have denied critical care in a single instance to appeal to have their names removed from the child abuse registry, if, like me, they had $2000 to pay a private attorney to prepare and file the appeal, and if it were clear that enough time had passed without any repeat incidents. It allowed these parents — the one-time offenders, like me — to volunteer to lead scout troops and otherwise work with children.

Over the next ten years, my experience was that parents of children with disabilities who insisted on appropriate education, who sought to invoke new IEP meetings, mediation, or due process procedures nearly always became targets of child abuse reports, or requests that they relinquish their parental rights in exchange for out-of-home educational placement or institutional placement in care. This happened to nurses married to physicians, to housewives married to lawyers, to irreproachably solidly-middle-class people of privilege, to the trusting, the vulnerable, the young and the poor, to people of color, to both the hard and the easy targets, alike.

It came to be a sad part of my legal practice to deliver to every parent of a child with disabilities who engaged me to represent their family, a warning that they would be watched like a hawk by mandatory child abuse reporters — their child's teachers and administrators and most Medicaid service providers, and medical doctors — for any slip-up. Aggressive demands for the appropriate services their child might well be entitled to by law would trigger this form of retaliation, so, it would be important to give those helping care for their child no pretext whatsoever. As a parent seeking to enforce the laws against disability discrimination and assuring disability services, each would need to conduct him or herself like Caesar's wife, walking upright, and always above suspicion. And, before they chose to engage me to represent them, we would talk about a plan for what to do, and what to say, when the child abuse investigator's knock came to their family door.

In another of the cases upon which Curt and I would work together representing the parents of a young boy with severe autism, we found ourselves headed to court to obtain a statewide injunction against the Iowa Departments of Education and Human Services to enjoin the practice of these two entwined arms of the State demanding that parents relinquish their parental rights as the price of the state providing needed services for their child. That injunction was granted, but these retaliatory practices had a way of creeping back again and again out of the darkness of human hearts. As a professional it is difficult to hear and accept a challenge to improve on the services one may feel one has been willing to give a lifetime of ambition to offer. It is hard to meet with — and welcome — what may seem like parental ingratitude.

Chris Foster from Davenport called to report in that same night. She had attended the conference at the Hotel Fort Des Moines that I had passed up. She gave a vivid account of Meg whining to Gerry Gritzmacher about having to incorporate Lovaas therapy at school, as all the participants sat in a circle designed to have everyone look for solutions.

According to Chris, Meg's body language was: *Not me.*

Chris described Gay Doyle's participation as talkative and willing to answer questions. State autism specialist Sue Baker sat stolidly silent the whole time. That offered the two of us a wealth of information about the relative powerlessness of Sue in the presence of Gerry. As a result of her observations, Chris sent Gerry a smoking letter of concern. If I could have stood up and hugged her through the phone, I would have.

Really, I was blessed with good allies — in a battle where now the tide was turning more and more strongly against us.

Sunday afternoon, Gay Doyle echoed all Chris's observations. So, by Monday, I was well and truly riled. "Meg, your remarks in Des Moines at the Parent-Educator conference — which Gay Doyle, Chris Foster and others reported to me — are at such variance with your support after reading *Let Me Hear Your Voice* last school year I am terribly disappointed. Ours was the IEP team that never was a team. No more notes — Ruffin tells me what happens at school now. Donna, please call me."

The Bridgewater autism resource team (ART) issued a bland brochure and a blander second letter of the school year. While they had added a subscription to Dr. Rimland's *ARRI*, as a new Bridgewater library item, and mentioned that Dr. Sallows had spoken at the fall Society meeting, Dot Gordon remained embedded in the team like a worrisome stone. There was a brief announcement that the Autism Society of America national conference would be held in Milwaukee this year in early July.

That sounded like a relaxing summer drive to me.

Meg tried, "Ruffin likes a *Where's Waldo* search book; he really enjoys this. Does, 'no more notes' mean from us, or is that for Donna?" I should have recognized she was offering me a chance to back up and save face, but I was far too hurt by the confirmed reports of her betrayal in Des Moines to see it.

Elaine asked, "Our nursery school needs to know who is picking Ruffin up after school on Wednesday. Public schools are dismissing two hours early, but we are not. If we don't know who is getting him, we will be obligated to send him back on the bus early when the public schools dismiss."

Fine, I thought. The IDEA's promise of transportation was just illusory, but I wasn't prepared to have a court fight about a Wednesday, here and there.

Elaine had more. "Ruffin had problems understanding sharing today. He wanted some big blocks and when the other boy who was playing with them wouldn't give them to him, Ruffin took them. We did work out a way for Ruffin to join the other boys. Otherwise, Ruffin played well with tractors and the boy's bike, pretended he was a cat, and helped make a giant toothbrush with the group."

I wouldn't be in good enough control of myself to attend that evening's school-sponsored parent network meeting. I wouldn't be able to listen and keep my mouth shut. Ruffin didn't seem to be feeling well enough to go anyway. By morning, it was clear Ruffin was sick again, and needed to stay home from school to avoid passing on a runny nose, a little cold.

Donna, and then Lisa showed up, to keep Ruffin from falling out of his routine.

When Ruffin was better and able to return to school, I was still resentful and demanding. "No more notes means no more than necessary for housekeeping from me. Elaine, I will pick Ruffin up from nursery school. Meg, I want to see the charting on Ruffin's IEP goals and objectives, Kim's charting on speech therapy, a progress note from the kindergarten teacher, and all the EYSE critical skills paperwork to prepare for our EYSE IEP meeting. I plan to write a comprehensive settlement letter for Curt to pass to ACSD's attorney so we can get the summer of 1996, and the next school year of 1996-1997 settled, hopefully, without more difficulty of a legal nature."

While Ruffin attended Elaine's class, Donna and I took the opportunity to confer at length. Meg had been upset — by my message in Ruffin's notebook. Donna had offered her own opinion that it sounded like I was more hurt than disappointed. She told Meg she didn't think I wanted to stir up any bad feeling, but, as Ruffin's mother, I couldn't just be everyone's friend. It was part of my role to advocate for Ruffin. Donna had told Meg, "Let it go," and after that Meg had seemed to feel better.

"Well," I told Donna, "I *am* hurt and disappointed, because we seem to be coming up short of Ruffin's IEP goals."

Donna assured me, "Ruffin is happy at school," and then admitted, "but his interactions are not up to par during the kindergarten lunch routine. In kindergarten shared reading, when I stood back a bit to see whether he could just follow along with directions to the group, he only got one item of the worksheet right. He even had to be helped to put his name on his paper.

"Two-step verbal commands are still very difficult for him. He was only able to manage to follow one-step verbal commands today. We need to be looking at how we can help him improve his ability to follow directions addressed to a group. Meg has identified another student as having the same issue and is thinking of working with the two of them together.

"We might need to call Evelyn about what to do, because it is really hard for me to see him struggle with this." I could see tears gathering in the corners of Donna's eyes. I could hear the tears in her voice.

"Ruffin raised his hand for help today — raised it all the way up. He said to the kindergarten teacher, Mrs. Linden, 'I need more directions.' But, you know, without giving her eye contact. Mrs. Linden came over trying to get eye contact from him by cupping Ruffin's face in both hands — she doesn't seem to know about the problems with eye contact in autism. I had to step in to intervene. It was too much. She really embarrassed him."

Back in Meg's classroom, Donna had demonstrated for Meg how Ruffin was unable to manage to follow two-step verbal commands and described exactly how Donna thought Ruffin was going to just sink in public kindergarten next year.

"Meg had a hard time acknowledging that, but she does want something better for Ruffin." Then Meg discussed another student with Donna. That child had failed to integrate into kindergarten successfully.

I thought I knew exactly who Meg had been referring to and nodded.

Donna went on. "The school doesn't want to see Ruffin back in preschool next year. Meg told me today that there are only 17 children enrolled in St. Pat's kindergarten."

"How does she know that?" I asked.

"Didn't you know? Meg's children attend St. Pat's rather than public school."

I thought that spoke volumes, and then, I remembered. "Meg's Catholic, isn't she? Maybe the choice is just religious."

"No, I don't think so," ventured Donna. "At least not entirely."

"What are you saying?" I asked.

"I'm not saying anything, because I haven't heard anything outright. But, you know, Meg's *working* for Miss Hobbs — between a rock and a hard place. Mary Jane, what Meg is saying is that *St. Pat's has only 17 children enrolled in their kindergarten.*"

Donna looked at me as if I seemed dense.

"Okay," I said, "I got that. If you can find a subtle way to let Meg know, let her know, I got her message."

"Good. Then you need to just go snoop around St. Pat's, poke your nose around and see what's going on there."

On Thursday, I wrote, as Ruffin's mother, his advocate, who was still nobody's friend, "Ruffin will go home with Donna today when she is done working so she can transport him to Lisa's for his afternoon work. Due to her new work schedule at TASC, Lisa is no longer able to provide Ruffin's Tuesday and Thursday afternoon transportation and I am out of town this afternoon at EYSE meetings in West Union.

"Sorry, Meg, I have never seen the book *Where's Cupid* in Ruffin's bag or in our home.

"Also, I need IEP charting, EYSE data on critical skills, and Kim's speech and language charting — whatever else will be used as data or information on EYSE ASAP. We need a report from Mrs. Linden and the other kindergarten teachers, the librarians — whoever else works with or sees Ruffin."

Meg replied, evenly, I thought. "We have a misunderstanding. I was not saying you had the *Where's Cupid* book at home — Ruffin was looking at it here and really enjoyed it, so I was just trying to tell you that. It's a picture book with very busy pictures and then each page has a list of things for the kids to search for. It is like the *Where's Waldo* books. There's also a computer game for this. Donna says she has some *Where's Waldo* so you can see what they're like. Sorry for the miscommunication."

Still struggling with my own resentment, I had lit into Meg. "I know what a *Waldo* hidden figure book is. People with autism have a superior ability and great fascination with finding hidden figures. *Of course,* Ruffin loves it . . . like he loves string . . . and tying all the door pulls and doorknobs together.

"The most serious miscommunication we have is that I have no response to my EYSE data requests.

"It was highly inappropriate of Miss Hobbs to have called Dee Ann Wilson about your part in Gerry Gritzmacher's presentation at the Parent-Educator conference. It was extremely destructive to have put out that scenario of the 'Lovaas problem' without presenting the many solutions which parents and cooperative professionals have come up with to solve it. That presentation was *poisonous* and *outdated*. It hurt me and my advocacy efforts. It hurt you. It will hurt lots of little children with autism.

"I spent a recent morning negotiating a solution without a fight for EYSE for a young girl with autism in North Fayette. Why can't *that* be presented? *That* be modeled?"

Donna and I conferred again at length Thursday afternoon. Miss Hobbs had called her into the office that morning to offer Donna feedback, being very pleased with her work. Mrs. Linden had reported she enjoyed having Donna in her room. Miss Hobbs had wanted to know when Donna thought she would be done working with Ruffin, and would Donna then be available to work at school?

Their conversation had taken another odd turn when Miss Hobbs asked what color she should consider painting her house. To Donna, it had begun to seem like a tentative job interview, including a painting job for Kevin on the side.

Miss Hobbs wanted Donna's opinion, "What do you foresee for Ruffin?"

Donna told her, "He's come along way. He's working hard, but he still needs help to fully develop. He works so hard. He deserves all the help he needs to make it all the way back. Into the mainstream. That's just what I think, what Mary Jane believes, and what Evelyn expects."

Then, Miss Hobbs had gone on to probe Donna's background growing up, and her education and feelings.

I asked Donna, "Does she, does the school want to hire you to work with Renee? Go ahead, maybe take all this at face value, as good. Not negative." I felt momentarily hopeful.

"No," said Donna. "No, Miss Hobbs wanted to know how it is you and I, such different women, ever became friends."

I had to admit that didn't sound good. "So, what did you tell her?" I asked. And I was curious, myself, too, to hear what Donna might have told Miss Hobbs.

"I told her you bought a house from me and Kevin."

Then Miss Hobbs had asked, "So, what credentials did you have that Mary Jane wanted to hire you to work with Ruffin?"

"'I was interested,' that's what I told Mary Jane. Interested in Ruffin and interested in autism and in being trained. And I told her about my work up in LaCrosse doing overnight supervision at the group home for St. Francis.'"

"And was that it?" I asked.

"No," said Donna. "Later on, in the morning, Meg gave me a copy of a scenario presented at some conference down in Des Moines, the one she went to. She said to me, 'This is how I feel.'

"Over the last couple of days, Meg and I have had quite a bit of discussion about the virtues of Lovaas's methods, about whether any drills are still necessary for Ruffin. Meg admits drills are necessary for teaching Renee."

"Okay," I said. "All this will help me, you know, advocate for Ruffin."

"I know," said Donna. "I think I need to take tomorrow off."

CHAPTER FORTY SIX

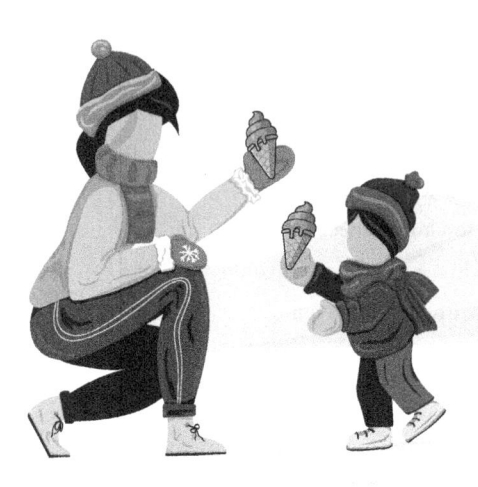

PLAYING HOOKY!

I called the school nurse the first Friday in March, the first day of the spring IEP-EYSE planning season. Ruffin wouldn't be in school. We were going out of town on business. Donna needed to take the day off, too. She wouldn't be in either.

Ruffin and I were going to West Union, to meet with Ray DeNeve, who had toys for him to play with quietly in the Bridgewater office there while I attended EYSE meetings for parents from our support group. An antique store in town sold excellent ice cream we could enjoy afterwards. Ruffin and I were going to play hooky!

That afternoon, I called Bridgewater's Dan Cooper who would be taking Ruffin's case over from Inge for his kindergarten year. I proposed what I thought might be appropriate for Ruffin's 1996 EYSE and placement for the 1996-1997 school year at St. Pat's. Our conversation, which was cordial, became the subject of an early March letter-for-the-record to Curt and Ruffin's educators.

Ruffin attended Sunday school and drew a picture of a spotted giraffe, a blue one, with a *Charlotte's Web* spider and a spotted sheep — all of them captured behind the bars of a zoo, also a picture of houses with steps and doors, under clouds and the sun, with faces looking out of every window, another picture of fences and roadways with their stoplights, and a person crossing the street in front of a stopped car with two faces in the car's windows. I was pleased to see all the faces at all the windows, all the people. Together, he and I did the finger play, from my own childhood, "*Here is the church, and here is the steeple. Open the doors and see all the people!*"

Chris Foster called from Davenport with the news that she had invited Bernie, yes, Dr. Rimland from San Diego, to come speak in early June in Moline, just across the Mississippi. The Society of the Quad Cities would sponsor his visit. No need to think about it. I wanted to meet Bernie, and to thank him in person. Ruffin and I would plan to make the six-hour round trip. Chris and Mike wanted Ruffin to meet Noah.

"Consider it a date," I said.

"Stay overnight, then, at our house," Chris offered.

There was a carnival that afternoon at the senior high, but it would be noisy. Ruffin and I could skip it. Seamus came over. He had landed the job to be St. Pat's maintenance man and custodian. So, we went back over summer plans for Ruffin and our tentative decision to send him to St. Pat's for kindergarten.

My written to-do list for Monday amounted to well over two dozen items, including finalizing EYSE plans for summer services for several North Fayette children with autism, corresponding with Prudential, billing my legal clients, attending an arraignment in court, writing to an attorney I had engaged to try to get my name removed from the child abuse registry, discussing Dr. Hagen's latest EYSE rule memo with Ray DeNeve, scheduling to meet with the St. Pat's school board about Ruffin's admission to kindergarten, walking Gay Doyle through Ruffin's theory of mind drills and listening to how she might adapt them for her own older daughter, getting Donna and Lisa paid, ordering Ruffin's and my tickets to hear Bernie speak, and calling several parent-attorney contacts around the country.

But, first, I brought Curt up to date on Ruffin's case — where I had no business representing Ruffin and myself. It was a smoking letter marshalling all the difficulties of this school year's shotgun marriage. I "doubted if a face-to-face meeting between Donna, Miss Hobbs, Meg, and the others would be fruitful or team-like."

I told Inge as much, too, when she returned my call.

Curt called to ask again for my best evidence that Ruffin had autism. Here we were, treading the same ground again. Catherine had written about her daughter Ann-Marie, "To a casual observer she now looked perfectly normal. They thought it helpful to diminish and downplay whatever problem I was rattling on about. On the other hand, their attitude inspired a certain defensive paranoia in me. Did they think I had made it all up? Yes, life is very boring on the housewife-mommy track. Maybe I'll con a few neurologists and psychiatrists and various other professionals into diagnosing my daughter as autistic. Create a little excitement around here."

Donna and I had a running joke that reflected our mutual acknowledgement of my own continuing anxiety in the face of Ruffin's diagnosis and fragile progress.

"You must be suffering from Munchausen by proxy." It was something Donna had seen in a movie on television.

"Yes," I said, the first time she had mentioned it. "It's a real thing. In the medical dictionary and as a plot artifact, you know, in *fiction!* I think it must be *vanishingly rare* in the world of real people here in our town."

"It must be as *rare* as Ruffin's *vanishing autism,* then," wisecracked Donna, and I cracked up on cue.

"I'm sorry, that is *not* really hilarious."

After pointing Curt to the early October letter signed by every member of Ruffin's re-evaluation team at Gundersen, I also sent him the pre-diagnosis May 1994 video I had originally sent to Dr. Caldwell showing Ruffin's earliest behaviors — toe walking, babbling, spinning of objects, with no attention span, and no functional language.

The written scenario Gerry Gritzmacher had presented with Meg — which Chris Foster, Sue Baker, and Gay Doyle had all attended — seemed to me, and to Curt, to represent a serious breach of the state's obligation to keep confidential matters that mediators had resolved between parents and their local educators.

This called for my writing a follow-up letter to Curt. "Enclosed please find the Gritzmacher Handout. Meg identified Teacher Betty Lou McVey to Donna as representing 'how I feel.' The speech and language pathologist is a dead ringer for Kim Pope, according to Dr. Tristram Smith's report of her comments in a spring 1995 meeting they both attended. The parent couple sound a lot like me.

Ray DeNeve called to follow-up on our recent EYSE meetings about summer services in his sector of Bridgewater. We discussed the possibility of his reaching out to two of Dr. Lovaas's other graduate students, Dr. McEachin and Dr. Leaf and their Autism Partnership for help with appropriate programming for older children with autism.

By then, I knew I could trust Ray and gave him a full heads-up on my re-engaging Curt to represent Ruffin, disclosed the August "hate mail" I had received, the libel threat on Dot Gordon's account, and the January-February child abuse report — because superintendent Charlie Johnson had been involved in the periphery of Evelyn's January visit concerning Ruffin's special education, and been a witness to retaliation in violation of *Section 504 of the Rehabilitation Act* and intentional interference with my relationship as a parent-advocate with other educators, including Donna.

Ray seemed both sympathetic, and unsurprised.

As the last sheet of the workday passed through the fax machine, Ruffin blasted in the door, trailing his book bag.

"Whoa, there, little buddy," I called. "I'll need to see that. Don't be dragging it upstairs just yet." Ruffin handed it over, and stomped upstairs to get ready for Lisa, to pull out a few of his favorite drill boxes and stack them up for her beside her chair.

Ruffin had brought home a nursery school worksheet — a matching task, tying soap to washing his face, toothbrush and toothpaste to brushing his teeth, and a comb and brush to brushing his hair, and his own magazine cut-outs of food items, pasted onto a brown paper grocery bag — lots of meats, which was surprising — since he still didn't eat many meats.

Meg had written, "I am gathering and collating the EYSE data. I will send it as soon as I can. I will need the home program data and charting, also." No problem, I thought. We just love shoveling data around here. Mrs. Wonderlich's junior high school volunteers would have something more to copy before they left for the day.

I got a call from Inge's secretary late that afternoon to let me know she would call me before the close of business. Donna and I conferred again waiting for Inge's call. There was a whole lot of shaking going on, a lot of fallout today from what I had written in the home-school notebook. Meg had come back to the classroom from the office furious, with Ruffin's notebook in her hand, wanting to know *how I had known* Miss Hobbs had called our state mediator Dee Ann Wilson to have Meg contribute to the conference scenario.

"I think *you* told me," Donna told Meg, and took Ruffin to the small corner of Meg's classroom behind a curtain where she was accustomed to work with him.

Ruffin himself had an up and down day according to Donna, wanting to go to recess, not wanting to go to kindergarten reading so much, being pokey, and then he had spat his food out at lunch. The other children had reacted to Ruffin's misbehavior.

Ruffin had told Donna all about our planned vacation.

"Yes," I admitted to Donna. "I need a break. I think I need my Mommy."

"Everybody is really stressed out," sighed Donna. "We all need this winter to be over."

I wrote Meg the next day, cranking up the heat. "You cannot identify 'critical skills' for EYSE consideration without my participation. There is no way to correct this procedural error now. As I told Inge at Bridgewater yesterday, I am willing to take EYSE in settlement of Ruffin's compensatory claim for 9 weeks of failed Head Start integration in the fall. Your attorney should be getting a letter today. Please send our old home-school notebook back to me tonight."

I also sent a letter to remind Miss Hobbs, "What is your present estimate of kindergarten class size for Ruffin's class now that kindergarten roundup is complete? Please let me know."

Then, I walked across Main Street to our support group meeting for some late morning pizza. I needed some support. Several of my clients, parents from Ray's sector, were there, reporting what each of their children would be receiving this summer as services, to encourage the rest of us.

"You just need to go *ask*."

I made a note to myself to tell Ray what a real difference his work was making.

But then I found out. Ray was way ahead of me. When Donna and I touched base that afternoon she told me *Ray* had just offered her a position to work with two of the youngsters with autism in his sector, as a behavioral troubleshooter. They would need to negotiate terms and salary. Donna was concerned it was a long, hilly drive south to North Fayette, but Meg had worked for Ray before and had nice things to say about him and would work for him again in a New York minute.

"I think you're sitting in the catbird's seat," I said to Donna, who was laughing with me. "You could be the subject of a bidding war between Ray and Miss Hobbs as early as this summer."

It was true. With Evelyn's training and her experience over time, Donna had achieved the status of a valuable resource.

But Donna's news about Ruffin's day had not been the best. Ruffin had balked a couple of times at doing harder tasks related to his learning some rudimentary concepts of time: today, yesterday, and tomorrow. He complained, "It's too hard for me to think. I don't want to." These time markers would prove to be very difficult for Ruffin to master.

In Meg's classroom, Ruffin had wanted to play chase and float down to the level of his favorite special education buddy. At lunch he had gone to sit next to one of his playgroup friends from early last summer, and the two of them had enjoyed a very social conversation — until they got into a fight over the ketchup. To me, this sounded wonderfully normal for a couple of 4-year-olds, but Donna seemed worried. Afterwards, Ruffin ate well, but became quiet and withdrawn. He refused to talk to Donna about yesterday, today, or tomorrow, and then relented. He just seemed tired and unfocused.

"Yes," I remembered. "He had some breakthrough babbling again last night."

Donna responded, "He was babbling in kindergarten shared reading, yesterday, talking to himself."

That was not good, I thought to myself. And then I was worried, too.

Inge called again, and I unloaded. "Why not have Curt just negotiate with Caron about what we might agree to do for Ruffin this summer and next year for kindergarten? It is going to be difficult for me to have to attend and participate in a face-to-face meeting that probably includes the people who sent me "hate mail" last August, just after mediation." I didn't have to explain that to Inge. She remembered it well enough from our mid-winter inclusion kerfuffle.

"I don't know who would have written that," she ventured.

"I'm not asking you who did, Inge. I'm not sure I ever want to know."

"It was totally inappropriate."

"Yes," I echoed, in the flattest tone I could summon. "It was totally inappropriate."

Then I rolled on into how I didn't really appreciate the school interfering with my employment of Donna. I explained to Inge how Donna had been feeling ill-used and pressured all fall and in January, had been importuned to go out drinking with the girls, a really unwelcome social invitation as far as Donna was concerned, and then seemed to have been called down to the office to be interviewed for a job next year as a classroom aide by Miss Hobbs.

"Maybe this is all standard small-town stuff, but as far as I'm concerned, it needs to stop. And Miss Hobbs should not be offering to have Donna's husband paint her house during these sorts of trips down to the office at school. She can find his business number in the phone book. If Miss Hobbs wants her house painted, she needs to call Kevin directly on business, and just keep Donna and Ruffin and me out of it."

Inge was quiet, listening, and unresponsive. Maybe she didn't consider all this quite as outrageous as I did. Maybe this sort of thing happened all the time at school. I wasn't there. What did I know?

In the face of her silence, I took another tack. "We might need to go back to mediation and get some help."

"We might," echoed Inge. To me, her voice sounded weak.

"Dee Ann might think Ruffin *doesn't* qualify for EYSE under the new rules, but she won't be pleased that the school failed to provide him with the first semester of the agreed-upon Head Start integration that was a part of our negotiated agreement last August. She won't be pleased the school waited a whole semester to let me discover that failure. Surely, she will consider Ruffin entitled to some 'compensatory education' for the loss of services we had all agreed last August he needed."

More silence from Inge.

"I think 3 hours a day, 3 days a week of playgroup and 4 hours a day 5 days per week of CARD drills would be fair compensation and would meet Ruffin's needs this summer. Otherwise, I am prepared to have Curt help me go to mediation, or to a formal due process hearing."

"We still need to have his IEP meeting this spring," said Inge.

"I know. I remember, Mr. Montague told me the first day I spoke to him, 'We like to have these meetings in the spring.' Please invite Mrs. Linden, Ruffin's kindergarten shared reading teacher. She told Donna in December that he will need a one-to-one aide in public school kindergarten next year, in her class.

"Evelyn thought when she met with us in January that what Ruffin needs is just a smaller class size of 15. That would be a less restrictive placement than saddling him with the embarrassment of a special aide. Why couldn't the public schools pay tuition for Ruffin to attend kindergarten at St. Pat's where classes that size are available? If we all agreed to leave Ruffin's weighting at 3.6, the public schools could pocket nearly $13,000 next year after paying St. Pat's paltry yearly tuition of $710."

"I don't think we've ever done that," Inge explained.

"Well, here's the thing," I said. "There's a wonderful story my favorite trial attorney Gerry Spence tells about trying a murder case in Oregon. He was proposing to try something a little different in the courtroom, when the Oregon prosecutor stood up and objected that 'Mr. Spence may do that sort of thing where he comes from in *Wy*-oming, but that's not the way we do it in *Or*-e-gon,' and then the judge, who was interested and intrigued, ruled, 'You're right, that's *not* the way we've done it in Oregon, but that's the way we're *gonna* do it.'

"Look, Inge, if we can't find a way to agree on Ruffin's being placed at St. Pat's, I am prepared to have Curt file a federal lawsuit to address the school's violations of the IDEA and the *Americans with Disabilities Act*, as evidenced — right there in black and white — in the terms of the nursery school contract I discovered in Ruffin's file on Valentine's Day, and to address any *Section 504* retaliation the judge *might* find the school has taken against me as an advocate for Ruffin and other children with autism during the school's handling of a child abuse report, and repeated requests for a physical therapy evaluation in mid-January."

"What's all that about?" asked Inge.

"O dear, you're really out of the loop here."

And then, I found a brief way to explain all that.

"Inge, Inge, Inge," I wailed, "I would really, really like all these matters of Ruffin's future education settled by the end of March because Ruffin and I plan to be gone the first two weeks in April, to visit Ruffin's grandparents for his birthday."

Inge responded very quietly, "It's good to know that."

Inge was a messenger. I wanted to be sure, before Ruffin and I left for North Carolina, that I had done all I could do to send my message.

Then I saw Meg had written to me, "Head Start visited. Notebook coming today." I fished out both our new and our older home-school notebooks and handed them to one of Mrs. Wonderlich's startled volunteers. I realized she must have been eavesdropping — not the right word — she couldn't have helped but overhear me — all the while I was on the phone to Inge.

"Could you please make a copy of these for Curt?" I asked.

"Sure, no problem."

"Be careful," I said. "What you are copying there could turn out to be evidence."

"It's important, then?"

"Yes," I smiled, "Very."

"I think I understand. This is important for Ruffin."

"Yes," I said again, and lifted the heels of my hands to the wet corners of my eyes and let her see I was crying.

I wrote Meg again on Wednesday for the record. "This is the second night in a row that Ruffin has stayed awake babbling. He may be tired again today. Ruffin and I will be on family vacation, leaving in late March for two weeks, so summer programming for Ruffin needs to be addressed this month so I have meaningful appeal rights. North Fayette district has already completed all their EYSE meetings."

Seamus dropped by with the paper. It was clear the school board was focused on building a new high school if they could manage to pass a bond issue. We were about to take the issue up when another parent-attorney interrupted us with a call. She thought she would be able to slip into a school district attorney training conference to be held in Florida and report back over *The Me-List* about a presentation on how to defeat parent requests that districts provide Lovaas programming. That made me happy.

That afternoon, I conferred again with Donna. Ruffin had asked her, "Will you tell me about your day?" It had taken Donna aback, put her right back on her heels in surprise. It was the first time he had ever made a personal inquiry about her or evidenced any interest in her life apart from their own day-to-day interactions.

"I think you are feeling the same sense of dislocation I felt back that first year in late November, the first time Ruffin told me, 'I love you.' Sometimes, until you hear him say it the first time, you have no idea what's been missing, what's still odd about him."

"Oh," that reminded Donna of something else. "In kindergarten shared reading, Mrs. Linden is mostly handing out worksheets now about phonics. Ruffin is really having problems with bringing up that sort of information. Next year, his teacher will need to know to wait for Ruffin to talk, that it might take him a little longer than other kids to really respond. But whoever his new teachers are, they really need to wait to let him try to answer and be willing to watch him think it through."

Then, after a pause, "And he's still not eating everything served for lunch."

"What do you think the problem is?" I asked.

Donna laughed, "I think sometimes — not every day — school lunch is just terrible."

"Yeah, I think I remember that. It must be true everywhere. You know, sometimes."

Donna returned to the most important issue, "The most difficult thing is Ruffin just loses focus and needs help, a reminder — several dozen times a day — to refocus. It's obvious. Mrs. Linden and Meg both know this is a problem for him. This is not how other kindergarteners are, and Ruffin's almost five now. Meg knows it is still difficult for Ruffin to learn whatever is being offered to a larger group. Behind our curtain, in our corner, he and I are working well on his theory of mind drills. That is going well."

After another pause, Donna reminded me, "Poor Meg. She's crazy busy. She has five IEP meetings scheduled between now and Monday, lots of notes to sort through."

"Well, Elaine let me know Ruffin met all his integration objectives today by playing tractors, balls, and wagons with varying small groups, and that in her class today they made butter, working in small groups by putting whipping cream in a jar and taking many turns shaking the jar until the cream churned. Then, they ate it!"

"Ruffin must have liked that."

"No doubt. Elaine's little class seems to be going well. It's not like kindergarten shared reading. It's a small group and the kids there are all his same age."

"I hear good things about Ruffin from Elaine whenever I happen to run into her."

"Good, all good. We can let well enough alone there then."

To follow up on our recent conversations about her daughter, on Thursday I sent Gay Doyle an article from Dr. Rimland's newsletter, *"Intervention: It doesn't need to be early,"* and some of the materials described in it from Dr. McEachin and Dr. Leaf of The Autism Partnership, including an announcement that Dr. Leaf would be speaking in Wisconsin, in mid-April about Lovaas-type interventions for older children, and "recent correspondence from Dr. Simon Baron-Cohen about his view of Lovaas's approach, the use of his own CHAT to screen for autism at 18 months, and the underlying research by Francesca Happe about theory of mind deficits in high functioning autism and Asperger's cases, together with Ruffin's set of theory of mind CARD drills — which seem to be working well for him."

I explained, "I think doing theory of mind exercises very early on would improve a child's ability to make more flexible use of Social Stories, Carol Gray's program, and other conventional social skills curriculum. Without a working appreciation of theory of mind, the more sophisticated conventional curriculum would be expected to fail or be adopted too rigidly."

Then, because I needed to know, I asked her, "Could you check and tell me again exactly when in early January you talked to Ruffin on the phone?"

I sent a similar letter to Ray DeNeve, since he was serving several older children in our support group who could benefit. As I was offering instructions to copy and assemble these mailings to our arriving volunteers, the phone rang. I was surprised to find myself talking to Gerry Gritzmacher.

"Tom McLaughlin in Norwalk is interested in running a Lovaas home program there. Could he call you to talk? I can't handle every call now about Lovaas. I have taken the assignment to manage our statewide efforts in autism now that we have this crisis of demand. I am going to be responsible for autism next year, going to keep the autism advisory committee chairmanship, and direct some parent-advisory responsibility to Linda Cronk."

"She's a really good egg," I laughed, "Much easier to work with than *moi,*" slipping into the little French I could remember from high school. "And I'd be delighted to *parley* with Tom. Just give me his full name and spell it, so I recognize him when he calls, and don't bite his head off."

Then, I let Gerry know I had re-engaged Curt to represent Ruffin and me and laid out in some detail the court action I had described earlier to Inge. I went right up to the edge of complaining about his thinly-veiled scenario of a presentation of Ruffin's and my dispute he had mediated with our school district — that he had trotted out recently with Meg in front of Chris Foster and Gay Doyle at The Hotel Fort Des Moines.

I didn't have to go all the way there before he offered me his apology.

"Apology accepted. But just don't think I'm sitting up here in the far northeast corner of the state, all snowed-in, and isolated. Understand, we parents are connected, all over the state, all over the country and, for heaven's sake, internationally, over the internet, and we are monitoring what schools do, and what they fail to do. Okay, now, have Tom call me. I'll do you a favor and talk to him, and we'll send him a great box of stuff. And watch your mail, you know, I'll be writing you, too."

Our volunteers assembled a package for a mother in Algona who was also seeking summer services (EYSE) for her child with autism there in far northwest Iowa.

A member of our autism support group, and organizer of our auditory integration training experiment of last summer called me. Her son's special education teacher had been warned by the administration to watch what he said to her. The turmoil around us seemed both palpable and pathetic.

Having completed all the EYSE meetings in the North Fayette district, I wrote to Ray DeNeve at Bridgewater, to each parent, and to each principal. "Enclosed please find my bills for advocacy services for six students with disabilities. These detailed billings are at my accustomed rates to reflect the market value of my professional services — but I have reduced the rate of each bill to $25 per hour — as I would reduce my rates for personal friends, family members, and to reflect my own and the parents' appreciation for settlements which have or may occur at the IEP meeting level."

In all my earlier discussions and correspondence with parents, I had represented that I would not seek payment from any of them, but made clear before sending confidentiality releases to any of them who had requested help or information, that I would prefer to assume the risk that payment would be conditioned upon their achieving some success in improving programming for their children, and then seeking payment from the school authorities as provided by the IDEA.

Having explained this now to the schools, I wrote, "Accordingly, please consider the reduced bills as claims for reimbursement from the AEA and/or the appropriate local school districts. My services to these children have been of real value to them and to the school authorities serving them. I ask that they be paid for — as is only fair to Ruffin and myself.

"In considering these claims for payment, you might want to consider the enclosed 1988 publication by Iowa's ALJ, Carl Smith, particularly the highlighted passage with respect to providing fair compensation to parent-advocates and consultants.

"With respect to the two cases which remain unresolved, should the matter of a free, appropriate public education (FAPE) go to due process, the bills for services to them reflect the degree of exposure the local school district and the AEA will be subject to at my accustomed rates — if due process hearing becomes necessary."

These were the same terms upon which Curt had handled his own claims for fees last August when he represented Ruffin and me at mediation. My letter about my claims for fees produced prompt agreements with their school districts for these two children's parents, as well.

According to her work diary, Gay Doyle had talked to Ruffin on the phone January 9th at 5:00 in the afternoon, and then called me back the next morning, January 10th. I was glad to have those dates nailed down to pass on to the attorney who would be trying to get my name removed from the child abuse registry.

A long discussion with Gay ensued about the ins and outs of her efforts to secure insurance coverage for her daughter, and a longer discussion about "recovery" and the openly skeptical position of Gerry Gritzmacher on that subject. If "recovery" or optimal outcomes from autism were possible in the academic literature from California and the "Maurice" family in New York, I thought similar results ought not to be impossible in Iowa.

When Ruffin arrived home, Meg reminded me it had been sweatshirt day. I had forgotten that — not that Ruffin had any great number of sweatshirts. One of the first things I had read about parenting a child with autism, or any disability, had been how important it was to attend to a child's grooming, and to dress him or her nicely, so other people would see a person who was valued and cared for, and be more inclined themselves to offer care and respect. Except for his tiny overalls, which he wore to the farm with Seamus, Ruffin's clothes were the nicest his grandparents and I could afford.

Ruffin went to Sunday school where he colored his worksheet about the four seasons. At home that afternoon he drew pictures of a blustery day with wind and snow blowing around a tall four-story house — then another of just the wind, snow and clouds, writing, 'I love you' front and back on the paper which he brought me for his refrigerator gallery.

CHAPTER FORTY SEVEN

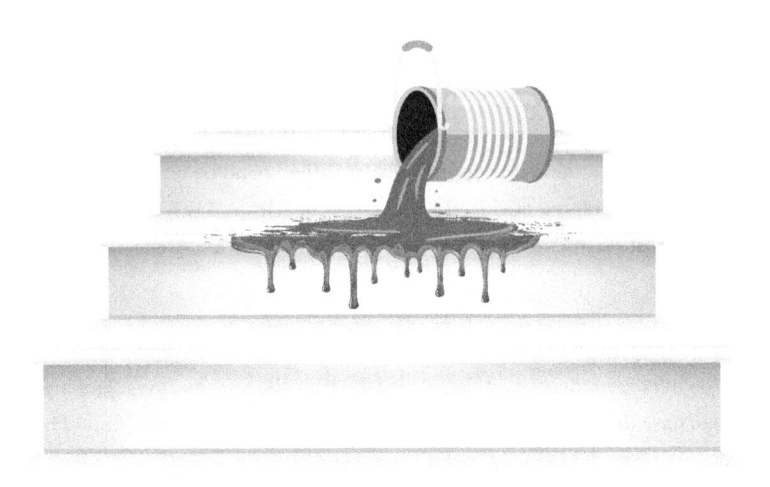

A BUCKET OF BLOOD

I met with the St. Pat's school board about Ruffin's admission to kindergarten Monday evening at the rectory. They seemed ready to welcome him, and Evelyn or Donna, if need be, should there be any behavioral problems, but based on principal Peter Smith's seeing Ruffin this year around the building, and given Elaine's good reports about his readiness, it didn't seem there would be any.

At home, Donna told me Ruffin had done terrific work. She had stepped back to receptive teaching on the concepts of "before and after," and then "yesterday and tomorrow." Ruffin responded by getting angry, saying to Donna, "I can do this."

They made up a clock game.

Then, Donna had Ruffin do some thinking about watching the weatherman on television.

"See the man in the small television — what do you think about it?"

"Get a wire and get the man out of the television," proposed Ruffin, a bit over focused on the mechanical.

At that point, Donna had asked him, "*You* ever been on television?"

Bang, and the light went on for Ruffin, "I was on a tape." Videotape brought it all together for Ruffin, by drawing on his own experience.

Meg had witnessed this little teaching moment. She had come over to test Ruffin on his IEP objectives.

"Wow," Meg exclaimed. "Didn't that really work? That might have been hard to teach before videotape."

Then Donna watched Meg do her own review testing. Ruffin stayed on target, but for items Donna saw Ruffin miss, Donna thought the problem was Meg's presentation was not clean or clear enough, and that Ruffin *knew* he didn't need to work hard to please her. Meg offered Ruffin too many escapes and rescues without holding him accountable.

It was true. Donna was imaginative, resourceful, and *tough*. Ruffin usually rose to the occasion with her. He was also responding well to a new statement-statement drill which required him to respond with an on-topic statement in response to a topic Donna opened for conversation.

Then, Miss Hobbs had come to Meg's classroom and had a conversation with Meg out of Donna's earshot — the two of them were talking, but not sharing any information. The most Donna had heard was the school would be sending me information for Ruffin's 1996-1997 IEP goals, and that "theory of mind" tasks would be included.

Joan called the next day to tell me Curt felt I had legitimate concerns that needed to be addressed promptly, so my early March letter to him would be going by overnight mail delivery to Caron so she could offer advice to Ruffin's educators.

A mother from Cincinnati, Ohio, called for insurance information. That got the volunteers busy. Then, a brain surgeon from New Jersey called to discuss beginning a Lovaas program for her child. I provided her with all our New Jersey contacts, and the volunteers prepared a box to mail out. A father from Chicago called for the same reason. I provided him with our Illinois contacts, and had the volunteers prepare a box for him, too. Another mother from West Des Moines called for the same reason. I provided her with all our Iowa contacts, and the volunteers prepared a box for her, too.

For our upcoming EYSE meeting, whenever that might be, I began working on a review of Ruffin's IEP goals, to see which goals he had met at home, in Meg's class, and at the private nursery school. Since we had no classmates at home, I couldn't speak to his interaction with them, but otherwise, Ruffin seemed to have met all his IEP goals at home — except he had yet to master the concepts of "before" and "after" or "event sequence recall from life," "yesterday, today, and tomorrow," "asking how questions," and "answering why one would feel a certain emotion," but these were emerging in his repertoire.

From the reports I had gotten, it sounded to me like Ruffin was not a behavior problem in either school, but there were significant problems with his understanding oral directions given to a group for seat work or oral response, and significant problems recently with self-stimulatory behaviors and stress.

Most of Donna's efforts during late November, December, and January had been devoted to pre-teaching the kindergarten shared reading curriculum so Ruffin could join his classmates by printing his name on his paper, doing seat work without "cheating" from another child's paper, and manage to get something out of his mainstream integration experience.

Mid-March, I let Meg know my schedule, and asked, "How did Ruffin do at kindergarten lunch and kindergarten library without an aide, or did he have one?" She had responded, "Ruffin went to guidance for a lesson with Duso the Dolphin about trying hard to stick to what you believe." That made me laugh out loud. Sticking to what he believed was hardly Ruffin's issue. He was *perseverative*. It might even be something he had learned at home or had inherited from me. Perseverance was the last lesson Ruffin, or I, needed guidance on!

Now, stop, and read on, I told myself.

"Ruffin got splashed at the Luther pool — didn't like it but was okay. He also took a shower and put his head under it. Did great! Mixed-up Day — clothes that clash, backwards — here."

O, dear, I thought to myself. You need to get with this casual Friday thing somehow. It had *never* been a thing in court, just not a part of my world.

The Link's spring issue arrived. There was one interesting passage: "Reduced class size in the regular education classroom. Most regular education teachers perceive class size as an issue of concern if they are expected to provide adequate support for the instructional and behavioral needs of students with autism. The preferred class size indicated by regular educators ranged from 15 to 19 students." That struck me as right on target with Dr. Granpeesheh and Evelyn's recommendations for Ruffin in next year's kindergarten.

Ruffin was absent the next Monday with a croupy cough he picked up watching the St. Patrick's Day parade that had streamed for hours past our front porch over the weekend. He and Seamus had been thrilled by the horses, the large teams of Percherons and Clydesdales, the little ponies dragging carts, the fancy quarter horses and rodeo rough stock, the fire engines and antique tractors and huge mechanical threshers like giant metal grasshoppers, the antique cars carrying the Dairy Queen and her princesses, the Pork Queen and her retinue, the local ladies and businessmen throwing out hard candy, chocolates, and cheese sticks onto the sidewalk. Ruffin had gone down the porch steps to gather his share.

Someone had offered Ruffin a kitten from a basket, which he had already taken to heart before I could get down from the porch. Now, we were blessed with a third cat, a long-haired grey one who looked to be too young to be away from its mother, seemed flea-bitten, and already mangy with ringworm. Ruffin had named him, concretely enough, as *Little Kitten*. He would be with us for over twenty years.

When I asked Ruffin what happened at school now, I did *not* get a litany answer of this, then, then, then, but got a very natural response. "So-and-so got sick and had to go home. She threw up on the floor and on someone's shirt. That little boy had to get a new shirt."

Also, I got lots of talk about Ruffin dreaming, using "books inside my head," and thinking. When I told Ruffin I couldn't see inside his head, Ruffin responded, "I can tell you and then you can think it the same."

Ruffin was also using paper and markers asking me to spell out words for him to write. He wrote *all* his letters by drawing their shapes — not necessarily by using the correct strokes. He wanted to label his house made of blocks with a sign, "Building for a Story," and asked how to spell "I love you" for his letters to my parents and his cousin Robert. He pointed these out to visitors and was pleased that they will "read it the same."

Ruffin was counting the days to vacation without being confused by the calendar day numbers. He asked to call my mother and talked back and forth with her for several minutes, recalling past events with her and planning future events at the beach. Donna's "yesterday, today, and tomorrow" drills had been helpful to him. I was hearing Ruffin use "yesterday" spontaneously to refer to the past, and "a long time ago" to refer to the more distant past.

Still, little red flags appeared on the horizon. Meg thought it would reassure me that Bridgewater's assistant director "'Moe' said yesterday he had had reports that Ruffin was doing very well." I was surprised since there had been *no record* in Ruffin's files of anyone communicating with Mr. Mosher as of mid-February when I had reviewed it.

Who was talking to "Moe" and where was that record?

"Elaine, Ruffin has been coughing and needs to stay out of the wind, but he also needs to keep mentally busy. If you can't keep him in for recess, call me and I'll come and get him, or come and stay in with him during recess. I am happy to have all the make-up days. Ruffin is reporting what others are bringing for show and tell.

"Meg, enclosed are the school's copies of all our CARD Therapy Notes. Signed notes are final notes. Unsigned notes are draft notes. Donna's notes from November to February reflect the intrusion into his CARD program of pre-teaching kindergarten shared reading worksheets, and the effect of the Head Start integration failure of the first semester.

"Where is the identification of critical skills paperwork? Where is the charting of critical skills?

"When is the EYSE meeting about Ruffin? Where is the IEP charting, Kim's charting, Mrs. Linden's report, the kindergarten library report, and when will I get them? *At the meeting is too late. I need this data in advance.*"

Meg replied, "I didn't get copies made today, but will send them tomorrow. You should be getting a letter today about an EYSE meeting. I think the date will be in late March."

Miss Hobbs *had* written me a letter dated March 12th, which arrived in the mail finally, after more than a week. "Your child, Ruffin, has been identified as potentially eligible to receive certain special education services during the summer break. The purpose of a meeting on March 25th is to discuss and plan EYSE services for Ruffin. IEP development for the 1996-1997 school year will take place after his Iowa City evaluation in April."

This was interesting, but not a sufficient meeting notice under the IDEA — since it failed to let me know who might be expected to attend. It would be a fatal procedural error on the part of Ruffin's educators.

But at least Miss Hobbs's letter offered me some indication that Ruffin's educators were getting ready to engage on the issue of summer services and next year's IEP, and that set me right to work — thinking as I did that money would be an issue — oblivious to the fact that my own plans for Ruffin to attend St. Pat's amounted to filing for divorce from my shotgun marriage to the public schools of last August. If Ruffin went on to attend St. Pat's through the eighth grade without an IEP, that divorce could cost his public-school educators $117,000 or more, over time.

I should have known that hurt feelings and disappointments would complicate any real consideration of "the best interests of the child." No, that was the *divorce* standard for the consideration of planning for the future of children — a higher standard than the IDEA standard of what was merely "appropriate to the unique needs of the child" as a student.

It was never *all* about the money, but for Curt to share with Caron I had prepared a balance sheet to show that sending Ruffin to St. Pat's under an IEP as a special education student in a private school placement by mutual agreement — as we were already sending him to Elaine's class — would net his public educators close to $13,000 each year. In the long run, placing Ruffin at St. Pat's looked to me like a win-win situation — Ruffin would have the benefit of an appropriate small class size, and both his public-school education agencies would do well financially.

And, with St. Pat's doing all the educating, the public schools and I would be out of each other's hair.

The next evening, as Ruffin slept, I worked on a chart to summarize Ruffin's progress on his IEP goals across all the environments, teachers, and therapists in his life.

The bus was late the next morning, so I took Ruffin to school. Meg handed me copies of her own charting of Ruffin's progress on his IEP goals.

Earlier that month, Meg had re-charted Ruffin's progress on *The Brigance*, marking him at above 5 years — often at 6 years or 7 years — on all his motor skills and behaviors, all his self-help skills, his general knowledge and comprehension, with the sole exception of the time concepts where she marked him as having about a 6-month delay, at 4 years, 6 months.

Meg considered him kindergarten ready in math, and even in most of his language skills. Interestingly, she marked him as most like a 7-year-old in knowing what to do in different situations, as a 6-year-old in knowing the function of various community helpers like policemen and firemen, and as a 6-year-old in knowing where to go for help.

But she herself had nothing from Kim about speech, or from Mrs. Linden about kindergarten, and nothing more to offer me.

Since there was yet another early out for teacher in-service, I went back over to school to pick up Ruffin again early in the afternoon. As Ruffin was pulling on his coat and boots, I fished out our notebook and saw Meg had written, "I've told Kim you need her papers. You'll have to call Bridgewater if you don't have them. The papers you have are what we use to determine proficiency in skills. Not sure what else you want."

This was both unresponsive and unacceptable. Ruffin and I stayed behind and waited as all the other children were bundled up and escorted out the door to meet their buses. I wanted to talk directly to Meg. She could see I was holding our notebook in my hand, and that I was not pleased.

Meg told me she had asked Kim repeatedly for her charting, but so far had nothing.

With Ruffin in hand, I walked the halls until I found Kim and told her I had written to ask for her charting several times in Ruffin's home school notebook. I told her I needed it faxed to me, because I wanted to share her work with Evelyn and Dr. Granpeesheh — since we all had a Monday meeting to discuss his summer services (EYSE).

Kim said she wasn't sure she had anything. She would need to look and get back to me.

I was furious and turned on my heel.

Even Ruffin could tell I was angry and asked, "What's wrong, Mommy?"

Once Ruffin and I got home, I reached out to Inge. She was Ruffin's consultant and case manager. When I brought up Kim's missing records, Inge told me she had gotten a hold of Kim, but not her records.

I was quite frustrated. Finally, I really lost it.

"Inge, I'm tired of doing *your* job, of rounding everything up so we — Evelyn, Dr. Granpeesheh, and I — can prepare for this meeting. You *know* why I don't even want to meet with Ruffin's team on Monday. It really will be a horrible meeting. And, if we don't have all Ruffin's data, it will be *useless*, too."

I was not prepared to go through the rigmarole of spending this spring chasing paper as I had done all last summer.

By now, I was in high dungeon, and warned her.

"You should know, too, what I know. Agency errors and omissions insurance doesn't cover any of you for *intentional* acts of retaliation against me, as Ruffin's advocate. Not to mention *intentional* violations of FERPA. No insurer covers the risk of *human meanness*. If I discover any one of you hold an interest in more than a homestead acre in town or more than forty acres outside town, I will do everything within my power to see that anything else that belongs to any of you is sold on the auction block — after court!"

That evening there was a knock at my door. Inge was there to deliver a thin manila file containing Kim's "Therapy Log."

When I pressed Inge for some information about the school's intentions about summer services (EYSE) plans for Ruffin to be able to pass on to Evelyn and Dr. Granpeesheh for them to weigh in on, Inge said she thought they wanted to consider continuing with CARD and were considering offering a playgroup.

By then, I was able to tell Inge that Curt's office let me know that Caron's position was she would be advising the school to do whatever Evelyn and Dr. Granpeesheh might recommend.

With what Inge had just delivered, I had a long fax that I could send to California — all the information we had gathered about Ruffin's educational progress. I let

Inge know that Evelyn and Dr. Granpeesheh would be meeting that evening about Ruffin.

"Okay, we'll wait to hear from you then," said Inge. She still looked like I had scared the bejesus out of her.

I said I was sorry it had to be like this, and I could tell she could tell that despite my best efforts I didn't feel one bit sorry. I was still upset.

I thought to myself, let her take that message back to the rest of them, and to Caron.

As soon as Inge was out of my driveway and headed down Main Street, I began faxing Dr. Granpeesheh and Evelyn.

"Evelyn: *By 12:00 noon March 25th, 1996,* I need a prescription from Dr. Granpeesheh and you on CARD letterhead for summer services (EYSE) per page two of my March 4th, 1996 letter — with one change — omit the name of RoJene Beard, who is not available, and substitute 'Lovaas Integration Therapist.' These attachments follow: My March 4th letter to Curt Sytsma; My legal notes — two pages; Ruffin's Progress on IEP goals in chart form; Meg's observations of February 9th, at nursery school."

Since the two early February kindergarten roundups, I had been researching IDEA case law concerning special education placements of children with disabilities into private and parochial schools. On these and related legal points, I offered Dr. Granpeesheh and Evelyn a summary of what I had unearthed, stripped of all the technical, legal citations:

If there is no contract between the private school where the student attends and the public school responsible for the child's education, the payment to which the private school is entitled from the public school is governed by the principle of *quantum meruit* — what the education was worth — and the private school is entitled to charge a reasonable tuition for the special education provided.

An appropriate remedy for the violation of a handicapped student's procedural rights under the IDEA is to make available to the student remedial educational services equal in time and scope to what the student would have been given had the regulations been followed.

When the mainstreaming requirement of the IDEA is at issue, the burden of proving compliance with the IDEA is on the school, regardless of which party brings the other to due process.

It has been held that the success of a student classified as gifted in regular education does not preclude his classification as an exceptional student with a specific learning disability so that he is entitled to special education.

It is proper and permissible to consider parental hostility to an IEP as part of the prospective evaluation required by the IDEA of a placement's expected educational benefits, and if the facts show the parents are so opposed to a placement as to undermine its value to the child, the child should be placed elsewhere.

Example: An IEP directing the placement of a child handicapped by a behavioral disorder and learning disability to a private day school, rather than to the alternative public school as recommended, was the least restrictive environment (LRE) that would be of educational benefit to that student, particularly considering the parents' hostility to the district's proposed placement.

A public school district may place a handicapped child in a private school. A handicapped student is properly placed in a private school where such placement is the least restrictive placement from which the student could receive educational benefit.

Unfortunately, in the cold light of morning, as I looked closely, I found, as I let Meg know immediately, "Inge did get me something from Kim last night — a 'Therapy Log.' But I am still missing all the following which are cataloged in her notes: October 11th, Notes regarding results and raw data on *Boehm Test of Basic Concepts*; October 30th, Notes re: results and raw data on *Bohem Test of Basic Concepts*; March 21st, TOLD-2 raw data. I need the description and empirical validation literature norming these tests ASAP before Ruffin's EYSE meeting."

Kim's log, such as it was — a list of activities and dates, bare of any particulars about Ruffin — proved to be disturbing in other respects as well. *"Kim needs to concentrate on the three-part verbal directive with each part having up to two critical elements for the remainder of the school year as all of Ruffin's other speech and language goals are mastered.* This is the memory-planning executive function exercise that Ruffin needs to be working on intensively in as many ways as Kim can set it up.

"Under the IEP, Kim has no call to be doing anything else. *No more sign, please.* If she can do three-part verbal directives with two critical elements from having Ruffin watch videos — great — but I find it difficult to conceive.

"Videos and conversation are available to Ruffin here at our home."

And, I had other FERPA requests I had raised before that were still unaddressed. "I still have nothing on critical skills, or from the kindergarten reading teacher."

That same day, Dr. Granpeesheh faxed, "It is imperative that Ruffin receive services throughout the summer months without interruption. It is appropriate that Ruffin receive the following: 4 hours per day, 5 days per week of one-to-one discrete trial therapy with a trained 'Lovaas' interventionist; 3 hours per day, 3 days per week of a supervised play group led by a trained 'Lovaas' interventionist and 2 afternoons per week in an unstructured play group with normal peers which is monitored by a trained 'Lovaas' interventionist.'"

This represented a total of 20 hours a week of drill, 9 hours a week of supervised play, and 6 hours a week of unstructured monitored play. Dr. Granpeesheh further cautioned that "any interruption of these services may lead to loss of presently acquired skills and as a result could be extremely detrimental to the progress that Ruffin has made in the past 17 months." She had conveyed what she thought in two separate documents, one suitable for his EYSE meeting, and another suitable for his later IEP meeting.

That same morning, the guided missiles of my messages to Inge, Meg, and Kim landed on Caron's desk in Waterloo. Caron called Joan to complain that I had been "threatening people — threatening to sue them and take their homes." Caron thought that I was "impossible," and making "impossible demands." Then, she assured Joan that ACSD, whom she represented and would be continuing to advise, was "planning on providing whatever Mary Jane's experts recommended for her son, Ruffin."

Caron asked that Joan and Curt tell me to "relax."

I told Joan I was pleased to hear that.

Caron must also have been consulting with Mr. Carew, the attorney advising Bridgewater, because Caron had also raised the issue with Joan that I was seeking out parents in the area to represent in special education cases, and that this was not "ethical," since I was representing to parents that my services were free of charge, but as the cases were settled, I had "turned around and charged the school for attorney's fees." Caron claimed that if this was a surprise to the parents I had represented, I could be disbarred for doing this and for advertising myself on the internet.

I told Joan plainly that if Caron and Mr. Carew thought I should be disbarred one of them would already have reported me to the bar association. I hadn't heard from them, and I didn't expect to, because I had all my files representing children with disabilities in Ray's sector of Bridgewater in good order.

Ray had invited me to several of these meetings, and I had entered the circle of special education confidentiality in every case at the written request of each set of parents on condition that they would not be expected to pay me anything as my clients. Ray understood that my loyalty would be to the parents, as my clients.

I had followed Curt's lead by throwing the greater part of my fees into the pot, to help reach each settlement there, and I found it more than a little rich that Caron and Mr.

Carew would be complaining about my reduced hourly rate of $25 an hour when the two of them were charging Ruffin's educators in the multiple hundreds of dollars per hour.

"Why, it probably costs at least a hundred dollars for the two of them to have a phone call with each other about Ruffin!"

There was silence from the other end of the phone, and I wondered whether I had shocked Joan, either with the information or my vehemence.

Then, Joan's voice came back over the line, "We have a letter from Caron to fax you."

Caron had written Curt back by *snail mail*. "We have attempted to reach you, Curt, several times this week by telephone but you have been unavailable. Please be advised that we do not have sufficient information, nor do we believe it prudent to respond to the allegations in Ms. White's letter of March 4th.

"We understand that the IEP meeting is to occur on March 25th, 1996. If Ms. White is unhappy with the outcome of the IEP meeting, we understand that she may take whatever steps are available to her under the law.

"Be advised that, if necessary, the district is committed to defending its personnel and the district from the unjust and unsubstantiated allegations and threats of the parent."

I called Joan back right away — since this was confusing. It was at sixes and sevens with Miss Hobbs's own March 12th letter to me letting me know the schools were *not* planning to have an IEP meeting for Ruffin until *after* the late April evaluation in Iowa City which Bridgewater had promised to pay for in mediation.

Joan said, "I don't understand all that because I wasn't at your mediation, but I'll have Curt call you tonight."

For Meg, it had been another version of casual Friday, Slipper Day — wear your bedroom slippers to class day — with a two-hour early dismissal.

I thought to myself, remembering what Joan and Caron had asked, whatever I thought about all these casual, truncated Fridays, relax, just relax. I found it hard to do. Maybe I was just an irremediable Type A. I knew a lot of trial lawyers were rumored to be that. Or maybe I was just a parent frustrated by unresponded-to FERPA requests. Where was the law when I needed it? Caron knew FERPA as well as I did and had seen to it that it was complied with last summer.

For the night, with Ruffin, I relaxed.

Curt called later that evening, as Joan had promised.

I asked him, "Do I have to go to Ruffin's IEP meeting?"

He assured me, "Whether or not you go, the team must still consider Dr. Granpeesheh's information. They must still provide Ruffin a free, appropriate public education. The issues will be the same."

I told Curt I would think over the weekend about whether I could manage to go to Monday's meeting.

What I didn't tell Curt was what I had been dreaming, repeatedly. It disturbed me.

But over the weekend I told Seamus about it, by asking, "Do you have a little pig or lamb or something you might be planning to butcher?"

"No. Why?" he asked. "Do you need meat?"

"No," I said, "I need blood. A bucket of blood."

"What would you need a bucket of blood for?" he demanded. I saw I had his attention now. "What would you do with it?" He wanted to know.

"I keep waking up at night with this dream. I sneak up on Miss Hobbs's porch — you know her house with all the gingerbread millwork on the far end of Main Street — around the corner from Donna's?"

"So, and what does that have to do with blood?"

"I think it's a sort of Passover dream. I have this bucket of blood and I just pour it all down that wide set of steps leading up to her porch. And then I wake up when I can't figure out how to get down off her porch without getting blood all over the bottoms of my shoes. I can't figure out how to get away clean."

"Well, that's weird, Mary Jane."

"I know, that's why I'm telling you."

"And you want me to get you a bucket of blood! So, you can do this? It won't do Ruffin any good."

"No, I just wanted to tell you."

"Tell me what? Tell me."

"It just seems to feel better already. I think telling you is nearly as therapeutic as actually doing it would be."

"Well, don't do it. It's crazy."

"I know. But just talking about doing it, maybe I won't ever have to dream about doing it again. It wakes me up at night."

"I can see that. You look terrible."

"But Ruffin's better, don't you think?"

"Yeah, Ruffin is better."

"Well, he's like a little lamb that the school just wants to slaughter! That's how I feel, and I need to decide whether to go to his school meeting, late in the afternoon on Monday. I don't think I have to, or, honestly, that I want to."

"If you do go, you need to go in a better frame of mind than it looks like you are in now."

"I know," I admitted. "I can't go like this."

"No," he said. "You can't."

"I know. My mom says the same thing. You and my mom always say the same thing. It's one thing I happen to like about you."

"Are you going home, then?"

"My mom says the same thing, 'Are you coming home, then?' Yes, I'm leaving on Thursday. I think I need to go to the beach. I need something to help me feel better."

"Look," said Seamus, laughing. "You have mail."

It was a small, square envelope, addressed by hand, nothing threatening. The mother from Algona had written me a card, a white wheelbarrow full of spring flowers to brighten my day. I handed it over for Seamus to read.

"We're *so* anxious for spring to really get here! That's why I picked this card. Anyway, I just wanted to thank you so much for getting that information out to me. You have been great. Our IEP went well, and we had no problem getting extended year services of 30 hours per week. We are disagreeing about preschool placement next year. The preschool consultant doesn't feel that 'untrained' people can involve my son in play with other children when it's very difficult for 'trained' teachers. That almost got me going. She also said Lovaas programs typically only take the higher functioning kids, so they don't have much experience with kids like my son."

Seamus was confused, as he pointed to that last passage. "Didn't our school tell you just the opposite?"

"Yes," I said, cynically. "Any port in a storm to be able to say 'No.' Go on, read the rest of it."

The note from the mother from Algona continued. "Then our consultant said, 'You don't know how difficult it is to get a child like your son to interact with other children.' Oh, really? Well, we got some services for the summer, so I'll worry about the next 'fight' later. He will only be in school 5 hours a week to start anyway. Thanks again for all your help. I was so glad to hear Ruffin is doing well!"

"That's a nice note," said Seamus. "It should help make you feel better."

"I seem to get a lot of them. And they do." I smiled, as I lied.

I found this note brought up a lot of mixed feelings.

CHAPTER FORTY EIGHT

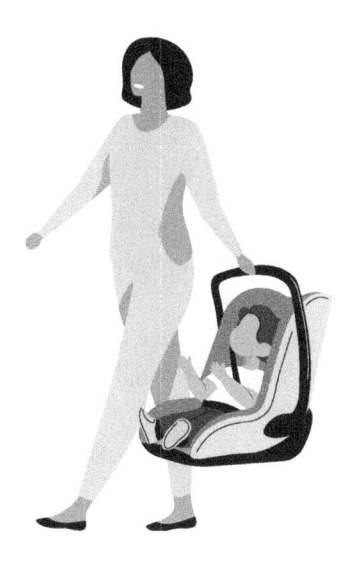

GONE. ON VACATION

I was acutely aware: this afternoon was the time set for Ruffin's EYSE meeting. I offered a lot of chatty housekeeping to Meg. "I'm in the courtroom this morning. When school is let out early, Donna can take Ruffin if I am not home. No recess outside today, please. Donna should stay in with him. She says that to teach the present 'theory of mind' drills effectively she needs two very intellectually and socially skilled classmates to work with her and Ruffin during morning drills ASAP, and during the summer."

When Donna ran Ruffin over to attend Elaine's class, she found Elaine was absent, sick at home with the flu that was going around town. Her aide had talked with the children about Easter. I thought to myself, only in my dreams was ours a Passover town.

It was time to decide whether to go to this meeting or not. I asked Donna if she would wait, while I called Curt one last time.

"Before you call him, I should tell you, Meg spent this morning 'pumping' me for my opinions about what Ruffin should be offered this summer and next year. They don't seem to have a clue. It was uncomfortable."

"No doubt. I'm sorry," I said, and then asked, "What, if anything, did you tell Meg?"

"That I hadn't been invited to their meeting."

I had to laugh at Donna's sheer audacity.

"It is what it is," she said. "I can wait while you talk to Curt and watch Ruffin if *you* decide to go."

Curt and I both felt, both agreed, tensions were higher by the day, and might not readily be defused by my appearance. I knew my own fury was something I could barely contain.

"I can't trust myself to go," I admitted.

"You should know what I've learned," said Curt. "Caron is not going, and Mr. Lord is not going."

"So, you're telling me this meeting is planned to proceed without legal advice and without the authority to commit district resources."

"That would seem to be the case. Caron thinks they will be offering Ruffin 20 hours of Lovaas over the summer."

"Ah, 20 hours a week, or 20 hours for the summer?"

"I don't know. She didn't say."

"Well, there's a big difference . . ."

As I began to get wound up, Curt suggested, "Let's say, you don't go. If you're not happy with the result of their meeting, we can go back again to pre-appeal mediation. For the moment, all the attorneys want to remain hands off and see what happens. None of them can get there."

"If I go, I won't be able to go — and not be an attorney."

"True," said Curt. "So, let's say, you just don't go. Remember, as Ruffin's parent, you always hold the one veto. You don't have to agree to whatever it is they offer you if it's not 'appropriate.'"

"I agree, then, you're right. It will be better if I don't go. I have no business representing Ruffin, or myself. I can't do it, you know, dispassionately."

"No," Curt agreed. "You can't. You can do a lot, but you can't do *that*. And just remember, if you don't go, there will be no waiver, no loss of your parental rights. I can convey your proposed plan and all your information to Bridgewater and the district, and then get their best offer on both the summer and Ruffin's fall placement for kindergarten."

"Good. I leave it to you, then."

"I think if we find we need to go back into pre-appeal mediation we'll see if we can't go before Gerry Gritzmacher, not Dee Ann, again, if the school's offer is not appropriate."

I turned back to what I could do with Ruffin there, still bundled up for a cold, windy afternoon. He and I headed back to St. Pat's where principal Peter Smith, and I went over the paperwork for Ruffin's fall enrollment in kindergarten. Based on how well Ruffin had managed Elaine's class, and Dr. Granpeesheh's recommendations, I signed it, and principal Smith signed it, too. He seemed pleased to learn Ruffin would be coming.

He offered me a written description of St. Pat's Kindergarten Title 1 Developmental Readiness Program. Then, he, Ruffin, and I walked out back of the schoolhouse to the playground where a small, heated, and air-conditioned trailer was stationed, and said hello to Mrs. Tinderholt, where she worked as the Title I reading teacher at "the neutral site." It looked a lot nicer than my garage last summer — and Ruffin had managed to learn quite a lot there.

How did the school's meeting go down in my absence and the absence of other people important to the formulation of an appropriate EYSE offer for Ruffin? In attendance were Miss Hobbs, Inge, Kim, and Meg. Materials available included Ruffin's previous IEP, faxed recommendations from Dr. Granpeesheh, information from Inge that she had received from me regarding my preference for summer programming, and Ruffin's cumulative file.

The group reviewed all objectives and quarterly progress reports. Ruffin had mastered some of his goals and some remained unmet. To address their irremediable procedural error of never having identified "critical skills," the group treated *all* of Ruffin's goals and objectives as "critical," along with Evelyn's newest "theory of mind" drills.

I suppose the results of the meeting suffered from my absence. The group discussed my ability to provide "typical family experiences" to address Ruffin's "social interaction maintenance." After Ruffin's remarkable developmental growth and rapid language development over last summer in our playgroup, when I read this, it landed as a real slap in the face.

To remedy my deficiencies, the group included a compliance objective — an earlier component of Ruffin's drill therapy — to be "maintained" — since his compliance was better with Donna at school than they imagined it was with me at home. True, no one was tougher on Ruffin than Donna. Meg was softer on him. Lisa was, too. And I was the biggest softie of us all because I was his mother — not just his advocate, but his refuge.

Since integration was an integral component of Ruffin's IEP, the absence of Elaine and the kindergarten teacher Mrs. Linden at the EYSE IEP meeting was also significant. Although Elaine had provided a kindergarten readiness report in January, the group needed an opportunity to discuss an update of Ruffin's integration and his social interaction. Elaine's input would have been important to the determination of Ruffin's summer needs.

As a result of Miss Hobbs's defective notice and this flawed process, a written offer was formulated for Ruffin. I was eager to see it, of course, and to review it with Curt and Dr. Granpeesheh and ask, "Would it be appropriate?"

If there was one thing I had learned in all my years practicing law, it was: it was always hard to get out the door for vacation. The same must be true for anyone, though.

Tuesday morning, I sent into school the UCLA Standards for Workshop Consultations by Ivar Lovaas, PhD. and Jacqueline Wynn, M.A., who had treated Catherine Maurice's children, highlighting a single passage: "It is possible to provide for certain immediate gains in the child's functioning using workshops. However, without extensive treatment experience supervised by persons who are showing expertise in areas such as peer integration, the gains will not be maintained and may not be useful as the client grows older."

I wrote to Senator Bill Frist, MD, of Tennessee about the IDEA Amendments of 1996. "I am the mother of a son with autism. I have a copy of the proposal for changes to the IDEA. It is very disturbing that the comprehensive system of personnel development provisions of the law have been omitted — particularly since current 'special education' teacher training does not effectively address the disability of autism."

I had the volunteers update my *Parent Perspectives* March booklet for Sue with a summary of what I had written earlier to Gerry Gritzmacher, including a full update of Ruffin's most recent developmental testing. We sent copies out to each AEA regional director across the state.

Underfoot, Ruffin was making pencil drawings of volcanoes, and coloring a leprechaun, tracing a path for him to a pot of gold at the bottom of an old unfinished worksheet he had dug out of his book bag. He was coloring his daffodils violet, following the crazy written directions of another worksheet, the work of an Easter bunny posed at the top of the page, holding a dripping paint brush.

Donna handed me her latest sheaf of notes, suggesting, "Take these with you on vacation. Your mom might get a kick out of them." I laid them on my desk and began typing them up.

"Ruffin is working on recognizing groups of 10 to 100.

"He is using a calendar to learn *before* and *after* in time, using the days of the week. He played a clock game with me. Ruffin was allowed to keep his turn until he missed. I managed to get a single turn.

"We also played a game on a board with 12 squares with clock faces. Ruffin would pick a card that had a time on it, like one o'clock, then he would draw in the hands on the clock with a wipe-off marker. I introduced the concept of a half hour and the practice of counting by 5-minute increments.

"Then, Ruffin and I worked on answering some who and how questions. I re-checked for maintenance whether Ruffin still knows his phone number. Ruffin stumbled on remembering his address, 'I don't remember.' I said: 'Yes, you can just think about it.' Ruffin: 'I don't know anymore.' Then I put Ruffin's address on an index card. Ruffin announced, 'I will be moving. I told my mom I want to live a short way to my grandma. I want to walk to my grandma's house.' I asked: 'Won't you miss your schools?' Ruffin: 'They are not new anymore. They are old.' I asked: 'Wouldn't you miss me?' Ruffin: 'I would visit you.' I asked: How will I work with you?' Ruffin: 'I will get to you.' Then, I asked: 'What about Danielle?' Ruffin: 'You will need to tell her so she will call me. I will walk to my grandma's.' This drill started out as a short drill on basic personal information. It just really snowballed into answering questions of who, what, where, and how.

"Ruffin was late for lunch because of his shared reading paper. He was to stay in his seat working until he finished along with other students who had also not finished. When finished, he was to join other students in a story book circle and card game. When the game was over Mrs. Linden asked to check all the students' papers. Ruffin's was not complete, and Ruffin did not earn an orange sticker and had a written message, 'Not finished!'

"Back in Meg's room, I asked Ruffin to show me his paper. He turned it over. He was upset. I asked him why he didn't want me to look at his paper. He said then, 'That's okay.' I then asked him how he was feeling. It took a while, but he labeled his feeling 'embarrassed.' I used theory of mind skills to have him discuss his paper, about untruths and dishonesty. I asked him what his mom would think about the teacher's message. He said he would erase the teacher's words and finish his paper.

"So, Ruffin was late for lunch. He missed getting a spot next to a student who is usually his best companion and had to sit at a smaller table of all girls who don't talk as much with him. When I asked if he missed sitting with his friends, he said, 'Yes.' I asked if he knew why he didn't get to sit with his friends. He did not answer. Then we talked about the reading paper that made us late for lunch that made him miss his place by his friend — one of his old summer playgroup playmates.

Ruffin's paper had his name at the top. He had completed all the capital G's and the lower-case g's and three letters of the word "goat," which he would have needed to have written completely twice to have finished.

Not so terribly awful, I thought, as Ruffin's mommy.

I reminded Meg Wednesday that Ruffin and I would be leaving on vacation. "I need to see a written summer services (EYSE) offer in time to exercise my appeal rights, if necessary, before I leave tomorrow morning. There is no phone at our vacation cottage."

I was getting some good theory of mind with Ruffin asking me, "Do you want that pillow? If you do, okay, but if you don't, I'd like to use it in my house." He was talking about his own, special flowered pillow which he treasured.

Ruffin was also using word attack skills — initial sounds of initial letters by verbal rehearsal to work at *Reader Rabbit* on his computer — he was about three quarters of the way through *Interactive Reading Journey* — a program in which he needed to earn access down the path by meeting performance criteria. I saw him using his word attack skills to make initial choices, then using a straight sight-reading skill to memorize and recognize the word thereafter.

Ruffin asked me, "Do you know what happened to the library?"

I asked, "Where?"

Ruffin told me, "At school."

Then Ruffin reported the library at school had a leaking roof, so library had been held in a classroom, by pretending it was a library. *No* expectation that I would really know about this if I just "used my thinking" — a more common demand of his of the recent past.

While Ruffin attended his last day before vacation, I wrote to Ray DeNeve of Bridgewater, Lorna Volmer of Heartland, and Gerry Gritzmacher in Des Moines. "Here are your copies of a Discrete Trial Drill Book compiled by The Autism Partnership, Dr. John McEachin, and Dr. Ron Leaf, who both studied and authored research papers at UCLA with Lovaas; the CARD Discrete Trial Drill Book compiled by Dr. Doreen Granpeesheh, who also studied at UCLA with Lovaas. Senior therapists like Evelyn Kung draw from these to construct an individually tailored 'drill book' for a particular child, in roughly the order shown on the Key Lovaas Programs *Flowchart*, also enclosed."

I had obtained these materials from the parent-professional group ACCESS in California, by trading them a copy of my written resources. ACCESS also provided videotapes of the several days of in-service provided to parents and professionals by

Dr. McEachin and Dr. Granpeesheh recently to their group. I passed all these to these state autism leaders with my recommendation. "I think you will find, as I do, that they would be most excellent parent-teacher training videos to use before someone arrives from out-of-state to do hands-on training, informal assessment, and working up an individually tailored program for a given child."

Our student volunteers arrived, ready to work, as Donna came in to wish us safe travels and dropped another sheaf of handwritten notes on my desk.

Report cards were sent home, just ahead of spring break. Ruffin had met all his integration objectives by dressing up as "animals" with two classmates and building blocks with a little girl with whom he had had a lot to say.

Miss Hobbs called just before school was out that afternoon to tell me directly there would be no EYSE offer made for Ruffin until *after* I got back from vacation. I suggested that there might be a fax somewhere in Myrtle Beach.

"No," Miss Hobbs cut me and that possibility off. "This is Caron Angelos's recommendation to us, to just wait. She has already spoken to Curt. As far as we are concerned, you can start your appeal now."

This was frustrating, of course. It also made no sense. Without seeing the school's EYSE offer there was no way of knowing whether it was appropriate, or if it were inappropriate — in what respects, and how exactly — which would be essential to what Curt, and I needed to know to even write an appeal.

I called Joan who let me know Caron claimed the recommendations from Evelyn and Dr. Granpeesheh at CARD had failed to fax through in time for the EYSE meeting. What? Hadn't I moved mountains to make sure they did?

"Joan, I don't think that is true. I faxed them. My own fax records show otherwise."

"Curt is who Caron talked to, directly, and I'm not sure he's coming in tonight. He's on the road. It's spring."

"I know," I said. "It's the season."

After reaching Curt, I decided not to delay leaving. "Who knows when we'll hear from them." By then I was whining a little.

"I think we'll hear from them soon enough."

"Okay, I leave the matter with you then."

"That's what I'm here for," said Curt. He knew it was hard for me to let go.

On Thursday, Ruffin was marked absent for spring break a day early, and correctly: "Gone. On vacation."

CHAPTER FORTY NINE

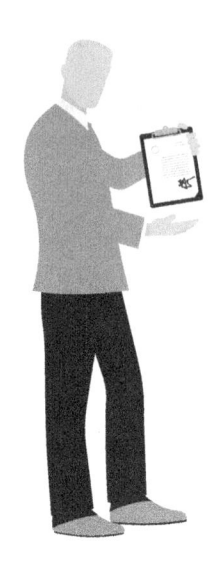

CURT FILES FOR DUE PROCESS

Continued delay in making an EYSE decision was untimely under both federal and state special education law. The regular school year would end soon in early June. So, Curt prepared a remarkably simple petition to the Iowa Department of Education on Ruffin's and my behalf:

"The issues involved in this due process request are:
1. Appaloosa Community School District (ACSD) and Bridgewater Area Education Agency (Bridgewater) have failed to carry out their duty of addressing Ruffin's need for extended year services (EYSE) in a timely manner.

"Because Ruffin, as a child with a disability, has a well-documented need for these services, failing to address the issue in a timely manner denies a free, appropriate public education (FAPE) to the child.

2. ACSD has failed to implement integration opportunities which are written in Ruffin's IEP. This is a violation of the U.S. Code, which states that services must be provided 'in conformity with the individualized education program.' 20 U.S.C. 1401 (18)(D).

"Because integration opportunities written in the IEP were not implemented, Ruffin is entitled to compensatory integration opportunities and services over the summer months.

"Thank you for arranging a due process hearing so that these issues can be addressed and decided."

Ruffin's educators had continued to scramble after their March EYSE meeting. I could see that in my later careful flyspecking of their records under FERPA. After they adjourned, someone realized the group had failed to invite all the people needed to formulate a specific and appropriate offer for Ruffin.

Mr. Montague had faxed Mr. Lord, "I have reviewed the regulations of FERPA regarding the question we discussed this morning about not having to obtain parental permission to show student records to a 'consultant' whom your district would hire for the purpose of improving instruction.

"I ask you to look at 99.31 — *Prior consent for disclosure not required*. Review the sections I have marked to see if you would agree that prior consent for the purpose we discussed is not required.

"You might want to contact your local district legal counsel Caron Angelos for her opinion on this. Another resource might be Kathy Collins, Iowa Association of School Boards (IASB) attorney."

Well, yes, I thought. Mr. Lord might want to consult legal counsel — since those provisions from the *Federal Register* were related to general human research studies in which the personal identifications of children and their parents were required to be closely held by researchers and needed to be destroyed after the studies were completed. And they dated back to mid-June of 1976.

Legally, I judged Mr. Montague's advice more than a bit of a "reach." But Ruffin's educators were prepared to reach out to consult the very person whom they had failed to invite to their summer services (EYSE) group discussion about Ruffin — Dr. Granpeesheh.

Miss Hobbs wrote to her. "I have just received your written recommendation for summer programming for Ruffin White. We are currently in the process of developing Ruffin's extended year individualized educational plan (EYSE IEP) and have several questions about your recommendation.

"On what data did you base this recommendation? What is the source of this data? What facts or circumstances resulted in your recommendation that Ruffin receive more services in the summer than he currently receives in the school year? You further recommend Ruffin attend a small class size kindergarten without a one-to-one aide. What is the basis for this recommendation? Should summer be an opportunity for transition for Ruffin, with reduced structured programming?" They sounded to me a lot like questions from Caron Angelos — like a cross-examination in the making.

Of course, these questions failed to address in any way the consideration of *compensatory education* over the summer to address last fall's semester of failed Head Start integration that Ruffin and I had been promised after a day-long and late-into-the-night mediation and IEP meeting last August. Or the issue of how a simple lack of structure over the coming summer might endanger Ruffin's successful transition into kindergarten that I thought we had all anticipated then — so he could begin to run loose in the universe.

Caron answered Curt's petition on April 1st, including as a sort of tattletale postscript, "Please also be advised that the parent opted not to participate in the IEP meeting for planning summer services (EYSE) and next year's IEP."

The Iowa Department of Education promptly issued an appointment order so Susan Etscheidt, Ph.D., Associate Professor of special education at the University of Northern Iowa in Cedar Falls could serve as our administrative law judge (ALJ).

The briefest description of her qualifications was enclosed with the order. Dr. Etscheidt taught at the institution where she had studied elementary education with a special education emphasis in 1973, and where she went on in 1976 to earn a master's degree in teaching the severely and profoundly handicapped. In 1984 she had earned her Ph.D. focusing on the education of students with emotional disturbances and behavioral disorders and began sitting as an ALJ in 1987.

She had issued only two previous written decisions after full due process hearings, one in 1991, and another in 1992. Between 1986 and 1992, during the summers, she had in-serviced special education teachers for the Iowa Department of Education. Between 1986 and 1989, she served on the Governor's Task Force on Autism and Developmental Disabilities.

Dr. Etscheidt echoed most of our school district's reply later that summer without taking up Caron's oddly tattletale attempt to shift the blame to me for failing to attend the March EYSE meeting.

HER DECISION OF June 3rd, 1996:

Attorney Caron Angelos, Local Education Agency (LEA) counsel, advised 'the school district has not yet completed working on a proposed extended year program' and that the plan would be ready 'for the parent's review by April 10th, 1996.' She requested no hearing until 'after April 15th, 1996, to allow the parties additional time to 'consult and negotiate.'

The next day, Dee Ann, who had mediated the earlier dispute between Ruffin's educators and myself the previous August, issued a letter to all the educators and attorneys concerned directing them to "forward to this office complete educational records and proceedings" within 10 days to her, and to Curt, for my benefit.

She also let everyone know that the pre-appeal conference on Ruffin's behalf filed last August, would "be considered dismissed," meaning, I supposed, that all our earlier issues of dispute were considered to have been settled and would not be re-addressed in the upcoming due process hearing. I took that to be an administrative button-up, Dee Ann simply reaching back to pick up a slipped stitch in her own knitting.

Although Curt already represented me and Ruffin, Dee Ann sent me a list of free or low-cost legal and advocacy service agencies to help present my appeal of the educators' lack of any plan for Ruffin's summer. This was required by federal law. Every agency on her list was in Des Moines — a day-long round trip from our hometown. Of the four, only Curt's group had any expertise in special education litigation.

Spring break had been lost to makeup days after our long brutal winter of heavy snow and subzero temperatures. Ruffin's fifth birthday on April 9th passed on the road back to Iowa, after our early celebration in North Carolina with my parents. We had fled again to Myrtle Beach to soak up the sun and some encouragement. And, as before, we needed to talk about money. I would be facing another expensive summer with limited opportunity to work for our living.

Still, it was peaceful there, and the days passed slowly under the sound of the rolling surf, with no phone in our rented cottage, long before cell phones were common.

Meanwhile, from her office in California, Dr. Granpeesheh drafted a reply to Miss Hobbs. As the ethical practitioner she was, she held it in confidence until she and I were able to consult with each other and I could give her my consent to release it. Dr. Granpeesheh's newest reply echoed all her earlier recommendations of March and offered me sound direction and a clear rationale for deciding for myself what to do about Ruffin's upcoming summer and next kindergarten year — regardless of the outcome of any due process hearing.

Our ALJ, Dr. Etscheidt acknowledged Dr. Granpeesheh's newest reply to Miss Hobbs's letter, pointing up what she found useful for herself in making her own later decision.

HER DECISION OF June 3rd, 1996:

In a letter to Nan Hobbs dated April 4th, 1996, and faxed April 15th, 1996, Dr. Granpeesheh provides a rationale for her proposal:

'The 20 hours per week of one-to-one discrete trial therapy is recommended to assist Ruffin with his difficulty to recall events and activities, process appropriate information and learn specific ways that will aid him in being successful within various social situations . . . As discussed during Ms. Evelyn Kung's previous visit, he also displays a delay in the pragmatic use of time sequencing reflected in his use of today, tomorrow, and yesterday . . . Ruffin also exhibits difficulty in focusing on an appropriate goal or direction due to the overstimulation that may be present in his environment . . . I have also recommended this one-to-one time to assist Ruffin in building his 'Theory of Mind' as well as any socialization techniques that are necessary . . .

'The three days a week of interaction in a supervised play group will implement these theory of mind and social skills acquired in the one-to-one time into a structured play group. Ruffin's special education and nursery schoolteachers both indicate that Ruffin still has difficulty in processing directions especially when the directions are given in a group setting . . . Overall, Ruffin still displays significant problems with understanding oral directions given to a group and it has been noted that this is the time in which Ruffin will begin to drop back into old self-stimulatory behaviors. I have recommended that a Lovaas trained therapist monitor this play group because Ruffin will need to be specifically directed in areas where he displays identified weaknesses and in turn, change those times into learning situations . . .

'The other two days that I have recommended in an unstructured monitored play group will then be useful for the generalization of the above learned skills in his interaction with typical children in peer play . . . (See Appellee's Exhibit A).

On April 8, the day before Ruffin's fifth birthday, while he and I were splashing in the surf, Miss Hobbs offered a letter of support for a $750,000 federal grant indicating that ACSD was "very interested in being involved" since "currently we are very limited in what to offer these students and parents."

The grant was authored by researchers in Heartland AEA and submitted on the day after Ruffin's birthday to the U.S. Department of Education to support teacher-training in TEACCH-style structured teaching methods throughout Iowa, *Development, Testing and Dissemination of Nonaversive Techniques for Working with Children with Autism; Demonstration of a 'Best Practices' Model for Parents and Teachers.* The unimpressive outcome of this wasted effort was described long afterward in a 2002 report to the U.S. Department of Education.

Curt and I and the nearly two dozen families in Iowa who had moved heaven and earth to mount home-and-school-based Lovaas programs for our children with autism since 1994 had no way of knowing that our efforts to help future Iowa families would be swamped by this $750,000 — some of it, of course, our own tax money.

The same day Miss Hobbs submitted her letter of support for Heartland AEA's federal grant, she also wrote to me, without having waited for Dr. Granpeesheh's reply to her questions.

The document I found waiting for me on April 10th when Ruffin and I returned to Iowa came with a cover letter. "To summarize, we believe Ruffin White does qualify for extended year programming. We are recommending 11 hours and 15 minutes per week for a period of 8 weeks of direct Lovaas drill. We include an additional 45 minutes per week of record charting and preparation time for the Lovaas therapist. We believe this is sufficient for maintaining and continued development of skills Ruffin will need to be successful in kindergarten next school year."

This was nowhere near the 20 hours per week Caron seemed to have been speaking about to Curt earlier. And summer was 12 weeks long. No mainstream or group or social experience of any kind was offered. It included three "critical goals and skill areas in which EYSE was recommended: Ruffin will comply with an adult request 90% of the time on second request; Ruffin will demonstrate the ability to process directions; and Ruffin will demonstrate the ability to recall specific information from the past, both short and long term."

Curt and I agreed this EYSE offer failed to meet the legal standard of "appropriate." It was at odds with Dr. Granpeesheh's expert opinion. And since Donna had not been invited to their March EYSE gathering, this offer's most unsteady plank was that no one from school had bothered to ask Donna whether she would be available to work for the school, or for me, or with Ruffin over the summer.

Curt and I began to cut a small, elegant case to press before Dr. Etscheidt from the bolts of material in my blue Binderteks, from the whole cloth of what we had. We needed to shape it to the specifications of his agency's existing published priority — EYSE — summer school for students with disabilities. We would aim at lowering the legal bar standing between summer school and *every* disabled child in Iowa, regardless of disability. We aimed to see that many more children would qualify in the future. This was the way Curt was accustomed to work — broadly, for wide effect — when he found himself forced to litigate.

Meg let me know what had been happening at school in Ruffin's absence. "We are starting transition activities for those whose programs will change. Because of this, we have started talking about next year and who is doing what so if the children talk about it at home, you will know why." Of course, mired in dispute as we were, no IEP conference for Ruffin for his 1996-1997 kindergarten year had even been scheduled yet, and his educators had no transition plan for him.

Meg had also written about Ruffin individually. "Ruffin went to recess, lunch, and library with kindergarten. What a great trip it must have been. He was *very* conversational today. Especially about being 5 now! When asked to tell about vacation separately from his birthday, he was able to separate the events and tell something about each as separate entities."

Donna had sent some notes, too. "When I asked Ruffin to tell me some of the things he did on vacation, he offered too much for me to be able to write you! Still, some of his sentences were somewhat incomplete, and he was also wanting to use his hands to gesture instead of using his words."

When Donna had asked, 'Did you do any work while you were gone?' Ruffin had replied, truthfully, "No, I didn't." We had lazed on the beach, built sandcastles, and watched the high tides sweep them away.

Donna and Ruffin had worked on printing Ruffin's first and last name on three different worksheets. And on a shared reading worksheet to review uppercase letters A through Z, on how to make the letters with proper strokes — rather than drawing them as pictures, as Ruffin was inclined to do. And saying the names of each letter as Donna pointed to them randomly — perfectly. Ruffin also completed dot-to-dot A to Z drawings of a cat, missing only the dot for N, and another dot-to-dot A to J of a winter sleigh, perfectly.

Donna had worked on some theory of mind tasks, too. 'Where is your classmate?' an absent child. 'How would you find out?' 'About where she is?' 'Who would you ask?'" They did some calendar work, changing the calendar from March to April and inserting new numbers into the calendar's stiff plastic pockets.

Joan attended two meetings that Friday and the next as a member of the special education rules council. Kathy Collins — the same attorney Mr. Montague had referred Mr. Lord to for legal advice so recently — represented the school administrators of Iowa at the same meetings. Kathy had approached Joan during a break to ask her if she thought that I "was going to end up being good for" Iowa Protection & Advocacy Services, Inc. — or if I would end up taking them "down with her."

Kathy made other comments to Joan, including, "Mary Jane is advertising herself on the internet — a 'no-no' for attorneys. She could be disbarred for hustling up business this way." And "The real problem with Mary Jane is that she can't handle her own child. How can that be the school's fault?" Kathy further pointed out that "Mary Jane was a mother who kept her infant son in a basket under her desk and fed him nothing but black olives and chocolate milk."

Fortunately, Joan and Curt were impervious to this attempt to interfere with their attorney-client relationship with Ruffin and me. Joan let me know the full details about these events much later when she offered me a written statement about them to the attorney whom I had engaged to get my name off the child abuse registry.

As for myself, I unloaded on Meg, obliviously, and frankly about the latest summer services (EYSE) offer from Miss Hobbs. "I am deeply concerned that ACSD and Bridgewater are unwilling to follow Dr. Granpeesheh's recommendations. No playgroup? Ruffin will suffer so badly if this is not provided. Dr. Granpeesheh got all the information that was provided to me, except Kim's speech and language therapy data which arrived too late for Dr. Granpeesheh's meeting with Evelyn Kung. Ruffin was also looking forward to playgroup this summer. What reason do you have for *not* meeting Ruffin's summer *mainstreaming* need?

"Also, *where* are you proposing Donna will work with Ruffin for 12 hours per week as offered? School? Or home? What rate will the local district and Bridgewater pay Donna? She charges *$200 a week* for this amount of CARD direct drill. Prudential Insurance is no longer paying — under an educational services exclusion. I am delighted to hear from Donna that ACSD and Bridgewater are both interested in purchasing her services for other children next year after Ruffin's program is complete in about August of 1996."

Lisa wanted to reduce her hours to spend the summer with her own children and a new crop of daycare babies. I decided I could take Ruffin Tuesday and Thursday afternoons for the summer, since I rarely had court hearings those afternoons. Seamus agreed to take Ruffin at least one afternoon a week for the summer. Donna just wanted to work Monday, Tuesday, Thursday, and Friday mornings through the summer. She didn't want to lead a playgroup but would need at least two typically developing children for her morning theory of mind drill sessions with Ruffin.

I called principal Peter Smith, to reaffirm his and my expectation that I would be sending Ruffin to St. Pat's for kindergarten. He let me know he had had no contact with ACSD about Ruffin, and asked, "What about transition planning with them during May?"

Since I didn't think any communication between ACSD and St. Pat's would be to Ruffin's and my benefit at that delicate moment I replied with some caution, "Ruffin is developing so quickly. Maybe the better transition would be in August with me, you, Ruffin's new kindergarten teacher, and Donna Schmidt." I explained briefly that ACSD and I remained at loggerheads and would be going to a due process hearing soon, promising, "I will do my dead-level best to keep St. Pat's out of it."

He quickly assured me, "Whatever happens, Ruffin will be welcome here."

And, yes, that did set my mind at rest. Curt and I would be able to fight as hard as we might like for Ruffin and the state's so many other disabled children who might benefit from a favorable decision from Dr. Etscheidt.

CHAPTER FIFTY

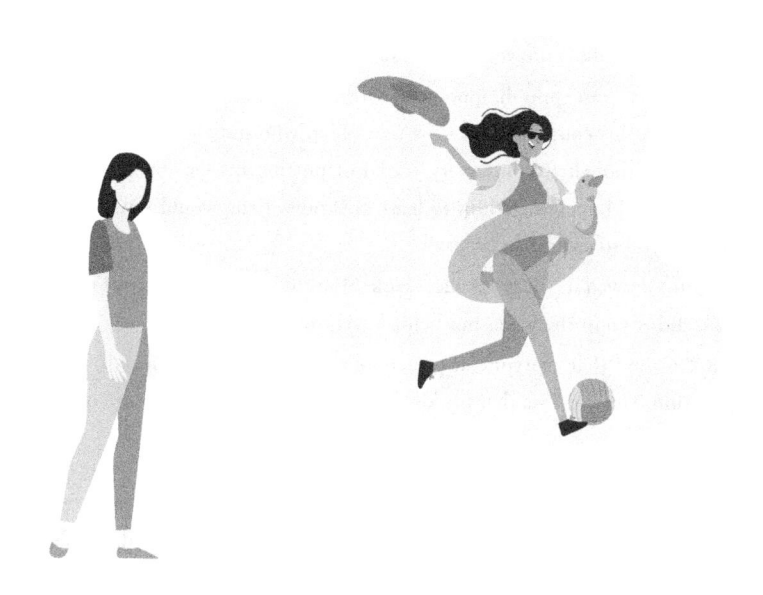

ANOTHER SUMMER ON THE HORIZON

I called Dr. Lovaas's friend, Dr. David Bishop since RoJene was already committed elsewhere for the summer. I updated him on Ruffin's progress, concerned that it seemed to have slowed over this year of continual conflict with the school authorities. Would he put a notice up in the Luther College psychology department for students there? I could offer $10 per hour for 3 to 4 days per week, 3 hours per day all summer to accompany Ruffin to a playgroup or local daycare. Any interested student could do some assigned reading on autism, write a paper about Ruffin, and have some training from Evelyn and Donna. Dr. Bishop mentioned that his little daughter would be spending her summer at Sunflower Daycare in Decorah which had programming for young children of different ages.

I shared with Ruffin's two schoolteachers, Meg, and Elaine, at some length. "Ruffin said that he swam at Luther Friday and took a warm shower and wasn't scared as he was when he was younger. He reports his new Luther friends are two girls — Jenny and Sarah — not big boys as before. Sarah is his favorite. He reports his classmate's friend is a boy. He described his life vest and the rafts that need a huge pump.

"Ruffin was upset and disappointed with his swimming because he feels he doesn't swim as well as his cousin Robert — a year older, who puts his head under and swims underwater. Although Ruffin is very scared of putting his face or head underwater, I think Sarah could encourage him to learn this now if she would say, 'Would you like me to teach you to swim *like Robert?*'

"Ruffin showed me he got a 'nice work' blue circle given to him at Luther by someone who didn't go in the water but helped everyone else out.

"Ruffin said that everyone at preschool thought (theory of mind!) that he had a nice vacation. He told Lisa that his kite from nursery school was 'made of wallpaper.'"

I had more stories to share. "Ruffin recently remembered vividly the events of his MRI back in October of 1994. 'I tried to save myself. I tried to pull the — gesturing — I gave him the word 'needle' — needle out of my arm, to throw it in the trash can. I was angry and scared.'" Ruffin was using two conflicting emotions to describe himself then. A perfectly accurate account of that past event.

Very commonly now, Ruffin would time-label events in his own past by "when I was 3, 4 or 5" — very accurately as to his age. He was beginning to use "tomorrow" some. And to use the word "actually" in a very theory of mind way to tell how things truly are — still a bit odd as if he didn't entertain the possibility that other minds may also know what might be true. This operated as a good verbal marker of his attention to the difference between appearances and pretend or silliness and the fact of matters.

About characters in stories, Ruffin could answer now "What does he *wish?*" with "He wishes he could marry her" — of the prince in a fairy tale. Then, he began offering his own wishes with "I wish . . ."

Ruffin went up to hear the children's sermon for the first time in church — saying that he wanted to "copy" the other kids now. He was still often up late at night — very, very talkative and unable to settle down — lobbying hard for another kitten and a television in his bedroom "like the other kids in preschool and my old school."

As always, I returned to advocating with Ruffin's educators. "Two students Evelyn is consulting on, a girl with autism in North Fayette, is printing her name and identifying many pictures, and a boy with autism in North Fayette has a speaking, functional vocabulary now of more than 100 one-syllable words and identifies many pictures, according to their mothers this weekend at our autism support group meeting.

"Enclosed is a review of Dr. Simpson's University of Kansas article from the most recent issue of *The Link*. Please note the 15- to 19-child class size recommendation which is in accord with Dr. Granpeesheh's recommendation for Ruffin for next year.

"I found the article cited in *The Link* — Gerry Gritzmacher sent it to me this winter after one of our telephone conversations. A copy is enclosed for Ruffin's educational file at ACSD and for Bridgewater — you need to send these file items to the ALJ for our due process hearing.

"This is data CARD did not have — CARD did not have the Lovaas 'Workshop Standards' document either. So, all these are *independently agreeing sources of expertise* about what Ruffin needs for successful regular education integration: CARD, Lovaas 'Workshop Standards,' and Dr. Simpson's article on behavior disorders.

"Do you want to spend another $6,000 on your Waterloo law firm, when it doesn't take an attorney or even a rocket scientist?" At this point, with Curt and Joan committed to litigate, and with my mind at rest about St. Pat's kindergarten, why hold back? I was powerfully frustrated.

Ruffin did some nice coloring and was assigned some memory work for Sunday school — the same memorization tasks I remembered from my own childhood during the 1950s. The preschool prayer: "God is good, God is great, and we thank him for this day. Amen." And the old-time religion *Jesus Loves Me* song: "Jesus loves me! This I know for the Bible tells me so. Little ones to Him belong. They are weak, but he is strong! Yes, Jesus loves me! Yes, Jesus loves me! Yes, Jesus loves me! The Bible tells me so."

Meg's class Monday was studying spring plants. But I wrote demanding, "I want to see Kim's session by session charting of her single unachieved IEP goal for Ruffin — multi-step commands for the remainder of the year. She hasn't charted *anything* on that goal to date. She owes Ruffin performance, whether she succeeds or not. Please advise her ASAP — I want to see her Tuesday charting — more detail than her 'Therapy Log' which discloses and communicates little."

I called Dr. Norman at UIHC. I remained fairly frazzled even after what I had tried to arrange as a restful vacation. He noted, "Mother called asking we invalidate releases she had earlier signed for school and AEA contact. She wants to complete new *Parent Questionnaires* due to changes over time." No way did I want evidence of my own human weakness of the fall to surface as evidence, anymore that I had wanted to show evidence of financial weakness then by borrowing from any bank in town.

"She will send her copies of recent records. She reports continuing disagreements with ACSD and Bridgewater, failure of the school to produce an acceptable programming offer and pending mediation and due process.

"She hopes we will be able to do good objective measures of Ruffin's progress since his last evaluation. She would also like us to consider formal or informal tests or tasks to assess 'theory of mind' per S. Baron-Cohen and F. Happe, and executive function.

"Also, she reported concerns about short term memory — low digit span and poor performance on three-step directions — also poor when there is a delay between directions and when the task is to be performed and time markers, very mechanical. He references things specifically to when he was a 3-year-old. Most other skills were in the 6- to 7-year-old range on *The Brigance*. Also, the Monday, Wednesday, and Friday integration group is closing.

"She is also concerned about poor quality social inclusion experiences with continued exposure to ECSE behaviorally handicapped students. Head Start students from last spring fell through this fall.

"School offered a 'shared group reading' activity that was too difficult for Ruffin (worksheets and phonics). This offered poor opportunities for social development and was so challenging that the Lovaas trainer was misdirected from her work to helping Ruffin keep up with this group.

"The CARD consultant redirected the trainer and said the failure experience would be good for helping Ruffin to learn that he had some problems and needs to communicate, and CARD person suggested integrating Ruffin into kindergarten PE — also to place Ruffin in demand situations where Ruffin should learn to recognize the need to communicate or relate.

"School agreed to fund discrete trial one-to-one teaching over the summer but will not be maintaining any socialization activities.

"School is also suggesting including Ruffin in regular education kindergarten (about 25 students) with a part-time associate as support. Mother is requesting a full-time one-to-one aide, but in a parochial school kindergarten where the class size is much smaller and with a 'very structured teacher.' She said school district egos have caused the school to reject this.

"Also asks about input and possible occupational therapy (OT) assessment regarding recent accidents which might, in her view, indicate perceptual motor problem (e.g., ran into a glass door and ran into a roof support 'as big as a tree'). Questions if Ruffin has normal protective reflexes as well. CARD has suggested summer obstacle course activities."

Donna came by to drop off her handwritten notes. Ruffin had had a difficult day. Miss Hobbs had come to offer Donna employment for 10 hours per week, at $10 per hour. Donna wanted to work as an aide with benefits. After Donna insisted, ACSD seemed to be willing to pay Donna $200 a week for 8 weeks of one-to-one instruction and to let Donna do this work at her home.

I told Donna I was thinking about Sunflower Day Care Center in Decorah for Ruffin's mainstream integration. Donna told me the schools wanted a settlement opportunity — but there was no movement yet on a kindergarten placement for Ruffin at St. Pat's.

I called Curt to bring him up to speed on all Donna's most recent intelligence, and to visit with him about calling Donna, Lorna Volmer from Heartland AEA, members of Dr. Norman's UIHC evaluation group, and my ally Ray DeNeve from the southern sector of Bridgewater as witnesses to support our due process case.

Mr. Lord faxed passages of Ruffin's home-school notebook directly to Caron in mid-April. "Unless you have a mainstream placement for EYSE you want to offer, I will begin interviewing playgroup leaders Thursday, so we have someone available for Evelyn to train in early May. Luther College is going to send me some students who know Ruffin from his adaptive PE class. Tomorrow when Curt and I speak with Caron and the scheduling folks for due process we will be proposing an attempt at mediation on summer services (EYSE) and an IEP for next year. The attorneys are scheduling with the ALJ tomorrow after lunch. Miss Hobbs could notify all of us if this proposal might work as a basic framework for the EYSE settlement. Is there a reason you have for *not* meeting Ruffin's summer *mainstreaming* need?"

Meg told me about Ruffin's day. She provided her charting of Ruffin's work on memory drills, repeating sentences of up to 10 words over the past week, with no charting for Monday, Wednesday, or Friday. Her Tuesday and Thursday charting showed success with only up to 4 or 5 words, and on Thursday after she discussed concentration with Ruffin, he was able to meet his IEP objective 3 times in a row — and then lost it again.

Donna reported the sort of conversation Ruffin was capable of by now.
Donna: 'What did you do yesterday?"
Ruffin: 'What did I did yesterday?
Donna: 'Yes."

Ruffin: 'I waked up. I got dressed. I went downstairs to have breakfast. I put my boots and my coat on. I went outside to wait for the bus.'

Donna: 'What was on the ground outside?'

Ruffin: 'On the ground?'

Donna: 'Yes.'

Ruffin: 'My bike.'

Donna: 'What else was on the ground?'

Ruffin: 'When I played friends?'

Donna: 'Think about the weather.'

Ruffin: 'The sun always follows my car. It always stays with me. It all follows my car. It stops with my car. It shines on me.'

Donna: 'Was there anything wet on the ground yesterday?'

Ruffin: 'Snow. There is still snow behind my house. We have three or four flowers growing.'

Donna: 'You have flowers growing in your yard?'

Ruffin: 'Lots of them. We need to put new seeds.'

Donna: 'What else did you do yesterday, after you got on the bus?'

Donna: 'Did you hear me?'

Ruffin: 'No.'

Donna: 'I asked you something. Weren't you listening?'

Ruffin: 'I can't hear you.'

Donna: 'I will repeat it for you. You need to listen when people talk.'

Donna: 'What else did you do yesterday, after you got on the bus?'

Ruffin: 'I go to school. I got my coat off. I then get in the room. Then I played. Then I had breakfast. Then I played. I washed my hands and then you called me, and I saw you.'

Donna: 'You saw me, and then what happened?'

Ruffin: 'Gym.'

CHAPTER FIFTY ONE

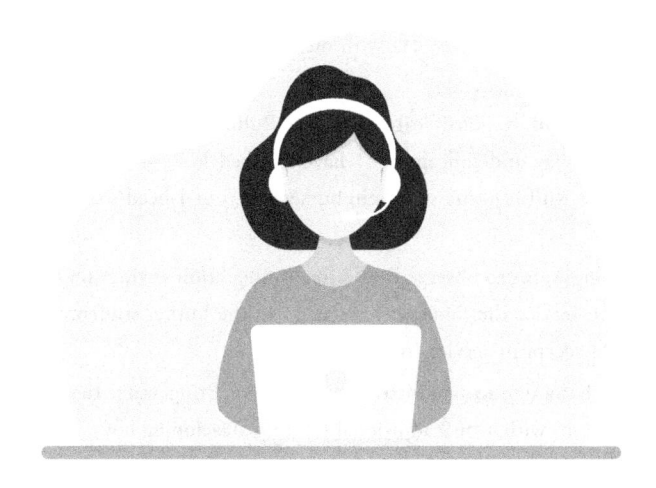

PONY UP, OR I WILL

I wrote to Meg in mid-April as my messenger. "We went to Decorah yesterday afternoon, saw chicks in the hatchery, and stopped in at Sunflower Day Care Center to check out their summer preschool group of 12 children led by a certified teacher. For a week in early July, Ruffin and I will be attending the Autism Society of America's annual national meeting. He has a day care program there for $50 per day.

"How about this for summer services (EYSE)?

M	T	W	Th	Fri
Donna	Donna		Donna	Donna
8-12	8-12		8-12	8-12
12-12:30 — Transport to Sunflower Day Care Center Decorah				
Sunflower	Sunflower		Sunflower	Sunflower
12:30	12:30		12:30	12:30
3:30	3:30		3:30	3:30

"Transport back to home. For 10 weeks of the summer.

"While at Sunflower, a Luther student in psychology trained by Evelyn Kung would help with integration and make daily written reports of Ruffin's behaviors and interactions at aide wages. Sunflower says they would be happy to accommodate having this Luther student on their campus.

"Wednesday would be a free day with me, or at Sunflower if I am in trial (at my expense).

"School would be responsible to transport Ruffin to Sunflower (maybe Donna would do this for pay and mileage — I haven't asked her) — or use a school bus. I would transport Ruffin home with reimbursement, but I need some flexibility because of trials.

"Evelyn Kung wants to observe Ruffin in all integration settings on Monday, May 6th and could in-service the Sunflower teacher and the Luther student aide that day. Sunflower would accept in-service from Kung.

"Sunflower has a one-to-one instruction room for Bridgewater that Donna could use for short sessions with 1 or 2 additional typically developing boys and girls.

"I learned it will cost about $90 per week for Ruffin to spend 40 hours per week at Sunflower. It's a daycare center, and there are lots of rules. Ruffin can be thrown out after 15 days of a trial period if he fails to adjust, and at any time thereafter if he were to be a behavior problem. That is, he has no disability rights under any federal law.

"Ruffin used 'worried' appropriately and spontaneously. Also, 'surprised,' 'fooled,' and 'tricky,' He described in detail the construction of a magic airplane he 'made in his head by thinking' which would operate on voice command — a magic airplane which he would like to purchase from the magic toy store. He is disappointed this store is not in Decorah.

"We picked out new wallpaper for Ruffin's room — Ruffin was interested in this.

"Ruffin was very chatty today — told me Kim read him a *Chicken Little* book. Kim's charting is better — but Ruffin can answer 'wh' questions, however complex from picture books. His IEP goal with Kim was to listen to an *oral* story and answer 'wh' questions — a much more challenging task.

"I need Kim's charting again today — and would she write even two sentences about what she does and is trying to teach?

"Kim needs to have Ruffin carry out 3-step 2-part commands in her teaching. This is where Ruffin's memory really fails him — when he must *do* something *and remember*. Maybe Kim is taking the first steps toward this activity, but let's get to it and get it done before the school year is up."

Ruffin and I went to St. Pat's playground after supper where he played with a boy from kindergarten. Ruffin lost his temper four separate times with him, telling him to do this (play by Ruffin's rules), telling him to run slower so Ruffin could win. The boy tried without success to teach Ruffin the rules of tag. Ruffin was too upset when tagged to play this game successfully. After one blow-up of Ruffin's, the boy relented and modified the rules to Ruffin's liking. After he found the level at which Ruffin could play without getting upset, they did have a nice time — mostly Ruffin imitating his use of equipment, the boy racing with him letting Ruffin win — running, crab walking, and rolling downhill. I was impressed with this little boy's skill and flexibility in handling Ruffin.

We read the *Chicken Little* library book with questions to focus Ruffin on "theory of mind." He understood most of the trickery and disguises of the story but seemed more interested in the mechanics of how the chickens and ducks survived the crash of the falling helicopter and who fixed the helicopter, and how.

"Donna — I am meeting with a Luther College student early this afternoon today for an interview. Could you stop by and meet her?"

My disturbing message was immediately faxed to Caron in Waterloo, who faxed Curt a letter of panicked protest, copied back to Mr. Lord, likely to appease and comfort him as her client. "Please be advised that we have learned that Ms. White is planning to interview, hire, and train a play group leader for her son. Please be advised that the ACSD has not authorized the hiring or training of personnel. In the event the ALJ rules that a 'play group' must be provided as a summer service (EYSE) for the child, the ACSD has not and will not delegate its authority to hire, train, or direct school personnel to the parent.

"Additionally, I am formally requesting that the parent provide us with a signed release allowing us to provide information to the Wisconsin Early Autism Center in Madison, Wisconsin, for the purpose of consultation with Dr. Glen Sallows — whom I had consulted the year before about Ruffin for last summer's services — concerning this student.

"Also, the classroom teacher is not the proper person to approach in the district concerning the summer services (EYSE) program. She has no authority to commit the district to any proposed plan.

"We also believe that it is inappropriate to use the child as a messenger for anything other than information concerning the child's daily activities. Please ask your client to communicate information of this nature to school administrators."

The next time Congress reauthorized the IDEA and amended it, parents were required to give their school districts a final opportunity to provide a free, appropriate public education (FAPE) *before* making unilateral placements of their children in private schools or other appropriate educational settings and then suing for reimbursement. Failure by the parents to give their school districts this final opportunity to provide FAPE themselves would result in the dismissal of the parents' reimbursement claim. Essentially — because it was only fair — I was giving this final opportunity to my school district: Get busy, pony up what Ruffin needs, or I will.

While I waited for an early afternoon phone call to schedule our due process hearing, I kept myself busy by trolling the internet. *The Me List* swarmed with all sorts of lists of Lovaas parent groups, recommending reliable consultants, sources for instructional materials, reports of legal cases with citations, and sample letters to write to school authorities, Medicaid, EPSDT, and insurance companies requesting in-home Lovaas services. Information was also posted about how to deduct Lovaas expenses as medical expenses from parents' taxes in IRS Publication 402, and the importance of maintaining or attaching a complete file of your expenses since the IRS computer algorithm would highlight any return claiming an unusually high medical expense deduction.

From his office-boat on the Chesapeake Bay, attorney Pete Wright published an online account of the newest federal rulings in favor of his client, Daniel Lawyer, a 6-year-old boy with autism who was found to need summer services (EYSE). The losing district had been ordered to pay his parents' $21,710.20 of attorney fees and to provide what the child had needed for the summer. I made a note of the citation of the case, 19 IDELR 904, for Curt.

Then I moved over to 'The Recovery Zone' organized by Ann Gibbons, of FEAT of Maryland, where I advertised the availability of Curt and Joan's booklet. I did some research in Perry A. Zirkel's textbook *Section 504, the ADA, and the Schools*. Here at the top of Zirkel's Hit List of *Section 504* 'No No's': "Retaliating against a student, staff member, or other person for filing a *Section 504* complaint."

Curt had filed Ruffin's pre-appeal last summer under *both* the IDEA and *Section 504 of the Rehabilitation Act*. Ray DeNeve had passed me the outline of special education law which another Iowa ALJ Larry Bartlett had lectured from and provided to Bridgewater administrators in 1994. My yellow highlighter sped over its many pages. I had to wonder what Meg and Inge would think about *Southside Public Schools v. Hill*, 827 F. 2nd 270 (8th Cir. 1987) holding that the termination or discipline of teachers who publicly raised issues about the management of special education programs may result in liability by the schools for violation of a teacher's right to free speech — leading to a $205,000 jury verdict, upheld by the Eighth Circuit on appeal.

Finally, my phone rang with the conference call. Dr. Granpeesheh, Mr. Montague, Mr. Carew, Curt, Caron, and our ALJ Dr. Etscheidt were all on the line and settled on May 3rd as the day to begin taking evidence. There would be another brief 15-minute call scheduled before that time for any pre-hearing motions. But, for now, we were asked for any objections to Dr. Etscheidt serving as our ALJ. No objection.

We had a brief discussion on how to exchange our respective exhibit lists.

The county courthouse would be contacted to reserve a courtroom, and there would be an alternate location in the public library where I had first looked up the word "autism" two summers ago.

We were offered mediation.

Curt spoke up, "We are always willing to go to mediation, but neither of the other sides is receptive at this juncture."

Caron and Mr. Carew agreed.

The three attorneys were informed, "You will need to notice that to me in writing."

That was all. We were done for the moment.

Curt called to tell me that when he had touched base with Caron before the conference call, she had been unwilling to waste any time on mediation. I was too volatile.

"Well, I suppose that's how I appear. It may be how I *am*," I admitted to Curt and had to admit to myself.

Curt immediately reassured me, "EYSE is my agency's top priority this year, so I have the backing to litigate that issue."

I offered Curt my personal legal assessment. "Caron has a terrible case on the evidence, on issues of both procedure and substance — and a real Achilles' heel on the issue of mainstream integration: bad on the facts, and bad on the law."

"It looks like we're all going to be pounding the table," Curt sighed.

I ran down the results of my fitful morning's legal research, while Curt made notes and appreciative noises.

Donna dropped by and I brought her up to date. She left me her notes of Ruffin's day. The most encouraging observation she made was of Ruffin at lunch. "Ruffin liked everything and ate everything on his plate. The first-grade teacher came in to read a book in the lunchroom. I am fading way back at lunch now. Ruffin went to lunch, got his tray, and left the lunchroom very nearly entirely on his own."

Elaine sent home Ruffin's cut and paste coloring page of a yellow sun, a bee, and purple tulips with curly green leaves. No name, however, on his paper.

Now that we had our hearing date, far away, in California, Evelyn spent half a workday gathering CARD's files and reports about Ruffin to be produced and reviewed for litigation. Unavoidably, this cost $260.

That afternoon, with Donna I interviewed Luther College psychology student Angela Robeson for her to attend Sunflower Day Care Center with Ruffin as an integration aide. She seemed interested, eager, and smart. Donna and I both liked her, immediately.

I had something to keep Ruffin busy. He was going to call his cousin, Robert. He did a good job looking for the phone number. I described where my address book was — downstairs, in the *foyer*, in the black leather computer case — go downstairs, find it, and bring it here. He made three trips before he succeeded. He brought up every black leather datebook from my law *office* going back to the year of his birth.

While Donna, Angie, and I visited, Ruffin had a long 20-minute conversation with his 6-year-old cousin Robert. They talked about the weather — storms here in Iowa and there in Cleveland. Afterwards, Ruffin regaled the three of us with news about the storm near Robert's house. It blew the roof off the church, blew down a tree on the road and sidewalk. Ruffin had asked Robert lots of 'interview-type' questions. Evelyn would have been pleased.

I was getting more and more theory of mind remarks spontaneously — "I wish, I worried, I didn't know you were there, You surprised me, You don't know" — this broke down when he was frustrated or rushed, but then he would say, 'I don't understand,' as a conversational repair.

In the home-school notebook, I didn't hold back. "Looking at Kim's chartings — looks like we have criteria on 2-part single-element commands. Donna, please review Kim's charting in the green folder. I'd like to see Ruffin move on to something more complex — I assume Kim knows whether the best next step is to move to 3-parts, or to add a second element. If Kim will say which way is most incrementally a move forward — we will play this game at home and on weekends.

"CARD says the file Caron and Mr. Carew ordered fills an entire filing drawer. They are taking it to a copy service for duplication. The school already has *much* of this material. *Your copy costs alone will likely exceed the cost of a Sunflower playgroup for this summer.*"

Of course, just as I expected, Miss Hobbs faxed my home-school notebook message to Caron with her own note: "MJW is at it again! I thought she wasn't supposed to do this anymore!" Yes, I thought to myself when I found this later in Ruffin's educational file, let's *not* communicate.

Then, I called Sunflower and arranged for Ruffin to attend 3 hours in the early afternoons of Monday, Tuesday, Thursday, and Friday, with flexibility to late afternoon, and Wednesday, all day, if necessary. I was able to schedule a 1-hour in-service for their teaching staff with Evelyn for May 6th in the mid-afternoon. If I hadn't made these arrangements, no arrangements would be available for anyone to agree to, or for our ALJ to order, since the schools weren't planning to do anything toward Ruffin's mainstream integration this summer.

After running my office copy machine sooty, I wrote Dr. Norman at UIHC about Ruffin's upcoming late April evaluation and our early May due process hearing. "Here is an indexed packet of documents for your comprehensive evaluation of Ruffin. We would like to have written reports of your findings ASAP. These are the principal documents that would be introduced as exhibits and discussed at due process — hopefully, the packet will prove handy for your quickest review of Ruffin's case."

Evelyn Kung would be arriving May 2nd to be available to testify on May 3rd. That evening, Curt and I would need to prepare her, and Dr. Granpeesheh by telephone.

Elaine sent home Ruffin's art project to cut out nine different small colored triangles, a small circle, and a stem to paste them within the outlines of a pre-drawn flower, and his school coloring project to draw a sun in the sky over a garden. Ruffin ignored the human figure of the gardener, and apparently missed the instruction to draw water sprinkling from the watering can held by the figure. He had carefully attended to and colored most of the flowers.

Ruffin and I went out to eat breakfast downtown, then went to Lansing's five and dime. Ruffin was still in search of a toy store with the magic airplane. He talked all the way to Lansing about what magic deeds this airplane of his imagination could do.

Donna and I sat with our calendars. "This Thursday is the day I need you to keep Ruffin after school. I'll be at the Bridgewater field office in West Union." Despite all the sniping over my own due process hearing, I continued to work amicably with Ray DeNeve for the parents of several of my clients with autism in Bridgewater's distant southern sector.

Monday, I ordered 50 subpoenas to issue for our due process hearing. I continued to swap gossip with our other home program families in Iowa and consulted at length with a doctor in Richmond, Virginia, who wanted to start one there for her little one. When Ruffin arrived home, he showed me he had been able to complete one of his two shared reading worksheets. One sheet was perfectly completed, the other was completely blank.

Elaine had sent home Ruffin's worksheet there with his name on it. He had followed her oral directions to color six different snakes their assigned colors by locating them in front of, over, in, around, on, or behind the log where they all lived. A challenging task, but Ruffin loved snakes, and knew his colors and his prepositions cold. On the back he had drawn his own spotted snake, named 'Spikey.'

Donna had pages of notes, as always, about Ruffin's day with her when she stopped by for an hour to visit. She had told Meg and Miss Hobbs she was disgusted with their failure to reach an agreement with me about Ruffin's summer program and kindergarten year.

"Was all this a prelude to having the DHS remove Ruffin from my home?" she had wanted to know.

Miss Hobbs was surprised when Donna mentioned *Section 504 of the Rehabilitation Act* and all the Reed Martin special education lecture-tapes she had been working her way through.

I gave Donna a copy of the *Iowa Rules of Special Education* about hearings and a copy of *Negotiating the Special Education Maze* to read and study. She had a late afternoon appointment with local attorney James U. Mellick for a few minutes to get advice about how to be a good witness and how to stay out of any trouble for herself.

Principal Peter Smith called. Could I meet with the St. Pat's school board again to explain what was going on? There were rumors around town. I said I would be happy to come explain, answer any questions, and address any concerns.

That same evening there was a public-school board meeting. What, if anything, did our school board know about our upcoming due process hearing?

CHAPTER FIFTY TWO

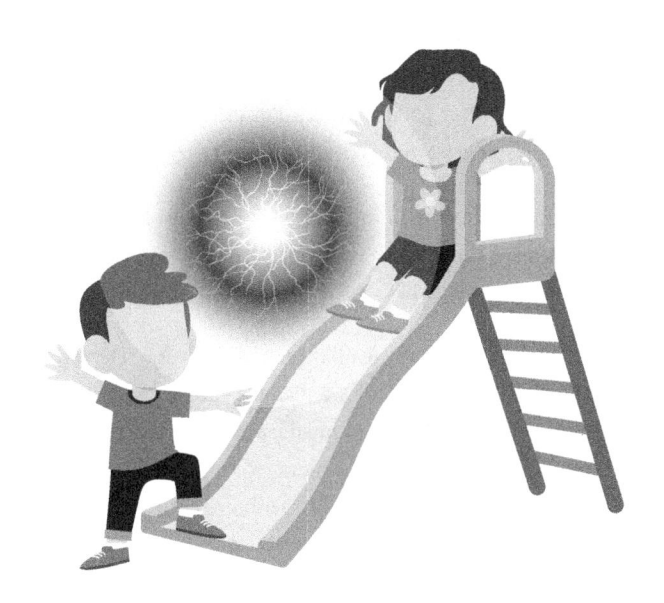

BEFORE DUE PROCESS

Dr. Norman and his University of Iowa Hospitals and Clinic (UIHC) team would not be able to issue their full written reports until mid-May — long after our due process hearing. He and his team wanted to stay above the fray. It was not their job to advocate or come witness for Ruffin. I found that cowardly and said so.

Donna told me Ruffin's educators thought it was just going to be seek and destroy with me about him until high school graduation, so they had determined to take an early stand. They were especially worried that I would continue to appear for other families at their IEP meetings. They knew it would be more expensive to litigate than to agree with me on any summer plans. Taxes were going to be wasted, too.

I agreed. Due process would be a waste of money.

Meg knew this was dirty pool. She did not approve. She had told Donna to warn me, "Be prepared." Meg was "disgusted and sick" and in disagreement with the school's legal strategy.

Donna's personal attorney, Jim Mellick, had told Donna, "Mary Jane is not going away."

"I didn't need to pay him to tell me that," complained Donna.

But Mellick also knew how St. Pat's was being pressured. He told Donna that one of the public-school board members, a prominent Catholic, was likely the source.

"Not good," I said. "But good to know. I'm meeting with St. Pat's school board tomorrow. Everybody seems fearful, even the university's evaluation team."

Late that afternoon I met with the St. Pat's school board in their school library to reaffirm my plan to send Ruffin there for kindergarten, according to the contract Principal Smith and I had signed earlier.

Thursday, I went back to West Union to work with Ray DeNeve and one of his southern sector teaching teams. While we planned summer programs for a couple of older children there with autism, Curt amended my due process complaint to allege Ruffin's educators were denying him the summer services he needed "because 1) the most recent offer fails to provide critical integration opportunities; and 2) fails to provide sufficient hours of one-on-one therapy, and 3) was not prepared in procedural compliance with the IDEA."

Curt also filed two pre-hearing motions on Ruffin's and my behalf: a motion to exclude any evidence "designed or intended to cast" my "personal life or parenting skills into issue;" and a request to take Dr. Granpeesheh's testimony by phone so that she need not fly to Iowa.

Caron registered another letter of complaint with Curt. "We have learned that your client has hired a Luther College student to work at a preschool in Decorah with Ruffin. Since ACSD is paying the expense for CARD to train personnel, the inclusion of any employee retained by your client would be inappropriate.

"Also, your client is continuing to send inappropriate information to the classroom teacher in daily notes. We must insist that the mother direct her comments about the child's summer services (EYSE) and next year's IEP to school administrators or legal counsel. The mother's conduct is extremely distressing to staff. The staff wants only to do their job and not to be embroiled in the mother's crusade. What must we do to get these notes stopped?"

Yes, Meg *was* distressed. But I thought the answer was obvious. Listen to Evelyn, listen to Dr. Granpeesheh, to Gundersen and to me, and make an appropriate offer of a free, appropriate public education. Keep your own written promises and be transparent. Step up and agree faster.

Friday, I wrote to Meg, Donna, and Elaine, and by early that morning Mr. Lord had faxed my latest note to Caron. "I have enrolled Ruffin at St. Pat's for next year as a unilateral placement given Miss Hobbs's position that she will not accommodate Ruffin with the appropriate class size.

"St. Pat's will — and they have all Bridgewater related and support services.

"I stand by all my previous offers to settle and am willing to do whatever it takes to cooperate in the preservation of public funding; that is, to keep Ruffin's weighted state dollars available to all of us. Without all our cooperation the matter of Ruffin's weighted funding will get rather muddy legally."

Caron sent us her list of ACSD's witnesses: Meg, Inge, Kim, Elaine, Miss Hobbs, Donna, Lisa, Mr. Montague, Dr. Granpeesheh, and Evelyn Chung, meaning, we supposed, Evelyn Kung.

Curt and Caron agreed to extend the designation of exhibits to the end of April.

Dr. Etscheidt ruled that Dr. Granpeesheh could appear by conference call with access to a fax for the presentation to her of exhibits about which she might be questioned.

I chose to open the hearing to the public, even after Dr. Etscheidt refused to exclude any evidence about my personal life and parenting.

But *sequestration* of witnesses would occur. Sequestration required that every witness who testified — except me, and Mr. Lord and Mr. Montague representing the defending agencies — remain outside the courtroom during the hearing, enter only when called to testify, and then leave the courtroom. The purpose of sequestration was to avoid witnesses sitting in to listen and learn how to conform their testimony to that given by earlier witnesses.

Dr. Etscheidt agreed that Ruffin's home-school notebook should be included in his official school record. Curt and I agreed to provide the schools with a copy of all Dr. Granpeesheh's files about Ruffin. The exchange of exhibits five days before the hearing would require long hours of work at the last minute, but litigation was always like that.

The official school record would need to be verified. I would need to perform new FERPA inspections of every educator's individual file.

The hearing itself would proceed very much like a civil bench trial — with opening statements, first by Curt, then by Caron and Mr. Carew, and would allow for final arguments by both sides, with a rebuttal on Ruffin's and my behalf by Curt. As the complaining party this time, I had the burden of proof, so Curt would have the last word.

Deadlines for the attorneys to file written briefs would be set after all the testimony and evidence had been received.

Caron wanted the late April UIHC full re-evaluation of Ruffin to be received in evidence. Perhaps the hearing record could be left open to receive it as soon as it was issued?

Under all the circumstances since our mid-August mediation, Curt cautioned everyone that the schools' litigation strategy should not be used as a tool for retaliation against me as Ruffin's parent and advocate, since that would amount to a *Section 504 Rehabilitation Act* violation.

In Ruffin's book bag, Meg shared her charting on Ruffin's memory drills for 10-word sentences and digits up to 5. Monday: No charting due to private nursery school. Tuesday: Sentences okay, but probably only 50% on numbers. Wednesday and Thursday: Ruffin was absent. Friday: Luther College visit. It must have been frustrating for Meg, trying to find time to chart those IEP objectives with Ruffin's splintered schedule.

But Meg was still writing, still sharing. "Ruffin went underwater accidentally today. He was quite upset until I suggested he ask you if he could call Robert to tell him he went under at Luther, just like he did with Robert at the beach. He has been telling us about that. He brightened up considerably. Then he and I had a splashing contest, and he was fine. Now he talks about it as a positive experience."

Elaine herself let me know, "Ruffin met all his integration objectives by playing cats with a classmate, farm set with the boys, and looking at a Disney photo album with the same classmate."

That same afternoon, Meg had gone to the nursery school to observe Ruffin there, to prepare herself to testify. I found Meg's more detailed account immensely reassuring.

"When I entered, Mrs. Mills commented that Ruffin had remembered to tell her that I was coming to visit after a prompt from his bus driver that he had a message.

"At the beginning of my observation, Ruffin was engaged in solitary play — the teachers commented that this was the first time in a long time that he had played alone. He was manipulating toys in the garage — driving a forklift up a ramp, pushing the lift up and down — using vocalizations for engine noises. He pushed the vehicle down the ramp and tracked it going down. When Mrs. Mills approached, he reported, 'I got all the town out.'

"Another boy approached and said, 'Let's play kitties.' Ruffin responded, 'Play kitties? Okay.' Ruffin crawled after the boy across the floor to the kitchen area — they pretended to eat the food there. The boy crawled away, and Ruffin followed. They went up the steps and then down the slide. Ruffin raised his arms over his head as he went down the slide in imitation of the other boy. They repeated this a few times. Then as Ruffin approached the slide, a second boy stepped between him and the first boy. Ruffin pushed him aside in an apparent effort to stay right behind his classmate. They were still crawling between slides and making 'meowing' noises. Ruffin went down the slide immediately behind his classmate and ran into him. Mrs. Mills reminded Ruffin to wait at the top of the slide, and he did the next time down.

"Mrs. Mills had a camera — and asked a group of boys to pose for a playtime picture. They all gathered at the top of the slide — fairly crowded. Ruffin joined in and had a big grin for the camera — very natural-looking.

"One time as Ruffin and his classmate touched as they went down the slide, they gave each other a static shock. They laughed and tried to repeat the shock the next time they went down. They were successful.

"Ruffin then went to the barn area and played with the animals there. He wandered to the climbing cubes and climbed on top. He called his classmate's name and waved him over. His classmate came, then Ruffin put his head down through the middle and crawled down in. He crawled out, over, under, in, and through. He and three other boys, including his classmate, climbed on the cube and imitated animal noises and actions.

"Ruffin went to the shelf and got the Santa puppet. He said, 'Ho, Ho, Ho.' And went down the slide two times with the puppet on his hand.

"Ruffin went back to the barn where five other boys were playing with animals and joined in. He put the sheep on some blocks, knocked it over, and repeated this.

"Ruffin returned to the barn area where his classmate was sitting at a table with a photo album. There was a lot of conversation about the pictures. Ruffin said, 'I like that, too,' among other things that I could not hear from my observation point. I did not want to be obvious by moving closer. I could tell there were sentences and turn-taking during their conversation.

"Ruffin turned to the shelves behind him, took out a puzzle and sat across from his classmate. He concentrated well on this and had no problems reassembling the puzzle. He put the puzzle away, returned to kneel beside his classmate and they again discussed the pictures in the album they were looking at.

"Ruffin walked away from the area and climbed on the cubes again. He walked over to a large tractor tire beside me. He crawled inside and called, 'Hello, anybody home?' I responded, 'I'm up here.' He got up on top — four other boys came over to the tire — Ruffin crawled back inside. They all followed him and imitated the way Ruffin curled up to fit inside as if to hide.

"The teachers announced clean-up time. Ruffin immediately crawled out of the tire and went to the wooden blocks which he began to stack and carry to their storage cart.

"It was my impression that Ruffin wanted to stay by the first boy, his classmate, but when he changed activities to one not of Ruffin's preference at the time, Ruffin was not content to stay beside him. It seemed that Ruffin was pulled by his desire to stay with his classmate, and his desire to do an activity of his choice. Ruffin did not seem unhappy but did not settle long at one play activity which he usually did more so than during this observation. Ruffin was very cooperative with teachers and peers. He would play with other children, but seemed most comfortable with the first boy, his classmate. His teachers reported no problems or concerns."

These critical mainstream developmental experiences were what Ruffin's educators were unaccountably unwilling to provide over the coming summer.

Monday, Ruffin was marked absent. He, Seamus, and I were in Iowa City for his re-evaluation by UIHC. Upon our arrival, I signed a release to myself for all Ruffin's medical records, to include transaction reports of all the phone calls made or received about him. His educators wanted this evaluation — which Bridgewater had agreed to pay for — as evidence. I wanted the information, too, to make the right decisions for Ruffin's future.

During the afternoon interpretive conference, Seamus and I were assured that Ruffin had been cooperative with all testing activities. His diagnosis remained PDD-NOS, not Asperger's because of his history of language delay. On the Stanford Binet, his IQ tested in the high average range: Verbal 107, Nonverbal 122, Full Scale 115.

An occupational therapist had checked Ruffin briefly for three different things: reflexes, guarding, and instability. His motion planning was within normal limits, at the 5-year, 5-month developmental level.

Ms. Wilding, the speech and language pathologist who had seen Ruffin twice before told us Ruffin was still wrestling with more abstract concepts in her directions to him like "either/or," "and/then," "next to" and "before." He did use "and/then" spontaneously. On the hour-long ASSET test she administered, Ruffin showed lots of inattention and was distractible. He offered a lot of echolalia with the increased language load. He would need simpler instructions. He had difficulty in specific language skills when trying to define things or state functions. When he ran into difficulty he simply echoed, but he had done well when asked to offer labels and categories. He had shown better pragmatic skills than academic skills, when giving definitions and meanings. He was exhibiting better formulation skills, with some fillers, in his sentences and grammar.

Ms. Wilding assigned Ruffin a language age of 4 years, 5 months receptively; 3 years, 10 months expressively; 4 years, 2 months overall language age — still a 10-month delay. During the last 8 months of our "shotgun marriage," Ruffin's accelerated language learning of last summer had slowed to a bare chronological crawl.

Dr. Norman told us the test he administered topped out at age 5. Ruffin's academic readiness for reading and math were both right at average, right on target within 2 weeks of age norms. He was able to follow 2-step directions and was better with upper case than lower case on his letters, with some reversals. Phonics, initial sounds, and identifying letters were shown by Ruffin's response to the word 'hippopotamus' — a word he knew the meaning of and could say now. Many of his numerals were written backwards, but he counted objects to 10 and was able to offer the next number after a given number, performed simple addition with objects, and was able to copy, color, and cut. But Ruffin needed a break during testing. Dr. Norman thought Ruffin would benefit from visual support. He supported Dr. Granpeesheh's small class size recommendation.

I made careful notes, because I was fearful that only my notes and my memory of this interpretive conference would be all we would have to offer as evidence to Dr. Etscheidt. But, because Bridgewater had paid for this re-evaluation and wanted to offer it as evidence, too, when we did get the full written reports, we were able to stipulate them into the record before Dr. Etscheidt took Ruffin's case under advisement to make and write her formal decision.

CHAPTER FIFTY THREE

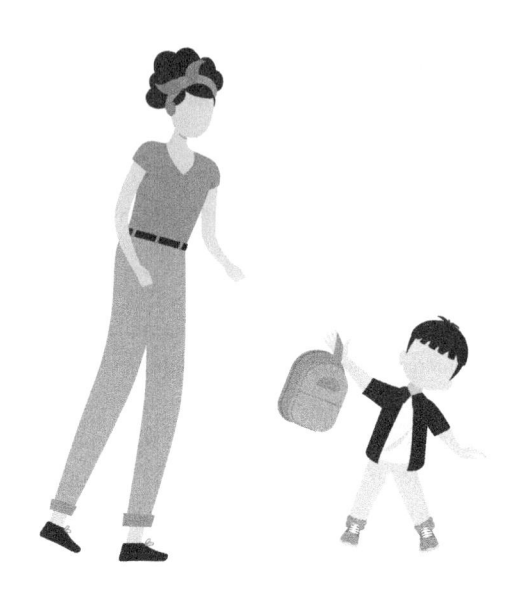

LEAVING NOBODY OUT, OR IN THE DARK

As always and as before, I wrote for the record, into Ruffin's home-school notebook. "UIHC will support Dr. Granpeesheh's class size recommendation that Ruffin be accommodated by a small class size (12 to 15) in a mainstream kindergarten class.

"This fall's reductions in Ruffin's one-to-one time with Donna, and of his association with typically developing age-mates really impacted Ruffin adversely. The two speech and language reports by Ms. Wilding that bracket this most recent school year are quite telling. I was surprised because I had hoped she would see a lot of progress as before, after last summer.

"Maybe if we had all done what we agreed to do — CARD in the morning and typically developing boys and girls in the afternoon (as Donna, Lisa, RoJene, Pine, and

I did last summer) Ruffin wouldn't be in this spot. Maybe he would be ready for kindergarten in the mainstream with 24 to 26 kids.

"The Bridgewater 'complete' educational record fails to include many of the most damaging documents I collected from Bridgewater back in August of 1995. I haven't seen ACSD's file production yet — I hope it will be complete."

In offering this analysis, by drawing these comparisons, and offering this sharp commentary, I was writing to our ALJ, Dr. Etscheidt. Miss Hobbs dutifully and predictably faxed that day's entry to Mr. Montague, Mr. Carew, Caron, Curt, and Dr. Etscheidt, leaving nobody out, and nobody in the dark.

Our new Luther student, Angie Robeson agreed to meet up with Donna and Evelyn on May 6th in the early afternoon — while our due process hearing continued. I wouldn't be able to join the three of them.

Donna dropped by with her most recent notes about midday. She told me Meg wanted to talk to the attorney, Jim Mellick, to get some advice for herself. I doubted Mellick would meet with Meg, since he already represented Donna. Representing two witnesses on opposing sides of our dispute would raise an impermissible conflict of interest for him. I felt badly that Meg must be feeling such a high level of concern.

I asked Donna to just step back and let Ruffin do whatever he might choose to do in Meg's classroom and elsewhere on the public-school campus, and just make careful observations for a written hearing exhibit.

Donna reported that in kindergarten shared reading Ruffin knew the sounds of his letters perfectly, and did a timely, assisted finish of the day's worksheet by working a bit quicker. This was the first day since he had been going to lunch with the kindergarteners that he had been able to eat everything on time.

"Ruffin told me all about his trip to the city yesterday. He said the big man there gave him ice cream that was silly." Dr. Norman had shown Ruffin an ice cream cone cut-out early in his examination and showed him the same cut-out later with a "bite" missing. It struck Ruffin as funny and memorable.

"He talked about his dad going with him. He added that he would get this television and would get married to his mom. When I told him he couldn't get married to his mother that he would get to pick a whole new person, one his own age, you could see he didn't really like that too much. But when I gave him a list of names including the little girl who didn't really love him from his kindergarten shared group, he thought this might be okay.

"He also carried a message to the teacher about the lunch tickets. Perfectly."

Caron had filed a dense twelve-page index of the school's records as her exhibit list. Now Curt and I could begin checking her list against my copy of Ruffin's educational file.

Curt and Joan drove up from Des Moines on the first day of May. I let Meg know, "Your attorneys can reach Curt here from now until Friday."

Principal Smith of Saint Pat's School assured me, "I feel confident that you and Ruffin will enjoy being a part of our St. Patrick's School family. We are very proud of our school and the opportunities that we offer. We feel there is a closeness at our school that many times can't be found elsewhere." I was encouraged by St. Pat's decision to stand by our written agreement and welcome us. Now, I felt free — emboldened really — to fight as hard as need be for meaningful change in the provision of summer services (EYSE) statewide, and for every student with a disability, knowing that Ruffin and I would have a safe place to retreat after the damage of litigation had been done.

Curt and I were deep into preparing for our due process litigation — one of my favorite things, but not Curt's.

Donna worked with Ruffin on emotional situations:
Donna: How would you feel if you were in a dark room all by yourself?
Ruffin: Scared.
Donna: Why?
Ruffin: Because I'm scared of the dark. I'm not scared of the basement. I'm scared of the noise when Mom lets the plug of the bathtub out and it goes swish.

Donna met with me that afternoon, bursting with news. Caron had asked to interview her at school. Donna didn't want to be interviewed without her attorney present. Donna and Mr. Mellick had told Caron they would talk to her and to Mr. Carew if the school agreed to pay Mr. Mellick's fee. This expense was not authorized by Mr. Lord and so, no interview with Donna took place at school before she left for the day.

Later that same evening, Donna called again. Ray DeNeve had just offered Donna a job as a liaison between Bridgewater and all the local school districts in his sector with CARD's Evelyn Kung. A meeting with human resources for mid-May was scheduled. Donna was excited, and I was pleased. Ruffin was going to claw his way back to the brink of the universe, a bit later, rather than as soon as I had expected last summer. Donna should have an opportunity to move up into a career. I knew her well enough to believe that even if this job interview were a "dangle" intended to influence her testimony favorably to Ruffin's educators, they were in for a surprise. As a witness, under oath or not, Donna was an experienced and wary truth-teller.

On May 2nd, the day before our hearing was to begin, Ruffin told me as I put him to bed about "the yellow important paper in my backpack" from nursery school about Mother's Day. He knew it was for a party where he would give me a secret present. Yes, he knew what a secret was — it was against the rules to tell me. He said he was awfully sad because he wanted to tell me. I told him it was a surprise, and okay if he didn't tell me. We talked more about his feelings. He wanted to name all the feelings he knew by then: angry, sad, happy, excited, embarrassed, surprised, worried, and scared.

Evelyn arrived.

Despite Dr. Etscheidt's rulings on his earlier motion, Curt continued to hope we wouldn't face the child abuse report issue, but I was more sanguine, and made sure we would have the witnesses we might need under subpoena in case we needed to call them. By subpoenaing the child abuse investigators as witnesses in our case, we telegraphed clearly to our adversaries: we were unafraid to address those issues.

UIHC wanted my authorization to release Ruffin's records to Bridgewater from his most recent visit, and for a year into the future. UIHC needed this to get paid. Caron filed an application for an order requiring me to release them, but I wanted to read the most recent evaluations first — to have the opportunity to correct any errors. I whined and moaned to Curt and didn't sign anything until after the hearing was underway and then limited my release to only the information immediately relevant to our due process issues — because at the time I really could not imagine any future relationship between UIHC, Bridgewater, Ruffin, and me.

I instructed Meg, "Send Ruffin home to my house, *not* to Lisa's. Thanks." Lisa would be testifying later if the school authorities chose to call her. Her name had popped up on their witness list. Hopefully, they would not be tempted to call her. She had never worked with Ruffin at school. No one from either side had issued her a subpoena. I hoped that meant she was unlikely to be called. This left her feeling relieved and free to work with Ruffin at my home while Curt, Joan, and I worked for Ruffin a few blocks downtown at the local courthouse.

CHAPTER FIFTY FOUR

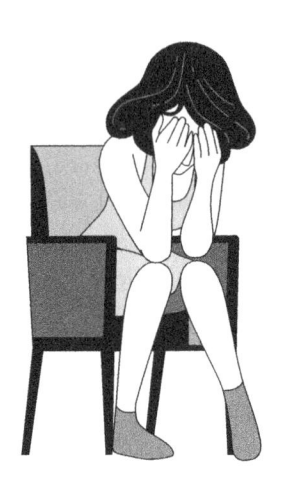

I TESTIFY

We all assembled before Dr. Etscheidt in the high-ceilinged wood-paneled upstairs courtroom familiar to me. I felt comfortable and eager to begin. Curt reaffirmed that the hearing would be open to the public at my request. I didn't think confidentiality served the interests of advocacy or of altruism.

Curt remained standing, nodding an acknowledgment to everyone in turn, and then offered a brief explanation of autism as a neurological disorder that caused a child to avoid human contact and to lack the skills for even rudimentary forms of learning. This was for the record in case of any later appeal since Dr. Etscheidt had been chosen to hear our dispute because of her own academic familiarity with autism.

Then Curt explained Lovaas's applied behavior analysis (ABA) as the only educational methodology that enjoyed an appropriate rate of success in educating young children with autism to satisfy federal disability education law. In this opening statement he went farther than he had ever gone before with Dr. Hagen by emphasizing that no other educational methodology supported an appropriate rate of learning in children like Ruffin.

Nodding again to Ruffin's educators and their attorneys seated across the double-wide polished oak counsel table, he offered a heads up to Dr. Etscheidt that we expected Ruffin's educators would argue that because he had made some educational progress before ABA began in the late fall of 1994, Ruffin must not even have autism. Then Curt explained Ruffin's medical diagnosis of PDD-NOS, as a form of autism, and pointed to the continuing support for his autism spectrum diagnosis most recently in the independent evaluations from both Gundersen and UIHC. He explained how and where Ruffin had been repeatedly tested and evaluated over the past 22 months.

Finally, Curt introduced me as a professional single parent whose 3-year-old had first been diagnosed in the summer of 1994, and the person responsible for having researched and implemented ABA methodology with Ruffin, a method which had doubled the rate of his development over the rate of growth proposed by his educators' original IEP. Instead of congratulations and interest, these stellar results with Ruffin's special education in my home had drawn litigation, and ugly, anonymous threats.

But the case presented to Dr. Etscheidt would be limited to addressing Ruffin's special needs for the upcoming summer. First, the educators had failed to follow the federal and state procedural rules in dealing with me as Ruffin's mother. We would also show that a full summer of appropriate services was critical to assuring Ruffin would remain ready to enter kindergarten next fall.

As a "back up" issue, we would show his educators had failed in significant ways to follow the August 1995 IEP they had agreed to after an earlier mediation — by failing to implement the agreed Head Start integration component during the fall of Ruffin's second year in special education. As a remedy, our position was Ruffin was entitled to "compensatory education" this summer for last fall's integration failure of 9 weeks' duration.

Caron and Mr. Carew opened for Ruffin's educators, taking the position that none of them had done anything to break federal or state rules, that despite my being a most difficult individual, Ruffin had always been offered a free, appropriate public education (FAPE), and that by failing to show up for the March summer services (EYSE) meeting I had somehow waived my due process rights as Ruffin's parent, and now had no way and no reason to object to whatever their plans were for Ruffin's summer.

That joined the issues so Dr. Etscheidt could see exactly where the parties were locking horns.

Before we left for the courthouse, Curt had looked grave. He had something to discuss. What could it be? I wondered. We had the evidence, tabulated in binders. We were going to be able to put our hands on it, without fumbling. Our subpoenas were all served and paid for. We had a bulging file of returns of service in multiple carbon copies. We had our witnesses, our experts lined up and prepped. We had our examination outlines. Our plans for cross. We had the law. Curt had written a pre-trial brief. The arguments were structured in his head. Sturdily.

Curt asked me if when I testified — did I think I could be a mother? Seem like a mother? Feel like a mother? Not be so hard?

As a mother at that moment, my mind travelled back to Dorothy, the chemist, the hard scientist, who had written as a mother, "It's difficult to hold back the tears, but so far no one I know has seen me cry outside the privacy of my own home." That would have been me, ordinarily. In this way, I imagined, I thought, I was sure I was like Dorothy. "I dislike women who cry easily and here I was becoming a first-class 'dripper.'"

But, as an experienced trial lawyer myself, I shared Curt's concern. And, as for myself as a witness, I knew what Curt would need to do, and how he would need to do it. "It's not hard," I had confided to him, as we stood together on my wooden gingerbread porch that early spring morning. "When you need to trigger those — when the time is right for those feelings — offer me a kind remark. I'll dissolve . . . utterly . . ."

And it was not hard for me. As I took the stand, just before lunch, I was able to cry, to weep, to leak through the better part of a day's testimony. And that afternoon, under hot eyelids, through hot tears, I broke down in rage. On cross.

It was not hard for me, once I started to cry, I couldn't seem to stop. It was humiliating. It was painful. And, very painful, I imagined, to witness. For poor Caron and grey Mr. Carew to press on against — grimly. But I was able to tell Ruffin's and my story as it is written here, but, of course, more briefly.

Curt's job was to focus my testimony on the EYSE issue, the summer at hand, by harkening back to the failure of Ruffin's current IEP to even address this summer, and to the spring IEP meeting season with its looming statutory deadline.

Curt asked, "As the March 25th, 1995, EYSE meeting date approached, did I advise you that the school district attorney Caron Angelos and Superintendent Lord would not be attending?"

"Yes."

"Did that concern you?"

"Yes."

"What were your concerns?"

"The educators on the IEP team would be attending without legal advice about making their EYSE offer to Ruffin, and the superintendent, the person with the authority to commit local district resources, whether people or money, would not be present."

I went on to explain why I thought my attending such a meeting would not be fruitful or productive and how I decided not to attend, after talking it over repeatedly with Curt. Yes, eventually, under all the circumstances, he and I had decided that I would not attend.

I recounted how, after that decision, Curt had assured me that the IEP team still had the duty to consider my autism experts' — Dr. Granpeesheh's and Evelyn Kung's — recommendations for what should be provided as Ruffin's summer education. And I explained everything I had submitted to the educators in writing, in advance of the meeting date, so all that material was marked and received into evidence.

Then, Curt and I doubled back to the much earlier mid-winter 1994 IEP meeting and how the EYSE issue and the identification of "critical skills" had been handled during Ruffin's first year in special education.

We laid out my position as I approached mediation before the beginning of Ruffin's second year of special education. I described all the mediation results and how the current IEP had been written after a long day's work of contentious mediation. I identified all our agreements, as those documents poured into the record.

I testified that I knew I needed to be involved in identifying Ruffin's "critical skills," and referred to our home-school notebook's various messages about this subject from time to time this spring, since I had understood, by learning the year before, that the identification of "critical skills" was an important educational and legal matter.

Both sides knew Dr. Etscheidt had asked for a copy of our home-school notebook. It had been taken into evidence early on. Curt and I trusted she would read it carefully before reaching any decision.

I described Ruffin's and my most recent trip to UIHC to see Ms. Wilding, and we introduced a copy of her earlier written report showing that over the summer of 1995 while I had directed his education in my home, Ruffin had been developing language twice as fast as a typically developing child. Ruffin *could* catch up with his typically developing cohort, and with the recent demonstrations of his normal to high IQ, he had *a special need* to do so.

Curt and I then introduced copies of the anonymous hate mail questioning my sanity which I had received just after the mediation agreement had been announced to Bridgewater employees by Mr. Montague, as well as the threatening letter that had arrived on its heels from an ISEA attorney written on Dot Gordon's behalf, alleging that I had libeled her as a member of Bridgewater's autism resource team (ART).

My discussion of these exhibits led back to the earliest instance in the fall of 1994 of the ART and Ruffin's educators questioning whether he had autism at all, and to their taking repeated issue with every medical team diagnosing or evaluating him since. Curt and I were going to meet that part of the educators' anticipated defense head on.

I explained how shortly after Ruffin's diagnosis I had begun networking with other parents and a parent support group, and how at least one other parent in our group had also complained of receiving anonymous hate mail after disputes at school. I laid out how long it took the settlement check promised me in August to arrive — not until six months later, not until the next February — because both educational agencies had repeatedly delayed performing on the financial obligations they had undertaken in our August mediation agreement.

Then, using the home-school notebook and letters I had written, Curt and I walked through the serious delay in Head Start mainstream integration during the past school year. Yes, Meg had told me a couple of months into our shotgun marriage for Ruffin's second year in special education, that she and I needed to amend his IEP because none of the Head Start children would be taking part. I explained that by that late date, the private nursery school — the only alternative mainstream placement for children of Ruffin's age — was already full and had a waiting list. I explained how, after insisting on it, I did get an IEP notice from Ruffin's principal Miss Hobbs letting me know, as required by law, exactly who would attend another mid-year IEP meeting to resolve this inclusion failure.

For planning Ruffin's upcoming summer, I said the input of my autism experts, Evelyn Kung and Dr. Granpeesheh, was needed to identify what should be Ruffin's "critical skills."

I whined that I was tired of going to IEP meetings where the bodies were stacked against me, and where no one else seemed to be familiar with the concept that year-round schooling was appropriate for students with autism. And, no, the arrival of the anticipated new EYSE state special education rule from Dr. Hagen in January had produced no new thinking, and no new action on the part of any of Ruffin's educators. Yes, I was frustrated.

Indeed, I was angry. I was furious because this spring, Ruffin's teacher had been packed off to a meeting in Des Moines which I had been unable to attend. But by nos-ing around, I had obtained and reviewed the presentation materials and heard accounts of the meeting from other attendees. The materials seemed to me to be derived from the earlier, very contentious confidential mediation with me about Ruffin's education the previous August, and were very harmful to public policy, to other young children with autism in Iowa, and to Ruffin and me, in my view. They echoed gossip I had heard about Ruffin and me around town.

Yes, as a remedy, I would be willing to accept 9 weeks of compensatory integration services during the summer of 1996 for the failed Head Start integration promised to Ruffin in the fall of 1995.

On cross-examination, I readily admitted I was not much of a housekeeper or a cook and that I hired a local woman to provide those services, so I could concentrate on how to address Ruffin's autism. Would this have been a question anyone would have dared to ask a single father? On this point, I was indignant.

I described how I had called Bridgewater for help the morning after Ruffin's first diagnosis, but that it was by reading and researching that I had learned that behavior modification was the only effective education and treatment for autism. I admitted to having spent the outrageous amount of $2,000 to $3,000 on books, videos, and academic studies in learning about autism and reaching this judgment.

Yes, I had investigated the TEACCH program from North Carolina, and explained my reasons why it offered nothing appropriate for Ruffin. I described ordering in Dr. Bernard Rimland's entire library of autism resources and reading them all, and what I had found there to be appropriate to try with Ruffin: megavitamin therapy, auditory integration training (AIT), and applied behavior analysis (ABA) as developed by Dr. Lovaas and offered now by CARD.

Indeed, I had willingly enrolled Ruffin in early childhood special education. And, yes, I had done so hopefully.

I admitted to the further outrageous act and expense of buying Ruffin a Macintosh computer when he was only 3 years old. Yes, after having submitted Ruffin to Bridgewater educational testing about that same time and learning from their school psychologist that Ruffin's *Bayley Scale* had been measured to be only 50, the equivalent of moderate mental retardation.

I suppose the effort on cross-examination was to make me out as a deluded mother unable to accept Ruffin's disability, a total kook who could not accept she had given birth to a child with disabilities.

I described how after reading *Let Me Hear Your Voice*, by Catherine Maurice, I had contacted Inge Nilsen at Bridgewater to ask for an Lovaas ABA program for Ruffin as a part of his special education, and how, after receiving a letter back from Bridgewater telling me no, in no uncertain terms, that nevertheless on November 4th and 5th, 1994 I had arranged for Evelyn Kung of CARD to come from California to help me start one for Ruffin at home.

As early as mid-October of Ruffin's first year in special education I had hired Donna Schmidt and Lisa Murphy, mere lay people, one a high school graduate and the other, a holder of a GED, and, yes, I had asked both of them to commit to carry out a two-year long home program for Ruffin.

Yes, it had always been my position that "I want you to meet his special needs, or I will do it myself." I supposed that was meant to make me appear arrogant. Which, of course, I was, although I had been reduced by that time to furious tears.

Given an open-ended question, I told how I set up and carried out my own summer program for Ruffin in 1995. No, the school had made no offer I would accept.

Then the time I was cross-examined about shifted forward, skipping most of the period of the educators' and my most unhappy shotgun marriage. Neither Caron nor Mr. Carew dared to broach the subject of the January child abuse complaint. It was passed over in silence.

Yes, on Thursday, March 21st, 1996, I did receive a manila envelope containing Meg's observations of Ruffin's performance on his IEP goals and her observation of Ruffin at the private nursery school. But nothing from anyone else, I added firmly. Inge had failed me as an advocate for Ruffin, and that's when and why I lost my temper with her.

I acknowledged CARD had sent me two unsigned letters on March 23rd for my review, and that I had secured two signed letters from CARD and four pages of summary plan prepared for Ruffin this summer which I provided to the schools for their summer planning.

Yes, I admitted I had already made some arrangements for this summer for Ruffin to attend Sunflower for play time in the afternoon on Monday, Tuesday, Thursday, and Friday, and for Donna to provide one-to-one CARD drills in the morning on Monday, Tuesday, Thursday, and Friday. Yes, I had offered Donna $2,000 to work with Ruffin during the upcoming summer. Indeed, I had decided to let Lisa go at the end of the school year because she had accepted infants she would be providing childcare for this summer who would interfere with her ability to provide effective one-to-one instruction to Ruffin.

Yes, I had asked Dr. David Bishop, a psychology professor at Luther College to advertise for a person to do Lovaas integration with Ruffin during his time at Sunflower. A graduating senior, Angela Robson, had agreed to work 3 hours a day for 3 days a week at $10 per hour, for a total of $900 for the summer.

The cost for the total mileage of 3,200 miles to take Ruffin to Sunflower and back over the summer would be about $800. The charge for Sunflower would be $27.60 a week, or a total of $276 for the summer.

I admitted this summer plan fell shy of Dr. Granpeesheh's written advice because I wanted to have a day with Ruffin for myself. I suppose I appeared both extravagant and selfish, while being unwilling to follow CARD's own prescription to the letter.

Called upon to do so, I gave a full account of what I had learned at Ruffin's most recent re-evaluation at UIHC that Bridgewater had paid for, but, no, I didn't yet have a full written report from the entire evaluation team. Of course, the schools and Dr. Etscheidt wanted to see that.

By the time I stepped down, weeping with rage, after the last questions, I thought I could see everyone else in this hearing room was more uncomfortable than me.

Dr. Etscheidt acknowledged my testimony, pointing out what she found useful for herself in her later decision.

HER DECISION OF June 3rd, 1996:
Ms. White testified that she has observed her son be 'spectacularly unsuccessful' in his approaches to other children in his integrated settings. She stated that although he may be 'swimming with the fish,' his interactions are not satisfactory.

Friday was not a usual day for a large group of litigants to show up at our local courthouse. Most trials began on Wednesdays. So, our group working there all day long on a Friday had not gone unnoticed. A handwritten letter had been mailed to our local gadfly opinion-writer for the newspaper. Since it was anonymous, he had passed it along, unpublished, to Mr. Lord, who placed it carefully in Ruffin's educational file — where I happened to run across it later that summer.

Dear School Board Member,

Are you aware there is presently a court trial going on at the Appaloosa County Court House that may last all week? It involves some lady who is suing the Appaloosa Community School District, or the school district is suing her. I don't know which.

I only know there are four or five lawyers working on it as I heard they get $150 per hour, and it could cost in the tens of thousands of dollars just for legal expenses.

I presently work in the Court House, and I overheard some lawyers from Waterloo talking about how long this was taking.

I did not see any school board members there, only Mr. Lord, our superintendent, and he seemed to be enjoying himself. He is not elected though, so he may not care.

When the press and public find out about this, the school board may look like fools.

I would not care, except I and my husband work hard to pay taxes to have it spent so foolish and stupid as on legal fees.

And now you are talking about building on a new addition. When the public finds out about this, you can forget that.

Signed, A Concerned Taxpayer.

CHAPTER FIFTY FIVE

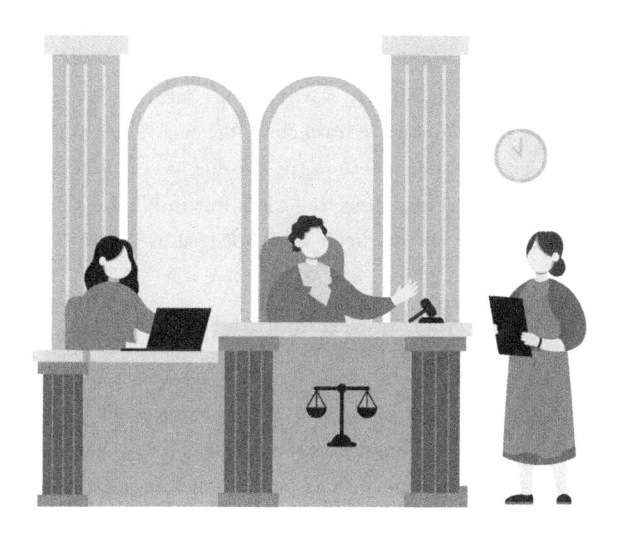

OTHERS TESTIFY

With my own testimony behind me, I could relax and just listen on Monday. Curt would have plenty of time to study Ruffin's records — at least the ones we had managed to gather — and sharpen his examination outlines over the weekend. Dr. Etscheidt would have time to review the many exhibits already received into evidence, but she probably needed to attend to her own grading, paperwork, and end-of-the-year academic roundup at her university. It was comforting to have Evelyn in town, to have her available to meet with Curt to get ready for the important part she would play in testifying for Ruffin.

Evelyn worked most of the day Saturday with Renee and her care providers, teachers, and aides at ACSD. This was a real testament to Evelyn's ability to continue to work with people with whom I found myself in sharp dispute.

Ruffin went to Sunday school, while Curt and I worked together in my office, and then visited with Evelyn to prepare her in anticipation of her and Dr. Granpeesheh's testimony. Evelyn spent all Sunday preparing to testify on Monday. CARD's participation in this process cost about $1,400.

I alerted Meg and the educators on Monday. "Since your Friday Luther College morning programming is no longer available, what will be done to meet your IEP performance obligation for Ruffin? What will be offered?"

The school's plan for Monday was for Meg's substitute to bring Ruffin and his ECSE class to the public library to learn about the circus. Since the county courthouse was in use for regular Monday motion day, our due process hearing had been bumped over to the small, low-ceilinged meeting room just inside the public library doors. It would be a circus, too. Dr. Etscheidt acknowledged as much. "Numerous witnesses testified, and voluminous educational records were received."

Dr. Granpeesheh testified over the phone from California for about an hour, optimistically, in her lively, still lightly accented voice. Dr. Etscheidt listened, but was ready to make her own, independent judgments. "Dr. Granpeesheh testified that Ruffin is at the end of the discrete trial section and in the middle of the integration year. She indicated that she was basing her recommendations on Evelyn Kung's two school observations of Ruffin. She testified that additional observation and information would be needed if there were conflicting data concerning Ruffin's performance in social settings."

Caron and Mr. Carew's job was to make sure there would be plenty of conflicting data introduced concerning Ruffin's performance in social settings. I wondered who they would use to do that. I didn't think Donna would be their choice. It would have to be someone else.

Continuing with her summary of Dr. Granpeesheh's testimony, Dr. Etscheidt found, "Dr. Granpeesheh testified that her recommendations for Ruffin's summer program included structured play (i.e., a play group environment where someone can prompt him and teach him how to do social activities like taking turns, sharing, etc.) in addition to the discrete trials. She testified that there was 'no way he could learn (social skills) unless he is immersed in a structured play group' with a therapist. She stated that the therapist must be highly skilled (i.e., she must know when to prompt in a social situation, the child's developmental level, and how to get the child to interact with other children). She testified that this type of therapy is more difficult than the one-to-one training, and 'ideally' only senior therapists are utilized for this component of the training. 'Lacking that, you do with what there is, basically. If there is somebody who has already worked with the child for over a year and has picked up good behavioral skills, then you have to go with that' rather than have the child wait.

"After the child has mastered the concrete developmental goals, he begins a series of social tasks. These tasks include the 'theory of mind' or perspective-taking skills. These are advanced, critical skills without which a child 'would be very concrete in their thinking.'

"Dr. Granpeesheh testified it would be inappropriate not to provide structured play sessions over the summer, as Ruffin will not maintain and generalize skills without the structured play opportunities. She described Ruffin's current need to be skill generalization: he needs to extend his learning beyond one-to-one into group situations.

"Also, the hours decrease for children who are finishing the Lovaas program. Dr. Granpeesheh indicated that the schedule for decreasing hours is very specific to the child but is usually over a 1-year period: 'the weekly hours can go from 40 to 20 — gradually decrease 20 hours — without hurting the child.' The final phase gradually reduces those 20 weekly hours to none. She testified that the program is individualized by the hours prescribed (i.e., if the child speeds through the first part of the program, the move to structured play can begin) and by the content (i.e., the drills are specific to the individual child's needs)."

Evelyn Kung testified that she was a graduate student at Pepperdine University in California and that she had worked for CARD for the past 4-and-a-half years, first providing direct therapy. She had risen to become a supervising therapist, supervising a group of direct therapists. Over her career, she had worked with some thirty children with autism.

Nodding in my direction, she testified that I had contacted CARD in late September or early October of 1994 and scheduled an early November workshop. She had received reams of paper from me before the workshop, during which she had the opportunity to observe Ruffin for some seven hours before developing an individualized program for him. This was her sixth trip back since that original workshop to advance and tweak Ruffin's program.

It was part of her practice to ask the parents for background about the child with autism, and in Ruffin's case she had also enjoyed the opportunity to talk with Ruffin's teacher, Meg Holub, and his Bridgewater case manager, Inge Nilsen, who had both attended the original weekend workshop. Of course, as Ruffin's mother, I had had input into the program proposed for Ruffin for this upcoming summer.

Ruffin should be ready to enter regular kindergarten in the fall, depending upon his summer progress. There would need to be good cooperation with his next classroom teacher, but she anticipated Ruffin would enter regular kindergarten in the fall.

Dr. Etscheidt listened, again, a bit selectively. "Ms. Kung testified that Ruffin has good imitation skills and will learn social skills from other peers."

Evelyn left as soon as she finished her testimony to observe Renee in her severe and profound classroom and to observe Ruffin at the private nursery school and then go meet with Meg. Then Donna took Evelyn over to Sunflower for the remainder of the afternoon to meet with Angie so the two of them could train her to work as an integration aide there with Ruffin for the summer. During brief recesses in our hearing, I was able to make quick calls from the phone at the library's front desk to assure myself all this came together as planned.

CARD charged $187.50 for Evelyn's hour-and-a-half long observation at the private nursery school that day, and $562.50 for her services to train Angie at Sunflower. My share of Evelyn's travel expenses was just $150, because she would visit four other Iowa families during this trip.

Elaine Mills testified that she was a private nursery schoolteacher who had graduated from Luther College in 1970 and then taught first grade for 11 years. She had earned an additional 30 graduate hours of credit over the course of her teaching career. She was a head teacher and currently certified by the State of Iowa. Although the private nursery school was not a public school, it was state licensed.

She was familiar with Ruffin as one of her students who attended her Monday, Wednesday, and Friday afternoon class. Miss Hobbs, the public-school principal, and the president of the nursery school had arranged for Ruffin's placement in her class, where he began attending back on August 30th.

She knew Ruffin also attended public school. At first, when he was placed in her class, she had been concerned that Ruffin was a special education student. But Miss Hobbs had promised the public schools would provide an associate to attend with Ruffin if necessary.

She and her president did agree to accept the public-school associate Miss Hobbs had offered, but only kept her less than a week since the woman had become more involved in helping other students in the class than in helping Ruffin. He needed no special attention in her small classroom of 15 students. Ruffin was just one of the kids. Truth to tell, she had more problems with other kids in her group.

I had wanted a computer added to her classroom, and Miss Hobbs had agreed to provide one, but she and her president had not wanted one there. That sort of technology would have been disruptive of their school's vision of fostering social development in young children.

This testimony was what Donna had warned me to expect of Elaine. She had confided that she longed to return to teaching in the public schools. The pay there was better and would have provided benefits that would give her family a greater measure of security. Who could hold that against her? Not me, but I couldn't help but be aware of the effects of these pressures in our small-town goldfish bowl.

Since I had already testified to last summer's arrangements for Elaine to co-teach Ruffin's summer playgroup with RoJene, and how Elaine had bowed out at the last minute, Curt and I saw no need to question her about why. Her bias seemed transparent to me, given her slant on the facts and her very agreeable demeanor during her examination by the school attorneys. Curt and I weren't left to wonder long who they would be using to introduce all that conflicting evidence of Ruffin's performance in social settings.

As for seatwork, Elaine always included small motor project time with coloring and pasting and the like, in which Ruffin participated. She gave verbal directions, and the children were expected to follow them. With Ruffin, it depended on the day whether he did or did not.

As to whether her method for giving verbal directions differed in preschool from her practice as a first-grade teacher, each year, with each class, she analyzed how she would have to approach giving directions. Any modification this year in her giving directions had not been caused by Ruffin.

She expected all the children in her class, except one, to be ready for kindergarten next year. Elaine identified her January report about Ruffin's kindergarten readiness, a report which she considered still current at the time of our due process in early May. She expected Ruffin to be ready for kindergarten in the fall — definitely.

Early in the school year Ruffin had exhibited some self-stimulatory behaviors but since then she had not observed any until last Monday when Evelyn Kung had visited her class. When Evelyn left, Ruffin immediately changed back to his normal behavior.

When Meg Holub visited her class to observe, her presence did not cause Ruffin to change his behavior.

As Ruffin's mother, I did not visit her class much, but whenever I did Ruffin paid attention to me, but not to class.

Elaine did not think Ruffin was imitating other children much, but he did play with both boys and girls.

Yes, Ruffin was absent for 3 days in March and 5 days in April. In the fall when Ruffin had been absent there would be changes in his behavior when he returned to school, but after absences in the spring, his good behavior had been maintained.

Dr. Etscheidt was persuaded by Elaine's apparent independence from either of the warring parties, and by her day-to-day classroom experience with Ruffin. Overall, I found myself pleased as well. Ruffin had managed to function within a mainstream group without alarming his teacher or his classmates.

CHAPTER FIFTY SIX

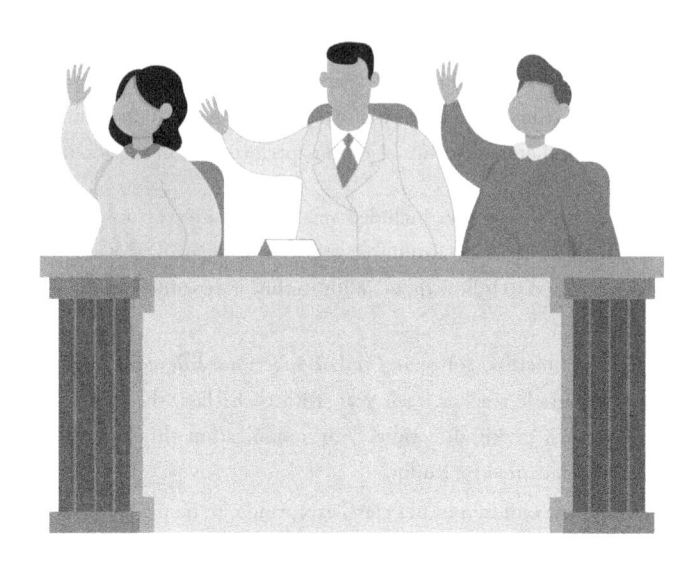

MID-HEARING

August Montague, The Man, as I still thought of him, testified that he was the director of special education for Bridgewater and had been for the last 19 years. He had a Bachelor of Science degree from the University of Northern Iowa where he had studied audiology. And, yes, a master's degree from the University of Missouri at Kirksville. He had taken other graduate courses at both the University of Iowa and the University of Minnesota over his 37- nearly 38-year career in special education. As a result of all those studies, and his considerable years of experience, he considered himself familiar with the special education of those with severe and profound disabilities, including autism.

It was his duty as Bridgewater's director to provide overall management and ensure that its employees followed all the special education provisions of the Iowa Code. He was familiar with all the federal rules of special education, too.

Bridgewater covered eight counties in northeast Iowa and served twenty-five school districts, four of which were among the largest school districts in Iowa. Administratively, he had divided Bridgewater into four geographical sectors, with each sector assigned to a sector coordinator. His chief deputy, Laverne Mosher, "Moe," was the sector coordinator for sectors one and two. The Man himself served in this role for sectors three and four.

Most cases were handled directly by the regularly assigned sector coordinator — but this had not been true in Ruffin's case. Mr. Montague testified that he had become involved in Ruffin's case in mid-July of 1994 when I had called him that summer. He advised me of the available services at Bridgewater. Then, he received copies of a great deal of information from me, which he had referred to "Moe" and down to Jack Wallace, an assistant coordinator working under "Moe."

Bridgewater kept a central file on Ruffin at our town's local field office. All the documents referred to by the other witnesses were familiar to him. Yes, in preparation for his testimony, he had reviewed Ruffin's complete, medical-educational file.

March of 1995 was the first occasion he had attended an IEP meeting for Ruffin, when there were indications there would be future litigation. Curt was there and a discussion of the state rules of special education indicated that some sort of opinion concerning summer services, EYSE, would be forthcoming from Dr. Hagen of the state department of education in Des Moines. Curt thought we should all wait for it to be issued.

New state rules of special education did become effective last summer in July, as anticipated.

He had also been present on August 18th, last summer, when a prehearing mediation was held. However, he was not at the evening IEP meeting that followed, but he understood from Inge Nilsen, his employee attending, that the issue of Ruffin's summer services (EYSE) had been put on hold, waiting for Dr. Hagen's opinion to issue. In January of this year, Dr. Hagen finally presented her interpretation of the new state rule addressing summer services.

Bridgewater's principal role in Ruffin's special education was to provide speech and language pathology services. Those services were always performed. Bridgewater had gone beyond its responsibilities to Ruffin by responding to the mother's demands for special testing and by paying for evaluations at Gundersen and at UIHC.

Bridgewater was not required to provide any services to Ruffin under ACSD's most recently proposed 1996 summer plan. Nor was Bridgewater required to provide anything under CARD's most recently proposed summer plan for Ruffin. Nor was Bridgewater required to provide anything by the recommendations from the UIHC arising out of Ruffin's most recent evaluation there. However, if any services were to be required by any group or by Dr. Etscheidt, Bridgewater stood ready to serve Ruffin.

Mr. Montague believed that ACSD's proposed program for Ruffin for the upcoming summer was in *substantial* compliance with state and federal special education law. Even though, yes, clearly, there had been *procedural* errors committed by ACSD, that is, by Ruffin's local principal and ACSD's special education director, Miss Hobbs.

If there were legal questions presented to Mr. Montague, he had a ready opportunity to consult with legal counsel, and to read and review special education laws and federal statutes. It was his obligation to provide accurate, up-to-date information to Bridgewater staff so they could follow state and federal regulations and all applicable EYSE procedures. He had no control whatsoever over whatever Miss Hobbs chose to do, or not.

No, he did not feel that the offer of a summer program to Ruffin had suffered because of his mother's requesting this due process hearing, or because of any of the earlier disputes with me.

Mr. Montague believed that the summer offer of ACSD to Ruffin would provide him with a free, appropriate public education. No, no, even though there were *procedural* errors committed, he felt that the process to develop Ruffin's EYSE IEP for the upcoming summer had not been impaired.

With these final beliefs and feelings of his, Dr. Etscheidt would strongly disagree.

Inge Nilsen testified that she was employed as an early childhood special education consultant with Bridgewater. She had a Master of Science degree from Ohio State.

She was Bridgewater's primary agent on Ruffin's team with the responsibility to facilitate staffing about Ruffin, and to stay in touch with me. Ordinarily, by law, local school districts were responsible for all special education notifications to parents, but in Ruffin's case sometimes she had done it — written the IEP notices and other notices sent to me.

Inge admitted she had only seen Ruffin twice in the hall this school year.

Nevertheless, she was a member of the late March group that met in Miss Hobbs's office to consider what, if any, educational program should be offered to Ruffin for the upcoming summer. She had agreed with the conclusions reached at that gathering in my absence, but, no, she didn't sign anything issuing out of that meeting herself. "Theory of mind" drills were considered for Ruffin at that gathering, even though she herself didn't know what "theory of mind" meant or entailed.

Earlier in March, she and I had talked on the phone. I had wanted the attorneys to handle the upcoming summer issues due to the hostility within the IEP team. I had told her that I wanted 4 hours a day of CARD drills, 3 hours of structured play for 4 days a week, and 3 hours of unstructured play per week.

She also vividly remembered that just before the late March meeting, she had received an incredibly angry phone call from me, and that I had sworn that I wanted this "fucking" thing resolved. This was true. I had stooped to swearing. The ugly degree of my lapse expressed the height of my sheer frustration.

Dr. Etscheidt was attentive, not so much to Ruffin's progress, as to the maintenance of his established levels of skill, whether behavioral or academic. Progress as a summer goal was clearly out-of-bounds as far as she was concerned, and not to be expected of him or his teachers. "Ms. Nilsen also testified that the team 'thought there was a danger of regression on this skill' of compliance due to the 'inconsistencies' between environments. She testified that the number of one-to-one CARD drill hours recommended were 'roughly equivalent to what he gets in the mornings at school . . . we thought it was enough to maintain what he has.'"

I had no intention of watching Ruffin tread water all summer.

Kim Pope testified she had been employed for a decade as a speech and language pathologist at Bridgewater. Her Master of Science degree was from the University of Northern Iowa in speech pathology, where Dr. Etscheidt taught.

No, Kim did not attend Evelyn's CARD workshop in early November of 1994. She claimed she had participated in his mid-winter IEP — the one just after Evelyn's workshop, when Ruffin's educational file disclosed that it had been Emily Knight, the school psychologist, who had read out Kim's written report in her absence. She was on Ruffin's IEP team because he had been assigned to her to receive speech and language therapy.

Kim recalled talking with me and knowing who I was and recalled receiving CARD drill materials from me and using them in some of her work with Ruffin.

At first, she denied feeling any hostility toward Dr. Lovaas and his methods. However, in early January, Mr. Montague had directed her to look at several due process cases describing the methodologies of other educators who opposed Dr. Lovaas and his methods, and that in January last year she had attended a conference put on by Dr. Lovaas in California.

The most recent summer offer for Ruffin represented something more than the usual school response to a parental request for summer services. The offer had been made as a response to his mother's advocacy by the group asking itself, "Have we asked what is it the parent wants? Can we offer what his mother wants in order that she not take us to due process?" The group had considered doing what I wanted to do to get themselves a happy parent.

Yes, the group had asked itself, "If offering some one-to-one drill time would not hurt Ruffin and might help — then why not offer some?" This was because Kim understood that ACSD and Miss Hobbs were working with a rational school district attorney,

Caron, who was not a savior like a white knight who wanted to fight to the death — because ACSD and Bridgewater couldn't risk losing this case and having a precedent set everywhere in favor of Lovaas.

She disagreed with Caron's legal strategy herself — since she believed there were no precedents in IDEA law, anyway, owing to the individual nature of each student. Of course, she admitted, law did get made in due process. Standards did get set in federal and state rules and due process. Of course, *procedural* rules were often enforced in due process. She knew.

When asked if Dr. Lovaas's UCLA methodology interfered with her work as a speech and language pathologist with Ruffin, she finally snapped back at Curt, "Can a couple days of training replace years of concentrated education to become a speech and language pathologist?" She had written a letter of her own to Dr. Lovaas calling him out for questioning the developmental procedures she had been taught at Northern Iowa, and the concept she relied upon herself — that different children had to be treated differently. Dr. Lovaas seemed to treat all children with autism the same. But she had never raised this issue from the floor at his conference in California that she attended.

Kim testified she had "a real strong feeling" that there was never just one way to treat every child, but admitted, educators did need to use Lovaas methods when they were appropriate. She herself had always preferred to look at the entire child to determine his or her program.

Since Emily Knight, the school psychologist, never testified, Kim was the only Bridgewater employee whom Curt asked about last August's hate mail, sent to me right after mediation.

"Did you write this?"

"I have never seen this before," Kim swore.

Ruffin's educators used the concept that if there was no regression in a child's skills, there could be no eligibility for summer programming. There had been meetings about Ruffin's critical skills during Ruffin's first school year, but there had been no critical skills identified during his second school year before the most recent March meeting about what Ruffin might need for this summer.

Kim had never known, much less imagined, that Evelyn and Dr. Granpeesheh of CARD would need her speech and language treatment notes for Ruffin before the EYSE meeting — not until Inge had called her one night. She had not tested Ruffin's speech and language development in preparation for her testimony. Although, yes, there were such test results — oops, right there in Ruffin's educational record.

No hearing, no matter how dire the matter at issue, no matter how close to the heart, to life, or to death, is without its moments of sheer hilarity, of revealed surprise, of stunning admissions pulled out of the mouths of witnesses like black, deep-rooted teeth. Under oath, Kim admitted to Curt, that all her previous testimony which she had offered with such cheerful confidence was the result of such long experience that it allowed her to treat all her students by "keeping all their records in her head."

Stop! I thought. This was enough. We were ahead, and Curt glanced over at me, read my look, and stopped.

Dr. Etscheidt seemed to be struggling to suppress what? A smile. A chuckle. I had never been good at reading people, but here was the snippet she wrote later, in passing judgment. "Mrs. Pope testified that there was no charting of the speech and language goals and objectives available at the EYSE IEP meeting of March 25th, 1996, but that she came to the meeting with 'clinical judgment' 'in her head' and that 'knowledge I have about a child is the knowledge that went to that meeting; those specific numbers of her charting did not go.'"

Caron was left to make a workmanlike attempt to rehabilitate Kim. She obviously worked with children with a variety of disabilities, trying to help each of them become good communicators. Kim tried to help even nonverbal students develop a means of communication. True, she finally admitted, she used test results to be able to compare standard scores over time.

At Ruffin's most recent EYSE meeting, Kim had tried to explain to the other group members present how Ruffin was functioning. Ruffin did a little bit better in compliance and following directions than other special education students — because of the unique one-on-one relationship he had enjoyed with Donna and his other home therapists. But all in all, she considered her own informal observations to be the most important thing in working with any child, and with Ruffin. Grudgingly, she also acknowledged for Caron, again, the importance of empirical data, such as serial standard test scores. As for Ruffin, Kim felt he probably needed no further services, especially this summer, because he already had a basic understanding of the language used in kindergarten.

Then, Kim admitted to Curt that she knew she was obligated to keep a working file, but she didn't have a copy of it, since she kept it largely in her head.

Ruffin had problems following directions, problems with memory processing, and with attention span. She and Ruffin's teachers needed to obtain Ruffin's attention first when working with him. He was then at about 90% accuracy in following 2-part directions. Ruffin would make eye contact, but really didn't have mind contact with other people. His verbal communication skills were very good for kindergarten and, really, she swore to us, she *felt* he would not lose this ability over the coming summer.

Under more questioning from Mr. Carew, Kim explained how one other person from Bridgewater, Emily Knight, a school psychologist, had also attended the Lovaas conference in California. Kim did learn about Lovaas there, but she felt Ruffin had made great strides from just learning in Meg Holub's ECSE classroom without Lovaas and before Lovaas. Of course, he learned more after Lovaas because anyone receiving direct one-to-one instruction for as long as Ruffin had would improve, but she herself continued to prefer a more naturalistic approach to teaching him — since we all learn language from the environment that we live in.

I found it difficult to credit anything Kim had said. Dr. Etscheidt wandered in finding her own facts and passing her own judgments. "Mrs. Pope testified that Lovaas one-to-one drills were recommended since Ruffin's mother wanted this and the team felt this method could meet goals that were set as critical. She testified that socialization was discussed but determined to be unnecessary as Ruffin was socializing quite well with adults and classmates in various integration settings. She testified that the group 'wanted to keep compliance going through the summer for when he begins kindergarten.' Mrs. Pope indicated that Ruffin's attentional ability affects his ability to process directions, more than memory deficits, or auditory processing difficulties."

Miss Hobbs testified that her experience in special education was limited to assisting in a special education class early on in her teaching career.

Yes, in special education she and her teachers needed to document Ruffin's file every time they made a move, or change, and planning decisions for Ruffin needed to be data driven. She claimed that Dr. Granpeesheh had failed to support her recommendations for Ruffin's summer hours of Lovaas with any such data. Apparently, she did not consider Evelyn's observations and reports back to Dr. Granpeesheh as data.

Miss Hobbs had to admit to several *procedural* violations of special education law in issuing various notices of IEP meetings throughout Ruffin's special education under her supervision, including those notices she herself had written and sent out.

Dr. Etscheidt found these admissions helpful in reaching her decision.

"Miss Hobbs testified that EYSE has always been 'an area of confusion as we sit in our meeting because there is no place on the IEP form to write critical skills. So sometimes we end up getting them marked; sometimes we don't.' She testified that Ruffin qualified for EYSE because 'he has some deficit areas that we want to maintain or continue to develop this summer.' Miss Hobbs testified that the three goals of their EYSE IEP offer represented a 'summation;' the 'common thread that goes through all his many goals.' She testified the recommended number of one-to-one Lovaas drill hours was 'based on what Ruffin currently has in school.'

Dr. Etscheidt accepted Miss Hobbs's reasoning on this latter point as determinative of the result — by relying on my own agreement to the current IEP — rather than on the expert opinion of Dr. Granpeesheh. This was an additional cost of the compromises I had made in last August's mediation before entering this school year's failed shotgun marriage with Ruffin's special educators.

Monday afternoon ended with Miss Hobbs stepping down. Curt, Joan, and I went to my home to meet with Donna that night to prepare her to testify. When I reached into Ruffin's book bag, someone from school had written in our home-school notebook, "Mrs. Holub gone. Mrs. Webber subbed." Curt and I surmised we would be seeing Meg on the stand Tuesday afternoon, then — after we expected to be able to rest Ruffin's case.

CHAPTER FIFTY SEVEN

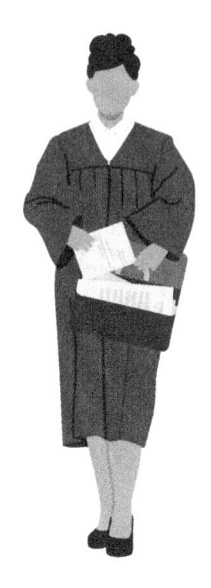

END OF HEARING

On Tuesday, Ruffin's absentee record kept by the school nurse reported that Donna had failed to come in to school, which was true, and that Ruffin had been absent, too, which was not — since our home-school notebook reported all his daily activities. Our hearing may have contributed to some confusion as to whether Ruffin was correctly reported to have been present or not.

As an exhibit in our due process hearing the schools had offered — and Curt and I had politely stipulated — to Ruffin's absentee record showing 39 absences and 3 late arrivals over his 2 school years of special education, 20 of which were due to various illnesses, and the remainder being for medical-educational evaluations at Gundersen or at UIHC, and for our 2 annual spring family vacations so Ruffin could celebrate his 4th and 5th birthdays in North Carolina with his grandparents. I imagined his record of absences would be of no moment since Ruffin fell below the age of compulsory school attendance. How could he be considered truant?

Donna testified that morning. She had earned a GED and had taken some college classes in phlebotomy at St. Mary's in Minneapolis. She had been trained by Evelyn Kung in early November of 1994 and had a pending offer of employment from Ray DeNeve of Bridgewater to provide Lovaas instruction. She was considering accepting that — after she completed her work as Ruffin's therapist.

She had first been engaged by me to work with Ruffin as a one-to-one therapist about a month before she had been trained by Evelyn for two full days during a workshop at my home. An important part of her work with Ruffin was to keep accurate charting, drill by drill, and day by day.

Using the techniques that she had learned from Evelyn, the changes she had seen in Ruffin over the time she had been working with him since November of 1994 had worked a miracle that was amazing to her.

Yes, she was a mother of a couple of children herself, a boy, and a girl.

She had been working on the elementary school campus for the most recent school year, pre-teaching Ruffin integration skills to help keep him looking like more typically developing students. She taught Ruffin ahead of time whatever the academic lesson might be in any class of typical peers he might be attending, and then she shadowed him into his various integration classes, following Ruffin everywhere he went, to help him engage socially. She kept notes of Ruffin's successes and failures, and of all her interventions to help him be more successful socially, whether they worked, or not.

She testified to Ruffin's various self-stimulatory behaviors and that he had become very adept at hiding them or disguising them, but they would still emerge when he had to strain his thinking to keep up with kindergarten academic content, especially in Mrs. Linden's kindergarten shared reading class which he had joined that winter. Kindergarten physical education, music, and lunch had been much easier settings for Ruffin to learn how to follow directions given to a group and were much more socially rewarding for him.

She had had recent conversations with Mrs. Linden, the elementary school kindergarten teacher where Ruffin attended shared kindergarten reading lessons about where Ruffin might be placed for kindergarten and whether if he were to attend kindergarten with her it would be difficult for him to learn there at public school without a one-to-one aide.

On cross-examination Donna indicated that it was not a part of her relationship with the school to share information informally with Meg.

And she had to admit she was still working on some of her own notes for me since our recent spring break vacation.

Most probably based on information she had let slip to Meg at school — Donna admitted Ruffin was less compliant with me than she expected him to be with her. She described dinner at my house as not always appropriate. Ruffin had eaten a glazed donut once rather than try his baked fish. Feeding Ruffin continued to present very difficult issues for everyone at home and at school. He still took baby bottles of chocolate milk. She had spoken about Ruffin's compliance issues with me.

Donna had seen some progress with Ruffin over the period since Christmas break, with Ruffin being more able to begin the sorts of tasks that other students in the kindergarten class were doing, but most of that progress was being made after teacher assistance directed to him individually. She described the goal of having Ruffin attend kindergarten shared reading was not that he learn to read, or write, but that he learn to follow directions given to the kindergarten group, and to have the opportunity of some integration with typically developing children.

Under Mr. Carew's cross-examination, she admitted that I had told her to "keep her fucking mouth shut at school" recently while the school and I were negotiating over Ruffin's summer program. It sounded terrible, just as it would, coming out on cross — and it failed to fully capture Donna's and my relationship of sometimes salty ribaldry. I told Curt it wasn't worth revisiting on redirect. Just let the word sit there on the record as a mark of my extreme frustration. I had said the same thing to Inge.

Then, when asked "What did the Lovaas people teach you?" a foolishly open-ended question posed by Mr. Carew, Donna took off on a long account of how Evelyn demonstrated exactly how to manage Ruffin with various techniques which she was now very accustomed to use with considerable success. Donna explained to Mr. Carew that she had never observed any other children at school engage in self-stimulation. It could look weird and would surely cause Ruffin trouble with other children.

Donna explained to Mr. Carew that it was not a part of her role to assist me in gaining compliance with Ruffin at home, nor was it any part of her role to take part in negotiating for summer services for Ruffin. It was hard, though, to keep her nose out of it.

Yes, she had asked for a $750 clothing allowance at the beginning of the school year, and I had agreed and paid her what she had asked, so she could buy what she thought she needed. No, my paying her that, or her wages, wouldn't affect her testimony. She was here to testify for Ruffin by telling the truth. Yes, sometimes she disagreed with me about certain issues. She had always spoken her mind in home-team meetings, and even at school when talking to Meg, Kim, and Miss Hobbs.

Certainly, by her observation — given that she knew me well — I had appeared stressed on the day of the scheduled meeting about summer services, yes, in late March when she understood that Curt and I had finally decided I would not attend.

Dr. Etscheidt wasn't impressed with any of the gossip. She was focused on what information Donna had to offer about Ruffin. "Mrs. Schmidt's 'kindergarten integration shadowing' observation notes indicate days with appropriate social interaction and days without peer interaction."

After Donna's testimony that day she went home to find that her seventh-grade son, Matt, had been sent to detention, and kept after school. Matt had been struggling to read since second grade and Donna and her husband Kevin had repeatedly approached Miss Hobbs and his elementary school teachers for help to no avail.

As the academic demands of junior high school came to bear upon Matt, he developed some typical secondary behavior problems that frustrated his teachers. Curt, who knew these issues well, suspected Matt might have undiagnosed dyslexia — and that Matt's detention during our due process hearing could have been motivated by retaliation against Donna for standing up as Ruffin's advocate.

Quietly, Curt approached Caron and explained what he saw in the situation. Caron advised Mr. Lord to get Matt out of detention and evaluated for dyslexia. Curt suggested Donna and Kevin pursue Orton-Gillingham methods of instruction that he knew to be effective. As a result, Donna and Matt spent the summer of 1997 living together three hours south in Cedar Rapids where Donna would be able to study these methods during the last year they were offered in Iowa.

After being trained, Donna succeeded in teaching Matt to read, raising his skills from the second-grade level to very nearly seventh-grade level. When the public schools were unable to follow through with further Orton-Gillingham instruction as they had promised, Donna and Kevin pulled both their children out of public school, homeschooled them and entered them into community college classes where they were both successful and went on to successful adult careers after college.

Late in the afternoon, it was Meg's turn on the stand. She testified she had a Bachelor of Science in elementary education and a Master of Science in early childhood education and work experience as a consultant and teacher of early childhood special education.

Meg had attended the November 1994 weekend CARD training with Evelyn Kung which had employed techniques of behavior modification, teaching one step at a time, and requiring mastery of each small step before moving on. She was supportive of Donna's efforts at school and praised her work with Ruffin as "great," based both on her observations of Donna's work with him in her room, and in Mrs. Linden's kindergarten reading class. She explained that Mrs. Linden, the kindergarten teacher, did not and was not required to chart Ruffin's progress there.

It was not Meg's role to respond to any of my special education administrative demands in our home-school notebook, and she did not. Miss Hobbs was Ruffin's administrator, principal, and the local district's special education director. Responding to me was Miss Hobbs's job.

For this summer's EYSE for Ruffin, the group had tried to pick the best vehicle for what they, the schools, wanted for him. She could not recall whether Ruffin's critical skills were discussed at that meeting. Yes, I had been sent a copy of the resulting EYSE offer.

Dr. Etscheidt focused on the matter of Ruffin's critical skills and the correctness of the school's procedure in considering them. "Mrs. Holub testified that she 'treated all the IEP goals as 'critical skills,' and data were collected for each. She testified that 'procedurally we did not identify the critical skills; we did not choose from the IEP goals any critical goal or skill.' She testified that they did identify critical skills during Ruffin's first school year, but in the August 1995 IEP meeting 'we missed doing that . . . restating that those would be (critical skills) or choosing new ones.' Since that most recent IEP indicated that 'EYSE issue has not yet been resolved,' Mrs. Holub 'treated all Ruffin's IEP goals and objectives as critical skills.'" That's how Meg testified to our late-night kick the can down the road decision about summer services (EYSE) after mediation.

"The quarterly progress reports of Mrs. Holub indicated 80% mastery in taking turns, 'okay' for spontaneous sharing, and 'okay' for imitating social play with an adult. She felt 'typical family experiences in the summer' would provide the social and group experiences Ruffin would need to maintain social skills. Ruffin does very well in the mainstream situation without extra supervision. She did not think he needed extra help with his social skills to enter kindergarten this fall. 'He does not need a structured playgroup to maintain or develop social skills; they are ingrained and will not be lost over the summer. The group selected one-to-one Lovaas due to its intensity and directness necessary to develop and maintain Ruffin's critical skills."

Meg's testimony about Donna and Lovaas represented a little resurgence of her courage, with the earlier shotgun-marriage IEP giving her a bit more cover to speak to what she learned at the first weekend workshop with Evelyn — for which, of course, she had written her *mea culpas* in Ruffin's cumulative file.

With Meg's testimony, our hearing ended, not with a bang, but with a whimper.

Dr. Etscheidt took the matter of Ruffin's summer education "under advisement" — meaning none of us would hear anything or know anything about how to proceed in educating or paying for Ruffin until she filed her decision in Des Moines.

Meanwhile, over the final few weeks of the regular school year, it was up to us — as wasps in a bottle — to continue to co-operate to provide Ruffin with his education.

CHAPTER FIFTY EIGHT

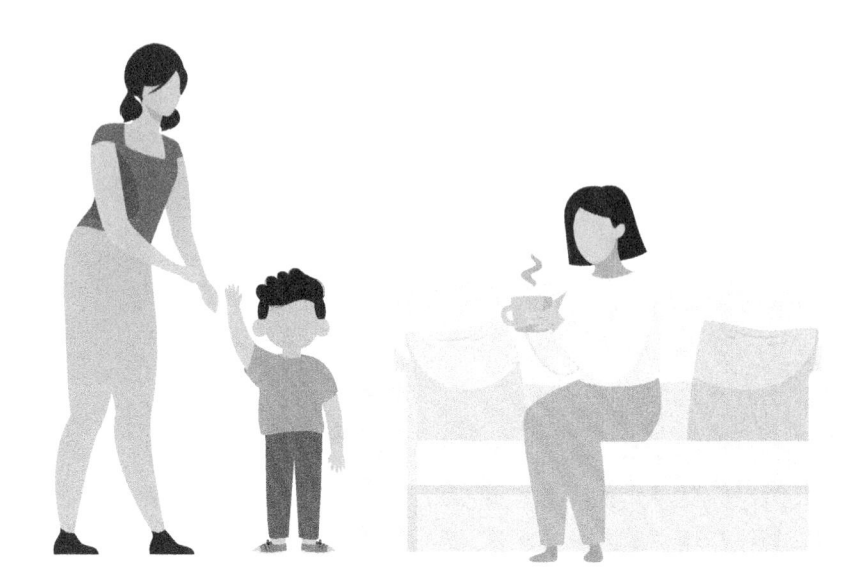

AWAITING SOME DECISION

Before she returned to California, Evelyn asked Meg, Donna, and Elaine to each complete a *Social Behavior Assessment Inventory* from Dr. Thomas M. Stephens' book *Social Skills in the Classroom*, 2nd Edition. She and Dr. Granpeesheh wanted to check for any discrepancies in their independent ratings of no less than 406 items of Ruffin's behaviors.

Meg rated Ruffin's social behaviors at an acceptable level for most of these items in her class which had grown to 10 special education students. This included Ruffin dealing with emergencies, following the rules for emergencies, identifying accident or emergency situations which should be reported, and reporting accidents or other emergencies to his teachers.

Elaine rated Ruffin social behaviors at an acceptable level for most of the items in her nursery school class of 15 regular education students. She rated some of his behaviors at a lower-than acceptable level, specifically: approaches teacher and asks appropriately for help, explanations, instructions, and so forth; greets adults and peers by name; offers help to teacher; pays attention in conversation to the person speaking; ignores interruptions of others in a conversation; lends possessions to others when asked; asks permission to use another's property; attends school regularly; brings required materials to school; completes assignments within required time; uses time productively while waiting for assistance.

Later, Elaine sent Miss Hobbs a little note, "Nan, Here's your copy." Howdy-do! I thought when I found it in Ruffin's educational file. Of course, Elaine's children attended public school.

Donna rated Ruffin's social behaviors at an acceptable level for most of the items from her perspective as his CARD-trained therapist supporting his integration with typically developing classmates. But she rated more of his behaviors at a lower-than acceptable level, than either Meg or Elaine. As always, and as I expected her to be, and paid her to be, Donna was Ruffin's closest observer, his truest friend, and his harshest critic.

While I worried about the coming summer, I took solace, as I always seemed to do in typing up Donna's detailed, daily treatment notes. She had banged away with Ruffin on various time concepts and his recall of recent events with mixed success.

"Drill: Expressively, using the words and concepts: Future, 20%; Present, 70%; Past, 20%."

This thought crossed my mind as I typed Donna's scribbles: Ruffin was naturally "mindful," centered in the present, as he should be, as a 5-year-old, but the past and the future would come to bear on him soon enough as they do upon all of us, and he would need to be taught these temporal concepts directly, just as Donna was trying to do. They would prove to be among the most difficult for him, as it turned out, and require educational focus for most of the summer and into the fall.

I focused on what clues there might be in Donna's notes to Ruffin's true kindergarten readiness. "Kindergarten shared reading: Seatwork worksheet, doing 4 simple directions perfect, but he could not get the 4th direction finished in a timely fashion. Ruffin needed to be told 3 times to move on to the next direction. He had most of the directions done but needed to have more information to complete the task.

"Also, he needed to be asked how the teacher would know this was his paper. He was able to tell me that he needed to put his name on his paper. He did this and joined his classmates.

"The kindergarten class was talking about a field trip to the hospital. Many students wanted to know if Ruffin would be joining them."

Ruffin seemed to have fallen into an interesting lesson at lunch. "He chose to sit by his friend and a little girl. I was told by the little girl that his friend had told Ruffin to move on ahead. I asked Ruffin if that was true. Ruffin said yes. I asked if Ruffin wanted to sit by the little girl. He said yes. Then I told him he should do what he wanted, and not let his friend, or any other student tell him where to sit.

"Then the little girl grabbed Ruffin and pulled him back with her. Ruffin seemed pleased. Ruffin needed a prompt to ask the girl's name and her favorite game. Ruffin was doing really well with this group talking and wiggling their French fries.

"Ruffin ate well and returned his tray perfectly. Ruffin recalled the girl's favorite game was tic tac toe, and that his friend liked to kick football, but you can't play football at recess."

Other lessons remained confusing. "Meg's class was responding to simple directions such as 'Stand in front of or behind or on the right or left of another student. Ruffin: in front and behind perfect, right at zero percent; left at zero percent. Ruffin was able to go to one side or the other but was unable to sort out right from left."

I chuckled at that, recalling that as a driver's education student, I had never been able to sort out right from left either — turning left into a median, flattening a street sign with the school car when our instructor directed me to execute a right turn at the upcoming intersection. Ruffin seemed to be "my child," in this respect.

One Friday, these were "Donna's Notes: Drill: Craft and Theory of Mind. Ruffin and I scribbled some lines on paper and then filled in each space with bright colored crayons.

"When I began to color my bright colors over with black, Ruffin made the comment, 'You are ruining your picture.' He then offered as his own thought, how he would not want to put black over his; and how I wrecked mine.

"We went through many exchanges of how I could fix mine, or if I could change mine into something that might look nicer. We also went into whether I could be thinking of doing something different with mine, about how I could be doing the same thing as him but thinking about something different.

"After finishing my picture and scratching out lines through the black surface, Ruffin could see that I hadn't wrecked my picture. Ruffin named the shape I had scratched out, and it became a duck. We added a bill, and then he began to cover his picture with black. He then scratched out and named his shape a bear, and we added more lines to make it more obviously a bear.

"Drill: 3-step directions: Color the big fish orange and blue, perfect; Color the little turtle brown and green, perfect; Color the big bird purple and yellow, perfect; Color the big rabbit black and pink, perfect; Color the big lizard green and red, 50%; Color the little lizard blue and orange, perfect; Color the big turtle yellow and brown, perfect; Color the little rabbit orange and pink, perfect; Color the little bird red and blue, perfect; Color the little fish black and red, perfect. Ruffin and I did this drill working off a Big and Little Critters Worksheet with 2-step directions from shared reading, marked 'Good job, Ruffin' with a star by the kindergarten teacher.

"With the big lizard, Ruffin needed my suggestion he reread and echo the directions. Ruffin was repeating the color names many times until he was certain he had found both colors. Ruffin's choice of coloring is very nice. He is finding certain areas for each color and not just scribbling his colors together."

I had to admire Donna's resourcefulness in creating this drill on the fly. It drew on Ruffin's very secure knowledge of the names of colors we had taught him earlier, his ability to read them, his natural love of animals, his skill at coloring to express his response with actions instead of words, all to develop his weaker memory skills into an early, successful attempt to attend to and follow complex 3-step directions. That many directions given at a single time proved to be a significant challenge — especially when given to him as one of a larger group of students.

Meanwhile, Curt and I prepared a settlement proposal to Ruffin's educators, hoping to settle all the matters of dispute before Dr. Etscheidt issued her ruling. I was willing to drop all my civil rights discrimination and retaliation complaints in exchange for the free, appropriate public education Ruffin was entitled to by law. Caron led us to expect an answer soon.

Ruffin had received a letter at nursery school. Scouring his book bag, he fished it out and asked me to read it to him. "Dear Ruffin, My name is Levi. I'm in kindergarten at St. Pat's School." This was an invitation for Ruffin to visit. "When you come to school, I will be your buddy. You may sit by me, and I will show you around. You will be able to see what we do each day and join us for lunch and recess. See you soon! Levi, Your friend at St. Pat's School." This, sealed with a horse sticker of a horse throwing a horseshoe, promised Ruffin something to look forward to soon.

I had an invitation, too, to a Mother's Day Tea to celebrate the end of the year for Elaine's class at the private nursery school. I would forego the Society's spring symposium in Des Moines that year. The AEA special education directors would be discussing autism and discrete trial training behind closed doors. Parents would not be welcome, nor recognized as stakeholders. Instead, I went to tea as invited, with Ruffin as my host. The children offered a special program, and Ruffin received his first diploma from Elaine. A photographer from the newspaper was there to take a group picture.

Earlier in the day with Donna, Ruffin had printed out a "Have A Happy Mother's Day" card with a garden of flowers, and a "Have A Happy Father's Day" card with neckties, so Seamus would have no reason to feel left out.

Driven by the calendar, I needed to nudge Ruffin's educators. "Private nursery school ends the middle of May, but ACSD runs until early June. What integration opportunities will replace Monday, Wednesday, and Friday afternoons? Maybe Ruffin could start Sunflower early? Also, now that Luther College adaptive PE activity is over — what will Ruffin be offered on Friday mornings?"

Meg replied, "On Fridays we will be doing gross motor activities in the room — today we did an obstacle course and practiced techniques for somersaults. We'll have gross motor play on Fridays, hopefully to include a trip to the park. I have passed your questions on."

An envelope arrived from Dr. Norman that Saturday with the full written reports of Ruffin's late April UIHC evaluations. I faxed a belt and suspenders copy of all of them to everyone who had been involved in our early May due process hearing. Finally, Dr. Etscheidt would have a complete record upon which to issue her decision. Maybe that would be coming soon, too, I hoped, before school let out for the summer.

That week, with still no decision from Dr. Etscheidt, I took the matter of Ruffin's year-end and summer education in hand. "Here are the UIHC individual reports for the cumulative file and circulation to Ruffin's IEP team, and to Elaine.

"Please bring Kim's attention to the relatively low expressive language score on the *ASSET* test Ms. Wilding used. Can Kim offer a written explanation of why her *TOLD 2* testing results are, or are not, at variance with Ms. Wilding's?

"Meg, can you regarding *The Brigance?*

"Donna, I want to meet with you some morning at my home on Ruffin's summer program.

"Starting Monday, May 20th, Ruffin's schedule will change to: Mondays through Thursdays with Donna AM at ACSD through lunch and Fridays with Donna AM, at Donna's home.

"On Tuesdays and Thursdays, I will pick Ruffin up in the early afternoon and Donna will transport Ruffin to Sunflower for integration. She will see that Ruffin gets situated at Sunflower during the week of May 20th and will train Angela Robeson hands-on during the week of May 27th.

"After ACSD lets out on June 3rd, Ruffin will go to Sunflower in the afternoon every day of the summer."

Here, Meg had written back. "About Ms. Wilding, I haven't had time to really study it, but from your earlier comments, I assume Ruffin didn't do as well for her as for me and Kim. What time or sequence of the day did Ms. Wilding test him? Fatigue and rapport enter in. Also, as noted before, he does better in a structured situation — less stress. Seems to clam up when pressured. We are trying to schedule an IEP amendment meeting to deal with the two-week lag between the private nursery school ending and our dismissal. Letter coming."

In Ruffin's book bag, Miss Hobbs had issued me an IEP conference notice to consider an IEP amendment the next day, just after lunch. She had invited and expected me, Donna, Meg, and herself to attend, with Bridgewater's Dan Cooper replacing Inge as Ruffin's special education consultant.

Kim's name was on the notice, but it indicated she would be absent. Although I would never know why, Kim was replaced on Ruffin's case by a new graduate speech and language pathologist, Lisa Shelton. I came to like her very much, and to admire her brief written reports of data, data, data — provided as early as the first week in May, during our due process hearing.

1. New task delivered while doing previous task, 8 trials, with cues =100%.
2. All tasks delivered at beginning of task, 8 trials, 3 failures, 4 with cues = 63%.
3. Recall of friends' names = 86%.

Then, surprisingly, Meg called right after supper, to follow up on Miss Hobbs's written notice to ask whether Donna and I would be coming. She assured me that sending Ruffin to Sunflower would be agreeable and that ACSD was willing to pay Donna, Sunflower, and Angela, and to provide transportation to and from Sunflower.

A little progress, at last, I thought. Of course, Donna and I would attend. Why not, if ACSD's answer to my request was going to be "Yes."

Still, I wrote back to Meg for the record. "Dr. Simon, the psychologist saw Ruffin first, Ms. Wilding saw him second, Dr. Norman saw him later, then Dr. Piven and the OT later still. According to UIHC, Ruffin's difficulty following directions seems to be *not* a short-term memory problem, but a language comprehension problem with respect to more difficult language.

"Ruffin has only been *using* language for 18 months of his 5 years — and Ms. Wilding is pointing to the communication areas where even high functioning children with autism or Asperger's have the most trouble: 1. They can decode words easily; 2. They can read without comprehension, and 3. They lack theory of mind as second nature. The resulting social naivete leads to real problems with classmates, and authority problems.

"This is what Dr. Granpeesheh and the theory of mind researchers are working on. Ruffin needs solid social routines to fall back on. We may be able to find out more about this at the Autism Society of America meeting in July — and about motor problems in autism."

I signed an IEP amendment, just after lunch, after a brief meeting. Miss Hobbs faxed it around to everyone concerned. It showed that Miss Hobbs *could* follow IDEA procedures when she set her mind to it — and when she needed to impress Dr. Etscheidt. It proved to have been a good move for her to make.

As for Ruffin, I just needed a workable plan. I lived in an unsettled mix of hope and continuing conflict. Maybe we would all hear something from Dr. Etscheidt soon.

CHAPTER FIFTY NINE

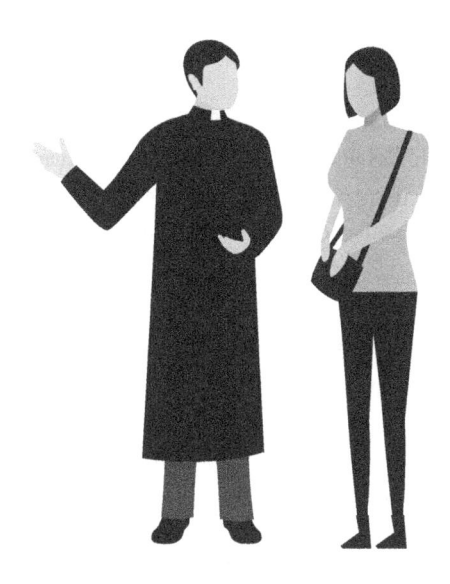

SORRY, TO EVEN BE HERE

I wrote to Meg, Donna, and Elaine that Wednesday. "While placing Ruffin *out* of public school is an amicable matter — especially at ACSD and Bridgewater's volunteered expense — placement of Ruffin *at* public school is not an option for the future given the actual and potential hostility during further litigation. Ruffin is too vulnerable to leave in the care of present administrators. Dr. Granpeesheh and the UIHC as our autism experts both rule ACSD out as appropriate to Ruffin's needs on class size grounds.

"Ruffin is entitled to a free, appropriate public education, and I am obligated as his parent to advocate for and enforce FAPE. I am entitled to do so without retaliation against myself or Ruffin or anyone assisting or supporting him and me. Meg's acknowledgment that this home-school notebook is an appropriate vehicle for the expression of all my concerns is welcome. Please pass this message to ACSD and Bridgewater administrations: I want everything addressed and settled — let's get the attorneys busy now on the whole ball of wax. Curt has my position and my authority to settle the civil rights and tort claims."

But Caron let Curt know our global settlement offer to resolve Ruffin's education and all the forms of retaliatory blowback had been declined. I was disappointed. I would have liked to let everyone — even Miss Hobbs — off the hook.

The school called late that morning about Ruffin's vitamins. He had not been given them before he left to visit his buddy Levi at St. Pat's kindergarten. That was not good. Donna had not been there to see to this — because she and I had been meeting together, planning. At least someone had called to let me know.

While Ruffin remained at St. Pat's, Donna and I worked until noon to prepare our latest report to Dr. Granpeesheh and Evelyn, and to plan Ruffin's summer. We went over all the CARD drills on theory of mind.

Ruffin had been bussed on to Elaine's class that afternoon for a stuffed animal show and tell, bringing his kangaroos, since Elaine had suggested that unusual animals would be most welcome. I went over to give Ruffin his vitamins and stayed to watch. Ruffin had been reluctant to separate from me.

Donna reported the next day, "I asked if Ruffin went to kindergarten reading here. Ruffin: No, kindergarten somewhere else. Ruffin then told all about his new kindergarten at St. Pat's.

"Ruffin: 'Matching game, ice cream and ice cream was hard to find. I got a few of them matches. But the skinny boy was good at me.' I corrected him to 'good to me.'

"Ruffin: 'He got a lot of cards. He was good at the game.' 'We had a recess with I saw the nursery school's door where we go out. There was a whole bunch of kids. I run through them, and I didn't fall. The game that was outside was tic tac toe.'

"Donna: 'Did you have lunch at the new school?'

"Ruffin: 'Not at school. No, at church.'

"Donna: 'Was it good?'

"Ruffin: 'Yes.'"

Meanwhile I had written Meg, "Curt says ACSD and Bridgewater rejected his and my offer to settle. I remain willing to have my attorneys settle all disputes and have given them the authority to do so with respect to all organizations and individuals." There was never any reason not to remain open to settlement, but it did take more than one to tango. Ruffin's educators wanted a judicial decision.

Caron registered a complaint about *this* book bag note. "The district is making every effort to maintain confidentiality in these matters. As I am sure you would expect, settlement negotiations are not discussed with non-administrative school personnel. It is the position of the administration that the classroom teacher and associates should not be privy to settlement negotiations or litigation threats. Perhaps it would be in everyone's interest if a daily note were provided for administrators as well as a separate note for the classroom teacher. Please ask your client if this procedure would be acceptable."

Well, I was not deeply sorry. Caron and ACSD's position seemed patronizing of Meg, who as "non-administrative school personnel" was doing the most of the school's work with Ruffin, and who probably cared about him more than the "administration." Also, I hadn't seen ACSD making any great effort to maintain confidentiality, except to protect itself.

There was no public school on Friday, due to teacher in-service, so Ruffin and Donna worked on his CARD drills at my home before Donna left for her final interview with Ray DeNeve at Bridgewater. The private nursery school had a last class picnic at noon, with each child bringing a sack lunch outside for a picnic and games.

Ruffin was eager to show me his memory book, in which he had printed his own name. Elaine had written out his personal favorites for him. Game: Pass the beanbags; Song: *I'm a Little Teapot*; Food: Corn; Colors: Purple and blue; Toy: The house and farm sets. Last fall she had measured his height at 44 inches; now Ruffin was 45 ½ inches. He had grown an inch and a half over the school year! He weighed in now at 48 pounds.

Ruffin flipped to the photo of himself taken the first day of school, then to his picture at Easter with the Easter Bunny, and one with several of his classmates now. Here was an early drawing with head, eyes, mouth, neck, and unformed body, circled by blue coffee-bean shapes, and then a drawing of his family — little Ruffin, Seamus, and me — standing in front of our Victorian, correctly shown with its three stories of windows.

On Monday, Meg's lesson plans included summer games and Father's Day.

That morning I talked to school psychologist Lorna Volmer at Heartland about information on their best practices and those on their staff certified in TEACCH methods to do hands-on training for a couple of teenaged brothers, children of one of our autism support group parents who had asked me to represent them to advocate for better services.

As a result, Heartland agreed some of their staff and Woodward State Hospital staff would visit Bridgewater and the family's local school district for a few days to provide information and training to the brothers' teachers, since their parents felt comfortable implementing TEACCH methods with their sons. The schools agreed to try them out over the summer with an offer of EYSE, as a new addition to the boys' IEPs.

It felt fine on a warm, spring day to have someone to help, and to be able to reach out and find help available. Given this opportunity to visit with Lorna, I also brought up the ACCESS organization of Orange, California with her, and let her know Ray DeNeve at Bridgewater, and Gerry Gritzmacher in Des Moines, had copies of all their available Lovaas resources.

Lorna never disclosed the existence or any of the details to me then of Heartland's grant application for $750,000 that would extinguish Iowa parents' efforts to incorporate Dr. Lovaas's ABA programs for preschool children with autism in Iowa's schools. It was unlikely that she would not have known about that effort, and likely she would have known — but, it would not have been helpful to our common efforts to disclose anything about that grant to me.

Seamus walked in at noon with the newspaper and opened it on my kitchen counter to the latest, bold letter to the editor, headlined, "Precious Life" by a local resident.

"I worry when my cat or dog is outside too long. We tend to worry over little things, and yet take no time to think, is the weather life threatening, when we place our young children on buses to go to school.

"It seems to me when it's foggy, and there is so much fog that we don't want to drive, we shouldn't let our children risk their lives in that same fog. Why do we allow others to make our decisions for us?"

In the Midwest, even the spring brought perils with the weather. This winter, I had felt less and less alone with my fellow exceptional parents being joined so openly in submitting our transportation complaints. But, as I thought about it, this open, local shaming seemed more effective than our useless complaint to the powerless advisory authorities in Des Moines.

Today was Ruffin's first afternoon at Sunflower. I planned to take him there and back and stay with him to be sure this was likely to work. With Ruffin in his car seat in the back, I took a quick dive into his book bag to learn how his day had been going earlier. Donna's treatment notes showed Ruffin was finally getting some traction on the various time concepts. Then, off we went to Decorah to meet with Ruffin's new caregivers.

Sunflower had a handbook of rules and policies as would any good childcare agency. They were licensed to serve no more than 83 children. All records and files of children were kept confidential. Sunflower did not necessarily close for bad weather but tried to remain open to provide care. That was part of their mission to serve working parents and their children.

They did have a written discipline policy which favored positive reinforcement and time out with discussion of behavior after time out release. Ruffin would be expected to behave despite his autism diagnosis. And "If Sunflower chooses to keep a child who has special needs requiring additional staffing for that age group, an additional per hour fee will be charged."

Sunflower had some small rooms, suitable for one-to-one therapies such as CARD drills or speech therapy. Their maximum staff-to-child ratio was 1 care giver for every 15 children. Ruffin's afternoon schedule, as a part of the 5-year-old Caterpillar group would be rest time, science, art, cooking, snack, large motor activity, and then a choice of activity centers.

The attorneys had agreed to submit all their legal briefs to Dr. Etscheidt that day. They lay in my fax tray as Ruffin and I returned home for dinner.

Curt had provided everyone a copy of *In the Matter of Peninsula School District*, a November 13th, 1995, 28-page ALJ ruling concerning twins with autism with Lovaas home programming year-round.

Peninsula was found to have violated procedural requirements and to have failed to propose appropriate placements for the "children who require intensive one-on-one programs of up to 40 hours per week, with training of instructors and parents, without extended breaks in programming to benefit from their education. The private services secured by the parents and provided to the children have been and continue at this time to be appropriate for them."

Reimbursement had been awarded to the parents of their past, present, and future expenses for the Lovaas consultants, including Dr. Tristram Smith, transportation, travel, lodging, wages, supplies, and materials for both home Lovaas programs. This had been a nice precedent which Tris had thought to share with us. I was grateful and called to leave him a thank you message.

I was anxious to have Dr. Etscheidt's decision, whatever it might be, so we could make firm plans for Ruffin's summer, so I could schedule my own hearings at work, schedule meetings with clients, and know what I could and could not count on in Ruffin's life and mine. I tried to imagine Dr. Etscheidt herself, working through the fat binders of evidence, the sliding stack of briefs. She would have the Memorial Day weekend to work quietly and focus. Or perhaps she was saddled with a thousand family obligations of her own? What did I know? Nothing. Of this woman who held Ruffin's future and the future of so many other children in her hands.

Miss Hobbs wrote to me, after clearing her draft with Caron and Mr. Lord. In the only real misstep that I saw Caron make in playing the game on her side of the net — representing ACSD — she approved a letter scheduling Ruffin's IEP meeting to plan his kindergarten year with a suggestion that I include "Ruffin's father and your minister."

I hadn't ever noticed Miss Hobbs at church. That could be me, not noticing, but maybe we shared a minister? I was confused, and then remembered Pastor Hansen had a couple of children in elementary school, both with cystic fibrosis, a physical disability that would have brought him into contact with her as the special education director. He and his wife had always been open about sharing information about their children to bring about a wider understanding of their condition. But there was nothing confidential in our small town, and, of course, nothing was sacred.

And I didn't imagine Seamus would provide much support in an IEP meeting. Seamus had little experience of public school, having attended only a couple of grades there after beginning in a small country schoolhouse, and then graduated from St. Pat's before the parochial system had closed their high school.

While Donna worked the morning with Ruffin, I walked down Main Street to keep an appointment I had made with Pastor Hansen in his pastoral office, where he kept his small library of religious books and prepared his sermons. First, I thanked him again for his help in watching Ruffin during our earliest medical evaluation last school year at Gundersen, and his kindness in explaining something of Ruffin's disability to his congregation.

He smiled, "I was happy to, as you know."

Then I passed over to him Miss Hobbs's latest letter — of which it was clear, as he read it while I read his face — he knew nothing.

Since he was in no way complicit in Miss Hobbs's suggestion, I quickly brought him up to date on my ongoing disputes with the public schools. Because I wanted it to go further, I mentioned I had already foregone $30,000 or more of IDEA reimbursement last summer in mediation. That seemed to me to be the limit of my forgiveness.

The good pastor was listening. This was a lot of money to talk about so openly. It was making him uncomfortable, but I knew that confiding my side was the time-honored method of setting loose gossip in our town.

I waltzed on to suggest that the various church members serving on ACSD's public-school board owed me and Ruffin a duty of confidentiality. And, since he, like me, wasn't born and brought up here, I suggested to him with quiet directness, "Don't even let them talk to you about this. And don't let them use you."

"They haven't approached me yet," he assured me, rather uncertainly, I thought.

"They might," I posited. "I'm here because I'm afraid they will. It would put you and your family in an impossible situation, I know. And I'm sorry. You know, to even be here." And I was.

Then, I explained what had happened to Donna's son, Matt, a seventh grader. I explained it the way Curt had explained it to me, as an all-too common, but illegal tactic, forbidden by federal law.

"These are not kind people," I told the pastor, who seemed ready to interrupt.

"And, yes, I am playing hardball with them, too," I admitted, giving him no chance. "I am fighting for Ruffin's life as a person, for his future, as an independent person. I have absolutely no intentions of letting up on these people, who, really, don't believe in Ruffin and what he can do, what he is capable of learning. You and your family and the church don't need any part in this. You don't need to find yourself ducking in the field of fire, getting caught in the crossfire of our nastiness. It's best Ruffin and I not put you, your family, or the church in any awkward situation. Actually, I feel it would be better for us to leave the church."

"No, well," he seemed confused for a moment. "I don't think it would be a good idea for me to attend any meeting at school."

"Understand," I said, "I'm not here to invite you, you know, as I did before to the medical appointment at Gundersen. Any suggestion that I invite you, or that they invite you," and here I paused for emphasis, "or ever confide in you, is highly inappropriate. Wrong."

"Yes, wrong," he echoed.

And we left it at that.

CHAPTER SIXTY

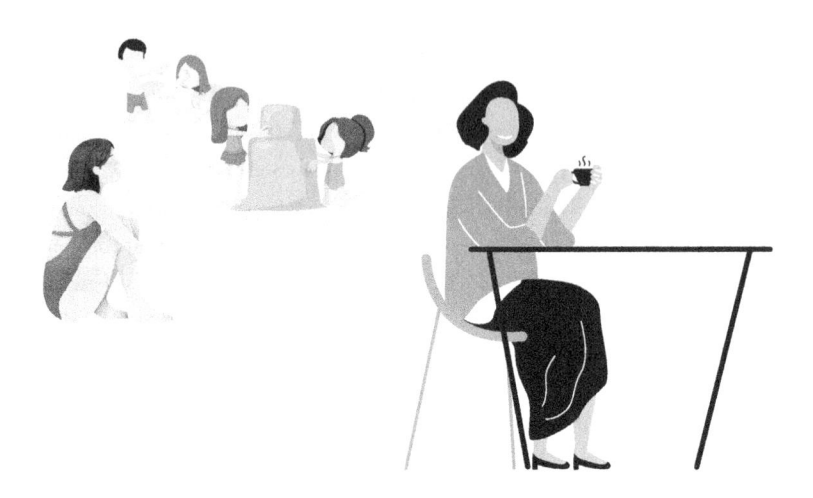

DECISION

There were no classes anywhere. It was Memorial Day, but unseasonably cold and threatening rain. These holidays always seemed to sneak up on our home program for Ruffin. Seamus was busy with his Vets group, barbequing chicken for a noisy eat-in over butcher paper in folding chairs, and a separate, longer line of people shivering as they waited for take-out. Ruffin and I could count on leftovers of everything except baked beans. The baked beans were running out fast. Over in Decorah, hunkered up in her rooms, Angie spent nine hours reading Ruffin's past educational and medical evaluations, and reading Catherine Maurice's book *Let Me Hear Your Voice*.

The next day Meg wrote from school, "We talked about pretending — on rainy days — nothing to do. Music — instruments, pass to left, named each one, and each child did a solo." As I read it, Meg's note sounded like the end of the school year, both weary and a little mournful.

Donna's notes were longer, as always, and considerably more hopeful. Ruffin had enjoyed a near perfect day. "Calendar Drill. Putting numbers on, perfect: Finding the day, perfect: Expressively: Reading, Yesterday was Monday, Today is Tuesday, Tomorrow will be Wednesday, perfect. We removed everything from our calendar with the understanding there would be only a few days of school left, perfect.

As an accidental irony, we were teaching Ruffin a bit of self-advocacy. "Drill on Unreasonable Request from an Adult." Donna had walked into Meg's class and asked Ruffin to dump all the toys on the floor. Ruffin was going to do it. She asked Ruffin to go pull another student's hair. Again, Ruffin was going to do this. Then, Donna told him that when a grown-up asks him to do something that is wrong, he should ask why, or say, "No I don't think I should," and be able to question adult authority. Ruffin had no clue since we were just introducing this.

When Seamus came over with the newspaper that Wednesday, he shook it open to a photo on the education page. There was Ruffin — as one among the future graduating Class of 2009 — with his nursery school classmates and teachers, seated happily in the front row, smiling, hands in his lap, head tilted to the right.

Meg brought back a bag of Ruffin's things from school. Sadly, I was on the phone, focused on a client's troubles when I answered the door. This was a bitter end to Meg's and my parent-teacher relationship which had begun so warmly in the fall of Ruffin's first year and developed into a partnership that had greatly benefited Ruffin — until Miss Hobbs had intervened that first December and had her way with us. The two of us, and our partnership, were no match for her overbearing and heavy administrative presence. Curt had commented he thought she had "a certain gravitas" in the way she carried herself. I disagreed. I thought she wielded a heavy hand.

Time to respond to Miss Hobbs's inquiry about Ruffin's kindergarten year IEP. I began, "Dear Nan," not that I felt that kindly enough about her to address her as "Nan" in person, but why not try to start our discussion of a new school year on a fresh foot? A clean foot to put into a fresh cow-pie, as it turned out.

"Your letter puts me in an impossibly awkward position in the absence of my counsel, who is out of state. His paralegal, Joan, can assist you or your counsel in selecting a date when he will be available to attend.

"Why do you suggest that my minister attend?"

"And, before we meet for anything, I need to make a FERPA inspection of all files and records relating to Ruffin."

I set out a comprehensive list of people to invite, including Ray DeNeve from Bridgewater and Lorna Volmer from Heartland "because she is acquainted with the accommodations which children with PDD-NOS or Asperger's Syndrome require to be successfully educated in the mainstream." Until my later inspection, I remained clueless that Miss Hobbs had supported Heartland's application for $750,000 aimed at putting a swift end to any use of Lovaas's methods in Iowa.

In closing my letter to "Nan," I remained focused on what Ruffin would need. "Would you please also advise me what the estimated kindergarten class size will be for next school year at ACSD now?"

Donna and Ruffin were off to Sunflower, where Angela took up guiding him and writing her first observations. "Rest time: Ruffin chose to read a book. We played Memory with two others. Ruffin won and wanted to quit playing. Donna taught Ruffin the lesson to be a fair winner and let others win, so he had to play again.

"Ruffin wanted to play on his own, but I made him find a friend to play with. He played with that boy for 5 to 10 minutes and then played alone again.

"Outside: We were playing a game of t-ball and each child got 3 hits. Ruffin took a 4th turn and Donna reprimanded him and made him sit by the fence for a couple of minutes."

Dr. Etscheidt's final decision was due — but it was a Friday. When it failed to arrive by the end of the business day, I thought to myself, if it were my decision to render, even if I had imagined I were finished, I would take the weekend to be sure.

Monday was Ruffin's last day of school, due to let out well before lunch. I needed to write to Miss Hobbs again. I called up a small note of encouragement, "Cows run away from the storm while the buffalo charges toward it — and gets through it quicker. Whenever I'm confronted with a tough challenge, I do not prolong the torment, I become the buffalo." *Wilma Mankiller.*

"Here is my claim for $2,492.97 for services which ACSD contracted with me to provide to Ruffin. The check may be made payable to 'Northeast Iowa Autism Therapists,' so that, as ACSD requested, when it is published in the minutes of the school board the payment does not appear to be going to me personally.

"Please present this claim at the next school board meeting and see that it is paid promptly within thirty (30) days. If this claim is not promptly paid, ACSD will be in breach of its settlement agreement of last August in pre-appeal mediation, and I am prepared to pursue whatever legal remedies may then be available to me because of that breach.

"Also, please share this letter with the board as you present the claim for payment. The actual cost of Ruffin's CARD services this year from Donna Schmidt was $8,000 ($200 @ week x 40 weeks' time). Lisa Murphy provided similar after-school CARD one-to-one therapy for most of that time at comparable cost. Thus, Ruffin's free, appropriate public education (FAPE) this year cost me between $14,000 and $16,000, but, of course, our pre-appeal mediation settlement agreement, if honored by the board, limits my claim to $2,492.97.

"Prudential, the other funding stream we considered available as we made our settlement agreement, is presently balking at paying for 'educational services' which should have been provided as a free, appropriate public education (FAPE) pursuant to the IDEA."

Dr. Etscheidt's decision arrived later that morning. She had ruled against ACSD and Bridgewater for violating my rights of due process. Since the child neglect report of January had remained confidential and never been disclosed to her, Dr. Etscheidt remained mystified about how last August's mediation "marriage" between Ruffin's educators and I had plummeted into such unholy squabbling.

Given Ruffin's progress, Dr. Etscheidt went on to make a modest provision for a summer program of one-to-one Lovaas drills, and community integration opportunities to be funded by the schools. But that was just Ruffin's and my individual victory.

For Curt and his agency, Dr. Etscheidt's decision represented a far greater victory and wider remedy that would redound for years to come for the benefit of every single child with any type of IDEA-qualifying disability educated by any school district in any AEA across Iowa. As a new legal precedent, it was important enough to be repeated twice in her written decision. "The extended summer program — which will allow the child to secure the benefits of a free, appropriate public education (FAPE) — has the same procedural and substantive requirements as the IEP developed for the school year."

This echoed sentence would work a fundamental change in the law, enlarging the obligation of special educators across Iowa to provide individualized summer programs and services (EYSE). For me, it made the game worth the candle, coming as it did near the end of Ruffin's individual program. By wisely suggesting and using the mediation process earlier when Ruffin and I still had much to lose, and using the due process proceeding aggressively later, when very little risk remained for Ruffin, Curt had assured I could preserve Ruffin's opportunity to run loose in the universe and still play a small role in bringing about the kind of change that would benefit many children with disabilities — not just those with autism.

As I read and re-read this important passage of Dr. Etscheidt's decision, I could not help but reflect on my first contact with Mr. Montague, on day one, just shy of two years earlier, and the excuse he had raised then to my frantic inquiry for services for Ruffin, who had been diagnosed the day before with autism — that it was summer.

That excuse would be illegal to offer anyone anymore.

Having set out her reasons, Dr. Etscheidt summarized her ruling in a formal way at the end. "Decision: The mother has prevailed on the significant issues concerning Ruffin's EYSE. The EYSE program offered by the schools denied Ruffin a free, appropriate public education (FAPE) because 'it was not prepared in procedural compliance with the notice and related requirements of the IDEA.' Specifically, (1) the schools failed to provide the mother with adequate notice concerning the EYSE IEP meeting which seriously hampered her opportunity to participate in the formulation of the EYSE IEP; (2) the IEP team did not determine Ruffin's critical skills at the time his IEP was revised, and (3) Ruffin's IEP team failed to consider vital information concerning Ruffin's needs in the EYSE determination process. Although the hours of one-on-one therapy are sufficient, the EYSE program 'fails to provide critical integration opportunities.'"

Since Ruffin and I were the prevailing party, the school authorities were liable to pay all the costs of litigation, including Curt's reasonable fees for representing us — as well as all the legal fees for the two attorneys who had represented them in their loss.

But the remedy Ruffin and I would receive was modest at best. Ruffin's educators would be given the opportunity of a do-over. "The IEP team is ordered to reconvene before June 10th, 1996, to: (1) Modify Ruffin's EYSE to include a current level of performance, goal and skill area and data collection plan for social interaction, and (2) Make arrangements for the provision of instructional service for a socialization goal."

I did not want to meet with these educators again, but for Ruffin, that summer, I would.

CHAPTER SIXTY ONE

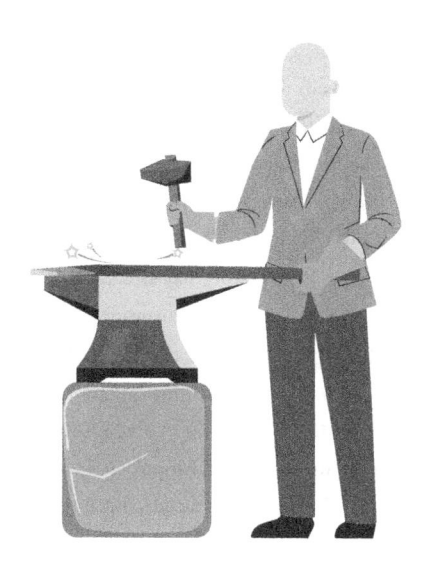

A NECESSARY LITTLE MOTION

Ruffin continued his education with Angie watching and writing from Sunflower. "Rest Time: A little boy took some of another little boy's toys, so he threw a fit. Ruffin told the first little boy to share. They were playing with the farm toys. Then Ruffin was playing 'pretend' — he was pretending the bucket was a tank with water for the horse. They really played *together*. I haven't seen this much from Ruffin before." She continued to describe Ruffin's entire afternoon at that level of detail. "Today he seems to be more interested in what the other children are doing (as compared to the other two days that I have observed). Ruffin was swinging his arms (possibly a self-stimulatory behavior) — but quit on his own." As I read Angie's first, long set of notes, I was heartened. Maybe this summer would really work for Ruffin.

Kim offered us a goodbye letter, passing Ruffin like a baton to us for the summer. She defended her failure to help him reach his agreed-upon IEP goals of last August. "In looking over the report from UIHC, I really don't feel that my testing is so vastly different. The only new test that Ms. Wilding gave was the *ASSET (Assessing Semantic Skills through Everyday Themes)*. I was not familiar with this instrument. After an investigation, I have come across only two copies of this instrument at Bridgewater. I did get a copy from one of my colleagues. She reports that 'It seems to be okay.' She didn't particularly care for the illustrations. The children she administered it to scored lower as compared with their scores on other more widely utilized instruments. In looking it over, I agree that the illustrations look very difficult for preschoolers to distinguish.

"I'm not clear on when during the testing day this took place for Ruffin. He may have simply been tired of the process and not performing at his optimum level."

Good riddance, I thought. Kim could bamboozle herself with these speculations, but I remembered the data, past and present. Ruffin's greatest language growth as measured by Ms. Wilding had come after last summer — when Ruffin had CARD instruction in the morning and playgroup in the afternoon with RoJene and Pine. This last school year's attempt to "marry" Lovaas and special education had been very hard on Ruffin, and it had been hardest to learn that all our adult troubles had slowed Ruffin's language development to an ordinary crawl.

Miss Hobbs began trying to contact me by phone the day after Dr. Etscheidt's decision, catching me as I tried to get out the door to drop Ruffin off at Sunflower and get to my scheduled court hearings in Decorah on time. With Curt still out of town, I had not had an opportunity to walk through Dr. Etscheidt's decision with him. I was flustered, furious, and hostile. Dr. Etscheidt was returning two wasps to a bottle to fight out the issues she had left unresolved. I could have been more gracious in explaining the strictures of legal ethics that limited Curt from talking directly to her as a party represented by counsel. I probably *was* scary.

After a flurry of conversations among legal counsel, Miss Hobbs issued a notice to Mr. Carew, Caron, "Moe," Curt, and me to comply with Dr. Etscheidt's deadline. "We are requesting your attendance and participation in an IEP meeting regarding your son, Ruffin. The meeting is scheduled for Thursday, June 6th, 1996, at 7:30 PM in the boardroom, ACSD high school building.

"Purpose of the Meeting: It has been determined that a break in Ruffin's program during the summer would impede his progress as he prepares to transition to kindergarten. Therefore, we are extending the instructional program for Ruffin through the summer months.

"In the ALJ ruling, we are mandated to include opportunities for social interaction in addition to the current summer service (EYSE) plan for 11 hours and 15 minutes per week of Lovaas drills over three goal areas. We will finalize plans for the Lovaas drills to include payment of Donna Schmidt and determine hours and location for the activity. We will also write a goal for social interaction and provide 3 hours per day 3 days per week for 10 weeks at Sunflower. ACSD will provide transportation to and from this program and pay for the Lovaas integrationist to monitor Ruffin. We investigated local community opportunities for social interaction with Ruffin's same-age peers. They are insufficient to meet the recommended 9 hours weekly for 10 weeks.

"The following information will also be considered with regards to Ruffin's summer service (EYSE) needs: CARD reports, teacher anecdotal records and chartings, speech pathologist reports, recent UIHC evaluation reports, and information from Sunflower. Over sixteen people from Bridgewater, ACSD, Sunflower, CARD, our home program, and everyone's purse-string administrators and legal counsel were noticed to attend, with an open invitation for me to "bring whomever you wish."

Unfortunately, Miss Hobbs issued her notice before checking with Evelyn and Doreen, or me and Curt for that matter, about whether any of us would be available. Evelyn responded to her later that afternoon, "I am sorry to inform you that both Dr. Granpeesheh and I will be unable to 'attend by telephone' the meeting you have scheduled to discuss Ruffin White's summer services (EYSE). Dr. Granpeesheh is out of the country, and I will be in class at that time."

Meanwhile, after I dropped him off that Tuesday, Ruffin continued to make a good adjustment to his new and challenging environment at Sunflower under Angie's watchful eye. She noted that Ruffin's Caterpillar class was "naughty, loud, and full of high energy so it was difficult to do anything when the entire class was either naughty or being reprimanded."

I still didn't trust myself to attend a face-to-face meeting with the school group. Certainly not alone, I would need Curt's support. With Curt on the line from Des Moines, I thought I could manage over the phone, by wearing a tethered headset, and being able to pace around if I needed to discharge my anger harmlessly into the deep powder-blue of my dining room carpet.

Mr. Carew, as always more distant and disconnected, had written, "I am advised that a meeting for Ruffin's summer services (EYSE) will be held. These Bridgewater people will be present: Jack Wallace, Inge Nilsen and Kim Pope. I do not plan to attend." Clearly, Mr. Carew wanted no further involvement in this losing matter.

I delivered six copies of CARD's current drill book for Ruffin to Miss Hobbs's office toward the end of the day for all their meeting participants. I also shared a note I had faxed to Evelyn. "Donna and I plan to have Ruffin work on these 42 CARD drills this summer. Would you kindly confirm whether these are appropriate? If you have other specific suggestions, please let us know. How much do we want Donna to accomplish this summer? Consider how much will then be left to accomplish after the summer is over. Dr. Granpeesheh's testimony at due process suggested that Ruffin should be capable of completing his CARD program in 6 to 9 months' time."

I was pleased to learn Angie had spent an hour dutifully reading all the research material provided to us on integration by UIHC and Gundersen. She would be a real asset to Ruffin's teaching team. In the absence of any agreement or arrangements, I continued Ruffin's education by having him work with her at Sunflower and then had Donna pick him up there and work with him at her home while I went off to court to begin a rare summer trial.

On the way home from Sunflower, Donna took Ruffin grocery shopping. He had to say what was next and give the order at the meat counter. When told to order meat and cheese, he needed a prompt to recall the cheese. At the checkout counter, Donna asked Ruffin, "What next?" as if she didn't know how to pay for her groceries. Ruffin told her, "You draw," meaning to write out the check for payment. He had jumped to writing out the check before telling Donna she should take her groceries out of the cart and put them on the conveyer belt travelling to the clerk.

When they got back to Donna's house, Ruffin missed putting the food away as the answer to 'What's next?' He told Donna, 'You eat the food.' Donna had to find many ways to ask *where* the groceries might be before anyone ate them. She began to have everyone — Matt, Danielle, and Kevin — put things away then, saying, 'What are we doing now?' Ruffin's answer was, 'Putting away.' Donna brought to Ruffin's attention, 'Then eating' would be next.

Donna and Ruffin had turned to cooking hot dogs. First, Donna gave him directions. 1. Take scissors and open the package; 2. Fill the pan with water; 3. Put in the hot dogs; 4: Cook. Ruffin was able to do step 1 and needed help to recall step 2, but then did fine on steps 3 and 4. We were moving along to teaching daily living and self-help skills Ruffin would need to live independently in the future.

Meanwhile, back in Des Moines, Curt filed a motion to clarify, supplement, or modify the decision. Having won an impressive victory for the greater provision of summer programs and services for every child in Iowa with a disability, now it was time to try to hammer the ding out of Curt's legal armor resulting from some of Dr. Etscheidt's remarks about the IEP meeting after last August's mediation when Curt had suggested the team kick the can down the road until Dr. Hagen could issue her new summer service (EYSE) rule.

Dr. Hagen had not managed to issue her reform to that rule until January — long after the Christmas break which had been used traditionally to measure the deterioration of "critical skills." In defense of his own reputation — which was valuable in settling so many matters without hearing — Curt found this supplemental motion necessary. As his grateful client, I strongly supported it.

Caron responded to Curt's motion tepidly. She had a greater interest in maintaining her good working relationship with Curt in her work with future clients than in bloodying her sword again in this losing matter.

My fax began to whir. Dr. Etscheidt had issued her ruling on Curt's motion. Although she denied it, she managed to enlarge her decision in a way that restored his reputation for integrity, by further excoriating Ruffin's educators. Whatever, I thought, as I whacked it with my two-hole punch for filing, as long as it exonerated Curt of any underhandedness. It had been a necessary little motion to bring.

CHAPTER SIXTY TWO

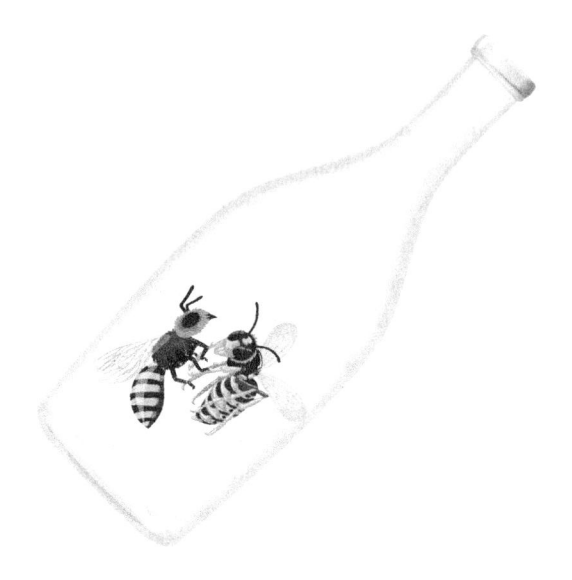

TWO WASPS IN A BOTTLE

Miss Hobbs let me know neither Evelyn nor Doreen would be able to attend our meeting, calling me in the evening the day before — late enough there might be nothing I could do about it. But Evelyn and Doreen were out in California, working on Pacific time, so I was able to have them put their freshest recommendations in writing. By mid-afternoon the next day, Evelyn had faxed them to me.

"Listed below are 59 appropriate drills for Ruffin. A more detailed description will be sent later, and I will need to discuss the specifics of each drill with Donna.

"Could I have the results of the Social Skills Inventory that Donna, Meg, and Elaine filled out regarding Ruffin? Those should assist in setting goals for many of Ruffin's social and emotional skills."

As a courtesy, and because I really wanted them to consider it, I faxed all this over to the school well before the close of business. All the school members of Ruffin's IEP team needed it in advance of our evening meeting.

Meanwhile, Kim had written a long report — the sort of thing she should have had ready for an exhibit at our due process hearing. No one from school bothered to share it ahead of time with CARD, with Curt, or with me.

To prepare myself I worked through Ruffin's last IEP, making a sheaf of notes about what I thought we would need to cover, focusing on the language goals that might be needed to bring both his receptive and expressive language skills up to the normal range as we had agreed, including all the CARD drills, Ruffin's ability to follow and perform 3-step directions, and the integration goals the school had failed to achieve over the last school year.

Also, Miss Hobbs had balked at paying CARD for Evelyn's work during our due process hearing.

Finally, Joan sent Caron a quick fax, assuring everyone that Curt would be on the phone for tonight's meeting. So, the stage was set for another long contentious meeting — fundamentally, between Miss Hobbs and me — as two wasps in a bottle.

Attending at the schoolhouse with a tape recorder were Inge, Jack Wallace, Kim, Mr. Lord, Miss Hobbs, Meg, Mrs. Linden, the kindergarten shared reading teacher, Elaine, Donna, and Caron. I chose to attend by speaker phone, trusting Donna to give me a full, visual report later of the inevitable and distracting eyerolling and body language. Angie sat in on one of my phone extensions. She was curious, having never attended an IEP meeting before. Curt was patched in from Des Moines, for support. Evelyn and Doreen were absent but had weighed in beforehand in writing. I felt I had enough — especially from Dr. Etscheidt's decision — to get what Ruffin needed.

By accepting rather than appealing their loss, Inge indicated the school factions were prepared to offer Donna $200 per week, or a total of $2,000 — nearly an exact echo of my settlement suggestion made weeks ago. I took this in with an odd mixture of both elation and dismay, while Inge explained the recordkeeping forms Donna would need to complete, passing them over to her. I could hear Donna rustle and murmur, "Thank you."

Inge then moved on to what the school factions were prepared to do to comply with Dr. Etscheidt's decision. They would adopt the arrangements I had put together earlier with Sunflower and Angie. Ruffin would attend Sunflower 9 hours a week for 8 weeks. Angie would be paid $10 per hour as an integration aide there. Angie looked over at me and smiled. I scribbled a little note and slipped it over to her, "Way better on your resume!"

The transportation Donna and I had provided to date would be reimbursed if I would submit a claim in writing. Going forward, every Monday, Tuesday, Thursday, and Friday, Joe, a bus driver whom Ruffin knew, would pick him up from Donna's at noon to ferry him over to Sunflower and would return him safely home.

To foster the mother-child relationship and Ruffin's compliance with me, I would be permitted to keep Ruffin home on Wednesdays, to teach him myself, as I had indicated I wanted to do in my recent testimony. Yes, I thought to myself, our theory of mind day, our computer day, our walk to the library, our trip to the pool at the park, our whatever Ruffin wanted to do day, with me.

As parent training, for a week in July, Ruffin would be excused from this summer schedule to allow the two of us to attend the Autism Society of America's meeting in Milwaukee. The district would pay for Ruffin's daycare and community fieldtrip activities there. He would also be excused for another week to attend RoJene's Pleasant Valley Day Camp. His camp fee would be reimbursed. Seamus and I had agreed we would both attend camp with Ruffin, as teachers. Seamus wanted to teach rope games. I signed up to teach poetry to an older group. This was all shaping up to be a fine and workable summer. I continued to listen, quietly and agreeably.

About this time, Kim interrupted Inge to hand in her freshly written report on Ruffin's language development, and to apologize. She was feeling ill. She would need to leave. Good riddance, I thought to myself, again, and asked if Kim's report could be faxed over to Curt and me.

Angie, who was watching me closely, on our end, indicated with a tilt of her head, a lifting of one eyebrow, that I seemed to be enjoying this meeting more than I had anticipated. Well, I thought to myself, maybe I was, but I hadn't seen Kim's report yet. Inge, who had it in hand most likely, replied, "Sure, we could do that," and hurried on.

We needed to write a summer social interaction goal for Ruffin with a couple of objectives that he would learn to follow group directions, learn turn-taking, sharing, and be able to participate in group sports before entering kindergarten. Inge called on Meg, who began to read out what she proposed.

On our end, I glanced over at Angie, who nodded. I reported, "Angie knows how to help Ruffin with all that. Evelyn and Donna trained her. She's a Luther College senior, majoring in psychology, a student of Dr. David Bishop, a friend of our Dr. Lovaas."

"Okay," acknowledged Inge neutrally enough, and asked Meg to continue. Ruffin would need to master "those CARD Drills relating to social skills as per a memo from CARD, attached as Exhibit A." I asked a few questions to be sure this represented Evelyn's latest fax of 59 drills, describing what Donna would tackle. It saved us a lot of time and left Ruffin's CARD program in Evelyn's and Donna's capable hands for the two of them to work out, from time to time, on their own, with Angie and me. The schools wanted no part of it, or any part in it.

"Works for me, here," I said, and meant it.

We took a break, so Kim's report could be faxed over. I considered it in the context of Ms. Wilding's two bracketing independent evaluations. Kim claimed Ruffin's speech and language skills were "adequate for classroom communications and academic progress."

When we reconvened, I offered my dissenting opinion.

"I find Kim's conclusion self-serving. According to our home-school notebook, she admitted recently that she has *never* worked on teaching Ruffin 3-step directions — our agreed upon IEP goal for him back in August. That is simply a failure of the school's promise to me, and to Ruffin, a failure to abide by our agreed-upon plans.

"In Ms. Wilding's earlier report, the one that arrived just after our August mediation, she found Ruffin had made up 2 years of language development over last summer when Donna, Lisa, Evelyn, RoJene, Pine, and I were responsible for his instruction.

"But, when Ms. Wilding saw him again this April, after our difficult and unduly hostile school year, after Head Start failed to show as promised, when so much of Donna's one-to-one work was re-directed into shared kindergarten reading, and after Ruffin working with Kim as his assigned speech and language therapist, she found Ruffin's language development had slowed — demonstrably — to something less than a bare chronological crawl.

"I put it to you that under your school instruction, Ruffin's language development slowed to the rate of cold molasses when we all know he has a prior record of providing a very robust response, you know, slicker than greased owl shit." Since I was on the phone, I had no idea how that landed, but I plowed on.

"What you owe him, and me, is some compensatory speech and language lessons this summer with a competent speech and language pathologist. Sunflower has small instructional rooms suitable for 60 minutes per week of one-to-one speech and language instruction, and a pool of capable language children to draw on for small group speech instruction.

"I will need Bridgewater to make that offer in generous measure or have your written notice of refusal of my request with your factual grounds and reasons."

Curt and Caron spoke up to clarify for the group that my request for summer speech and language services would need to be considered, and, if refused, be supported by a written *refusal notice* under the IDEA. Disagreement could lead to renewed due process litigation. At this point, Curt mentioned that the schools also needed to pay CARD's past-due fees and Evelyn's latest bed and breakfast bill. Caron agreed that was only fair.

I hoped the schools had had enough of litigation. The beginning of this meeting had begun to sound like it. We might all be headed back to due process before Dr.

Etscheidt, but I thought probably not — since speech and language therapy fell into Bridgewater's hands to provide or not.

By then, I knew Bridgewater was the more amenable party among my adversaries.

As it turned out, I didn't have to wait long. Bypassing Mr. Carew and Curt, as the new director of Bridgewater, "Moe" called me early the next morning. He would be talking to his subordinates about exactly how to meet Ruffin's need for summer speech services.

Later, my fax whirred in a letter from "Moe." The unmet speech goal that Kim had failed to address during the school year would be addressed this summer by someone else.

My impression was that "Moe" was more amenable to taking advice from Mr. Carew than Mr. Montague had ever been, or that "Moe" had simply taken the bull by the horns himself and wrestled this problem of Ruffin to the ground without asking or having to pay for Mr. Carew's opinion. Wise, either way, I thought.

I called "Moe" to thank him and agree to his most recent proposal. He would be interviewing a new speech and language pathologist that afternoon. He seemed relieved when I assured him that I was more than willing to move forward and would sign an EYSE IEP addendum.

CHAPTER SIXTY THREE

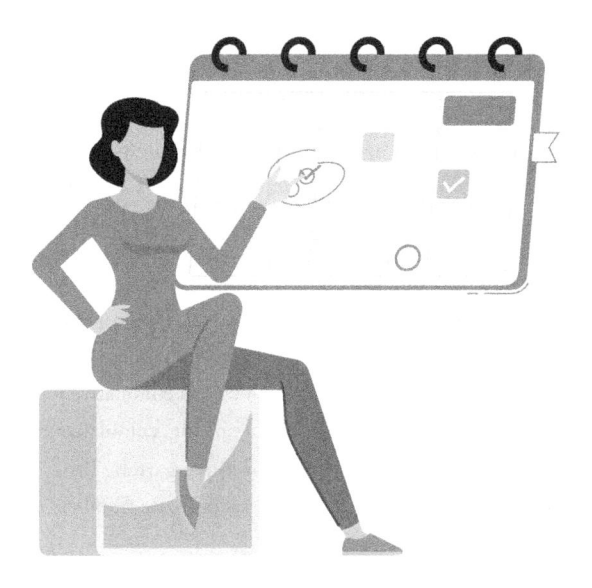

SHE WHO SETS THE AGENDA

Mr. Lord ran an IEP Notice, a letter to CARD, and another to me past Caron for her approval before sending them all out. It was remarkable how Dr. Etscheidt's decision brought Ruffin into focus. The school authorities were requesting an important annual IEP meeting on July 1st to plan his kindergarten year at ACSD in the class of the kindergarten teacher, Mrs. Linden, who "has been involved with Ruffin and understands his needs," and who would "continue to receive in-service, and consultation as needed." But Ruffin's "need for further discrete trial method" would be "discussed," and "all speech and language services terminated."

To address Ruffin's admitted "difficulty processing verbal directions" and his social skill development, he would "require the services of the multi-categorical resource teacher," Nora Sikes, who would "consult" with Mrs. Linden. Keeping Donna at school as Ruffin's one-to-one aide, as Mrs. Linden had told Donna she wanted, was "not necessary" because it would "stigmatize" Ruffin — as if pulling him out of class into the resource room would not.

As an option, St. Pat's had been written off because "no special education program is available there to support Ruffin's needs." Obviously, I would not agree, but this was information — seeing these pre-determined choices laid out so openly.

Along with both agencies' purse-string administrators and legal counsel, over twenty people from Bridgewater, ACSD, Sunflower, St. Pat's, CARD, and our home program were invited, with an open invitation again for me to "bring whomever you wish."

As I pondered all this at home, I wondered how the proposed recommendations and non-recommendations had been developed? At *another* "meeting before the meeting?" Of whom? The notice was not even shared with CARD. Instead, Dr. Granpeesheh and Evelyn were sent a separate, opaque letter giving only the meeting's time and date.

Another letter was addressed to me, signed by Miss Hobbs, setting June 20th as the day I could make my FERPA inspection. She claimed, "I no longer keep any personal file on Ruffin but put everything I receive directly into his cumulative folder. The other files you have requested (Lord, Holub, and for school nursing, cumulative) will all be available.

"Currently I have 77 children enrolled for kindergarten. There will be one class of 20 students, and three classes of 19 students. Again, these numbers may change."

By Friday, June 7th, Ruffin's summer education continued officially, with Donna still providing him CARD drills at her home making good use of her daughter, Danielle, and still providing transportation to Sunflower. "Today is the first day I have heard of the magic airplane. Ruffin explained this as his dream to Danielle and how it is made of wood, and that it is strong and can get its big, giant muscle out."

"At Sunflower," she reported, "Ruffin was toe-walking and flicking his fingers and using a high-pitched voice. He returned from the bathroom, and someone was sitting in his spot. He pointed it out, but when the teachers redirected him, he sat somewhere else.

"When lining up for lunch, Ruffin needed to be asked to join the group by the teacher. At the table, I gave him no prompt for conversation. Ruffin offered information to a teacher about a piece of pizza with black olives. He raised his hand when needing something. The boy across from him pointed out that there was a brown spot on his apple. Ruffin made a comment back, but no other conversation.

"All the other children talked back and forth, even a little girl from the other table managed to get in on the table's activity. Ruffin was looking at the ceiling and around the room. I offered him a prompt. The teacher gave more information and did introductions of the students. He ate well — pizza, carrots, apple slice, watermelon, and white milk. He could care less if any other children were in the room."

Angie's report was a bit better. "Some older kids came in and gave a puppet show. Ruffin laughed at all the appropriate times. He first sat up front with all the kids, then moved closer to the substitute teacher. He was playing with the puppets appropriately with the other kids. There were 5 kids in total in his Caterpillar group. Ruffin was talking throughout the puppet show and did a better job than some of the other kids. The puppet that he controlled asked, 'What is your name?'

"Play Time: The class played with puppets. Ruffin invited a little boy, 'Come on, let's skip.' That child then asked him to play checkers. Ruffin did not know how to play, so I made a paper checkerboard to teach him first. Then they played. Ruffin was fairly alert to the game, although the other child reminded him when it was his turn. He is still a little slow with checkers, but with practice will surely improve.

"Dr. Rimland flew in from San Diego that Saturday. Ruffin and I went to hear Bernie speak, to meet him in person, and offer him a warm thank you for all his earlier help. As planned, we visited the Foster family in nearby Davenport.

Although Ruffin had complained of a headache and a stomachache in the car, he perked up with Noah's older sister who played with him patiently for a couple of hours. It was a puppet show (Ruffin's first question was to ask the name of her puppet) and an "I'm thinking of with clues, so you guess" game, with the two of them taking turns. One clue was always the letter with which the answer began. Ruffin was able to offer this sort of clue easily.

In our absence, there was another Saturday gathering of "Moe," Al Neidecker, and Jack Wallace. By Monday these three upper echelon Bridgewater administrators were writing me another letter, enclosing Meg's typewritten present levels of educational performance (PLEP). It was a slipped stitch we had dropped during our earlier summer services (EYSE) meeting.

"Ruffin is demonstrating age-appropriate social skills in integration settings at this time. Consultation with both the kindergarten teacher and the private nursery school teacher indicates that Ruffin functions at age level in their classrooms without extra reminders or cues from the teacher. For EYSE, Ruffin will be placed in an integrated setting with some shadowing to maintain these skills at the appropriate level *and to assist in gaining more skills.*"

On Monday, I ordered a copy of Catherine Maurice, Gina Green and Stephen C. Luce's newest book *Behavioral Intervention for Young Children with Autism, A Manual for Parents and Professionals*. Catherine's new book contained a useful chapter on mainstream integration of young children who were on their way to running loose in the universe.

Miss Hobbs directed the school board secretary how to make all the payments to Donna, Angie, and Sunflower for the summer. I banged out a businesslike letter seeking over $500 of reimbursement for Donna's and Angie's attendance during recent IEP meetings and for Donna's training Angie, along with a second letter about Angie's work with Ruffin, seeking over $250 of reimbursement for what I had already paid her. Two weeks or more after Donna and Angie had begun their summer work and training, Miss Hobbs contacted them both, sending along Ruffin's EYSE goals and some forms to report on his progress. Sunflower billed the school board. Mr. Lord initialed his approval to issue a check.

Some things were beginning to run like butter without my having to work every detail like a fiend. Step by step, following the path laid down by Congress in the IDEA, we were getting there.

Meanwhile, Ruffin continued learning at Donna's home, two steps forward, one step back. "Emergency: calling 911; What to do if he is lost? Perfect; What to do if he is hurt? Perfect. Ruffin was whining and didn't want to share, but once we got into the game, he settled in. When asked why he was unable to do a task Ruffin admitted that he had not been listening. He was not interested in keeping track of when it was his turn, nor any new directions."

At Sunflower, Angie continued to observe Ruffin and his classmates closely.

"Ruffin was trying to play with a little girl, but she was preoccupied. Ruffin turned to play with another little girl. He was talking to her, but she was being snotty. Ruffin said, 'If you need help then just call me — 911.' Finally, he was included in the girls' play — as the doctor. (Note: these girls are cliquey, and I would have a hard time being included in their play. It is noble that Ruffin kept going back, trying again and again to be included)." As I read this note by Angie, it brought tears to my eyes. Donna and I would never have any trouble working with her. Like the two of us, she was pulling for Ruffin.

When he and I arrived home, Ruffin and I piled in my car and drove down to the Mississippi river town of Lansing where a small circus had set up three tents, with lots of sticks and strings to fascinate Ruffin, and splintery bleachers, where we sat eating hot dogs and French fries while a group of aerialists performed, shimmying up and down poles to reach the trapezes and swing. There was a lubricous elephant, a striped zebra, and a caged lion. The air was warm and full of flying insects. I was able to tell Ruffin what I had planned we would be doing the next day.

Ruffin and I got up and left with Seamus long before dawn to drive to Des Moines for an early morning argument in the Iowa Supreme Court for Mr. Ezzone. Although we had finally collected on his judgment, the losing parties had balked at paying the hundreds of thousands of dollars of interest that had accrued between the jury verdict and our successful appeal.

In the large, ornate courtroom, Ruffin was able to sit quietly with Seamus during our 45-minute argument. He knew the people in black robes were "judges." Once our case was safely submitted, Ruffin, Seamus, and I toured the state capitol building with Mr. Ezzone who invited us out to see his own latest construction project, and then back to his home to see his antique radio collection. It would be hard to say who was more fascinated, Seamus or Ruffin. Mr. Ezzone offered to show Ruffin how to play his personal one-armed bandit — from which Ruffin easily won three nickels. Then we went with Mr. and Mrs. Ezzone out to their favorite neighborhood restaurant where Ruffin's milkshake was poured into a tall, fluted glass balanced on his head by a waitress standing on our table!

The three of us left the Ezzones for an afternoon visit to the Blank Park Zoo. A leisurely ride around the park on the kiddie train let us view, and Ruffin name, all the exotic animals without having to walk too much in the heat of the day. On the way home, we stopped for a picnic supper in New Hampton, the small Iowa town where I had tried the *Ezzone* case some four years before. For me, the day completed itself in a perfect circle.

Meanwhile, Miss Hobbs was revising an earlier draft letter to me. "I have contacted Lorna Volmer about attending. She will discuss this with her supervisor and will notify us. I am inviting Mary Carter, chair of Bridgewater's autism resource team. She, too, has experience with PDD-NOS and children with autism." After vetting her revisions with Caron, Miss Hobbs re-dated all her earlier letters to me, to CARD, and the IEP notice, and sent them out by fax.

Ruffin, and I spent our Wednesday morning at the park and the afternoon at the pool. Ruffin noticed one of the boys from Meg's class and one of his little girlfriends from last summer's playgroup. He seemed to do well with these children whom he knew but had a harder time meeting new children. He yelled insistently across thirty feet of distance, "What's your name, kid?" This awkward approach scared or turned off most other children and frustrated Ruffin who argued with me that because he had asked the other child's name, the child should be willing to play, and to be his friend.

While I prepared for a full working day of juvenile court, Ruffin and Donna worked on various "theory of mind" exercises by making good use of Donna's visiting nephew, who was about a year older than Ruffin. "Ruffin was not able to direct how the others were to jump on the trampoline, so he became angry and sat along the side. I prompted him to join in on what the others were doing, instead of sitting on the side angry."

After court, I began a letter to Mr. Lord and "Moe," "conveying information for circulation to Ruffin's IEP team members in advance of our July 1st meeting, including all our home and summer program data, and "'Supported Inclusion,' Chapter 16, of Catherine Maurice's parent-professional handbook, by Susan C. Johnson, Linda Meyer, and Bridget Ann Taylor. (See p. 332 for Mother's assessment of Ruffin's prerequisite skills for inclusion)" along with several other articles about inclusion by Midwestern scholars.

I also thanked "Moe," copying to everyone concerned, "I appreciate that you have asked the Department of Education how a parochial school placement can be arranged for Ruffin, and about the extent of support and related services Bridgewater can provide to him in that setting."

Finally, copying in everyone concerned, I wrote most carefully to any future ALJ, state judge, federal judge, or appellate court to memorialize all my concerns, propose a coherent agenda, and marshal the educational file evidence into a single, written record. As it turned out, this letter formed the basis of the discussions that occurred in a day-long July 1st, IEP meeting — the first of Ruffin's eight IEP meetings which came the nearest to being conducted as Congress had intended when it passed the IDEA.

CHAPTER SIXTY FOUR

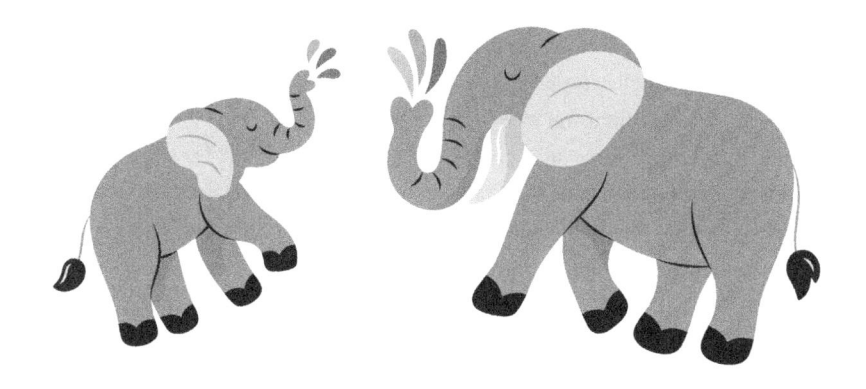

DID YOU KNOW, MOM?

Angie reported in mid-June, "I told Ruffin all the other kids knew his name. Why didn't he know their names? I asked him if he knew my name — No! He said he needed to ask his mom and would tell me at swimming lessons."

"My Notes: After Sunflower, when Ruffin came home, we went outside. We met a neighbor child JJ, and the two of them played together after I set them up — by asking Ruffin if he knew this child's name — Ruffin then asked. JJ knew Ruffin's name, probably from school. He is six years old. His mom came out and introduced herself. JJ stayed for about an hour and a half and the two played well together, except when Ruffin came inside in tears once when JJ 'wouldn't play with me.' As things fell apart from time to time, I directed them to the backyard, upstairs, to take a break, have a snack. A new location or activity was enough to get them going again."

Then Ruffin worked on his computer and colored — an elephants and peanuts picture — commenting, "Did you know Mom, elephants eat peanuts? Elephants are gray," going on and on with every bit of trivia about elephants you would have no interest in hearing about, unless you were his mother.

I went in Monday to sign the new summer services (EYSE) IEP addendum which had been typed up to reflect our early June meeting and my negotiations afterwards for speech and language therapy with "Moe." Under Mr. Lord's watchful eye, I signed it, noting, "I agree with the EYSE services as *ordered by due process* and will make my child available to receive them." Which, thanks to me, I thought to myself, had been ongoing these last two weeks. I also noted, "Ruffin will receive additional services per Dr. Granpeesheh's recommendations on Fridays at parent expense." The Saturday PLEP by Meg had been added. Angela and Donna were named as Lovaas interventionist and therapist, respectively. This document also noted that Ruffin would be receiving speech therapy from Bridgewater.

I was looking for *all* the receipts, so Mr. Lord showed me that he had signed agreements with Angie, Donna, and Sunflower. Then, I reminded Mr. Lord that I needed his answer to my early June demand to be paid for the expenses I had advanced to enable our summer services (EYSE) agreement.

"That's still hanging fire," I said as evenly as I could manage.

"I'll get back to you on that," he promised, flipping through a pile of Ruffin's papers, digging down to find my correspondence. "This it?" he asked, handing it over.

"Yes," I nodded, as I handed it back.

Later in the day, he faxed me. "After careful analysis I have made the decision to present it to the Board of Education for their approval for $2,492.97. To pay for the two camps, we will need a paid bill showing your expenditures." All of which I found perfectly satisfactory. Obviously, Mr. Lord was invested with a great deal more power to commit resources than Miss Hobbs and was much more pragmatic about what appeared in the small print of the newspaper. And he was just much easier to deal with as a person.

According to Donna's notes, although he was counting easily to 100, Ruffin was continuing to struggle with time concepts and any recall of past events and other matters of "common sense." "Multipart Directions — Ruffin was to give me directions for making a bowl of cereal. You should have seen Ruffin's face when I began to pour the opened bag of cereal on the table and asked him what I was missing and told him how important it was to listen to and give all the directions."

Ruffin was still struggling to learn Angie's name, too. "Rest Time — There seem to be groups formed, but Ruffin is not a part of any one of them. I asked Ruffin what my name was. He said it starts with an A. Then another child said my name.

"Ruffin asked to play with the fly puppet. I told him, no more fly puppet. He could pick a different one. Later when I asked, 'Do you remember your classmate's name?' Ruffin said, 'Angie, I can't remember.'"

The next day, he couldn't remember Angie's name when Donna asked. He also got tripped up by some of the trickier conventions of language. "A boy was drawing with a 'hot pink' crayon, so Ruffin wanted to feel it. I explained how the boy just meant 'bright pink.'

Angie also continued to redirect Ruffin from his default preferences. "Note: Ruffin did not want to play *Candyland* — he wanted to play with the *See n' Say* (which spins!)."

At Sunflower — the next day, Angie asked if Ruffin remembered what her name was — "so Ruffin asked me, 'What's your name?' After a while he said, 'I give up.' I told him during rest time to think hard and afterward he should be able to tell me my name. I told him it made me sad that he couldn't remember it. During rest time I read the notes in the green folder, and noticed he worked on my name this morning with Donna. Ruffin made lots of guesses for my name. He asked if it started with J, K, or A. Then started to think of names beginning with A. Then after a while I said the next sound in my name was N. Ruffin made more guesses. Another child came by, and we worked on her name, too. I asked, 'What's your bus driver's name?' Ruffin replied, 'It's too hard.' I told him my name and asked him to remember it. Another little girl joined us. I asked Ruffin if he knew her name — he did! Good job!"

"At snack, five minutes after Ruffin asked his tablemate's name, he couldn't remember who she was. He guessed, wrongly, three times. I kept asking, 'Why don't you remember her name?' Ruffin is terrible at names — we need a lot of work here.

"Later on, I gave him some new directions and he didn't pay attention. I asked him to repeat what I had said — he couldn't. He fell back with his chair because he was tipping back." All in all, I could tell Ruffin must have had a much harder day than mine.

After Angie left Sunflower for the day, Ruffin stayed on for a new 45-minute session with Lisa Shelton, the new speech and language therapist "Moe" had assigned to replace Kim. Lisa included a daily note in Ruffin's travelling folder. She turned out to be a therapist after my own heart. "Notes of SLP — 3-part verbal directions with up to 2 critical elements — each task delivered separately — perfect for 7 trials; new task delivered while doing previous task — perfect for 7 trials; all tasks delivered at beginning — 14% — 1 out of 7 trials." Over the summer, Ruffin would improve markedly under her precise tutelage.

On our Wednesday, Ruffin and I walked downtown for breakfast, dashed into the pharmacy, and then headed for the public library. Ruffin chose several books. When we got back home, Ruffin's new neighborhood friend JJ came over. The boys played without dispute in the back yard until it was time to go to the library's reading program. It was on trees with lots of hands-on samples of branches, pinecones, and wood sections. Ruffin sat up front with JJ, passing each fragrant sample along, after a sniff. Ruffin greeted his St. Pat's kindergarten buddy by name. We stopped in at JJ's home for cookies, more fragrances of cinnamon and nutmeg, to inhale and name. The boys then got back together, playing until late afternoon. Then Ruffin helped me grocery shop — was responsible to push the cart, and very helpful. JJ returned to play outside.

None of this would have been possible last summer.

After what had happened to her son Matt during our due process hearing, Donna decided not to work for either ACSD or Bridgewater, but to take another opportunity to work for a young newly diagnosed child with autism in LaCrosse, whose family was being served by Dr. Glen Sallows of the Wisconsin Early Autism Project. The parents, a couple of married physicians, had also been in touch with me. I was pleased to be able to write a strong letter of recommendation for Donna to Dr. Sallows.

I inspected Ruffin's school records. During our due process hearing I had been unprepared for an argument that Ruffin had been absent often, or tardy on my account. I needed to see Ruffin's attendance records, the evidence as it had been kept. I would compare the schools' attendance records with our home-school notebook. First, I collected a copy of the school calendar for 1995-1996. The attendance records had been kept by Ruffin's school nurse, in her file, which had never been provided as a part of my earlier FERPA inspections.

A most surprising discovery lay in the school nurse's file — a long-ago December 21st, 1994 memo by Miss Hobbs from Ruffin's first, early months in special education. It explained a lot and supported the worst of my early concerns that Miss Hobbs talked the talk to my face and had walked away on walking the walk behind my back, whether we were talking Lovaas, auditory integration training, Head Start, or now — the newest issue of kindergarten class size.

Her long memo opened a wide window onto Miss Hobbs's personal consternation, resentment, and injured pride. "To be honest with myself, I do question Ruffin's diagnosis. (As it seems do others on the team who are involved with this student.)

"I also question Ms. White's parenting skills and wonder to what degree lack of involvement with him in his first critical years of life may have had on his language delay. However, I would never tell her this.

"This Lovaas program sounds a bit ridiculous. I feel sorry for Ruffin. He is 3 years old, attends school all day, every day 5 days a week. (That in itself is a bit unusual.) From what Ms. White has told me, he then goes home to 3 hours of Lovaas each night where he is drilled on labelling items, labelling feelings (another point of disagreement we had on December 16th, as I suggested feelings are learned through watching others, practice, and a variety of experiences.) Donna Schmidt and Lisa Murphy are 'therapists' having attended the 12 hours of training she paid for last month. Seamus provides 'physical education' by playing with him.

"This all seems inappropriate for a 3-year-old. When does he get to play and explore? When does she parent? As Ms. White addresses the progress Ruffin has made, she would lead you to think his progress is based totally on Lovaas at home and would negate the 30 hours per week he spends in school.

"Finally, I agree with the team that Ruffin is currently provided with a free, appropriate public education. From what I have read, that is what IDEA is about. 'According to the U.S. Supreme Court, the IDEA was not enacted to maximize the potential of students with disabilities, but rather to open the door of education to these students.' *Students with Disabilities and Special Education* 1994, Data Research, Inc. p. 7.

"I am giving copies of these notes to Superintendent Lord and Meg Holub, simply for their information, and to reinforce that I have in fact done this activity on December 21st, 1994. This is not my normal procedure for my personal work journal; however, these are unusual circumstances."

As I read through this sorry, but honest and revealing document at this late date, seated there with Ruffin's file, in her own empty conference room, I wondered how matters might have gone differently if Miss Hobbs and I could have shared our feelings and misgivings more forthrightly, and more openly, face to face and transparently, rather than my having to write endless letters to request the services Ruffin needed and she having to write this memo to collect her thoughts and defend herself to Meg and to her superintendent, Mr. Lord.

I remembered that when I had learned that first summer how Ruffin would have a woman principal, I had been thrilled. When Miss Hobbs had first shown Ruffin and me around her schoolhouse, even opening the door to the bathrooms, she had seemed weighted with gravitas, dignified, just as she had impressed Curt recently. A powerful Ocean Liner, as I saw her during our first August IEP meeting.

But what did I really know of her personal and professional struggles to persuade her superintendent and our school board to bring the district's disabled students home from Decorah to our town, to a new program of her own making? With all my request letters pouring in, all these meetings and fuss about Ruffin, the exceptional parents' embarrassing donation of missing and needed teaching materials, what uncomfortable scrutiny might she and her newest project have attracted? I wasn't thinking about the difficulties of her position, as an educated, middle-aged single woman, accountable to an elected board of powerful local people, bankers, farmers, and main street businessmen and women. I was focused on Ruffin, and myself, and on children across the state, across the world like Ruffin, on networking with parents like me, and on making Ruffin's education work — hopefully, toward his entering the mainstream by kindergarten.

So, with her district at risk as the primary responsible funding source, by our first fall and early winter Miss Hobbs and I had become swept up in the sort of misunderstanding and miscommunication more common to dueling medical malpractice experts or to spouses squabbling over custody, visitation, and support — truly toxic emotions to bear down on Ruffin.

But, by sharing her notes with Mr. Lord and with Meg, Miss Hobbs had converted her private resentments and misgivings into an educational record — which had somehow been concealed until after due process — a record which Curt and I had been unable to read or offer to Dr. Etscheidt as the damning evidence it was.

I also found a yellow stickie on Ruffin's cumulative file folder: "96-97 Placement St. Pat's kindergarten." Perhaps that was a more recent sign to pin my hopes upon?

All this detritus in Ruffin's school nursing file offered me a fair amount of insight about what ACSD had been thinking and communicating about, and crucially, just exactly how long this had been going on without ACSD focusing on Ruffin as an individual or responding to change. How utterly disheartening it all was. How grateful I was for Ruffin's packrat of a school nurse.

That Saturday, I submitted a "for the record" protest to Dr. Etscheidt based upon "Section 41.31(2) (256B), 34 CFR 99, 300) *Access to educational records* which provides: 'Reviewing records. Each agency shall permit the parents of an eligible individual . . . to inspect and review *any education records relating to the individual that are collected, maintained, or used by the agency* under these rules.' Although I specifically requested *all* files kept on Ruffin, I was never given access to this file folder — in which I found Miss Hobbs's early memo.

"This memo was not produced. Accordingly, I request that it be produced to you and certified to your record, belatedly, along with any explanation ACSD may have to offer as to why this memo was not produced to me for inspection, or to you.

"It appears that this memo did circulate among IEP team members, and that it was 'culled' out of Mrs. Holub's personal file and Mr. Lord's personal file (both of which were supposedly produced to me on June 20th, 1996 — neither of which contained this memo).

"It also appears that both Miss Hobbs and Ms. Nilsen kept handwritten notes of EYSE conversations with me which were not produced to either you or myself. (Three examples are enclosed, one dated March 5th, 1996, and one dated March 21st, 1996, both by Ms. Nilsen, and one dated June 4th, 1996, by Miss Hobbs, all found June 20th, 1996, in Mr. Lord's file).

"It does appear that forms of personal communication are going on 'behind the cumulative file,' that are not just personal musings, but are being *used*. Accordingly, I request a full re-inspection of the files from which these exemplary materials originated, and the inspection of any other similar 'personal' files kept by any ACSD or Bridgewater employee."

Since this was not a formal motion, I didn't really expect a response from Dr. Etscheidt. After all, Curt, Ruffin, and I had *prevailed* in due process. We had *won* the services Ruffin needed despite the school authorities' careless underhandedness. But I wasn't beneath being a tattletale, running with a complaint of injustice to the sitting authority. What remedy was there to offer to us now, after the fact?

Mostly, I wanted these sorry facts out on the table before Ruffin's IEP team met again. Caron and Mr. Carew deserved fair notice of who, what people, and what sorts of agencies they were representing. Having this information would give them considerable leverage in advising their clients and bringing them around to compliance.

CHAPTER SIXTY FIVE

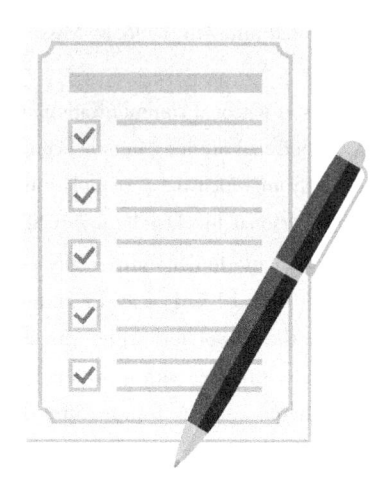

READY FOR SUPPORTED INCLUSION?

Ruffin's summer continued at its unsteady pace. "Angie, Ruffin is not having a good day. Time to push turn taking and compliance — since he doesn't like feelings of frustration. Ruffin could tell me your name today. He also said he liked you. Donna."

"At Sunflower, Ruffin got to plant a tomato plant and peas, but seemed to be suffering from today's heat."

"My Notes: When Ruffin arrived home, he was eager to tell me about talking with Joe, the bus driver. Then he had a few minutes when he "wanted to be by myself." He went out to swing and came back in a good mood.

"His new friend JJ came over. They played in the sandbox, the tent, the garage, the bedroom, the sidewalk on their Big Wheels, ate popsicles, and traded bubblegum.

Ruffin made JJ say 'please,' and play T-ball. JJ was very adept at changing the rules to simplify them for Ruffin who was frustrated by the competition involved in running bases and didn't get the concept of tagging JJ out with the ball.

"JJ proposed rather than play real ball, that they 'take turns practicing.' An excellent solution. Ruffin loved it, and JJ was content with it."

With Ruffin down for the night, I sat curled on the couch to rate Ruffin on a checklist I had found in Chapter 16, "Supported Inclusion" of Catherine Maurice's newest book. Did Ruffin have the skills now to truly benefit from an inclusion placement? Using okay, E+, E, or E- to indicate skills I saw as "emerging" based on Donna and Angie's daily treatment notes along with my own, this is what I thought I saw:

1. Language skills
    a. (E-, okay, 1-step) Follows 2-step directions when presented to a group
    b. (Okay) Communicates needs and desires
    c. (Okay) Answers simple questions
    d. (Okay) Asks simple questions
    e. (Okay) Engages in simple exchanges of conversation
    f. (E) Recalls experiences

2. Social skills
    a. (E+) Takes turns during activities
    b. (Okay) Waits quietly
    c. (Okay) Reciprocates greeting from peers and adults
    d. (Okay) Participates in circle activities
    e. (E+) Initiates play activities with peers with or without adult prompts
    f. (Okay) Imitates peer play

3. Academic skills
    a. (Okay) Learns through observation of others
    b. (NO) Completes seat work independently
    c. (E) Raises hand to seek adult assistance
    d. (NO) Learns targeted objective during group instruction
    e. (Okay) (Has learned kindergarten curriculum in one-to-one) Completes grade-level academic curricula

4. Behavior skills
    a. (E) Responds to delayed contingencies (reinforcement is delivered to child following a period of time rather than immediately after the targeted behavior, e.g., the mother contracts with her child for ice cream after school if the child follows directions. The reinforcer is provided after school so as not to draw extra attention to the child during school)
    b. (Okay) Exhibits disruptive behaviors at near-zero levels in all environments
    c. (E+) Stereotypic behaviors under stimulus control; that is, the child engages in stereotypic behavior, if at all, only under certain stimulus conditions (e.g., alone; during playtime at home) and not under other conditions (e.g., in public places like the classroom).

Making a final check of Ruffin's book bag, I saw that Ruffin's teacher at Sunflower, Kay, had sent a little note that she was getting married, so there would be a couple of substitutes taking her place during her weeklong honeymoon. Ruffin had brought home a page from a coloring book, *Wedding Day Morning*, showing the bride and her maid of honor getting dressed. He had colored their skin green, their flowers orange and yellow. O, dear! I thought to myself as I headed upstairs to bed.

By that Friday late in June, Miss Hobbs was hard at work on another agenda for our upcoming early July IEP meeting, circulating her draft to Caron, "Moe," and Mr. Carew for comment. Either "Moe" or one of the attorneys had reminded her to add an item: "To review parent request for Ruffin to attend parochial school and discuss options with regard to parent request" and had suggested she edit out some of her more condescending language, "In an attempt to make you more comfortable in this process . . ."

Honestly, we were all preparing for an uncomfortable meeting.

Monday, on court day, I made several copies of the second most interesting discovery I had made in my most recent inspection of Ruffin's educational records — that letter by the anonymous female courthouse employee who had written the newspaper to try to reach the school board during our due process hearing. I was determined to reply to her and make several copies to leave on the law library's study table, in all the women's bathrooms, and deliver to all the courthouse offices. I was certain then, it would reach her, and stir up quite a bit of trouble — whether it would be good trouble or bad, I could no longer be a fair judge.

"Your handwritten letter was found in Superintendent Lord's personal file of my son's confidential educational record when I inspected it recently.

"There was no evidence there that any school board member has seen or read your letter. Our newspaper has a policy not to print anonymous letters. If you resubmit your letter with a signature, it might be published.

I explained the history of legal proceedings in plain language as I would to a jury.

Addressing her concerns about attorney fees, I explained, "Because the district lost the due process hearing, the district will not only have to pay the fees charged by its attorneys from Waterloo, but also the fees charged by my attorney, Iowa Protection & Advocacy Services, Inc. A special law requires this to encourage the district to 'do the right thing' in the best interests of special needs children, without putting parents through a court fight. The taxpayers are also responsible for paying Mr. Carew, the Dubuque attorney for Bridgewater Area Education Agency, who attended the week-long hearing with an associate. The district may also have to pay my legal fees for representing my son if I choose to submit them.

"Your estimate of the attorneys' hourly rate at $150 per hour is probably about right for the Waterloo attorneys or Mr. Carew. Iowa Protection & Advocacy Services, Inc.'s fees and mine are less — at about $125 per hour. Your estimate of 'tens of thousands of dollars just for legal expense' is probably right in the ballpark — since Iowa Protection & Advocacy Services, Inc.'s fees, for one lawyer were about $8,000, before writing his 50-page winning brief.

"When it was clear to everyone that the district was likely to lose, my attorney and I offered to give up our attorney fee claims and just settle for what I had sought for my son in the first place, but the district rejected our offer. The district wanted a decision.

"The Administrative Law Judge who made the decision is a professor of education at the University of Northern Iowa, Dr. Susan Etscheidt. As a result of Dr. Etscheidt's recent decision, every child with special needs in Iowa is more likely to be entitled to some kind of a 'summer school' program next summer.

"There are 15 such children now in our district. There are 5 children who bring in about $13,680 each to the school district, and 10 children who bring in about $9,120 each — a total of $159,600 of state dollars per year to fund the 2 special education classrooms here in town. The district needs to get busy planning to provide next year's 'summer school.' And because each child with special needs should spend some time 'included' with typically developing children, some of them should be invited to join in on the fun — summer-school-type activities — crafts, music, and games.

"At my last meeting with the district, I raised the issue of who was ever going to exercise common sense for the taxpayers. You may find it unfortunate that a court would appoint another lawyer to do this. I think, however, if most taxpayers knew the facts, taxpayers could speak — as you have written — very eloquently — for themselves.

"As a result of the intensive, early education my son has benefitted from, he is remarkably close to overcoming his medically diagnosed disability. His success will result in savings of about two million dollars ($2,000,000) of taxpayer money — the estimated cost of a lifetime of special education, supported employment, and group home living — all of which he was predicted to need by his doctors and Bridgewater two years ago.

"If you would like any further information about the district's disputes with me, please do not hesitate to call. "

To this explanation, I also stapled *Treatment Resources for Children with Autism*'s recent cost-benefit analysis, prepared by a group of autism-parent certified public accountants from Plano, Texas, drawing on government data.

I heard that word got around, but no one rang my phone to ask questions.

CHAPTER SIXTY SIX

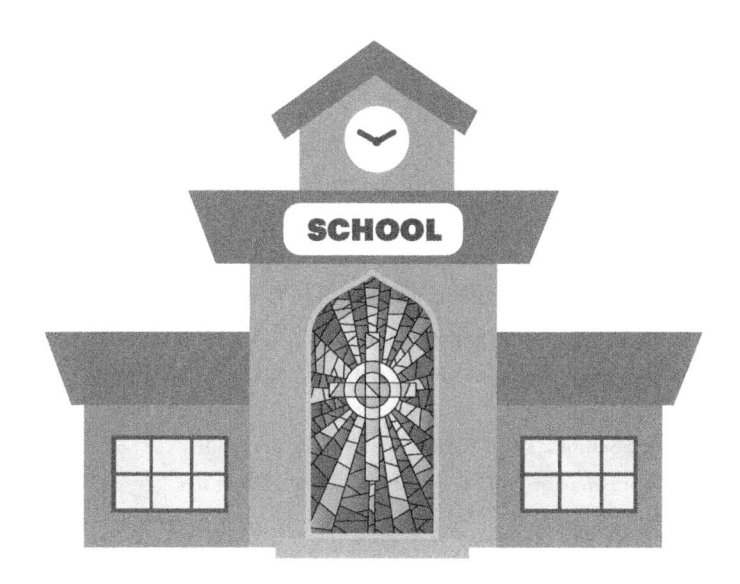

FINDING THE LRE

The next morning, I warned everyone concerned, "*If our upcoming July 1st IEP meeting is guided by Miss Hobbs's proposed agenda the team is likely to violate the IDEA's least restrictive environment (LRE) placement requirement.* Perhaps a neutral person could manage the agenda — someone not associated with either one of the possible placements? A Bridgewater employee not previously deeply enmeshed in controversy — Dan Cooper as Ruffin's case manager for the upcoming year — would be a logical and entirely customary choice.

THE FOLLOWING AGENDA MIGHT AVOID VIOLATING THE IDEA AGAIN

1. Review the current IEP, by reviewing data from: Mother, Donna Schmidt, Angela Robeson, Sunflower staff, Lisa Shelton, SLP, and team members with last year's end-of-year school data: Meg Holub, Mrs. Linden, and Kim Pope, SLP. Then invite comments from ACSD and Bridgewater, including autism resource team (ART) member Mary Carter.

2. Discuss recommendations for small class size from Gundersen, UIHC, CARD, and in the educational literature on inclusion circulated. Then invite comment from Evelyn Kung, who will be available by phone for a limited time.
3. Identify goals and objectives.

Then I set out my own proposed goals and objectives for Ruffin.

"We need to find the least restrictive environment (LRE) in which Ruffin can be reasonably expected to meet these goals and objectives with the team's consideration moving from the least restrictive (with 'support' and 'related' Bridgewater services) to more and more restrictive environments, starting with:

A. St. Pat's kindergarten of 13 to 15 students, by inviting St. Pat's staff to comment on which of Ruffin's needs could be met there and listening to the mother's belief that St. Pat's routine grading and evaluation practices can assure her of Ruffin's progress and meet all goals and objectives except the language and CARD drill goals. These might be met with Bridgewater 'support' or 'related' services from Kim Pope or Lisa Shelton. Discuss Donna Schmidt's and CARD's continuing availability for consultation in case any language or behavior problems arise, and then moving to:

B. ACSD kindergarten of 19 to 20 students, by inviting ACSD staff to comment on which of Ruffin's needs could be met there among the 77 kindergarten students with whom he would be regrouped for both reading and science. The kindergarten teacher Mrs. Linden should describe her admitted need for a one-to-one aide for Ruffin. Who will do this since Donna Schmidt is no longer available? Discuss speech and language services from either Kim Pope or Lisa Shelton. Nora Sikes should be prepared to describe her individual plans for Ruffin in the multi-categorical resource room and how she will meet his needs, goals, and objectives. Completion of the CARD drill program should be discussed.

"Please advise me who the 'we' of your most recent letter includes, and please provide your draft PLEP now."

"Discuss the mother's concerns about mutual hostilities compromising the educational value of programming to Ruffin in the public schools."

Then, I sent the announcement of Catherine Maurice's newest book to Ray DeNeve. "This resource contains the Bancroft New Jersey Lovaas replication site drill book and several good articles on inclusion techniques." I knew I could trust Ray to pass it along to "Moe" as encouragement, and as a sign of peace.

The next morning my fax whirred out a reply from Mr. Lord. "ACSD does not cull Ruffin's cumulative records. As superintendent, it is my personal right to determine what records I keep and what records I destroy. The discarding of memos is not culling." Mr. Lord failed to offer this thin and defensive explanation directly to Dr. Etscheidt — but he made a much more important agenda concession. "We will begin the meeting with your agenda and then cover any necessary additional items from ours."

During our July 1st IEP meeting, Seamus and Ruffin planned to spend the day together, out at the farm, exploring and cleaning. Ruffin would get filthy and have a lot of fun.

I called over to the school early and learned that Caron and Mr. Carew had arrived.

Eager as I was to launch into my agenda — the one Mr. Lord had acknowledged we would follow — Mr. Carew interrupted to ask that we have everyone identify him or herself on the record for the court reporter I had sent over. In attendance were Inge, Meg, Miss Hobbs, Donna, "Moe," Mary Carter, from the Bridgewater autism resource team (ART), Mark Kamm, the president of the St. Pat's school board, Mrs. Martha Byrnes, the kindergarten teacher Ruffin would have at St. Pat's, Angie, Mr. Lord, Al Neidecker from Bridgewater, Kim, Emily, Mrs. Linden and Lisa Shelton. Curt and Evelyn were listening quietly on the phone.

Mr. Carew also tried insisting that we discuss the items set out in Miss Hobbs's notice, but I simply moved back to the agenda Mr. Lord had acknowledged and began reporting what Ruffin had been doing that summer.

The first concern I raised was Ruffin's difficulty in learning people's names. "Ruffin is not very good at this. I know how offended some of you have been that I haven't always known all your names, so I know that's a difficult social problem. If I don't get the names of your organizations right, I know that upsets you."

Another concern I raised was Ruffin's continuing problems with the calendar. "This is a true weakness that Meg had noticed, and that Donna is working on mightily, but we are just not getting a whole lot of progress on time and calendar concepts."

I wanted to acknowledge Bridgewater and "Moe's" decision to add speech therapy to Ruffin's summer program. "Lisa Shelton is making steady progress on the multi-step commands which Kim had identified in her testimony at due process as a critical kindergarten skill. Maybe we'll get that done this summer, which would be very helpful in being able to offer Ruffin group directions, having him be able to remember them, and carry them through."

But as early as I could I needed to reassure St. Pat's that Ruffin was very *nearly* kindergarten ready. "Looking at the readiness checklist that Miss Hobbs handed out during her February kindergarten roundup, I thought Ruffin probably had all those skills, except 'being able to wander the neighborhood for two blocks' and 'being able to tie his shoes.'

"Recently, I've been following Ruffin for about a block's distance and letting him go to his neighborhood friend's house. He doesn't have to cross any streets to get there but it's a good long city block and then around the corner, so I would say he's doing that now.

"Overall, Ruffin is making good progress this summer. My final concern is his ability to take group directions and how he is going to be able to do paper worksheets. We need to find the most appropriate place for him to be able to succeed in doing that.

"As I talk with you, I really do want to entertain offers. Offers are what I'm looking for, and I think I've put my requests in my correspondence since mid-June and continuing up to now with Mr. Lord. You are free to reject my requests for what I want as a free, appropriate public education for Ruffin." Of course, for the first time ever at an IEP meeting, this was wholly disingenuous on my part.

Miss Hobbs responded to my opening, "Could I put you at ease right now? We're prepared to make an offer of a 15-child classroom at ACSD." This was a further concession, but somehow it failed to put me at ease.

"That's the first I've heard of a 15-child classroom because it looked like to me from our correspondence that you were committed to a 19-child classroom."

Miss Hobbs seemed to acknowledge that, "Okay."

That, too, failed to put me at ease. Why Mr. Lord and Caron would allow Miss Hobbs to speak for the district in this meeting mystified me.

"Based on some of the things I've discovered recently in Ruffin's school file, I have some concerns about people being nice when they really have other feelings. I don't think this is a place for that. I didn't come here to be patronized or nullified. I want to hear what you think and if you think wrongly, I want to contest with you so that we get at it, but I don't want to find things in Ruffin's file where people have said things to me that they truly do not believe. This is a time for us to be real and that may include some anger. If you're angry go ahead and be angry. There are certainly some issues upon which I feel some anger.

"In this meeting I really want you to think of me, if you can, as committed to my son and to myself, and I want to make the right choice for him."

Although I couldn't see it because I was at home on my phone, I could imagine someone — who? Miss Hobbs? Mr. Lord? Caron? — gave the nod to Meg, as always, to have her try to run interference by trading on her closer relationship with me to take on the hard work of mother-wrangling, of putting me at ease.

"This is Meg. Mary Jane, I'll address what you just said. We all believe that you are committed to Ruffin and to obtaining what you feel is the best program for him. We respect that and we believe that. We also feel that you do not believe that we are that committed because we disagree with you. You feel that there are other things going on here that are not going on. You have accused us of having been coerced into recommending things that we do not believe in, and that is not true."

I thought to myself over all the items I had found in Ruffin's file. Meg had expressed enthusiasm for Ruffin's CARD program in our home-school notebook, and then been required to recant that, in writing, to recommit herself to the school's program and to Miss Hobbs. I had called her out on that, embarrassed her, hurt her, and then sent Donna into school to virtually replace her during Ruffin's second year in her classroom. I could hear the hurt in her voice.

She went on, with her assignment, "We respect your right to disagree with what we feel we recommend as the best program and we have a right to expect that respect from you too. Maybe you don't believe it, but that's the way it is and if you can disagree with us — we know you disagree with us, and we respect your right to do that — you also have to respect our right to do that, too."

Meg was a problem, but whatever happened in this meeting, Meg would be a *past* problem. Ruffin was going to have a *new* classroom teacher. The real problem now and for the future remained Miss Hobbs. So, it was time to come right out with it, and I did by putting my finger right on the sore spot.

"Just recently, I discovered Miss Hobbs's December 21st, 1994 memo, a copy of which went to you, Meg, which questioned Ruffin's Gundersen diagnosis of autism, pointing to me as the cause of Ruffin's difficulties and making a number of other comments which indicated to me the school district's 30-year lag in thinking about autism and its 20-year lag in thinking about special education."

That left Meg scrambling. "All right, but back off from that a minute to realize that in this system as in most systems it is set up as it is supposed to be set up. Miss Hobbs, whatever you believe about her, is an excellent administrator."

Well, I might have begged to differ. I would have agreed with Dr. Etscheidt, but I managed to do that silently. Now that she was on a roll, it was better not to interrupt Meg.

"It is not Miss Hobbs's job to know all the procedural things about special education."

Except that as the district's special education director, it was, but, again, I didn't say so. Caron and Mr. Carew knew: Miss Hobbs's procedural faults had cost both the local district and Bridgewater dearly in our recent due process hearing.

"Miss Hobbs is learning, and she knows a lot about special education, but as Ruffin's IEP team it was the team's job to make recommendations to Miss Hobbs and then for her to follow up on those. We were the team that made — Miss Hobbs did not make the recommendations. She listened to us, and we made the recommendations."

Ah, there it was, Meg's admission of what I had suspected had happened *again*. This IEP meeting had been preceded by the usual "meeting before the meeting" that Curt and I had repeatedly condemned as a wide-spread and illegal practice.

Miss Hobbs, or one of the attorneys cuing her to interrupt, saw the danger of another procedural error.

"Let's continue to work through our agenda and we're still with you, Mary Jane. Do you have anything further to add? It looks like Donna Schmidt is next."

Since my court reporter had the admission I needed to prosecute a second successful due process, I agreed cheerfully enough. "Yes, let's all hear from Donna now."

Later parts of the meeting, and the real discussions they prompted, were the sorts of things I had hoped would help St. Pat's the most since I had already chosen to place Ruffin there, somehow, some way, if I could also get everything else I thought he needed.

Theory of mind issues went right to the heart of Ruffin's remaining social difficulties, so we needed to discuss those for the benefit of those attending from St. Pat's. I spoke up again, "So, I hear some theory of mind remarks and he is picking up theory of mind type language and grammatical structures, but there is a pragmatic disconnect between whether he truly has a connection with another person and truly understands what that person is thinking and doing. That's the problem I think he's going to have with his classmates, particularly as they become more judgmental — maybe not this kindergarten year, but by first grade."

As always, as Ruffin's mother, I seemed to be the only person thinking into the years ahead, but I was wrong. Donna was curious, too, and asked Evelyn a question.

"Is Ruffin going to move on — develop — beyond all this modeling? Is he going to actually have thoughts, theory of mind, like you and I do, or is he going to be left mechanically modeling?"

Evelyn responded, "Ruffin is going through a developmental stage, a kind of period, when he has to feel the social consequences of his own awkward behaviors. Just because he has asked somebody's name and they're not his friend, he will try to play with them. It's not very natural to him, but he will. Ruffin is picking up a lot already, but he's going to need more practice and more prompting, but he seems to be more aware of how people respond to him."

I tried to reinforce what Evelyn was saying, by offering, mostly for the benefit of those attending from St. Pat's, "You must be clear in explaining to Ruffin why the social consequences are different from what he expected. He won't intuit it. He won't get it naturally."

Evelyn explained a bit more of what she had in mind to help Ruffin develop in this particular area. "Right now, you are prompting Ruffin through set-up situations and offering him models to imitate, but eventually I will ask you to set up a situation where Ruffin is going to fail, but you are going to be there to work Ruffin through it and try to help him figure out what happened. You know, 'Why did they walk away, even though you do know their names?' 'Even though they are your friends?' He will need your external prompting."

Then, I spoke up, again. "Ruffin also has an expectation that 'please' is a magic word. If one person says 'please,' the other person must say, 'yes.' The person asked does not have the option to say 'no.'" As soon as the words were out of my mouth, I had to wonder how many people in our meeting must have had the same thought cross their minds, 'The apple doesn't fall far from the tree.' No one would have dared voice that observation. Meg simply asked Angie whether she had anything to offer us.

"With games, Ruffin doesn't like to lose. That's a really big problem. He walks away from a game if he's won." Which, I had to admit to myself, was exactly my plan here — to walk away from the local public school, having won at due process. On the phone, I couldn't read anyone else's eyes but Angie's. I couldn't tell what any of the other participants might be thinking. On balance, I didn't need that distraction. I needed to focus on listening.

Then, because Evelyn held a long view of Ruffin's future development, and in light of her unique experience and expertise, Evelyn told what I found to be a chilling story to underline the importance of teaching social and theory of mind skills *now* to Ruffin.

"I just saw an adult with autism this weekend who is very high-functioning and has a regular job but got fired because when other people walked into his office, he didn't say anything. He would just sit there. He might say, 'Hi.' Other people thought he was rude. And he didn't understand when somebody else was mad at him. People never felt comfortable with him sitting there in his office. It was causing problems at work, and he got fired for it.

"I tell this story as a way for you to see how crucial the transition is for a person with autism into the world. We need to teach social skills and theory of mind. Early."

CHAPTER SIXTY SEVEN

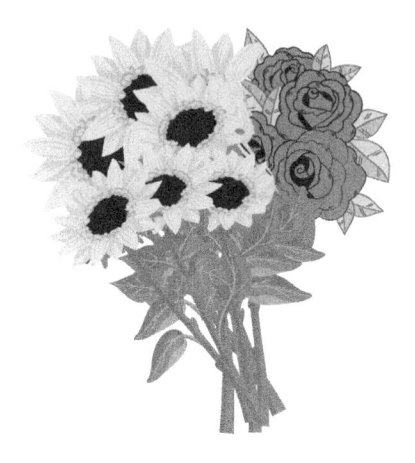

A ROSE BY ANY OTHER NAME

Donna discussed Ruffin's problem with names. "As for his recalling any names — he and I really worked hard on his learning 'Joe,' the name of his driver. We sang songs about Joe and did all kinds of stuff to help Ruffin with his memory. We got 'Joe," but, poor 'Angie,' we've tried having Ruffin sing songs and everything, and he can't seem to learn her name. Maybe 25% of the time he can recall her name now, otherwise he takes a guess and a stab, mentioning other children's names at Sunflower.

"Ruffin has brought up one child's name from Sunflower, but his conversation was more about his shoes." Yes, I thought, his were the first Ruffin had seen of Velcro closures. He had been very intrigued with those shoes and managed to tell me all about them. Donna knew, too. "Ruffin was learning to tie his shoes, until he pulled a fast one and got his Velcro closure pair. He was about 70% of the way to learning how to tie his shoes."

With Meg seeming to have taken the baton of leading the meeting, she checked the agenda Mr. Lord and I had agreed to and called on Angie. "Do you want to talk about what you've seen this summer?" I was pleased to hear her treating Angie, a recent college graduate, as a trusted source, if not a professional equal. Yes, I thought, this was the sort of exchange I had always hoped for in an IEP meeting.

Angie gathered her notes and spoke up. "When I ask Ruffin what my own name is, he usually offers "Jenny" as the answer, or some other name."

Donna piped up again at this point, "When I ask Ruffin what your name is, I get 3 guesses, 3 different responses, 3 different names, and one is a boy's name, so, I'm sorry, Angie."

Angie admitted there really was something in a name. "I tell Ruffin it makes me sad that he doesn't know my name sometimes. And I've been hearing 'Jenny' a lot of times. I think Ruffin doesn't hear my name right. He has the "J" sound of it. If my name were 'Jenny,' it wouldn't be a problem, but that's not my name and so it is."

This is where Evelyn's autism experience and expertise came into play. "If you can gather pictures of the other children and teachers, that's usually the best way of teaching names to children with autism."

I tried to make this very concrete for those attending from St. Pat's. "Whoever his classmates are then, we need to take some Polaroid photographs almost the first day of class, so that whoever is responsible for making sure that Ruffin learns their names has those photographs to work with."

"Yes," Evelyn echoed to reinforce this message. "Can I make a suggestion for Angie right now? If you can, get a tape recorder and get each of the Sunflower kids to speak into it and then give the tape to Mary Jane and Donna so they can have Ruffin listen and try to figure out who is talking. We want to learn how much Ruffin's listening to the other children, whether he's actually listening to and discriminating the sounds of their voices."

Donna asked a good and clarifying question about Evelyn's proposed exercise. "Evelyn, do you want us to present Ruffin just the audible voice recordings, or present the visual aid, the photographs, with the voices?"

Evelyn picked up on that. "Present both the voice recordings and the photographs and have Ruffin identify the voice to the person's picture. It's harder if you just present the voice recordings. Presenting both together would help Ruffin a lot in getting him ready to tune in more receptively to his environment."

From her place at the meeting table, Donna was able to assure Evelyn, "Everyone is nodding their heads 'yes' here."

Meg echoed Donna, "We got it."

Evelyn reinforced this again, "And that means photographs and voice recordings of all of you, too, who work with Ruffin."

For the first time in the meeting, "Moe" spoke up and in an exchange with Al Neidecker they managed to locate a camera Bridgewater had bought for the autism resource team (ART) to bring into Angie at Sunflower by having Lisa Shelton pick it up from the Decorah office where it was stored.

CHAPTER SIXTY EIGHT

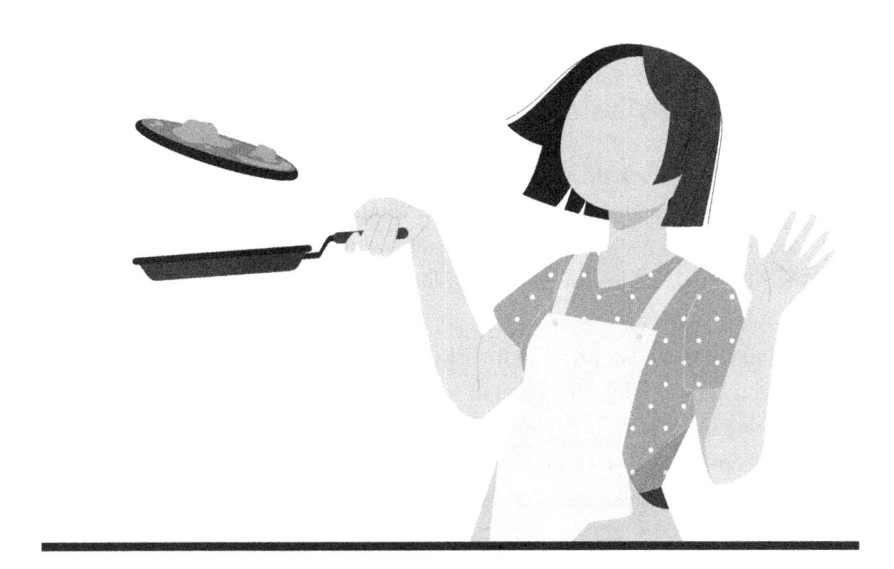

THAT'S THE PLEP

I was feeling surprisingly good about this annual IEP meeting now. We had been discussing what Mrs. Byrnes would need to know to prepare to teach Ruffin at St. Pat's. I took up the agenda again as Mr. Lord and I had agreed to it.

"Let's hear from Lisa Shelton, the Bridgewater speech and language pathologist who has been working with Ruffin this summer."

Lisa was ready. "I've had 4 sessions with Ruffin. We're working on a single objective: following a 3-part direction, with each part including 2 critical elements such as size, shape, color, or something of that nature.

"I started out by giving the 3 steps individually at first. I have Ruffin do the first, then the second, then the third separately. After he has completed all those correctly, I give him the directions for the first task and while he is completing that, I present the directions for the second task, and then as he is working on that, I present the directions for the third.

"Once he was able to do that correctly, I would alert him, 'Okay, I'm going to go through all 3.' That's what we are doing now, and Ruffin can respond correctly at about 45% on average.

"I can see this skill of his carrying over into kindergarten if we continue to progress this summer. He might continue to need this sort of instruction again in the classroom. Right now, he and I are working on the development of this skill one-to-one, and I would like to see it generalize into next year's classroom."

With that, Meg took the agenda back. I knew we were headed for a recitation of her pre-written meeting-before-the-meeting present levels of educational performance. With Ruffin such a moving target, her PLEP suffered from Meg not having seen Ruffin since late May. It would be historical, but I hoped it would be useful information for those attending from St. Pat's.

Meg moved down her prepared list. "Ruffin can hypothesize 'why.' When shown a picture and asked, 'Why is this person sad?' or 'Why is this person happy.' I have loved listening to Donna's drills about 'How would you feel if I stepped on your new toy?' Ruffin can respond to this type of question without a visual prompt or a visual cue or anything. He can engage in those kinds of conversations about emotions very appropriately."

With all the tensions of this summer's issues behind us, with all the conflict of the due process hearing behind us, it was wonderful to hear Meg open up again and share details about Ruffin that would help us next year as he moved on.

Meg offered some thoughts for next year. "When we approach the time concepts, of today, yesterday, and tomorrow, we may need to use a visual calendar. Another way to probe for these concepts, or that I have heard other kids use spontaneously is to ask, 'How many sleeps?' meaning how many times did I have to sleep and get up, so 'It was three sleeps ago.' Anything concrete like that, that we can offer Ruffin might help him put time in focus.

Winding it up, Meg reported, "In the final goal I have addressed Ruffin's participation in discrete trial format training with generalization opportunities. Donna has all the charting on those drills, and Evelyn has some reports she had turned in as Ruffin's supervising therapist, working for Dr. Granpeesheh of CARD. Ruffin progressed in his CARD program according to both Donna and Evelyn, and I can add that Ruffin did generalize those skills learned in his one-to-one drills. Donna would bring Ruffin out into the various classrooms and have him participate, and she and I would observe him generalize."

Evelyn responded, as she usually did, with praise, "Good."

Meg acknowledged that with what sounded to me like some relief, "Okay, so that's the PLEP."

CHAPTER SIXTY NINE

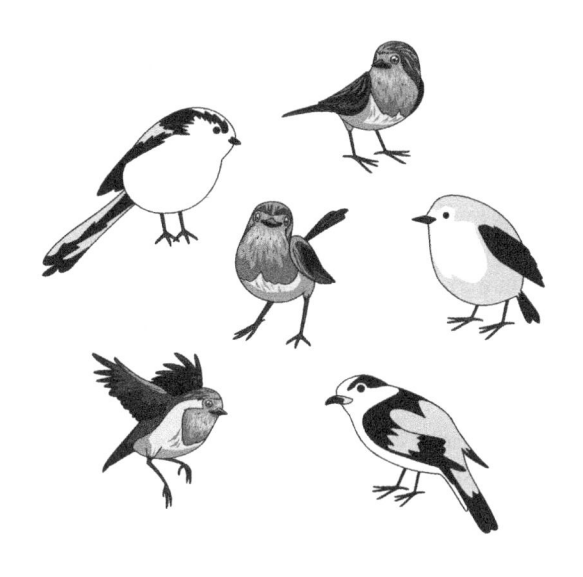

KIM AND EVELYN

Meg called on Kim who announced, "I'm going to comment from the last speech and language report that I wrote in early June." She had tested Ruffin on a couple of standardized instruments toward the end of last school year. This would be a repeat of very old news from our recent summer services (EYSE) meeting — old news that should have been available well-before our due process hearing.

I hoped someone was handing around copies, particularly to those attending from St. Pat's. With Kim defending the success of her own work with Ruffin, her report would sound very reassuring. At this meeting, that would work for me, and for Ruffin.

Kim rattled through a list of average and high average picture vocabulary scores and then explained a more interesting auditory discrimination test.

"Some of these word pairs get quite difficult and a lot of the words used are those that children of Ruffin's age don't have a clue about their meanings. The word pairs start out very simply. 'Red' and 'dead' are the first one. 'Bed,' 'bred;' 'pig,' 'big' and by the end, it's 'Conoco,' 'comical.' Ruffin got that one. 'Madder,' 'matter.' Ruffin got that one, too. 'When,' 'win;' 'leave,' 'leaf.'

"He had to have listened very carefully to do this correctly, and again, Ruffin did quite well. He was very interested. Everybody has said this over and over, if Ruffin is very interested in what you are doing and you have his attention, he does perform quite well. If you have lost him somewhere along the line and he is not interested, his performance really sags.

"Earlier on the oral vocabulary subtest, I offered him a word and asked Ruffin to tell me the meaning of the word or to tell me all the things he knew about the particular word. The first word I gave him was 'Bird, tell me what you know about a bird.' And this was his answer, 'A bird has wings, and a bird has feathers to fly and wings, and it has a beak, and birds can sing, and birds have claws to hang on trees.' He was going on and on. Ruffin was just telling me wonderful things about birds and all his responses were like that, continually."

It was a parade of the earlier elephants. I wondered if Kim appreciated that this was a common enough symptom of Asperger's Syndrome — one that could get to be a rather troublesome social behavior.

"With the next test, something interesting happened. I needed to get a basal performance. With Ruffin who was 5 years old, I might want to probe for a basal measure by beginning at 4-and-a-half, or start a little bit lower, and then skip up through the test. With Ruffin I tried to skip a level. He and I didn't need to do all those early pages, but Ruffin said, 'No, let's go back. I want to do that one. I want to start at the beginning.' Ruffin did not want me to skip any of the pages, so we did the whole thing."

This, too, represented a rigidity of behavior associated with autism or Asperger's Syndrome which I knew was common enough and could sometimes prove troublesome. This didn't surprise me, and it put a very human face on Ruffin's developing personality and abilities for St. Pat's and Mrs. Byrnes.

I warned, "Well, Ruffin doesn't like to skip ahead."

Kim agreed, but knowing little about autism that I could hear, fundamentally misunderstood. "Ruffin did not want to skip. This testing was not work for him. He was very successful at it, and he was enjoying it and he liked to do it."

Meg understood, and she appreciated Ruffin's rigidity as having shifted the power dynamic between himself as the child and Kim as the adult. "Ruffin is turning into a teacher."

This little testing situation was about rigidity and control. Sometimes in life, sometimes in a classroom, the schedule slips and a teacher might find the class running behind, running out of time, and might need to be flexible. I wanted Mrs. Byrnes to be alert to the possibility that in these situations, she might need to find a way to help Ruffin become flexible.

So, I spoke up again for Mrs. Byrnes' benefit. "Ruffin doesn't like to skip ahead. He does not want to skip things. He wants to do it all and do it right."

Kim then mused on her papers and decided not to offer her written comments that I was able to read later — strongly opposing Ruffin's summer CARD program. That had been decided by Dr. Etscheidt.

"I can just skip this part and sum up."

So, finally, she did. "I really consider Ruffin's speech and language skills to be adequate for oral communication and I do believe they would also be adequate for classroom communication and academic progress."

After reporting what she could have reported well before our spring due process hearing, Kim was *history*.

Before Mrs. Linden could be called on for her report, Mr. Lord interrupted. "First, we need to introduce an individual who has come in."

A woman's voice responded, "I'm Nora Sikes, the multi-categorical teacher." No thank you, I thought. All we need is another special education teacher who arrived late, and who had missed all these earlier reports. I didn't want Ruffin to be teased by his classmates for disappearing regularly into a resource room. He had worked too hard. We had worked too hard for him to simply wash up there. What were these people thinking?

Mr. Lord shouldered on with his interruption. "Evelyn is on the line. Is there any chance we could take a break, while keeping Evelyn on the line? How much longer is it going to take to get Evelyn off the line?"

Mr. Lord didn't like paying Evelyn for her time or expertise. CARD would charge $146.25 for her to attend this IEP meeting by phone for a total of 2.25 hours, a relative pittance compared to what he was prepared to pay Caron at $150 per hour for this meeting which would run on and on for a total of seven hours — $1,050 at least — with Mr. Carew also sitting in clocking at least the same, or double that for Bridgewater, since Mr. Carew had also brought along his junior associate.

I asked, "Evelyn, how much longer do you have to be with us?"

"About fifteen minutes, because I have another meeting to attend."

Kim had wasted more time than she was worth. Time to move along, so I consulted my agenda and suggested, "Let's hear from Mrs. Linden briefly and then, Evelyn, I'd like to hear from you about what you've heard here, and what you recommend."

Mrs. Linden spoke up. "Ruffin joined us 4-and-half-hours a week in the morning during a language session when I was teaching alphabet skills. Now, Ruffin did not join us for learning those academic skills. He joined us for socialization and practicing making transitions.

"In the time he was with us I saw definite improvements in basic transition time within my classroom. This is a big thing for kindergarteners: to know that when it's time to move, you move."

This rubbed me the wrong way, immediately. I didn't want to send Ruffin, or any child, to school so he or she could be easily "herded."

"It was hard for Ruffin at the beginning, but by the end of the year he was doing very, very well at moving when he needed to move and even looking forward to going to activities he enjoyed more. He knew that at the desk, activity was going to be more academic, more writing. He knew when we went to the circle corner, the activity would be a story, with more movement, and he enjoyed those times.

As always, ever ready to go the extra mile, Evelyn spoke up briefly to let us all know she had rescheduled her next meeting so she could spend more time with us.

Finally, Meg called on Evelyn. "You want to react to any of this?"

Hardly a warm or enthusiastic invitation, so Evelyn spoke with greater caution than she was accustomed to do in our home-program brainstorming and technique critique conference calls or quarterly meetings.

"Some of what I've heard sounds familiar. Ruffin has made a friend, a neighborhood friend, JJ, who is going to help him a lot. Next year, Ruffin needs to continue in a small class of 13 to 15 students because in a bigger class he will still have his attention difficulty and his desire to do what he wants to do as opposed to what the class is doing.

"Of course, he will learn as he goes through the school year, but right now at Sunflower, although Ruffin has been there about a month — longer than most kids his age would take to learn the names of the people in his group there — Ruffin doesn't know many of their names. It is an exceptional difficulty for Ruffin that the population of children there has changed day by day. The reason we need to keep his next class small is so that he will be able to adjust well, considering that he still has difficulty in a setting like Sunflower.

"If Ruffin were to be placed in a bigger class, that would not be appropriate for him. We already know from all the people we have just heard from that Ruffin's performance is different in different settings. If he were placed with a large group, he would require an aide. Somebody would have to deal with him individually, and Ruffin would continue to respond differently than a typical child.

"Ruffin is very bright. He can compensate for some of his difficulties. He is already doing that, and he is interested in learning. Still, his attention is going to be a big problem going forward, as will be having him use all the appropriate social interactions we expect from a typical child of his age. We are going to be teaching social skills for a long time into the future. A lot of his social skills will be memorized routines, or scripted at first, but Ruffin is already generalizing. One thing about Ruffin that he does well is that he has generalized all the things he has learned by working one-to-one.

"Ruffin did well during the speech testing Kim did because he enjoys that one-to-one academic setting. It was very structured and very much like what Ruffin knows he's supposed to be doing in his one-to-one drill sessions. There's a beginning; there's an end, and it's almost a game for him.

"Our plan should be that by the end of Ruffin's kindergarten year, we will be done with his special education, so I don't have to be a part of it. His planning group can just go ahead and place him in any classroom as you would a typical child."

That was my goal for Ruffin. After the difficulties of mediation, due process, and this sort of drawn-out meeting, I thought the rest of this group would have found this goal and Evelyn's projection of it attractive enough — getting Ruffin out of special education.

Meg took back leading our meeting then. "Okay, Evelyn, other than the appropriateness of a small class size, do you have any other recommendations, for example, with respect to whether his one-to-one therapy should continue, or anything else?"

"There are still some drills I think would really benefit Ruffin, to help him develop socially."

Yes, I thought. The difficult set of 59 social drills Evelyn had sent for me to share with this group ahead of time. I asked, "What about having a speech and language pathologist work with Ruffin on the remaining uncompleted CARD drills? The ones addressing definitions, attributes, and some of the weaknesses identified in Ms. Wilding's last report from UIHC. Could that person work on Ruffin's social routines in a relatively short one-to-one pullout session?"

Evelyn responded to my concern. "Maybe 20 minutes, twice a week."

Meg spoke up to try to clarify. "So, a little bit of one-to-one wouldn't be bad, but you don't want it occurring — "

"In front of other kids." I had interrupted her.

And Evelyn echoed me, "I don't want it in front of other kids."

"Right," acknowledged Meg.

Evelyn underscored her point, again, "We want Ruffin to be treated as a typical peer, as a typical child. Definitely."

Miss Hobbs was confused. Wasn't this supposed to be a special education meeting? She asked Evelyn directly, "So, are you recommending any pull out, or not?"

Evelyn was definite. "I'm not recommending *any* pull out at all. Earlier when we had less experience at successful integration, especially as we began a child's first integration experiences, teachers tended to pull a child aside. If Ruffin doesn't *value* the company of his classmates, if he hasn't spent time with other, typically developing children to the point he really comes to value them, to the point he really *wants* to be with them, every pull aside will seem rewarding to him, and set him back socially.

"Our children with autism in intensive treatment master the identification of objects and concepts because they've been doing it one-to-one for at least a year before entering group instruction. Getting them to follow along, to be able to raise their hands, to be able to ask another child for help, to be able to discern when asking another child for help would be cheating or when it would be appropriate are critical classroom skills."

"By the end of his kindergarten year what we want to see is that Ruffin values his classmates socially, and understands his social status with his peers, so that if a teacher pulls him out to do one-to-one work because he wasn't paying attention, that Ruffin wouldn't like that, and that being pulled aside would be something he did not enjoy.

"What we want to try to avoid if Ruffin is not paying attention, *especially the first half of his kindergarten year*, is having the teacher pull him out one-to-one to have him concentrate academically. The danger is Ruffin would learn to like being one-to-one with his teacher, and that he would learn to like being separated from the other children. It may be harder for Ruffin to sit with the other children, but he needs to try, and to be challenged to do it *now*."

CHAPTER SEVENTY

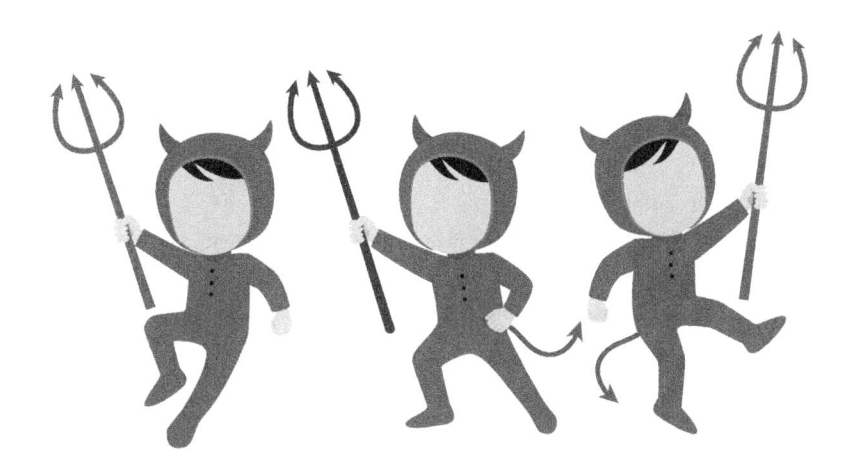

THE DEVIL IS IN THE DETAILS

Moe spoke up, after Evelyn left, "We need to establish who the basic core team is here. Without a doubt the core team includes the mother."

Yes, I thought. I wanted to be a part of *all* the meetings — including the "meeting before the meeting" the schools always seemed to have. But I, too, wanted to work with a smaller, nimbler group. I could do without Kim, Emily, Mrs. Linden, Nora Sikes, Miss Hobbs, and even Mr. Lord. I kept my thoughts to myself, as "Moe" went on ticking off his own core dream team.

"We have Ruffin's teacher for next year and we don't know whether that will be Mrs. Linden who was Ruffin's integration teacher at ACSD or somebody else that Miss Hobbs would identify, or whether it would be the St. Pat's kindergarten teacher, Mrs. Byrnes, if Ruffin ends up going to St. Pat's."

Interesting, I thought. "Moe" was considering that as an option.

I didn't imagine ACSD would place Ruffin at St. Pat's for any one of a number of reasons — professional pride, unwillingness to create a precedent that would allow other highly valuable special education students to exit their programs. But, despite his move to collapse the meeting to a core team, "Moe" seemed to acknowledge that it would be my choice, and my choice alone, to walk away from public school.

Many other names were mentioned and discussed, but Peter Smith, St. Pat's principal, went unmentioned.

"Moe" was ready to wrap up. "Other than that, I am open."

I spoke up, "And Evelyn."

Mr. Lord objected, in an indirect maneuver to replace Evelyn, who was expensive. "Isn't there an autism resource person from Bridgewater's ART?"

At that point, "Moe" offered, "Mary Carter from our Bridgewater ART is the person who has autism skills. We could keep her on Ruffin's team. She would be happy to come, but you need to understand, she has a whole area in Dubuque that she covers."

Mary Carter might be an improvement on the local autism resource team (ART) members who were nowhere in evidence now, but Mary had never met Ruffin that I knew. About Mary, I reserved judgment, but it didn't sound like she would be available during the winter. The drive from Dubuque to our town was particularly wicked.

Then, Miss Hobbs weighed in, supporting her own preferred plan for Ruffin. "We suspect Ruffin's memory problem is going to be something that will need a lot of work, and that's why we are recommending the multi-categorical program for him, with Nora Sikes as his teacher. That's why she's here. Mary Jane?"

Given Evelyn's advice not to pull Ruffin out for one-to-one instruction which he would find more rewarding than the company of his classmates, and which might brand him as "special," this called for another episode of crossed swords.

"Obviously if he goes to St. Pat's, his principal will be Peter Smith."

Time again, for Meg to step in to protect Miss Hobbs and back me off. "We're getting into legalities with church and state here. At St. Pat's we would need to monitor Ruffin's social skills acquisition and his progress somehow. We want someone assigned to that role, but it could be a Bridgewater speech clinician, too, if Ruffin were getting speech services."

Well, exactly, I thought. Far better that Meg voice this solution than I do it.

I responded, very neutrally, "I don't think we can decide who the team will be until we find out where we are going to place Ruffin. At some point we need to decide who the team is."

But really, I was curious about hearing from someone else. "I wonder if we could hear from Mary Carter."

Nobody objected to that, so we did.

"Obviously, I do not know Ruffin. I just met him recently," said Mary Carter, a new voice. I wondered when and where that meeting might have been. No one had bothered to let me know in advance or have me consent. I would never find out.

"So, most of my impressions are from what I've heard today and from the information I was sent before this meeting. First, I'm really impressed by how much Ruffin is doing with his academic skills. His kindergarten teachers will be really pleased by what he already knows coming in, and Ruffin will probably be able to be a peer helper to other students.

"I'm in agreement with what Evelyn has said. Two things I note here are Ruffin's problem with following directions within a group because of his attention issue and the issue with ongoing social interaction. It sounds like when Ruffin is in a familiar classroom with familiar children he does better. To be positive, Ruffin will be going into a kindergarten classroom where a lot of the other kids won't know each other. They will all be starting from the same place.

"We have found with our students with autism that putting them into integration situations briefly is nearly a *disservice* to them because they don't know the other students very well. They're sitting by new students, and it is hard for our students with autism to feel a part of the situation, no matter how hard the teachers try, no matter how hard the other students try.

"From what I read, I wasn't sure whether Ruffin was initiating socially, because I didn't see a lot of that happening myself. But from what I'm hearing here today, when Ruffin is comfortable, he has a lot of conversational language.

"Teaching Ruffin social interaction may present some problems. Providing visuals and cueing him to directions given to the group will help. Ruffin also seems to have a hard time starting and finishing projects or worksheets. That, too, may need some cuing from the teacher at first. I agree with Evelyn that Ruffin is probably going to be best served in a smaller classroom of 13 to 15 students to give him one more year of boost before he can manage a regular-size first grade classroom."

Very helpful, I thought, trusting that Mrs. Byrnes was listening.

Then I returned to the completion of Ruffin's CARD program. "If you look at the latest set of drills that Evelyn has set out for Donna to get accomplished — and Donna's not available after the end of August — we are going to need somebody to pick up and try to do that one-to-one discrete trial work. Ms. Wilding's concerns about definitions and attributes could be worked on in a number of those CARD drills. Would a speech and language pathologist be able to work on those and on the social skills guidance issues?

"I looked at the public school's social skill curriculum and their skill screening assessment instrument, both of which I borrowed. They assume the kind of theory of mind development most kids have at age 4 and age 5. *Ruffin doesn't have the underlying theory of mind for any of this curriculum to make an impression on him.* What Ruffin will need are explicit rules.

"To teach Ruffin, 'This is a routine we use when we are faced with teasing,' we offer, 'It's a good idea to try these things,' giving Ruffin some explicit rules, because he's willing to seize on rules: 'I have to ask their names;' 'I need to ask to play.' Ruffin needs to learn the rule that if somebody says, 'No,' the rule is to go ask somebody else. Maybe you will support me on this. Ruffin is going to need those kinds of structures to get through social situations."

"Let's say he's gotten to a fork in the road where he is encountering some difficulty. He needs an absolute rule that will probably keep him out of social trouble. The problem is that most social interactions are more complex than any of the rules. If Ruffin does develop some theory of mind skill this summer, maybe he can be more flexible in learning social skills, but at this point Ruffin's going to get into situations where he isn't flexible. I can't see her, but I would guess that Mary is nodding her head now."

According to Donna, who reported to me later, Mary was.

And I knew I probably had "Moe's" agreement on this point, too, since this was the same argument I had made earlier and successfully to him after our last meeting when he and I had agreed to bring Lisa Shelton on board as Ruffin's new speech and language pathologist for the summer. Now, I was making my argument to the full IEP team.

It was "Moe" who spoke up. "And I would agree, Mary. These kinds of things are going to have to be done within Ruffin's speech and language program. We're going to have to try to avoid a one-to-one pullout speech program. That's not the kind of speech program any of you are recommending.

I certainly agreed with "Moe," and welcomed his leadership. I liked the concept. It was Meg's and Evelyn's concept, too.

CHAPTER SEVENTY ONE

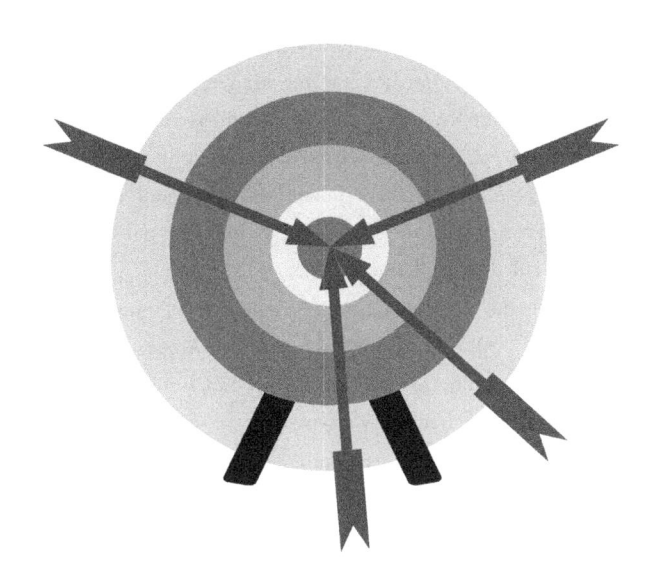

AIMING FOR FULL INCLUSION

Moe spoke up again in our long July 1st meeting, strongly favoring full inclusion for Ruffin. "I would like to see speech as something that would happen incidentally to his total kindergarten program. There may be deficit areas that Ruffin will have to work on, but I agree that pulling Ruffin out of his regular kindergarten program would not be to his benefit."

Meg was ready, too, to turn to a discussion of that tricky word, that difficult concept of "inclusion." "So, okay, we were given some research on inclusion and on small class size. Does anybody want to comment? In one of those research articles, there was a checklist of the attributes that children with autism should have before they were included . . ." Yes, I thought, without interrupting, at the end of the chapter on inclusion in Catherine Maurice's newest book. "I read through that checklist, and Ruffin obviously qualifies for an inclusive setting as his placement. He has a lot of the skills, and many others he will need are emerging."

Now, I spoke up, since I had scored Ruffin myself on that checklist. "Yes."

Seeming to have missed Mary Carter's points, Emily wanted to muddy this up. "We are looking at Ruffin as someone entering kindergarten. We don't expect those children to be able to count from 1 to 100. We need to keep in mind: 'What do we normally expect of children? We need to compare Ruffin to typical kindergarteners. If Ruffin is attentive only half of the instructional time, that sounds terrible, but if another student also appears attentive for only half of the instructional time, it might be the activity was one that failed to challenge the class.

Meg offered Emily the support of another concern that I thought Mary Carter had also already addressed. "And there's that observation in Angie's notes about Ruffin at Sunflower. It was hard for Ruffin to enter that peer group, but it was because it was very tight. It would be hard for anybody new to enter it."

Well, yes, I thought, if Ruffin's inclusion failed, we could always blame his teacher or his classmates. This simply brought home to me again: I needed to choose Ruffin's new teacher and his classmates with care.

This was hard work for these educators. Inclusion wasn't a new special education concept. It had been around since the 1980s, but our local district's special education program was still in its infancy. Full integration or inclusion of young children developing through autism was new and cutting edge in the 1990s. Not many children with autism had ever developed sufficiently due to intensive, early intervention to even need a program of full inclusion into any mainstream classroom.

Finally, Meg was ready to turn to writing some goals and objectives, but Mr. Lord interrupted. "How long is this going to take?"

Miss Hobbs stepped in to offer a shortcut. "I thought Mary Jane had written some pretty good ones."

But Mr. Lord, who was paying overtime for his employees, was looking for something else. "Is this meeting going to last another 30 minutes and be done, or is it going to last another 3 hours?"

I assured Mr. Lord, "It's going to take more than 30 minutes."

Mr. Lord offered us a lame attempt at levity. "I know, I'm being facetious."

CHAPTER SEVENTY TWO

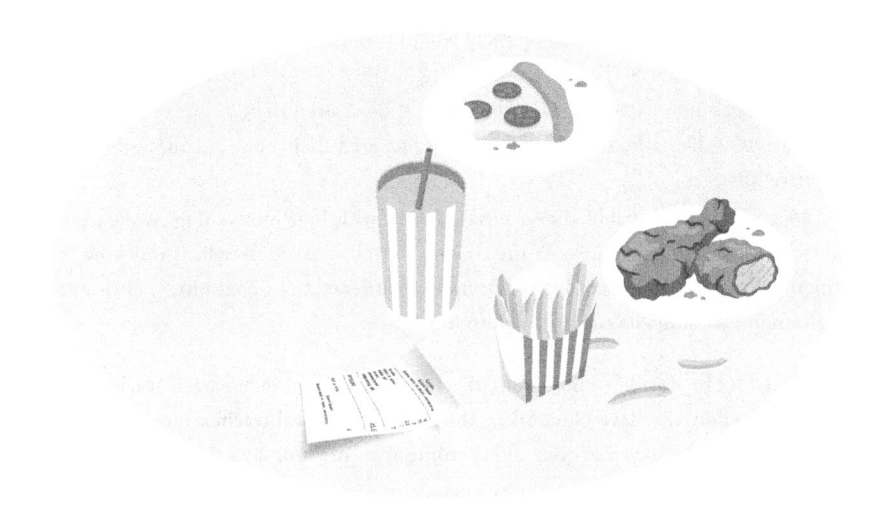

AFTER LUNCH, WHOSE OX?

When we broke for lunch, I told Angie she could go if she liked, called Donna to tell her the same, called Evelyn to see if we could have her back on the phone later in the afternoon before we wrapped up, and called St. Pat's where I told their school secretary, the wonderful red-haired Maureen Mahoney, that I could tell the way the wind was blowing through this morning's meeting, and that if Mrs. Byrnes and Mr. Timm had better things to do this afternoon, I thought they had heard all that they needed to know to be able to manage Ruffin in kindergarten. Maureen was sympathetic and assured me she would let them both know.

I called Curt and told him he should go do something useful for the afternoon. I could handle the rest of the meeting. It would be boring. I would need to wait it out. I thought I could wait it out.

Meg took up leading the meeting again for the afternoon. For me, it was like eavesdropping on "the meeting before the meeting." I found it instructive. It was a long lesson of several hours as the remaining group struggled to construct an offer of a free, appropriate public education (FAPE) for Ruffin at public school.

With this group struggling to formulate an offer that I would need to consider and either accept as "appropriate" or reject as "inappropriate," it was not in my interests, or Ruffin's best interests for me to contribute to writing a plan that might pass legal muster. Whenever I was remembered or asked what I thought, I replied with an appropriate neutrality, "You go ahead."

I wasn't going to speak up. Let them forget I was even there. I was determined to go on listening like a fly on the wall as they prepared their best, but inevitably inappropriate offer.

Meg and Emily squabbled over several issues, with Inge intervening, as she usually did, with a helpful suggestion. As the fly on the wall, I asked myself, is this how they work together in my absence? Well, writing was harder work by committee. At this rate, an afternoon wouldn't be time enough to finish this.

Miss Hobbs was worrying about the burden on her kindergarten teacher, Mrs. Linden. "Couldn't we have Nora Sikes, the multi-categorical teacher, monitor Ruffin's social skills goals in the classroom and do some assessment of how Ruffin is doing?"

Likely this was a push toward burden-sharing? I would have wagered that Nora Sikes was a Bridgewater employee. It sounded like that was the issue when "Moe" answered, "The only trouble I would have is: if you are going to give Nora Sikes that role, then the question is: 'Are you placing Ruffin in regular kindergarten, or are you placing Ruffin into some special education program?' To have another person monitor Ruffin's social skill goals and objectives on a day-to-day basis, you might want to add some support staff. Would you want to do that with an additional classroom aide? An aide assigned to the kindergarten?" Who, I imagined, would be a local district employee, at Miss Hobbs's and Mr. Lord's expense?

The issue went unsettled. This IEP process always seemed to boil down to matter of resources. Whose resources? Whose ox needed to be gored on Ruffin's behalf?

"Appropriate" and unique was what St. Pat's had to offer Ruffin — without accommodations or any changes to their existing program: a class of 14 kindergarten students, always accompanied by a single teacher, going as a single group to reading, science, art, music, library, lunch, and recess, and graduating as a group into first grade with the same teacher again next year. Ruffin would have his grade-ahead buddy, and that child's mother as his Chapter One reading teacher if he needed her. And, if necessary, early morning latchkey, should I begin my court day three counties west of here, and every afternoon latchkey until suppertime.

All of it, under Seamus's watchful eye, with no skin off anyone's nose.

CHAPTER SEVENTY THREE

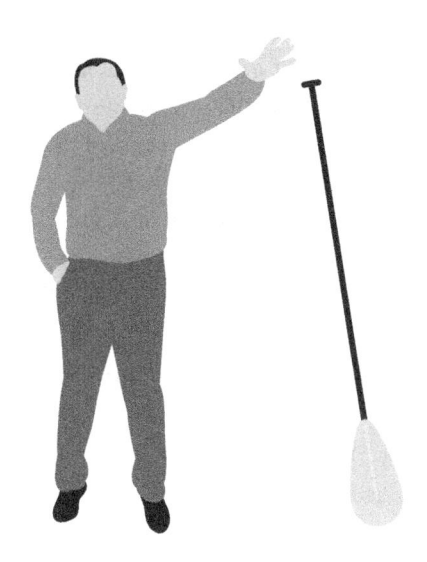

CARD: HOW TO FINISH?

It was still July 1st. Meg moved the meeting's discussion on. "We have some concerns about language." For several minutes Mr. Neidecker, Kim, and Emily dictated suggestions to her for how low their plan for Ruffin might go. Their hopeless, aimless tangle exceeded even my strategic patience. Meg seemed to need help.

I offered, "Everything you want is in the CARD drill books, the books Donna has from Evelyn. The drills Evelyn has written will cover all your language goals." My distant interruptions were not penetrating the ongoing impenetrable discussion. "If you look at Ruffin's deficits which Ms. Wilding identified using the ASSET, those are addressed by the drills that Evelyn has currently assigned for him."

Finally, this penetrated Meg's consciousness.

"Okay, we'll use those drills. The ones we identified in the EYSE amendment early this summer after due process?"

I answered, "Yes. Evelyn was going to send us some further drills if she saw Ruffin making further development."

Meg still had faith in Ruffin as a little engine that could. "If he's already achieved them all, that will be good." And she was relieved now, having completed her role as the scrivener, "Finally, I've got what you all were trying to tell me. We can go ahead."

Not really. We had turned an important corner, but we weren't done yet. I spoke up again. "Dr. Granpeesheh testified at the due process hearing that Ruffin ought to be able to complete his CARD drill program in 9 months' time at most. Counting from May, he should finish by the end of the first semester of kindergarten. And, of course, he needs to finish his current summer language goal."

Meg asked, "Kim, can you read me that summer goal?"

Since Kim had never done anything with it all through last school year, and wasn't working with Ruffin that summer, Mr. Niedecker ventured something lighthearted. "Lisa has it memorized."

Emily thought she could make a joke, too. "Lisa was just waiting for you to call on her."

Lisa offered, politely, "If you like, Meg, you could just copy it?"

Emily could not keep out of it. "Nice charts there, Inge." Emily would be referring to Lisa's genuinely nice, data-rich charts, in several carbon, color-coded copies.

Meg acknowledged them, too, "Lisa got so technical."

That, and she was a hard worker, was why I really liked Lisa. I wanted to say so, since she was young, and new to this terribly jaded group. Probably, it would be the kiss of death. "They're very nice for me," I said. "I get the yellow copy."

Meg summed up then. "For the record, 'Ruffin will be able to carry out a 3-part verbal directive with each part having up to 2 critical elements at 85% accuracy, unmodeled.'" It was the same goal proposed and agreed to for Ruffin nearly a year before.

Emily prompted by asking, "By?"

Meg asked Lisa, "Do you think Ruffin is going to have this skill this summer?"

Lisa answered, "I think so."

Meg went on then, "So, Ruffin ought to be able to generalize this skill by January."

Miss Hobbs was upset by the date though. "These are all January goals. We're going to have to reconvene Ruffin's IEP team again in January."

Sorry, I thought. Once he got going, Ruffin had always been a moving target. No plan made for him so far had survived so long as a semester. But Miss Hobbs measured her students' lives out in yearlong coffee spoons.

Kim did, too, apparently. "Ruffin could make these same goals by the end of next year."

It was "Moe" who stepped in to disagree, to urge the group to consider Ruffin as an individual. "If Ruffin is going to meet all these language goals in January, you may want to get together and say, 'Hey, here he is.'"

Meg seemed unsure. "So, his speech goals run only through January?"

Mr. Neidecker sounded to be firmly in Kim's and Miss Hobbs's camp. "And, if he's met this summer's one language goal by August, you're home free on that one. You can always quit."

I didn't care for the sound of that. "Evelyn says he might complete his full CARD program in 6 months. He might do it in 9 months. But if you can document that Ruffin's mastered all his drills . . ."

Mr. Neidecker interrupted me, "We're done."

I insisted, "Once you've reached the appropriate percentage for mastery."

Inge was curious. "Do we look at Ruffin's CARD drills then as a kind of exit criteria? Mary Jane, as I read your articles, are we looking at decreasing levels of the Lovaas methodology with him?"

"I think what you want to do — if you're going to exit from CARD — is Ruffin needs to complete the full drill program. Then, hopefully, most of these social and language skills that can be addressed by Lovaas's methodology will have been achieved.

"Then, we will be at a point where we are looking at regular autism programming, asking, 'What kind of accommodations does Ruffin need?' He may always need a pocket calendar. Most of us do."

"Moe" stepped in here, "And those are appropriate accommodations."

I continued to lay out my personal vision for Ruffin. "Those are very appropriate accommodations. If Ruffin's really functioning.

"But obviously, I would like to see Evelyn assigning drills and seeing to their completion until she is satisfied. If you look at Ruffin's current drill book, these are all the things he could learn to do which would help him with abstract thinking skills, self-organization, theory of mind skills — all those skills which are foundational to all the school guidance programs for typically developing students, all those skills which are foundational to all other teaching strategies so they will work with him.

"Then, his teachers will have less accommodation to do in the future."

Over the phone, I could make no eye contact, but I sensed: I had convinced "Moe."

It was "Moe" who reached out to take the steering oar. "Are we talking about bringing on a one-to-one trainer to complete Ruffin's remaining drills? This is the time I need to find out whether this is going to happen. We have talked about completing Ruffin's CARD drills on or before January. Who is going to do that?"

Meg moved like the small boat she was. "Yes, we need to assign that. CARD drills are a special education program, not just an accommodation, am I right?"

"Moe" assured her, "CARD drills are a program, right. That program, whether it's done before school, or after school, or during school, is going to get done, and we've got to take the time to do it. This begins to answer your question about the least restrictive environment, and will lead you to consider what Ruffin needs, who is going to do this, for how much time, and where — as we set this CARD drill program up."

Meg's protest evaporated. "Okay, there you go. Obviously, we need to look for a CARD therapist. We know our favorite therapist, Donna, is not available. What do we want to do?"

Miss Hobbs volunteered Meg. "You're trained."

I found that rich. Meg had needed to write a *mea culpa* for having attended our first CARD weekend training two years ago on her own time, on a weekend.

Meg must have found it rich, too. "Yeah, I am trained. It will cost you."

Miss Hobbs tried to make light of that. "Always does."

Mr. Neidecker piled on, "Pay now or pay later."

This was ridiculous. The State of Iowa would be providing over $13,000 a year for ACSD and Bridgewater to educate Ruffin. These agencies had the money they needed to pay for what Ruffin needed.

Miss Hobbs began ruminating on whose personnel would be finishing Ruffin's CARD program, and who would be paying to do it. "Moe" made it clear that he and Bridgewater were willing to put their money where his mouth was and expected Miss Hobbs to do the same. "I would say speech therapy is another issue in and of itself. Speech therapy should be offered to Ruffin in combination with the completion of his CARD program. The two therapies ought to be in support of each other. As I said earlier, if you are offering a general education environment to Ruffin you are also going to want to support him in other ways. We want CARD-taught skills to become an integral part of the total general education classroom environment. We want to know that the things Ruffin learns in his CARD program are also going to be implemented in his classroom, so Ruffin begins to generalize."

"If we provide Ruffin his CARD program after school, and then supplement that a couple of times a week with some small group speech therapy activity, we are likely to get the best result of all. We ought to be able to reconvene in January and say, 'Gee, you know, we really seem to be finished. Ruffin has achieved . . ."

I broke in like a well-raised Southern girl to finish "Moe's" sentence to show that I understood him and agreed. "All these language goals. He's got all this stuff!"

Miss Hobbs was not going to cross swords with "Moe." "Makes sense to me."

Meg asked then, "Are we going to continue speech and language therapy for Ruffin in the fall?"

Despite her recent written recommendation to discontinue Ruffin's speech therapy, Kim was cornered. "As far as I know we can."

The team had been led by "Moe" to some promising conclusions. "Moe" continued to prompt everyone along then, by indicating that he was willing to commit Bridgewater's financial resources to Ruffin. "Why don't we set up two 20-minute speech sessions a week then?"

Meg was writing, dictating to herself, "So, 40 minutes a week."

Kim didn't seem to want any of it. Maybe her feelings were hurt. She had been replaced over the summer since she didn't like to work over the summer. Her answer was short and clipped, "Ask Lisa."

As the newest employee in the Bridgewater group, Lisa didn't want to get in the middle of this. She seemed to want to keep her distance, just get along, and find her own place quietly. "It doesn't make any difference to me."

"Moe" stepped in to settle it. "Write it as two 20-minute sessions."

Meg raised the obvious issue. "Okay, then we need the CARD drills. Who is going to do those?"

Miss Hobbs stepped up, "Well, we're going to."

Not so fast, I thought. Where Ruffin went to kindergarten would be my choice. I hoped to be leaving Kim, Emily, and Miss Hobbs in the dust. Mr. Neidecker didn't sound like fun to me. And, because Ruffin was moving up out of the realm of early childhood programming, Meg and Inge would both be history, and unavailable.

Although trained by Evelyn two years ago, Meg was busy developing her own classroom program, ready to welcome new students. "I'd like to state my position . . ."

I interrupted her before she could bow out. "I would be very happy with Lisa finishing Ruffin's CARD program."

That surprised Miss Hobbs. "Is Lisa interested in doing it though?"

Having Lisa accept this assignment would shift the cost from ACSD back to Bridgewater, since Lisa was a Bridgewater employee. And it would affect Mr. Neidecker's resources in the sector he was responsible for, which flummoxed him. "We could lump the CARD drills together with the speech therapy package, if Mary Jane likes — just lump it all together."

I needed to speak up again. "Lisa could do Ruffin's CARD drills in after school sessions. We need to ask Evelyn what time would be appropriate for Lisa to set aside to get them all done."

"Moe" needed to conserve Lisa as a resource. "Lisa is under a full-time contract. To take her away from other students she will be serving is not appropriate. If she's going to be seeing Ruffin twice a week, I can't assign her to do his CARD training after school."

So, I put it to the group, "Who are you thinking of having do Ruffin's CARD drills after school?"

Miss Hobbs offered some of the people whom Evelyn had trained to serve Ruth's daughter Renee.

I didn't want to poach on Renee's program, so I suggested something else. "I think if what you're offering is CARD drills after school you need to find somebody and have Evelyn train that person."

Then, Miss Hobbs made a swift administrative move to get Ruffin's CARD program out of her bailiwick and her budget. "I'm wondering if this is all under speech, if this is even an ACSD issue . . ."

I was ready to take up her idea — to get rid of her as Ruffin's administrator. "Moe" had proved so much easier to work with over the summer, and during this meeting. So, I agreed with her. "It is speech, and a Bridgewater responsibility. I'm in agreement with you."

"Moe" stepped up and took both administrative and full financial responsibility then. "All we can do is see what we can do to get a hold of somebody who can do Ruffin's CARD program as a part of his speech program and see if Bridgewater can contract for it. I can make the offer of who it is going to be, and that will be either acceptable or not acceptable to you, Mary Jane."

I was pleased, fairly sure that "Moe" and I could make a deal, just as we had for the summer.

CHAPTER SEVENTY FOUR

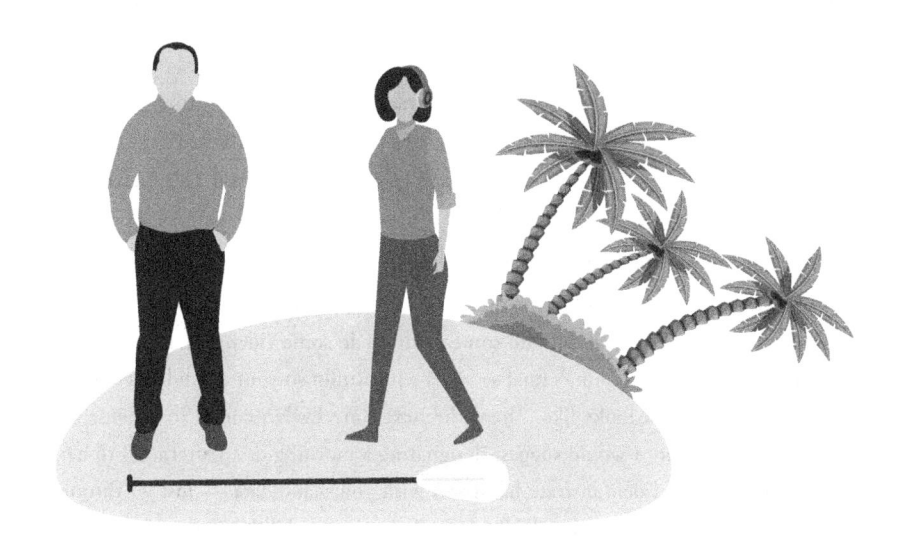

WHO? "MOE" AND ME

Seamus could show up at any time with Ruffin. It was getting late in the afternoon. Then I would need to watch him, attend to him, and keep him busy. Miss Hobbs seemed anxious to be done, too. Meg shuffled her forms to read them out at length. I could be patient enough with my coffee and can of whipped cream, trying to keep my cool.

"Moe" reminded Meg, "The Lovaas drill sessions need to go on the forms."

Meg proposed then, "Let's call it 'One-to-one discrete format training.'" No, no, I thought, "we" would never want to commit the names CARD or Lovaas to paper, not ever. Not even after "we" could all say it, all mouth it in this meeting.

How endlessly silly this was!

It looked like my whipped cream can was just shooting the last of its compressed air. I dropped it as quietly as I could into the garbage. If Seamus did arrive before this meeting was over, I would send him right out again with Ruffin to bring me a fresh can. I told myself: Patience, patience, patience will get you there. Seamus would say, I imagined, "No, I'm not going to bring you more whipped cream. All you need is patience." And leave me with Ruffin . . . Meg broke into my sour reverie. "We don't know the amount of time to offer."

"Moe's" mind was running down another track though. "Can someone give me an idea of how long the person assigned to do this would have to be trained?"

Meg could. "Well, Inge and I were trained with Donna. It was a 2-day session."

I confirmed, "Right."

Meg asked me, "Was it 12 hours?"

I speculated, "We are looking at the end of CARD's full program. Whoever is going to be trained by Evelyn should do some reading, do some video review in advance. We could video some of Donna's final sessions with Ruffin so your candidate could see what this type of work looks like. Then, the next time Evelyn comes to provide services to other children, I would suggest designating a morning or an afternoon to have Evelyn work with and demonstrate hands-on with your candidate — just go through and demonstrate each assigned drill. With Ruffin's present skill level, that ought to be sufficient. You should check that, of course, with Evelyn."

We had wasted the early time Evelyn had been with us, so, now that we'd worked this far through the agenda, it looked to me like we needed to call her back. "Based on Dr. Granpeesheh's testimony at due process, she was anticipating an August to January period. The question your group needs to ask Evelyn is: 'What does that opinion of Dr. Granpeesheh's mean? How many weekly hours of service will get Ruffin finished by January?' Ruffin has 16 hours a week now of direct one-to-one services. What is Dr. Granpeesheh thinking of — specifically. I — we — don't have the answer to that."

So, I thought, we had picked that dropped stitch up on our needles, but nobody knew whether to knit or pearl. The group was stymied, but I couldn't let it go to become an ugly ladder in everybody's pantyhose.

Meg herded us on, continuing to tick down her list. "The next question is: 'Are there potential detriments to the individual if served in a general classroom?' Mary Jane, we stated in our letter to you that we didn't feel there was, and you wrote back and said you didn't think it would harm Ruffin at all to be in a general classroom."

I responded, "Right."

Time to bite the bullet. I wanted to talk about which schoolhouse would offer Ruffin the best environment to succeed in kindergarten.

"I am interested in finding the least restrictive environment. I want to look at St. Pat's as the least restrictive alternative. Looking at our written statement of Ruffin's need for the fewest changes possible of teachers and student groups — at St. Pat's Ruffin would not have *any* changes at all. Reading instruction is not fruit-basket upside down. Science instruction is not fruit-basket upside down. Ruffin would stay with the same student group for every subject of instruction. There is no mixing of the St. Pat's teacher and student groups. If there is any mixing at all — whether at recesses or lunch or anything like that where the two kindergarten classes do activities together — the total kindergarten population at St. Pat's is only 28 students. Ruffin's universe of mixture would be just 28 students.

"I assume from our discussions today that the state Department of Education and Bridgewater are both required to provide Ruffin a free, appropriate public education if I were to choose to place him at St. Pat's — even if what this group offers him might pass legal muster as "appropriate."

"If, for whatever reason, I were to place Ruffin at St. Pat's, Ruffin would still be entitled to speech and language services and discrete trial training and still have the consulting services of Evelyn Kung, right?"

And I knew this was right, based on my earlier legal research that special education services were required to be provided in private and parochial schools for students, like Ruffin, with special needs.

"Moe" responded, speaking for Bridgewater, "We can make no commitments as to what St. Pat's would do as far as providing somebody in the regular education kindergarten classroom to monitor Ruffin, record observations, and collect data. You and I have talked about the fact that Bridgewater can't commit to whether St. Pat's would do that."

On balance, I didn't really care to have Emily or anyone else from Bridgewater monitoring Ruffin or having his classmates twig on to him being watched, or have Emily over at St. Pat's bothering Mrs. Byrnes, or making her uncomfortable about being observed. Emily would make more trouble than she was worth. That's what I thought. That's what my experience of her had been for the last two years. Another good riddance!

Not that I said any of this when speaking back to "Moe."

"I understand. I've talked to St. Pat's about what they can and can't do, and what they can and can't report to me about Ruffin's social skill development.

"But, as I make my decision, I have to wait for this group to present me with a written offer. I must either accept or reject it. If I reject it, if I choose to challenge this group's offer as inappropriate, we will all be back to a reimbursement claim for St. Pat's tuition — to resolve by mediation or litigation as we have done before.

"If I don't want to go to the trouble of challenging this group's offer, if I choose to move ahead and place Ruffin at St. Pat's, in their regular kindergarten with a single teacher and 13 other students, Bridgewater would still have to provide a free, appropriate special education at St. Pat's — at least the speech and language services we all agreed he needs, and the discrete trial training after school."

Then, I turned to Miss Hobbs with a question to clarify what I had heard on the exceptional parent grapevine. "As a point of information, ACSD doesn't have a latchkey program anymore, does it?"

Miss Hobbs admitted, readily enough, working parents be damned, "Not anymore." ACSD's latchkey program had flopped because most local parents depended on grandparents and close relatives for childcare. I, myself, really needed latchkey.

Then, I went back to negotiating directly with "Moe" over the heads of the remaining group.

"Let me ask this question: If we had some discrete trial training after school as we agreed Ruffin needs, is the St. Pat's latchkey program a place where Bridgewater could pull in a couple of typical latchkey peers for a group speech situation? Might there be some latchkey kids who would want to participate?"

"Moe" considered that for a moment. "That's possible."

Once she knew the way the wind was blowing, Emily was ready to go with "Moe's" flow. "Usually, St. Pat's latchkey operates in one classroom with a single teacher and all the children who are staying."

This called for a gulp of cold coffee before I could splutter, "Right, right, right, right. If we need a setting for small group speech and for discrete trial training, I wonder if St. Pat's latchkey program — which is not strictly a parochial school program — just their after-school program — if I can persuade St. Pat's to accommodate you, would Bridgewater have any problem operating in that latchkey environment?"

"Moe's" mind was wrapping itself around the possibility. "Before I commit to that, I need to understand. I thought we were talking about Ruffin needing two 20-minute sessions a week for speech and language services — to be done as pullout during the school day."

Based on my legal research, I asserted, "Yes, and Bridgewater can do that at St. Pat's." "Moe" understood I was referring to the little Chapter One reading trailer parked out back, on the playground. "At the neutral site."

And then, "Moe" just barreled on, "And we were talking about Ruffin needing discrete trial training. If that can be grouped with other latchkey children a couple or three times a week, there are peers who would be part of latchkey and we could work something out. I'm more than willing to sit down and see what we can work out with St. Pat's."

Yes, I thought so, too. We — "Moe" and I — had got there. I didn't say thank you as I should have, but I was able to acknowledge what I had heard. "That helps me understand what would be available to Ruffin."

CHAPTER SEVENTY FIVE

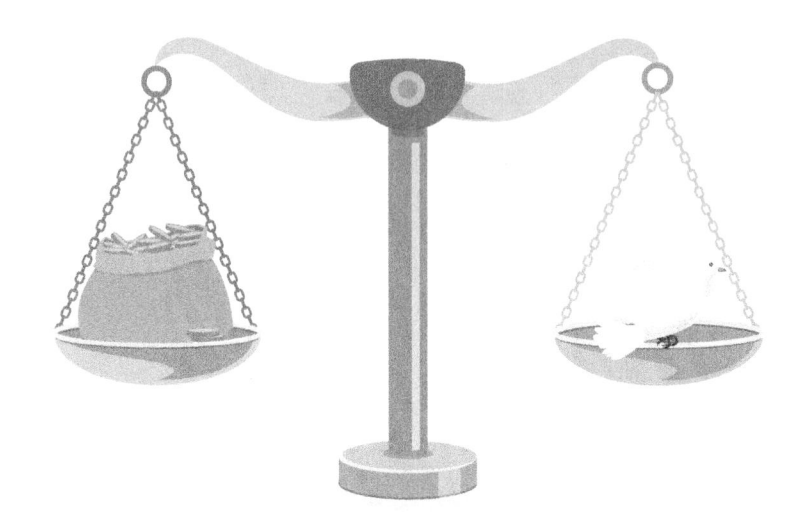

MONEY IS CRUCIAL AND SO IS PEACE

It was Inge who sent us down the rabbit hole of money again. "Maybe we haven't identified a regular education placement. We've identified several accommodations. Do we really have a special educational instructional program here?"

"Moe" answered firmly, "No. Ruffin's program is going to be delivered in a general education setting — in the mainstream with accommodations and strategies *added* so that Ruffin's needs are met."

Inge observed, flatly, "That is level one programming."

"Moe" agreed, "That is level one programming."

I understood this as a reference to how much state money Ruffin would be able to draw down from Des Moines, to pay for all the accommodations and strategies this year's IEP might promise him.

Miss Hobbs understood, too. "Do we need to address Ruffin's weighting?"

Trying to be helpful, I spoke up. "Ruffin is weighted at 3.6 now and I would offer no objections if the group of you wish to continue his weighting at that higher level in order to pay for these longer meetings and all these accommodations and services that we agree he needs."

Mr. Lord understood more than I did about the money. "If you send Ruffin to St. Pat's, we do not get the extra dollars, so Ruffin's weighting would fall to 2.6."

"Moe" shared Mr. Lord's understanding of the money. "That's right, we will not get the extra dollars — if Ruffin goes to St. Pat's."

I was stunned into a simple echo, "You won't get it."

Mr. Lord made it clear, "Nobody."

"Moe" drove home his point to me, "Nobody will get the extra dollars."

It sounded like "Moe" was the administrative expert on this issue. "I don't think you can continue to weight Ruffin's programming at the current 3.74 level. You could weight him more than 1.64. But I would say Ruffin is at level 1 programming."

These weighting numbers were a little different from those that Ray DeNeve had explained to me earlier. They seemed, if anything, to have inched up a little, but I understood they represented the factor to be applied to multiply the allowance of state funds for a typically developing student in regular education.

Miss Hobbs, who sounded disappointed, checked to be sure. "So, 1.68?"

"Moe" affirmed the bad news, "1.68."

Inge continued to press, "Maybe higher because as Mary Jane mentioned, Ruffin may always need some level of accommodation — whether it is a pocket calendar or a calculator or whatever . . ." There must have been a nonverbal signal to Inge, from "Moe," that I missed, because Inge concluded, "So, Ruffin's program will be resourced at only 1.68."

I wasn't about to let the short tail of the money wag the dog here. My sole concern was Ruffin's future. "Please, complete your written offer so I can study it. I will need time to talk it over with the people who help me make decisions for Ruffin."

"Moe" went back to waffle a little as discussion of this issue died. "Ruffin will have a regular class with supplemental assistance. I don't know." So, I didn't know either and wouldn't know until I saw the paperwork on which Ruffin remained weighted at 3.74 — a most fortunate circumstance for his future.

We entered the late afternoon with my request for time triggering some obvious disappointment and impatience. Miss Hobbs, for one, seemed disgusted, and grumbled, "I just have to express I would be a little uncomfortable not finishing now. Ruffin is waiting. It made sense to me when Ruffin went over to the private nursery school last year, and to Sunflower for this summer, but now . . ."

Mr. Lord interrupted whatever unspoken feeling Miss Hobbs was suffering. "When you get done writing that, I want it — so we make sure we've got everything written down there that is supposed to be because I don't want somebody going halfway home and finding we forgot something. I want to go in the other room, make 15 copies of it and pass it out to everybody."

Everybody was everybody but me. But I didn't care. I didn't care. This was not about my hurting their feelings. This wasn't about *them*. This was about Ruffin, and, yes, for me, it was *personal*.

Mr. Lord thundered on incoherently, "Best of your recollection." Then he made another announcement. "I just received correspondence from Evelyn Kung as I went in to call her to ask if she could visit with us again at a quarter to four, so I made everyone a copy."

We took a quick late-afternoon break to review Evelyn's fax, putting her earlier recommendations into writing for whomever might be involved with Ruffin next year.

Meg continued moving through her set of written forms, taking down the last of the legalities lightheartedly, since we were getting close to the end. "I'm going to invite you to all my IEP meetings, 'Moe.' These are the pages I always have the most trouble writing."

"Moe" assured her, since Ruffin was not yet 14-years-old, "You will not need to plan for his vocational experience yet."

No, I thought to myself, not now and not later. I envisioned Ruffin graduating and heading off to college — like most students with his measured IQ and parents who expected it of him.

Meg finally asked me, "Mary Jane, did you get a copy yet of what I have written?"

I answered from my end of the phone, "I don't think so. Do you want to take another little break while you fax it to me? And, let me just summarize what I will be expecting," I said, as I rattled off a long list.

Meg assured me she had everything in order. "Right."

I checked, "Does the school have a copy of Ruffin's current CARD drill book?"

"Moe" answered me, "Discrete trial training is found on page 11."

Meg continued reading what she had written there, "As defined by CARD."

"Moe" and Meg rechecked, saying back and forth to each other, "Got it."

Yes, I thought, the district and Bridgewater both "got it." A Pyrrhic victory at this late date in Ruffin's special education.

Finally, Meg wanted to be sure all the lawyers still attending were satisfied. "Mr. Carew, did we answer all your questions?"

Mr. Carew would not be drawn into putting his cards on the table where I could hear about them. He kept them close to his vest. "I've talked to Mr. Mosher about my questions."

"Caron, did you have anything?" Meg asked and must have gotten a negative head shake. "Mary Jane, did you have anything?"

I was curious about Mr. Carew's hidden hand. "No, I guess I can talk briefly to Mr. Carew after we are done."

Meg seemed pleased. "Okay, that will give me a chance to write up a transition report."

Besides running the copy machine, Mr. Lord had succeeded in his efforts to get Evelyn back on the phone.

Evelyn asked cheerfully, "How is everybody?"

"Moe" answered wearily since we were late in the day. "Just wonderful."

I went right to the point. "Evelyn, can you tell us — Dr. Granpeesheh testified at the due process hearing that if Ruffin were to complete his entire CARD drill assignment that might take 6 to 9 months from May of 1996. I don't know what she was basing that estimate on — as far as how many hours per week of one-to-one discrete trial training would be required?"

Evelyn worked for Dr. Granpeesheh, but she wasn't Dr. Granpeesheh, and couldn't really be sure. I let Evelyn know what had been going on in our meeting during her absence. "Bridgewater has committed to do some after-school discrete trial sessions to finish off Ruffin's theory of mind and organizational skills."

Evelyn seemed pleased. "Good."

I also let Evelyn know, "We have an after-school program at St. Pat's that might be the setting for this."

"Moe" let Evelyn know, "We're looking for a recommendation so we can proceed to hire somebody."

Evelyn wanted to defer to Dr. Granpeesheh and suggested, "Dr. Granpeesheh will be in later today. I can talk to her and see what her recommendation for Ruffin is. She has looked at everything we have about Ruffin, so when she gets back, I can talk to her. That's not a problem."

I thought Evelyn ought to know that whoever "Moe" might hire might need training. "Since we know that Donna is not going to be available after August, one of the things we've been talking about, is whether the next time you come to Iowa to work with some of the other children you could train another Bridgewater employee to finish off Ruffin's discrete trial program."

Evelyn understood. "Yes, no problem."

I had another question to ask for "Moe's" benefit. "And how much of a training session would that new person require? Assuming the new person does some reading, looks at some videotapes, and visits with Donna before you arrive here — would you need more than a morning or an afternoon?"

Evelyn was surer about this answer, which fell more closely within her responsibilities. "A morning or afternoon session would work, especially if the new person has done some reading, watched some tapes, and talked to Donna. I could visit with your new person for a few hours to go through the specifics of exactly what to do and go through all the assigned drills so the new person could see how each works. A morning or an afternoon session would be enough."

"Moe" seemed pleased with that. "Okay."

Evelyn did too. "No problem at all."

Of course, I needed a record. I had to ask, even in this atmosphere of good feeling, "We'd appreciate a written recommendation from you and Dr. Granpeesheh. I think the school might feel more comfortable having that."

Mr. Lord instructed, "Fax it to me right away."

"Moe" was willing to take a back seat. "Evelyn, if you would fax that out to Bill, Bill will get it out to all of us." I remembered Bill was Mr. Lord's given name.

Evelyn responded evenly, "Okay, that's fine. I'll make a recommendation for the number of discrete trial services for Ruffin."

"Moe" let her know, too, "We're thinking about completing his full CARD program between now and January."

Evelyn took that in evenly too. "Okay. I'll talk to Dr. Granpeesheh about that."

"Moe" seemed pleased. "Great."

Evelyn checked again, "Is that good?"

"Moe" replied, "That's good. Thanks, Evelyn."

I let her know I was pleased, too, and that she was really free to go.

It was four o'clock. I couldn't expect Seamus to keep Ruffin much longer. But Mr. Carew had a procedural question. "'Moe,' if Evelyn is going to fax that, are you willing to meet whatever recommendation she makes? And does Mary Jane want to call the IEP team together again to discuss the recommendation?"

I thought it would be fair to offer a legal shortcut. "As long as the recommendations that Evelyn's made arrive and Bridgewater is willing to meet them, I can make a knowing and intelligent waiver of calling everybody back together again. Does that help you, Mr. Carew?"

Mr. Carew chirped back, quickly enough, "Yes, it does."

I would leave it to Mr. Carew to explain our little dance with each other. There was no need for any legal amendment, but Meg was worried. "What do you want me to write about that?"

"Moe" replied, "I would just say: 'See recommendations forthcoming.'"

Emily couldn't follow our little dance, either, but she wasn't worried. As always, she had the answer. "And the amendment will be made once the letter from Evelyn arrives."

"Moe" seemed to be getting irritated with Emily, too. "No, as soon as Evelyn's letter comes, I want to get it."

Then "Moe" asked me, "Lisa needs to know where Ruffin is going to go. My question is, and Mary Jane, I don't want to tie you down, but I need to know. How soon are you thinking about getting back to us so all the people here know whether you are going to take the offer we will make for a free, appropriate public education or whether you are going to take Ruffin to St. Pat's?"

I answered, but I didn't want to be hasty. Would I reject their offer, place Ruffin, and sue for reimbursement? Or was St. Pat's $710 of annual tuition small potatoes, a game not worth the candle — particularly if "Moe" was ready to see that Bridgewater did its part? I needed time to think. "I would like to have 10 business days."

Meg seemed relieved. "Can I tear this now, take it apart into copies for the file? Are we done?

"Moe" had the last words then, "Oh, yeah."

It had taken all day. Oh, yeah.

At home, I turned to Ruffin's travelling notebook to write to Donna and Angie, who had both left our marathon meeting at noon. "ACSD offered a 15-child classroom with adaptations and Bridgewater offered CARD drills after school and 40 minutes per week of speech and language therapy.

"Donna, you were complimented in your absence as 'our Lovaas therapist.'

"Angie, you must have been impressive. The superintendent, Mr. Lord, asked if you were graduating and would be available in the fall.

"If you two are *not* paid for Monday morning by Mr. Lord, please let me know."

Seamus dropped Ruffin off in a great hurry. There was some swelling under Ruffin's right eye — a fall? Neither Seamus nor Ruffin gave any report of what, if anything, might have happened.

The next morning, like a little pony, Ruffin went back to his steady trot of summer learning with Donna, Angie, Lisa, Seamus, and me, all putting him through his paces. After just a 3-day break, it proved a bit difficult to get him headed back in the right direction, even under Donna's determined guidance. Angie had better luck after Donna got him going.

Meanwhile, Dr. Granpeesheh responded to Mr. Lord, who quickly shared her fax with "Moe," and me. "Based on Ruffin White's progress in his current program, I recommend that Ruffin receive 6 to 10 hours per week of one-to-one discrete trial therapy to assist him in his integration into a regular kindergarten class in the fall of 1996. These hours should occur outside of the classroom hours and should focus on helping him to adjust to his new classroom setting as well as to work on any deficits that he may still possess in his overall functioning."

Lisa Shelton, M.A., SLP, the new Bridgewater employee, who had begun working with Ruffin on that final pesky IEP goal turned in her trial-by-trial data each day using a simple + or – for each trial's result and noting with a superscript c whether Ruffin had required a cue, and then calculating Ruffin's daily percentages. That day she charted 10 trials at 80%. Her reports also began to carry anecdotal comments. "We spent time talking about the pictures and the fact that we are working to learn his friends' names. He was able to name six children from his first look at their photographs. Wow! I'll send their photographs home so you may use them. Please put them back in his bag daily."

Here was enthusiasm, to which I offered reinforcement. "Very encouraged by the name game, the photographs of his classmates (the visual helps us know what he really knows and should be using). I am so pleased to see more progress on multi-step commands."

As soon as Ruffin got home, he crawled on the couch for few minutes — rested, snacked, and then JJ appeared at our front door. They played in the neighborhood with all the children in the corner house — several little girls, 3 to 6 years old. They played "spies" and "hide and seek" and "rescue 911" and "sending you to jail."

JJ persuaded Ruffin to try ravioli for supper, and he was keen to teach Ruffin more words. "Rescue is just another word for help. They mean the same." Ruffin was very impressed with the fact that two different words could mean the same.

On July 7th, I informed St. Pat's principal Peter Smith, Mr. Lord, and "Moe," "Ruffin will attend St. Patrick's lower grade school next year for his regular education placement in the mainstream. I understand that Bridgewater will meet CARD's recommendation for 10 hours per week of Lovaas programming after school and provide Lisa Shelton's services as a speech and language pathologist for 40 minutes per week. My understanding is that the public-school authorities will pay any fees charged by CARD for their services for the 1996-1997 school year. Enclosed is my check to St. Patrick's in the amount of $710 for Ruffin's tuition."

It was a good compromise — better than the shotgun marriage I had made last year. I needed Ruffin to be in a safe place with a small class with what Evelyn and Dr. Granpeesheh recommended for him — a stable unchanging group. I needed the flexibility of latchkey so I could return to full-time work. Suing ACSD for $710 reimbursement of yearly tuition was not a rational choice. In my world, it was half the retainer I charged to begin a divorce — just the small price of peace, of knowing Ruffin's needs would be met without fuss by a group of educators who were prepared to welcome us, and whom Ruffin was prepared to meet.

CHAPTER SEVENTY SIX

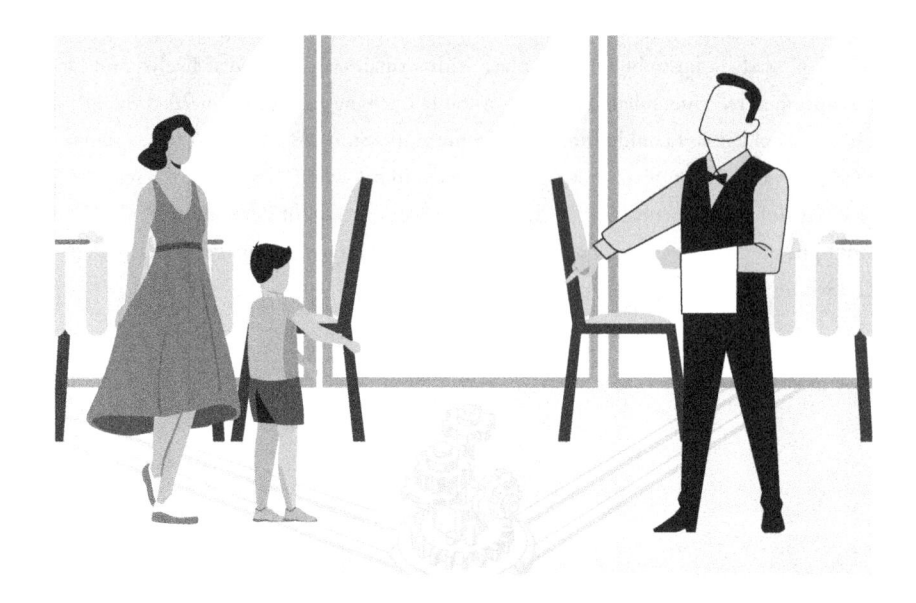

HERE, ABOVE THE WORLD

Ruffin and I travelled to Milwaukee as planned. Since Ruffin was of kindergarten age, he would be able to join several field trips to nearby parks with swimming, fishing, and crafts, and tour the Milwaukee County Zoo, the Discovery World Museum, and Circus World with an arranged one- to two-adult to child-with-autism group. That sounded like fun for him and offered me a chance to see what was going on with Bernie and Ivar's 1960s baby — the nationwide Autism Society of America.

The second anniversary of Ruffin's autism diagnosis passed quietly while we were there. We would miss the local CARIN' meeting to plan the installation of adaptive physical education equipment at our public schools and parks, but I let Ruth know that I would be happy to report back anything of value we might learn in Milwaukee. We would be back in time to help install the equipment.

Whenever the offerings at the conference seemed irrelevant to Ruffin's and my personal situation, he and I stationed ourselves behind a small exhibit table, with a video screen playing clips of Ruffin's treatment program as it had played out over the last two years. We had copies of Curt and Joan's booklet on offer. Many visitors to our table recognized its comb-bound spine and plain grey and black cover and stopped to introduce themselves. Most were parents. A few were teachers. Ruffin exhibited his own patience, good behavior, friendliness, and technological savvy by operating the video, obviously enough, starring all the earlier versions of himself.

We continued to run into all sorts of people, both the helpful and the unhelpful, the pleased and the skeptical — including Ms. Wilding, Ruffin's speech and language pathologist from UIHC, and Dr. Byrna Siegel, soon to surface as one of Dr. Lovaas's courtroom adversaries.

One night after one of our table-visitors suggested it, we made our way up to the revolving restaurant on the top floor of the hotel with its panoramic view of the city. Seated at the very edge of the glass-walled rotating floor, Ruffin was fascinated. Our server was captivated by Ruffin's questions and escorted us both to inspect the responsible machinery at the center of the floor. We were clearly past the earlier episodes of Ruffin's poor public behavior that had led me to pay for but abandon a hot meal uneaten. Here, above the world, I could be proud of Ruffin's competence, his questions, and his surprising and burgeoning charm.

Back home, Donna was able to take a well-earned, first family vacation since the fall of 1994. Angie substituted in. "I was writing the date on this paper, when I messed up and said, 'Oh, today is Monday, July 15th, 1996.' Ruffin remarked, 'The fireworks will come again.' I asked, 'When will they come again?' Ruffin: 'July, I think.'

"We talked about Milwaukee. Ruffin: 'I can't remember what I did.' Then, he brought out a black tiger from his backpack. 'I got it from a machine outside that maked it.'

"When I asked, 'Did you eat dinner anywhere special, in a tall building? See the city?' Ruffin replied, 'I did, and the floor goes round and round.'

"Break time: Five minutes. Ruffin: 'I hope five lasts long.' On Sunflower's playground, Ruffin wasn't scared of anything. I talked about his being scared of the water. Ruffin said he had figured out a way to do bubbles. 'Put air in your cheeks.'

"There was a tic-tac-toe board on the playground, so we played. He did an excellent job! He really understood it because he kept 'blocking' me.

"After break, he hid the Play-Doh, 'tricking me.' Today's teacher asked, 'What's behind your back?' Ruffin: 'Nothing.' The teacher smiled, 'You're lying.' Ruffin smiled back. Later, I was laughing, so Ruffin did, too, and asked what I was laughing at. I said it was good to laugh. Ruffin: 'Not all the time. It is not good to laugh at someone.'

"Ruffin was talking about the breeze. Ruffin: 'There is hundreds of breeze in the shade and no breeze in the sun.'

"Ruffin got a drink — did great — got his nose wet and didn't seem bothered by it.

"A man was jogging by, and I told him I jog every day. He asked why. I said to stay in shape, healthy and strong. Then we talked about muscles, blood, and bone. Ruffin: 'Red takes it away and then blue takes it back.' This was about our blood.

Ruffin: 'Do you know how metal melts?' He sure seemed fascinated by all the wonders of the world."

By mid-July Ruffin began to enjoy swimming and calling Angie's name to get her attention. In the park, "a boy was crying. Ruffin: 'Who is that crying? Someone is afraid of the slide. Maybe it is a little too high or maybe he doesn't like slides.' Ruffin was probably right."

At Sunflower, "he seemed to prefer to play with the kids rather than by himself and this is behavior that I don't always see. A little girl left for the day and was giving everyone a hug and Ruffin approached her and gave her a hug. This was a sign of affection that I have *never* seen from Ruffin.

"Ruffin made a paper double scoop ice cream cone with his favorite flavors. The teacher demonstrated the activity first. Ruffin did a nice job — this activity seemed not too difficult for him even with all the directions given at once — he was able to follow them.

"Maid Rites for lunch. Ruffin 'tattled' on someone for not trying their food — I've never seen him do this before. He usually worries about himself. At lunch Ruffin was talking with the other kids who were sitting near him. At snack he doesn't usually talk, but he does seem to be talking a lot more. He just seemed more socially aware today."

Ruffin and Seamus spent most of the day Sunday helping me clean my new downtown office building. We washed the windows, and then Ruffin played quietly with his new space shuttle Legos.

Ruffin's sense of time continued to improve slowly. He and Angie "played a snowman game: 'Can you make a snowman in the summer?' Ruffin: 'Winter.' I asked, 'What else happens in the winter?' Ruffin: 'Snow falls, people play with coats and mittens and snow pants and boots.' I asked, 'Anything else?' Ruffin: 'Trees die and plants.' I asked, 'Who comes to visit in the winter?' Ruffin: 'Santa! When it's dark.' I asked, 'Can you tell me about Santa?' Ruffin: 'Long, long beard, round curly beard, He's fat. He has toys — if people are good. And red clothes.' I asked, 'Does he drive a truck?' Ruffin: 'He flies on a magic sled with deers.' I asked, 'Who leads the deer?' Ruffin: 'I don't know.' I asked, 'Have you heard of Rudolph?' Ruffin: 'No.' Then, I sang him *Rudolph the Red-Nosed Reindeer.*"

Later, at Sunflower, there was "Origami. Visiting Japanese students taught this activity. First, they shared their names which were a little different. They spoke extraordinarily little English which made this challenging. Ruffin did an exceptionally good job of imitating what his partner had folded and liked this activity."

At Sunflower, "Ruffin played with two girls from Louisiana. He told them his grandma lived near them. She lived near a mountain. He told them to stay for a long time so he would have friends to play with."

While Ruffin was busy, I followed up with "Moe," who was looking for an employee to do Ruffin's one-to-one CARD drills at St. Pat's latchkey next fall. He agreed Donna could train that employee, and that Evelyn would be available to consult since she would be coming back to continue to see Renee, Ruth's daughter. He would like Donna, Evelyn, and me to continue to work with his southern sector coordinator, Ray DeNeve, too.

That evening, I put a copy of *Let Me Hear Your Voice* in Ruffin's book bag for Lisa to read. She replied quickly. "Mary Jane, that was a great book! Thanks for loaning it to me. I'm ready for more information to read. On 8 trials of 3-part verbal directives Ruffin is perfect, and on 8 trials with all the directions given in advance, Ruffin is 88%. His recall of friends' names was 82%."

On July 26th, a Friday, Angie took Ruffin out to Dunning's Spring, a small forest park with a high and wide waterfall outside Decorah on the banks of the Upper Iowa River, just a short walk from Luther College. It became one of Ruffin's favorite places to visit in summer, with the cool air pouring off the water. It was likely a place Dr. Lovaas would have visited many times years ago when he had been an exchange student from Norway at Luther just after the Second World War.

"Donna's Notes: Ruffin talked about what he had been doing while I was gone. He was genuinely happy to see me and to spend the morning with me. I felt the same way toward Ruffin. He recalled his trip to Milwaukee after he asked me a question about what I had been doing.

"We talked about time sequences. I asked questions that covered past, present, and future tense and although his language was not shaped correctly, Ruffin was able to get close enough, I understood what he seemed to be thinking. I offered him Meg's term 'sleeps' for time. He understood this and made a comment, 'That's all it is?'

"We read the book *Don't Look Back*, covering theory of mind 1. making decisions; 2. solutions; 3. fear; 4. defeat; 5. courage; 6. letting go to move on; and 7. excitement with a new adventure. Ruffin gave me a real-life story for each.

The end of July, Donna had an appointment. No big deal, Ruffin could stay home or at the office with me. Now, he was so easy to care for, able to say what he might need or want, busying himself on his computer, inviting me or my new legal assistant Robin over to see what he was doing, or what he might have done.

I was flush with happiness that summer, having announced my decision that Ruffin would attend St. Pat's. Ruffin was thriving. I was caught up in the work of remodeling my new office and busier than ever with Robin's help, planning to rent a couple of the back rooms to Ruth when she opened her accounting business there after graduation. She, Robin, and I would keep a room there of special education resources for exceptional parents to visit, and as a place for us to meet and strategize.

"Angie's Notes: I think Ruffin may be tired of working with all his adults. Interacting with the kids is not such a chore anymore. He prefers to be with the other kids now. It was time to get dressed after swimming and Ruffin would *not* go. He would not listen to me. He jumped into the pool again and finally stepped out when I warned him I was going to write his mom a note. It was good that he wanted to stay here with his friends, but usually he does a better job of listening. Although most of the kids don't listen either, so I guess that was normal."

By early August, Evelyn prepared a new 29-page drill book for Ruffin. Donna and I met to go over it while Ruffin occupied himself. He was able to play quietly and productively while we made plans and assembled new teaching materials.

"Angie's Notes: All of a sudden Ruffin came over to me and said, 'Do you know what? My grandma has a pool, and it is deep.' I said, 'So, you need to learn to swim.' Ruffin: 'Yah!'"

I followed up again with "Moe" asking whether Ruffin's latchkey aide for St. Pat's had been hired. A couple of days later, Mr. Neidecker called to tell me that Lisa Shelton had been assigned to do CARD drills with Ruffin for the fall semester. I told him about CARD's most recent drill book update. He agreed to contact Donna to make financial arrangements about training Lisa.

St. Pat's had mailed out their school supply list. It was a treasure hunt to go the local five-and-dime on Main Street to buy the kindergarten box of 8 regular crayons, 5 number 2 pencils, a long box of Kleenex, Elmer's glue, plastic safety scissors, a rest-mat, a blank cassette tape and then walk back to my office to pull all Ruffin's pre-school health and immunization records. Finally, we washed out a 5-quart ice cream bucket and arranged everything in it for easy carrying.

St. Pat's also sent their Parent and Student Handbook. Their latchkey program would run from after school to 6:00 in the evening, a full three hours after school — plenty of time for Ruffin to work on Evelyn's assignments.

The philosophy of the little school was expressed:

STUDENTS ARE:

The most important people in our business.

Not dependent on us; we are dependent on them.

Not an interruption in our work, but the purpose for it.

Not cold statistics, but flesh and blood human beings with feelings and emotions like our own.

Not the ones to argue or match wits with.

People who bring us their needs, and it is our job to fill those needs.

Deserving of the most courteous and attentive treatment we can give them.

The lifeblood of this and every other institution.

In mid-August, Angie sent me a personal note. "Professor Bishop invited me to meet O. Ivar Lovaas at the end of the month. I'm pretty excited!"

Then, she went on to report, "Kay asked if Ruffin wanted to swim. Ruffin said, 'No.' Then after three of the other children went to change clothes, Ruffin came to me and said, 'Changed my mind.' Then he raced off to find the other children."

"Angie's Notes: Ruffin was talking more today. He asked Kay who the line leader was. By asking that question, Ruffin got to be the door holder. He liked being a helper. Everyone gave Kay a group hug and Ruffin was one of the first to join in."

By late August, Ruffin was at home with me on a Wednesday when Lisa Shelton sent me her final charting for the summer. "Here is a quick summary of Ruffin's summer sessions. It's clear the 3-part verbal directive with each part having up to 2 critical elements is very difficult for him. He's just beginning to reach 80% accuracy in his final two sessions, against his goal of 85%. His recall of friends' names is up to the high 80% to low 90%, but, of course, now he's going to have a classroom of new friends."

Fortunately, St. Pat's had let me know there would be only 13 students in Ruffin's new kindergarten class with Mrs. Byrnes. The other kindergarten class with Mrs. Kelly would only have 13 students, too. So, St. Pat's would be a total kindergarten universe of 26 students.

Principal Peter Smith assured me that his plan was to keep these classes together next year for first grade, and that his two teachers would move up to first grade next year to continue teaching each of their groups. The only other teachers Ruffin would encounter were Mr. Christopher the physical education and computer teacher, Mrs. Kamm the librarian, and Mrs. Ryan the music teacher. He would need to get to know Mr. Smith, and Mrs. Mahoney, the school secretary. A small, stable universe, as Dr. Granpeesheh and Evelyn had recommended.

For the moment, I had Ruffin to myself. Angie was off to graduate school and Donna was shopping for school supplies for her own children. The Autism Behavior Therapy Alliance would be holding a conference in Minneapolis — a three-hour drive north — with O. Ivar Lovaas and Catherine Maurice both speaking. I was invited, but couldn't go, because that Monday was Ruffin's first day of kindergarten.

It would be Seamus's first day back at the school where he had graduated, too. I could step back from my role as Ruffin's advocate. I didn't think Ruffin would need much advocacy from me this year, at least not with anyone at St. Pat's. The school was such a good fit, and everyone there seemed to be quietly on board. But, having Seamus there, daily, working during the latchkey hours, would give me an eye on how Ruffin was doing and managing without my having to ask bothersome questions of anyone but him.

Fall, my favorite season, came early as it always did in Iowa. I was looking forward to the beginning of school as if I were a small girl returning myself. Ruffin was looking forward to Fridays of show and tell, to morning milk, to afternoon milk on Mass days, snacks from home of fruit, veggies, and cheese crackers. Together, after school, we hung his monthly activity calendar on the refrigerator, so we could remember the color assigned to each of the upcoming days through August and September, beginning with August 29th, as a sunny "yellow day."

I was hopeful that this school year would be easier, since I would only need to work with Bridgewater on the aspects of Ruffin's education that remained "special." With Donna's support, Lisa Shelton began her work with Ruffin in St. Pat's latchkey, providing notes of her work, which were always cleanly clinical and data-driven, drill by numbered drill.

Mr. Neidecker let me know when Evelyn would be coming back to Iowa to spend two-and-a-half hours in the afternoon with Ruffin at St. Pat's and meet with me later that evening. "I would also like to ask your permission for Lisa Shelton to contact Ms. Wilding regarding suggestions for speech and language programming for Ruffin. We will continue to make a good faith effort to meet the CARD recommendation of 6 to 10 hours a week of Lovaas training. As we discussed, however, there will be times when Lisa may need to take sick leave, attend an IEP meeting, or go to an in-service."

I had to reply to him, sternly. "You are not authorized to have Lisa Shelton contact Ms. Wilding. Ms. Wilding has performed a valuable service for Ruffin by exquisitely documenting the success of a method she does not and will not endorse. We have already agreed in Ruffin's IEP that Lovaas is the programming methodology appropriate for him. It is supported by empirical data. Other independent researchers have replicated it widely now. Most importantly, it has been individually replicated with Ruffin. See, for example, the Gundersen reports from the fall of 1995.

"If Lovaas is not broke for Ruffin, why experiment with fixing it? I am unwilling to consent to do so.

"Over the last two years, both Gundersen and Mayo have changed their practice with respect to recommending Lovaas as a method for use with preschool children with autism, and now advise parents about it, provide photocopies of literature from Dr. Lovaas's UCLA Clinic and generally are willing to support parents' requests for insurance, Medicaid, and school district funding. Despite repeated opportunities to review the present medical standard of care, UIHC continues to refuse to do so. As recently as our conversations at the summer Autism Society of America conference in Milwaukee, Ms. Wilding has made it clear that she and I continue to disagree about Lovaas.

"In his cumulative file, Lisa Shelton has access to all Ms. Wilding's previous written evaluations of Ruffin, but as Meg Holub cautioned in her testimony at our recent due process hearing, any evaluation or recommendation concerning Ruffin that is more than a few months old is out-of-date, due to his established pattern of continuing developmental progress.

"Ms. Wilding's last evaluation of Ruffin in April of 1996 is obsolete. Since that time, Ruffin has made a good adjustment to his St. Pat's classroom. His worksheets come home correct and complete, and he claims and names four friends. He is showing good progress in math skills — adding, subtracting, and using simple fractions in his home computer work with Edmark's *Mighty Math Carnival Countdown* and The

Learning Company's *Interactive Math Journey*. He is recalling past events, planning future events, and holding extended conversations on topic, showing, and expressing theory of mind, albeit still somewhat mechanically — these skills are currently targeted in his CARD drills — and following simple 3-step commands without getting lost in the process.

"As you know, Lisa Shelton worked with Ruffin 90 minutes per week all summer long on a single, neglected 1995-1996 speech and language objective of following simple, 3-step commands, moving Ruffin from 14% success to 85% success. This is the equivalent of the mastery of a *single* CARD drill task.

"Enclosed please find Evelyn's latest 29-page programming outline for Ruffin. As you will see, Ruffin and Lisa Shelton have a great deal to tackle before January of 1997.

"After our July IEP meeting, Mr. Mosher called to let me know that Lisa Shelton would be made available to take Ruffin's CARD assignment. I was delighted that she was so assigned, and that her other IEP meetings and in-services were not going to present a problem. I have a contemporaneous record of this conversation.

"Given my sources of information in the community, I understand that, based on the number of children requiring services and their special needs, Bridgewater's plans were to hire three speech and language pathologists to serve us here — Kim Pope, Lisa Shelton, and one more — but that only two were actually hired, and the work of three speech and language pathologists was then assigned to the two of them.

"From those same sources, I understand that if Lisa Shelton were to attend other IEP meetings and in-services, she would have one or the other such conflicting commitments every Monday and Friday. Effectively, this would cut Ruffin's scheduled services to 6 hours per week at most, and thus, far less in practice — accounting for snow days, holidays, and illnesses. This is not acceptable to me.

"Whether my sources are correctly informed or not, Ruffin's needs according to his IEP have not changed. Ruffin's IEP has not changed. Until I am comfortable agreeing to any changes, I continue to rely on Mr. Mosher's agreements with me as to how and who will implement Bridgewater's obligations to Ruffin under his IEP. Lisa Shelton has now trained with Donna Schmidt for a week to be able to provide his CARD program.

"May I suggest that Bridgewater hire and train an appropriate person to be available as a substitute for days that Lisa Shelton is ill. I understand that Donna Schmidt may have identified an appropriate person, but, of course, you would need to get her hired and train her.

"Once such a person has been identified, hired, and trained and has demonstrated her proficiency in teaching and charting to Donna Schmidt, Lisa Shelton, Evelyn

Kung, and myself, I would be willing to consider having her substitute for Lisa on any Mondays and Fridays she might need to be free to attend an IEP meeting or in-service, provided that all her other absences are covered.

"I trust you understand where I am coming from — you may not change programming without a properly-noticed IEP meeting or solve administrative difficulties Bridgewater has known about since early July at Ruffin's expense. I hope the suggestion I've set out in this letter will assist you in finding a workable solution to what remains your staffing problem."

For the time being, Lisa Shelton continued to show up to work with Ruffin during latchkey.

CHAPTER SEVENTY SEVEN

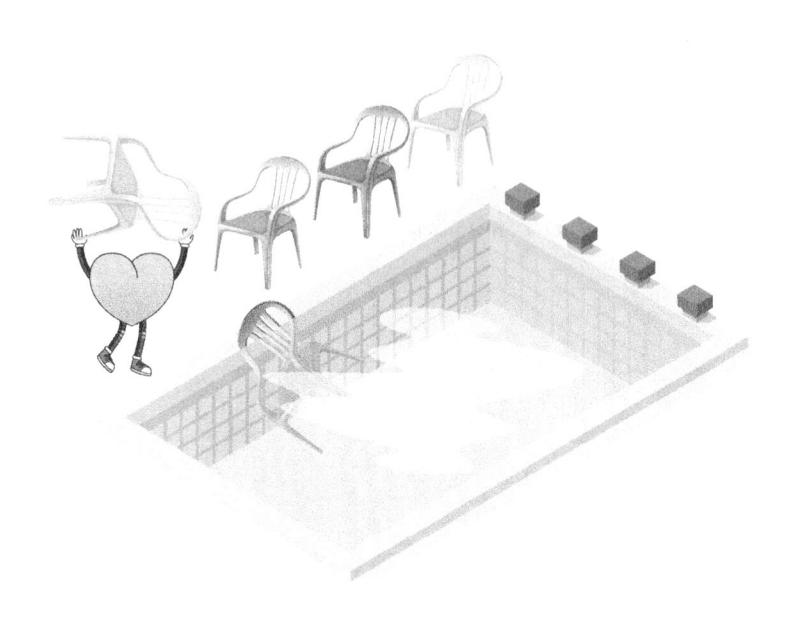

A HEART MAKES CHAIRS SWIM

"Lisa Shelton's CARD Latchkey Notes: Ruffin initiated conversation 7 times. He recounted a huge portion of recess, including his feelings and a portion of his school day, saying, 'I wish . . .' He also asked 5 questions.

1. Names today, yesterday, and tomorrow and the month (with visual cues) 3 out of 4 trials, 75%. He missed today's month of September.
2. Sound and letter recognition, perfect.
3. Address, phone, parents' names: needed an auditory cue for address and phone.
4. Rhyming words: 10 out of 10 trials. If I gave 2 words that didn't rhyme, Ruffin came up with words that would rhyme with each.

5. Staying on a topic: Our topic was cars. Ruffin stayed on topic for 3 minutes during the conversation. Ruffin asked 1 question during that time.
6. Analogies: 9 out of 10 trials, 90%.
7. How do you know? 'When is it time to go to bed?' Ruffin: "Cause it will be dark.' 'When is it time to eat?' Ruffin: 'When Rose comes.' And with a cue, 'When I'm hungry.' 'When is it time to take a bath?' Ruffin: 'When my body is dirty.'
8. See something incredible: Ruffin: 'I see a tree growing on a car.' 'I see a bulb making rain.' 'I see a tree upside down.' 'I see a kitten flying.' 'I see a big, huge giant fan blowing people away.'
9. What's missing (used 3 pictures): 5 out of 6 trials, 83%.
10. Counting Objects (tactile stimulation): Ruffin went to 43, with cues needed for 28, and 30.
11. Rote Counting (visual cue): Ruffin went to 100, but needed cue for 40, 45, and 75.
12. Months: Ruffin went through all 12 months perfectly, with only visual cues."

It seemed to me Ruffin and Lisa were doing well. I missed Ruffin's and my Wednesdays together, but I could see Ruffin was on a roll again at school and after school in latchkey.

In mid-September, Ruth asked me to attend Renee's newest IEP meeting. She had spoken with Mr. Neidecker about having Lisa Shelton work with Renee. He had told her, 'We're going to get a substitute for Lisa within the next week, a permanent substitute." I appreciated Ruth's call. It was important that she and I stay in touch about our children — so we would not be played against each other, given the scarce resources of Lisa, Donna, and other trained personnel.

That Friday, a letter arrived from Mr. Neidecker. "Our plan would be to employ Donna Schmidt to train Wendy Norton as Lisa's substitute and to phase her in under Lisa's supervision." This was followed by a detailed schedule. "Be assured we plan to provide services as set forth by the current IEP and recommendations as set forth by CARD until January 1997 and then future needs will be considered. We are pleased that Ruffin has made such a good adjustment to his St. Pat's classroom, and we look forward to continuing to serve him in accordance with the IEP." A sensible and acceptable answer.

On balance, I felt that the more individual people, therapists, and teachers that Ruffin could relate to, the better. Although Anne Sullivan had been an early inspiration, I didn't want Ruffin to become a life-long dependent on Donna as Helen Keller had been upon her companion and teacher. My goal was an independent life for Ruffin — for him to move freely among others, for him to be able to learn from anyone and on his own — wherever he might choose to run loose in the universe.

Except for Lisa Shelton's latchkey notes, it was possible by mid-September to abandon Ruffin's home-school notebook which had been so important during his first two years of special education. I heard nothing disturbing from Mrs. Byrnes, and Ruffin was able to communicate what had happened at school well enough for me to feel certain he was doing fine there.

By late September, Lisa's latchkey notes made repeated references to Ruffin's wanting to be with his friends, rather than sit with her. "Ruffin was very distracted by the kids outside, said he was 'Sad, 'cause I just want to play.' After telling him we would go outside for a while he said, 'I'm happy 'cause I get to play with the kids before they go in the gym. 'What goes with what? 9 out of 10 trials. In the middle of this task the other kids came in, and Ruffin immediately said that he wanted to go with them. It took many prompts to get him to finish this task."

As I read this latest entry, I could not help but feel sad for Ruffin and enormously encouraged that he wanted to be with his classmates as friends. It would be something to raise with Evelyn.

Evelyn was due back the next Friday. She spent a full afternoon with Ruffin at St. Pat's and dropped by early that evening to visit with me.

That Sunday, I wrote my first and last note ever to Mrs. Byrnes. "Evelyn Kung was pleased with Ruffin's progress since May. She saw good things on the playground and in the classroom and you certainly have a sharp eye for noting his small difficulties. Evelyn expects this will be her last visit. I am so pleased Ruffin is with you and Peter Smith at St. Pat's. I feel confident it was the right choice for him."

Meanwhile, Ruffin drew and colored a card for Evelyn that looked to me like a rainbow tree with uplifted branches beside a rainbow circle. We sent it to Evelyn with a note. "Dear Evelyn, (with a heart), This on the top half of the page is a half-cave and to the left is a round circle (with another heart), Ruffin." With my postscript, "Ruffin dictated this message to you and said where to put the hearts. Mary Jane."

The last Monday in September, "Lisa's CARD Latchkey Notes: Ruffin initiated conversation 4 times, including specific names as to what kids had brought for 'orange day' and included events for tomorrow and yesterday. Ruffin asked 6 questions. If/then social cues: 'If you're going on a long trip with your mom, what should you do?' Ruffin:

'Bring a pillow and blanket in case it is cold. Bring food.' 'What's the first thing you do when you get in the car?' Ruffin: 'Put your seatbelt on.' 'If the girl next to you is poking you while the teacher is talking, what would you do?' Ruffin: 'Tell the teacher.' 'What do you tell her?' 'She is poking me.' 'When you're all done with lunch, what do you do?' Ruffin: 'Put spoon, tray, and fork where they clean the dishes. If you don't finish your food, you put it where they clean the dishes anyway. They wash the dishes for next time.' I see something incredible: Ruffin: 'I see a big giant apple crawling on the roof, smoothing the whole-wide world.' 'I see three little bears digging in sand.' 'I see a heart making chairs swim under water.'"

Robin, Ruth, and I settled into my new office building, where letters and legal papers began to pour in. Angie sent us a note from graduate school. "I got to talk to Dr. Lovaas at the Minnesota conference. He knew who you were. The lawyer who spoke gave your name as a contact for someone who might know about court cases and Lovaas funding.

"Graduate school is great. I'm giving a presentation in one of my classes and I wanted to show a Lovaas video on behavior modification. I mentioned to my professor (a woman who studied with Lovaas from Washington State) that I had a home video of treatment. She thought that would be more interesting to see because of its personal practical use.

"I'm writing to you because I wanted to ask your permission." I was delighted with Angie's letter and happy to give her permission.

The last Thursday in September, a Bridgewater audiologist tested Ruffin's hearing at St. Pat's and reported her results with "no recommendations at this time." I continued to wonder if auditory integration training had made a difference, or if Ruffin were simply, finally outgrowing his susceptibility to ear infections. Whatever the reason, the news was good.

Wendy Norton joined Ruffin's team at the end of September, as Lisa's substitute, and as a Bridgewater employee. She was never as precise a note taker nor as organized a teacher as Lisa. She was not trained as a speech and language pathologist, but, to me, she represented the wider community, the people of our town whom Ruffin would need to interact with to enjoy an independent life here and beyond. Evelyn agreed this was a challenge Ruffin needed to learn to surmount.

From "Wendy's Notes: Wh Questions: 'What do you do with aspirin?' Ruffin: 'Eat it.' 'Why do you take it?' Ruffin: 'When you're sick.' 'Who gives you the aspirin?' Ruffin: 'I do.' 'No, only adults take aspirin. Children take Tylenol.'

"What is ketchup made of?' Ruffin: 'Blood of cows.' 'No, ketchup is made from tomatoes.'

"Time Concepts: 'What did you do when you got home yesterday?' Ruffin: 'I checked to see if JJ was home. We played dragons in the backyard. We couldn't go out front. The dragons are pets, just pretend.'"

Wendy was working on her own by early October. I could see Ruffin was still learning, always doing better at home with me in the evenings, and on the weekends.

I got another call from Dr. Lovaas who was attending his 45th graduation reunion at Luther. He needed the names and phone numbers of parents and attorney advocates I had been working with across the country. Robin and I had nearly a thousand on file. He and I were able to discuss Ruffin's recent progress. Dr. Lovaas assured me it sounded like Ruffin was going to be fine and seemed especially pleased with Ruffin's friendships.

CHAPTER SEVENTY EIGHT

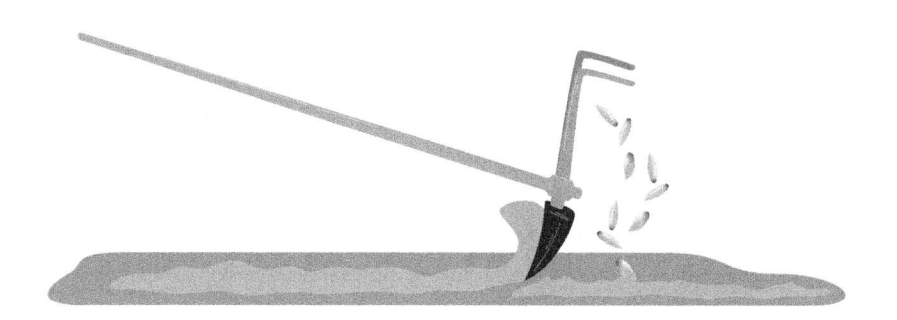

PLOWED UNDER LIKE A SEED

Kathy Collins, the Iowa Association of School Boards attorney who had complained to Curt and Joan about my legal practice and my parent-attorney posts on *The Me List,* made my reputation statewide as an attorney-advocate — perhaps inadvertently — by writing about the results of our due process hearing in her regular column: *CYA — Consult Your Attorney.* For years afterward, until I retired in 2015, school administrators and AEA employees across Iowa recognized me by name, and recalled my role as Ruffin's mother, whenever I turned up at IEP meetings with parents or wrote on their behalf — or simply suggested parents mention they had called my office — before presenting their requests that their children's special needs be better met in specific ways.

"The practice of 'special education law' is crazy," I whined to Curt.

"Yes, it is," he agreed.

"And yet, you continue to practice it," I said with some wonderment.

"And you will, too," said Curt with confidence.

And, so I did for more than a decade.

I sat down to write Dr. Lovaas on a slow Friday. "I pass on a few items about how matters are developing in Iowa," enclosing Curt's recent letter to UIHC concerning their continuing failure to prescribe intensive discrete trial training. "Unfortunately, at UIHC we are starting with some folk who hold to the view that your method is abusive of children and turns them into non-functional robots, so using Byrna Siegel's views and authority to bring them along seemed a useful half-step forward to try." I also sent him Collins's announcement about Ruffin's and my recent successful due process case for summer services.

"One of our regional educational authorities Heartland AEA near Des Moines has applied for a $750,000 federal grant to undertake a study to empirically document the efficacy of current special education programming in Iowa for young children with autism or PDD, including some model TEACCH programs.

"Sadly, this much money would be enough to treat every newly diagnosed child in our state. Very sadly, although all the witnesses at Ruffin's due process hearing testified that his progress was 'a miracle,' his school principal submitted a letter in support of this grant. Seeing is *not* believing — for those who have to provide the resources.

"P.S. Have you heard that *Smart Money* magazine is writing an article about how to access insurance, Medicaid, and school district funds to pay for your program?"

I had tried to end my letter on a light note, but overall, it was a description of sad failure. Curt and I had never been able to find a powerful, committed educational or medical partner to work with on the inside of the special education fortress. That fortress remained well-defended.

From "Wendy's Notes: What would you do if? 'What would you do if you and your mom went to a store, and you got lost and couldn't find her?' Ruffin: 'I would ask a policeman, where is my mom?' 'If you did see a policeman, what would you tell him?' Ruffin: 'I don't know. I'm lost and I can't find my mom.' 'Then you would need to tell the policeman your name and your mom's name.' Ruffin: 'Yeah, Mary Jane White, and my name is Ruffin White.' 'That's good if you can find a policeman, but what if there isn't a policeman.' Ruffin: 'Ask a grown-up for help, one with good eyes that is not a stranger.' Wendy and Ruffin went on to discuss other situations. 'If you were playing outside and a stranger asked you to go for a ride in his car?' Ruffin: 'Tell him no.' 'But what if he would give you lots of candy?' Ruffin: 'No.' 'What if they needed help to find a puppy?' Ruffin: 'No.' 'What else should you do if this happens besides say no?' Ruffin: 'Go inside my house with my mom.'

I thought we had lost the war in Iowa, but we were going to win the battle for Ruffin.

Wendy's Notes: "Ruffin needed a cue to ask to play with a classmate. I suggested Ruffin play tag with the others, but he did not want to. He said he runs out of energy too fast. Ruffin showed me the boat he made in school. I asked where he might want to sail to. Ruffin said, 'To an island to find buried treasure.'"

As far as I was concerned, Ruffin was a treasure.

I contacted Dr. Lovaas again in mid-October. "Gary Mayerson, an attorney-friend of mine in New York, has advised me that Dr. Siegel has been hired by his school district to testify in opposition to his request for Lovaas programming for his preschool son. This will be before the same federal judge, Constance Motley, who decided the very favorable *Malkentoz* case on April 15th, 1995, in New York. Attorney Mayerson also advises that Dr. Siegel has been hired by several school districts for the same purpose. This was very dismaying news to me. Perhaps it is not news to you.

"Here is Heartland Area Education Agency's April 10th, 1996, application for the $750,000 grant submitted to the U.S. Department of Education. These folks 'would like to demonstrate that our training and follow-up (based on TEACCH-like programming) results in the same amount of change as was reported by Lovaas.'

"It is not clear to me whether this grant has been awarded, or whether it remains in a preliminary stage, and whether anyone at the United States Department of Education would listen to or read a critique of its experimental design. I would be most interested in your or Tris' thoughts about how this application might be responded to."

Ruth needed to be aware, too. "Miss Hobbs wrote an April 8th, 1996, letter of support for this $750,000 grant.' It is dated a month *before* she testified in Ruffin's case about our district's commitment to Lovaas programming."

Chris Foster, Susan Smith, several other Iowa mothers, and I touched base by phone in late October. We felt we were floundering in our advocacy efforts without an enthusiastic and strong partner on the inside of the educational establishment, and the $750,000 grant to Heartland AEA concerned us greatly — not only for children in Iowa, but for children across the country.

Robin assembled and mailed hundreds of letters I prepared to all the parents on our nationwide list who had requested and received a copy of Curt and Joan's booklet. "If this grant proposal does not seem to be a fruitful way to spend $750,000 of your tax dollars, you need to let your voice be heard by writing a letter to Ms. Gail Houle and Dr. Thomas Hehir at the addresses given below."

"From Wendy's Notes: Describe a person: Ruffin needed some cues. 'Describe a teacher.' Ruffin: 'What's describe?' 'It means you talk about the person.' Ruffin: 'They teach. She's good to teach children, and when you're not quiet, she rings the bell.' 'Describe a mother.' Ruffin: 'She helps you, takes good care of you, gets you clothes when you're a baby.' 'Describe a janitor.' Ruffin: 'What's a janitor?' 'He takes care of the school.' Ruffin: 'You mean Seamus?' 'Yes.' Ruffin: He mops the floors and gets them all shiny, fixes things. He gets the balls off the roof.'"

An early intervention conference, *Behavioral Education Strategies for Children with Autism or PDD* was held in late October at the Hyatt Regency, Houston, sponsored by Families for Early Autism Treatment FEAT-Houston, Inc. with O. Ivar Lovaas providing the keynote and afternoon demonstrations and general sessions by Bridget Taylor, M.A., Edward C. Fenske, M.A.T., Ed. S., Gina Green, Ph.D., Jack Scott, Ph.D., Andrew S. Bondy, Ph.D., and attorney Michael O'Dell. I would love to have gone, but I really couldn't manage it.

But a few years later, attorney Michael O'Dell and I teamed up to try a due process case together in Dimmitt, Texas, for a cotton farming family there. Ruffin was about seven at the time and came along. He got to drive a huge multi-million-dollar cotton harvester around while the father of the family and I prepared his testimony there in the harvester's cab which was roomy enough for the three of us. We were the "prevailing party" in introducing Lovaas methods into his young son's IEP and celebrated our victory by eating homemade ice cream all the way home back to Iowa. The family's mother had made and packed us a couple of gallons in a cooler for the back end of our trusty Volvo station wagon.

Ruffin continued to battle to master concepts of time as we approached the second anniversary of Evelyn's first visit to us in Iowa. "Ruffin recalled that on Thanksgiving we eat turkey, and that he lost his tooth yesterday while biting down into some hard Halloween candy. Ruffin responded appropriately 11 times to questions from other children and asked 4 of his own. Ruffin needed a cue to ask others if they would like some popcorn. Ruffin asked another boy if he had Direct TV. They were talking about Saturday being cartoon day."

Dr. Lovaas and I spoke again for the last time on Monday, November 4th. The upshot of his call was that he was aware of the Heartland AEA grant problem and was working on it.

We were fighting a rear-guard action by now in Iowa. That fall, Sue Baker, Iowa's Autism Services Consultant had been recognized by the University of Iowa Board of

Regents with a Staff Excellence Award and interviewed. Sue had identified, "The number one request currently is to respond to a new service delivery model highlighting behavior modification for very young children," including "providing resources to enhance expertise for new service models for early intervention." She also mentioned the need for developing videos to provide "specific hands-on examples of teaching units that illustrate" among other approaches "discrete trial format," the code words she was permitted to use to avoid ever breathing the name "Lovaas."

Ray DeNeve of Bridgewater had written to Dr. Hagen, copying his suggestion blindly to me. "This letter is written to request your support for getting the State of Iowa an individual trained in the Lovaas Method who could serve as a resource to all the AEAs. While there has been much discussion regarding the methodology of working with children with autism, I feel that there has been enough study done on the effects of the Lovaas Method to warrant such a position.

"Many of the school districts and the AEAs are faced with excessive costs in obtaining services from out-of-state providers because no one is available within the State of Iowa. It is extremely difficult for a single AEA to have a person with these qualifications on staff full-time. There is not enough work for a person full-time within an agency. One person statewide to work with the AEAs would be a conservative start. Later, a second option that might be desirable would be UIHC initiating a program to train individuals in the Lovaas Method."

Wow, I thought, reading Ray's letter from inside the front lines to inside the citadel of powerlessness. From what I knew of Curt's and my previous two years of raising this issue, Ray's lobbying would fall like a pebble into a still pond with no ripples of any consequence. It left me feeling profoundly sad.

From far away, New Jersey parent-attorney Lisa M. Parles let me know about a mid-December conference in Long Island, New York, to exchange information between parent groups supporting intensive ABA services. Parents and professionals in New York's Department of Health's Early Intervention Program would continue to gather in sufficient numbers over time to issue a 1999 highly-influential and detailed *Clinical Practice Guideline, Report of the Recommendations - Autism / Pervasive Developmental Disorders, Assessment and Intervention for Young Children (Age 0-3 Years)*, a document that would be maintained and updated in 2017, offering continuing guidance to families and professionals in the practice of ABA and the work of Dr. Lovaas.

Most areas of the Midwest continued to remain difficult territory for parent-advocates to plow. Advocates for Lovaas in Kansas were plowed under, too.

The Des Moines Register published an article on November 17th about Heartland AEA, headlined "Low-key school agency may be *too* low-key." "The public agency has 500 employees and is spending 39 million dollars this year. It is governed by a board of directors whose names never appear on an election ballot. It has a chief administrator with a $117,000 salary package — higher than the governor's."

Two days later, Evelyn faxed me, "Hello! Two things that I need to ask you about. 1. Bridgewater still has not paid the bill for the due process hearing and the last few workshops, so accounting wanted me to find out who I should contact. Can you let me know? Thanks! 2. Dr. Granpeesheh would like to know if we could have a short videotape of Ruffin playing and having a conversation with someone. We would like to show how he is these days (Isn't it wonderful?) I keep telling her how wonderfully he has done. If it is a good tape, she would like to use it in a video."

Dr. Granpeesheh did use several clips in a documentary about Ruffin and three other CARD children, *Recovered: Journeys through the Autism Spectrum and Back,* now readily available on YouTube.

By late November, in my new downtown office with Robin, I began taking calls from parents asking me to help represent them at IEP meetings for their children with disabilities. It was the season of Thanksgiving, and I was grateful for Ruffin's steady progress, but frustrated by our failures in advocating for system-wide changes.

But we could still do our small part — by advocating for individual families.

CHAPTER SEVENTY NINE

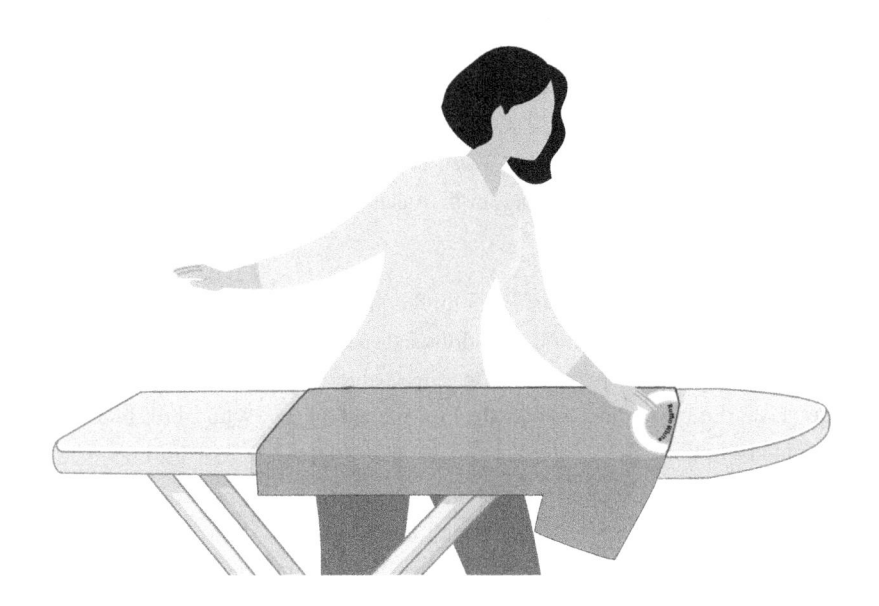

THE DIGNITY OF BRAVERY AND AUDACITY

By early December, Wendy's report on Ruffin's "Why do you like? drill was, 'Do you like moving?' Ruffin: 'Yeah.' 'Why?' Ruffin: 'Because it's fun. I wonder where we'll go on the next move. I go from place to place. It's exciting not knowing the house you're going to move to.'"

Then, Wendy asked, "Do you like latchkey?' Ruffin: 'Yes, yes, yes.' 'Why?' Ruffin: 'Because you get to play all the time. Not have to work.'"

As soon as I read this, I called Evelyn who suggested we all step back and test Ruffin's progress by letting him navigate entirely on his own during latchkey.

"Today is the first day that Ruffin spent all his time in latchkey. This gave him a chance to react to any situation that might occur and to see if he knew what to do. When

I told Ruffin that he would get to play full time now, he had a *huge* smile on his face. Nice timing too, since there were a lot more kids for Ruffin to choose from. Wendy."

An IEP notice issued near the end of February inviting Lisa, Mrs. Byrnes, principal Peter Smith, Wendy, Evelyn, and me to a meeting in early March, right after school in Ruffin's classroom at St. Pat's. Lisa circulated her report of Ruffin's formal language testing a couple of days ahead of time. At 5 years, 9 months, Ruffin demonstrated "average or above-average" language ages of 6 years, 11 months to 7 years, 1 month and "had achieved all his IEP goals" including "drills as defined by CARD and following 3-part directives."

Based on Lisa's report, we amended Ruffin's IEP which ran through July of 1997, to change the direct services for CARD drills and speech and language therapy to indirect services only. Ruffin's participation in general education was for "all classes all of the time." I was thrilled for him, and for all of us. We had done it. With a little button-up, we would be finished.

Belt and suspenders, we agreed "Ruffin will be monitored for CARD drill-skills and speech and language skills when Evelyn Kung is in town." She would be back often to see Renee and others in Bridgewater. We were left with a single annual goal: "Ruffin will demonstrate age-appropriate behaviors" with two simple short-term objectives that Lisa would check if either St. Pat's or I had concerns: "1. Ruffin will maintain age-level language skills, and 2. Ruffin will maintain age-appropriate social skills."

Which, of course, since he had been prepared to do, Ruffin did — under Seamus's watchful eye at school — without any further advocacy or meddling from me.

That kindergarten year, Ruffin quickly made a new best friend, Joe, who visited many afternoons, weekends, and overnights, especially after Ruffin and I settled into a new house that Donna and Kevin helped us rehabilitate to its 1908 glory.

Ruffin's life continued as the ordinary childhood most typically developing boys and their parents enjoy. He and I held regular spelling test rehearsals at breakfast downtown. We joined field trips here and there locally, summer horse-riding camps for trail rides along the Yellow River with Seamus, and parades by riding high on the St. Pat's school float. By our fireplace, I read every one of the over a million words of Harry Potter's magical adventures aloud to Ruffin and Joe. Every year, Ruffin placed veterans' flags around the courthouse perimeter and guarded them overnight for Memorial Day with Seamus.

Once, when Ruffin was about seven, on a visit to my parents, we made an add-on detour visit to Peter and Pam Wright's home on the shore of the Chesapeake Bay, where Pete docked his paperless law office boat. Despite his own dyslexia, Pete had represented Shannon Carter and her parents on their long trek to the United States Supreme Court for the opinion that had supported our right to seek reimbursement from the public schools. Pam had trained as a school psychologist. They were delighted to welcome Ruffin, look him over, and assure me that he seemed to be developing and growing up well.

Ours was a story blessed with privilege and luck, but lest it seem these were the keys to our success, I would say both were helpful, but not strictly necessary. My personal heroine is my grittiest client, a waitress living in a trailer in the boot-heel of Missouri. She called me out of the blue one morning, seeking information. Her older daughter, her toddler had just been diagnosed. She had a new baby, too, and a husband who had just left them — the metal walls of the single-wide were too noisy with all that crying and screaming.

After I heard her out, and she heard me out, she wanted to know how much it would cost to mount a home-program. Without hesitation, I told her that she would need $100,000 over the next two years to try to treat her daughter.

That produced a half a minute of silence. Then she ventured, "I have several of those offers for credit cards sitting here. I was going to toss them. So, it would take about five." That sounded brave.

She also had a mother, a grandmother, several aunts, and a couple of sisters, so her plan developed. She would train them as her therapy team and "keep the money in the family." By the time I travelled down to Missouri a couple of years later to attend an IEP meeting for her daughter to enter mainstream kindergarten, she had used the last of her credit to retain a bankruptcy attorney.

Ruffin began attending summer science camps after sixth grade at Edgewood College in Madison, sponsored by the Wisconsin Center for Academically Talented Youth. For this pre-taste of college life, Seamus and I drove him a hundred miles east to his first overnight dorm room. By mapping and measuring the height of the campus trees there, he became fascinated by GPS and triangulation, and was not a bit homesick.

Then in the first semester of seventh grade, we hit a bit of a bump in the road. We weren't alone. Most of Ruffin's longtime St. Pat's classmates moved to public school to avoid a troublesome new teacher. As I had begun to suspect from our early morning, last minute spelling test rehearsals, Ruffin struggled with the troubles typical of boys with dyslexia. On his own, he had already begun to experiment with the latest voice recognition software, IBM Via Voice, as an easier way to "write" his longer assignments at home.

After reviewing Donna and Kevin's experience with Matt, and the Orton-Gillingham methods Curt had recommended to them — and rehashing the public schools' miserable failure to implement that method — I turned to searching the internet. I discovered a private Orton school on the East Coast, The Gow School in South Wales, New York.

Before Christmas, Ruffin and I visited the campus. Gow was marvelous, but large, since it also offered a full college program. Tuition there exceeded my annual income by several multiples. The admission group at Gow recommended Linden Hill in Northfield, Massachusetts, as a smaller campus, just for middle school boys.

That year, Linden Hill had shrunk to a tiny student body and skeleton teaching staff. A student sexual abuse scandal the year before had led to the messy discharge of their headmaster and several teachers. The full investigation was available to read online. Sexual abuse would be the risk of leaving Ruffin alone at any boarding school.

The new headmaster and a small surviving group of older teachers — who had all trained at Gow — welcomed Ruffin — and my years of experience of advising parents of children with disabilities. Ruffin's tuition would be reduced there, if I would help guide prospective parents to skilled local advocates to help them secure tuition reimbursement from their school districts — a result much easier to negotiate in the two federal circuits out East than back home.

For his second semester of seventh grade, I drove Ruffin out to his second overnight dorm room. We bought the requisite blazers and khakis into which I had ironed his laundry tags. He would wear a school-colored tie. There, Ruffin learned to listen to his laptop read to him, and how to speak — slowly, in phrases, please — into a headset microphone so his own words would rise up in seconds flat upon a screen. He learned to mimic Steinbeck and Hemingway, and to print his papers, by pressing *Print*.

That winter, he also learned to ski — a flashing solitary — down night-lit Berkshire's black diamond trails, and to hike Monadnock. He learned to play within a baseball team, the year his teachers' favorite, unfavored Boston Red Sox won the series. Baseball and golf became his own preferred sports of discrete events that allowed him ample room for individual feats of skill, while avoiding the social fluidity of soccer, or basketball.

My law office was situated a hundred miles east off the future route of the Avenue of the Saints, someday to be developed as an interstate from St. Louis, Missouri, to St. Paul, Minnesota. So far, there were only small signs erected toward the hopes for this federal project along our mostly two-lane blacktop rural highways.

Not too many out-of-state clients ever just wandered in.

A couple, a solo legal practitioner and his wife, a registered nurse, whom I had represented a decade ago were driving the Avenue of the Saints through Iowa and called ahead to schedule an appointment by detour. After years of working together in autism advocacy and litigation, this would be our first face-to-face meeting.

They arrived with their then middle-school-aged son who went into our backyard to play. And did play. With absorption. Quietly. With his sister. The two parents sat with me for coffee, and then slid a $10,000 check across my kitchen table.

They insisted I take it.

First, they told me they had sold their home and all their things in Arkansas and planned to sell their car to fly out of Minneapolis, to emigrate to Italy, to become Baptist missionaries there, where they would not need this money, they assured me.

I was aghast at their sheer audacity.

Then they told me a second story, both of them — talking over each other — vividly recalling the first occasion years after the diagnosis of their son's autism when they had a half hour together, just to sit and share coffee. He had been about eight. How heavenly that had been, they remembered, with gratitude. And attributed this small miracle to Lovaas ABA, an intervention I had recommended to them in our first phone conversations.

Their son had developed into a good traveler. He had begun treatment well after 60 months, after age 5 — when it seems the window for fully normal development often closes irrevocably. He did not experience a fully optimal outcome. Our petition for certiorari to the U.S. Supreme Court seeking to establish a right to personal injury damages for educational malpractice had been turned back on Tenth Amendment grounds. The Eighth Circuit ruled that educational agencies enjoy sovereign immunity. Same as any King, they could do no wrong. Nevertheless, their son had developed into a good traveler. A good enough traveler, they would undertake their new venture fearlessly with him and their young daughter.

And where was Ruffin, they asked. They had been hoping to meet him. Would he be home from school soon?

I explained his absence.

"Well, let this help with that."

I folded their check. I bowed my head, too, acknowledging the dignity of their check, of their deliberate detour.

We exchanged hugs all around and said our final goodbyes.

When they were gone, I sat at the kitchen table for a while, without working, racked by my own sobbing.

CHAPTER EIGHTY

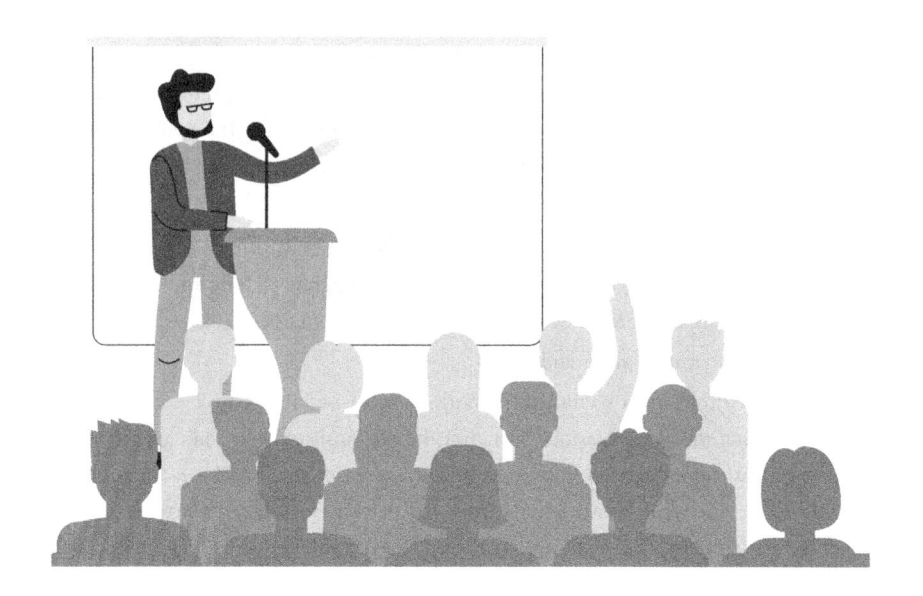

RUFFIN CUT LOOSE IN THE UNIVERSE

Did Ruffin want to go back to Linden Hill for eighth grade? Yes, he did. He enjoyed the small classes of no more than three boys, reading *The Red Pony* and *The Nick Adams Stories*. He worked hard with his one-to-one math tutor. The headmaster had called one in for him as soon as his classroom teacher sensed Ruffin was bored. He loved swimming now and visiting Mark Twain's home in Hartford where he wrote those two books we had read with Joe. He spent his thirteenth birthday, the first I ever missed celebrating with him, at the Massachusetts Institute of Technology. Now he wanted to study engineering.

Ruffin still had his IDEA entitlement and Bridgewater had left his 3.74 weighting for special education unchanged since kindergarten. So, well before the end of his seventh-grade year, I recontacted the public-school authorities to ask what Ruffin's schedule as an eighth grader might look like at home.

I spent a day at the local schoolhouse, attending classes, and observing. The advanced English class was advised that the SAT and ACT tests were expensive. Community college admission didn't require them.

When I complimented the chemistry teacher on the large collection of glassware, he explained, "We like to keep them in these cabinets. They are too expensive to allow our students to use. They could break them. I usually teach by showing videos of the experiments. It's less dangerous."

Before noon, I had walked into the Office, asking the school nurse for a couple of aspirins. I didn't have the energy it would take to try to reform this.

I did have a long, detailed independent evaluation of Ruffin done back East by a reading specialist recommended by Linden Hill. In it, she described the exact nature of Ruffin's multiple dyslexias. In a separate assistive technology assessment, she had also introduced Ruffin to several newer forms of accommodation, including *Dragon Naturally Speaking*, that could help Ruffin tackle a rigorous high school curriculum.

Ruffin would need a foreign language to apply for college. The reading specialist warned that it would be an uphill battle for Ruffin to master a second language like Spanish, French, or German. But he had some unique skills that would help him easily discriminate Chinese characters. As pictures, to him, they were *not* chicken scratching. For him, a language like Chinese — so difficult for the rest of us — would be easier.

I called for an IEP meeting that summer, so Ruffin could be formally placed at Linden Hill that fall. He had cheerfully submitted to two days of Bridgewater's own testing while he was home for the summer. We were delighted to find that the Bridgewater reading specialist used *Dragon*, too, to write her own briefer evaluation.

At thirteen, Ruffin was of an age to begin to learn how to advocate for himself and seemed willing to come to that morning's IEP meeting. We entered the schoolhouse he had never attended, where we were ushered into a large, long room, big table, big chairs, nicely air conditioned. Planned to be a long meeting, then.

Caron the Good was back to represent our local district as their attorney. An additional school psychologist, a Bridgewater employee from outside our district, a young woman with large blue eyes, took a seat beside me. Her name came up right away, and I promptly forgot it, as introductions went around the table. Why she was there was not immediately apparent. She had been invited in to help wrangle me. The meeting was full of people — body-stacked — in the middle of summer vacation.

The morning session dragged interminably through various reports of present levels of educational performance, the PLEP — through which I stifled myself. This was required by law. Ruffin was bored and mystified, and never called upon to speak.

Finally, a halt was called for lunch.

Ruffin and I went home. At our kitchen table, Ruffin offered up that he thought the meeting was going on too long, and to no good effect that he could see.

"Well, yes, they are dogging it," I agreed.

Then Ruffin surprised me by insisting I go back alone for the afternoon session and "kick some butt." No, he didn't plan to go back.

Although he wanted me to "kick butt," Ruffin didn't want to see it. He wanted *me* to go do that, so he could go back to Linden Hill.

He knew full well who was who. I was his parent.

As Joe blasted through the back door, I headed back to the meeting.

The afternoon dragged on. I began to interrupt a bit, interject, suggest, ask outright, to push and prod the group along. All the while, I met with greater and greater, first with increasingly-smooth — and then frank — resistance.

Dragon was too expensive a software program to purchase for a child. Yes, it was an ADA workplace accommodation for the Bridgewater reading specialist who had carpel-tunnel, but Ruffin couldn't use a laptop in a classroom. That equipment could be broken. Then what?

No, he couldn't study Chinese. No one in our town spoke it. There was no one who taught it. Since our local district and Bridgewater could offer Ruffin something "appropriate," no, they were not prepared to discuss paying to place Ruffin at Linden Hill. It was a private school. And out-of-state to boot.

Finally, I was reduced to impatience. I slipped in an expletive, deliberately, as an intensifying adjective. The young school psychologist, the so far otherwise-quiet Blue Eyes beside me, spoke up to admonish me.

"We don't allow that kind of language here" — meaning, I supposed "in school."

I turned on her sharply. "I'm not the child here. We're none of us children here. We're all adults here. I expect to use whatever adult language is necessary to press my point here. Surely, *you've* watched HBO? Surely, *you* have been to the movies? Don't pretend *you're* suffering shock here! — have never heard this type of *fucking language*!"

The lower rims of her eyelids suddenly brimmed up with tears. Honestly, I could have cared less. This meeting was more important to me than it was to her. Or than she was to me.

As a further pattern-interrupt, to show I could have cared less, I gripped the open water-bottle I had brought to fortify myself — stay hydrated, stay calm — and pitched it — end over end — down the length of the long, narrow body-stacked table. I had been *reduced* to this. I was *furious* that I had been reduced to this. I was utterly and completely livid that Blue Eyes was expendable, as she was, to the future of my son . . .with water now on everyone, on all the scattered papers.

I needed to move. Shouldn't I be the one tearing up throughout this meeting when for myself, selfishly, more than anything I wanted Ruffin back home? I stood to take greater control of myself, and of the course of this meeting that seemed to be headed nowhere.

Caron, the single real decision-maker here, and I moved out into the hallway. I told her this was an ugly meeting that was only going to get longer. And uglier. I urged her if she had money to offer, she needed to offer it up.

She protested that she didn't have any money to offer — not without calling Des Moines.

I insisted, "Get on the phone and get after the money. Now, before this gets any uglier."

So, in that way, in the hallway, Caron and I resolved matters quickly.

Then the two of us went in to announce the end of the meeting. All the bodies were sent home for vacation.

Caron drafted a financial agreement within a day or so. All the available special education state money for which Ruffin qualified under his heavy disability-weighting would be passed along to me, less a small three percent, accorded our local district for its administrative oversight of Ruffin, who would be technically registered as 3.74 of their public-school students from here on out. But I would be free to spend what there was — about $20,000 a year, paid over nine monthly installments — for what I would represent in writing to be, what I took the risk for Ruffin to be — magic word here — *appropriate*: Linden Hill.

That was nowhere near the whole amount of tuition and travel costs of attending Linden Hill — full tuition there was over $45,000 a year. That would have been our full legal entitlement under East Coast (Second and Third Circuit) and West Coast (Ninth Circuit) legal precedents — but it was enough I could continue to afford to stay home and work in the Midwest (Eighth Circuit) after driving Ruffin back to Massachusetts that fall.

Time was money, too, as Curt had taught me. There was good value in sweeping off the table what money was readily available — what money there was at the far-away state level, without further delay for Ruffin, or much more ugly fuss.

This single horrible meeting proved to be an enduring victory for Ruffin. The financial agreement Caron crafted was simply re-dated and up-dated — with increasingly available state money as was allocated in far-away Des Moines — for the remainder of Ruffin's education — through his high school graduation.

Every year I would sit through an IEP meeting in the spring, rejecting every offer to bring Ruffin home, handing over my signed papers, which the group would gather up with a sigh of relief. Then, I would bring out the brownies or the marshmallow treats and everyone would let their hair down and want to know, "How is Ruffin doing?"

And I could relax for another year and tell them.

Ruffin completed eighth grade at Linden Hill. The campus closed every third weekend for students to visit their families, and while the teachers spent time with their own and regrouped. But it was not enough time for Ruffin to travel home, so I went to visit him regularly, and unannounced, too, whenever I could — to keep my eye on what I could, sleeping in a vacant dorm room. In all, over thirteen months' time, I made over a dozen trips to northern Massachusetts.

Ruffin and I got to know the mountain towns and motels of the Connecticut River Valley. Seamus was able to get away once for Ruffin's graduation when all his early awards were reprised, and his final ones announced.

Linden Hill School Awards, Seventh Grade, May 20, 2004: The Peter R. Walter Gentleman's Award, "presented to the boy whose personal manner is an unpretentious, positive influence;" The President's Education Award from Rod Paige and George W. Bush "in recognition of Outstanding Academic Excellence;" The Pinewood Derby First Place Speed Award; The Most Improved Skier Award; The Green Team Intramural Team Spirit Award.

Linden Hill School Awards, Eighth Grade, May 26, 2005: The Headmaster's Award Silver Bowl, "presented to the boy who has demonstrated a quiet determination to achieve academic growth;" The President's Education Award from Margaret Spelling and George W. Bush "in recognition of Outstanding Academic Excellence," Leadership & Cooperation in Study Hall Award; Team member for the Rube Goldberg Team, sponsored by MIT April 9, 2005; Soccer Award, 2 poems to literary magazine, Outdoor Recreation Award, Softball Award.

After visiting a dozen private high schools around the nation — hoity-toity ones on the East Coast, a Quaker school in Iowa, an Episcopal hockey school in southern Minnesota, schools on the shores of various of the Great Lakes, including a wonderful new technology and ecology school in Wisconsin — Ruffin finally met his match at St. John's Preparatory School on the Benedictine campus of St. John's University in Collegeville, Minnesota, a seven-hour drive north of our home in Iowa.

Ruffin had spent an hour in Mr. Fraley's physics room where experimental apparatus filled the floor-to-ceiling shelves covering every available wall of the classroom before he presented a power point with embedded videos to the faculty admission committee. Ruffin was able to show how he would learn, how he could download audio books into his MP-3 player, and how by continuing to train his *Dragon*, he should be able to complete any written assignment. What he handed in would look like anyone else's paper. He imagined he would enjoy listening to his reading assignments here while walking in the surrounding woods.

The older monk who served as headmaster announced St. John's had never admitted a student with Ruffin's disability history. I was sure we were on the way to being ushered out, as we had been everywhere else.

"But why not?" ruled the monk, raising both hands, and both sleeves of his black robe, as if this would be a lark! The science teacher, Mr. Fraley, with over four decades of experience teaching physics, had passed him a note beforehand. "I want to teach this one."

Now, let Ruffin here speak for himself from an early college-admission resume.

"Head of School Honor Roll every semester of high school.

Academic Honors:

"National Honor Society, Saint John's Preparatory Virgil Michel Chapter — admitted 10th grade. My personal service project was to promote awareness of the environmental impact of a "paperless" school using assistive technologies and voice recognition systems. I tutored younger students in the use of these helpful software programs. One of these students could not type easily, having lost an arm. Another student, like me, has some learning disabilities with spelling and handwriting challenges.

"Sophomore & Junior years, St. John's Preparatory — on the tech crew for theatre (3 plays @ year + coffeehouse + dances), setting up sound and light systems, handling wireless mikes, wireless receivers and routing their signals through a sound board, regulating frequencies, using advanced sound cards and diagnostic tools with programs for theatre cues and more advanced tuning for sound effects. I planned directional speaker placement and used a computer to calculate sound delays in the various theatre spaces at school and in downtown venues by measuring various distances and accounting for the speed of sound."

Each summer through high school, Ruffin returned home to renew his friendship with Joe, his relationship with Seamus, with all the farm animals and with a favorite hammock strung up on a couple of old trees on Seamus's farm. He attended science camps at Iowa State and the University of Iowa. Now, let those teachers speak of him, in their references for his college applications.

"Explorations! 2007 at Iowa State University — Rocketry 101: Ruffin worked hard all week and really applied his knowledge of rocketry to each of his projects. He always worked responsibly and was respectful to his classmates. He was dutiful in his homework assignments and accurate in his calculations of the data collected. He was very diligent and helpful in the collection of flight data. His rocket designs were very well thought out and successfully completed. Doug Richardson, National Board-Certified Teacher

"Explorations! 2007 at Iowa State University — Robotics using Not Quite C: Ruffin was a challenge for me to have in the class. He operated at a level that had me scrabbling for answers to his questions. I have no doubt that Ruffin will do great things. He was talking to me constantly, asking me for clarification on seemingly minute details, all to understand everything thoroughly. And for this I am amazed. I hope that this thirst will continue to inspire him in the sciences and throughout. This thirst for knowledge will allow Ruffin to fully understand any concept he desires, in his life. Matthew Goodman, Graduate Student in Materials Science and Engineering

"Poser 4 Computer Graphics and Animated Figures at Belin-Blank Center University of Iowa, Summer 2005: It was a pleasure to have Ruffin in my class. He clearly possesses the technological skills that enabled him to quickly grasp the concepts of this very demanding piece of software. When situations began to get frustrating (who knew that animating mannequins could prove so challenging?), Ruffin was able to think through problems and create solutions with very little assistance from the instructor. He even took the time to record his own soundtrack to accompany the animation. Ruffin's final piece, entitled *"Bad Joke,"* is a great example of Poser's capabilities, or, rather, Ruffin's capabilities, since this software wasn't written expressly with young filmmakers or animators in mind. Instructor Gary E. Glenn

"Building Radios at Belin-Blank Center University of Iowa, Summer 2004: On the first day, I saw Ruffin taking an especially long time to make his coil. Then I saw the beautiful result and realized why it was taking so long. He obviously takes a great deal of pride in his work, which produced some very nice results. His radios worked right off the bat. It's even more amazing that he could do this right after his surgery (appendectomy). Excellent job, Ruffin." Lyle Lichty, Professor, Cornell College

"Everyday Physics for the 21st Century at Belin-Blank Center University of Iowa, Summer 2003: Ruffin was a nice addition to this year's class. His best work occurred while working with his team in the physics Olympics competition. His catapult was one of the best in the class. Ruffin has good problem-solving skills. I enjoyed teaching Ruffin, he added greatly to the class. He asked good questions and offered several stories during discussions. I encourage Ruffin to continue with his pursuit of scientific knowledge and seek other opportunities to demonstrate his excellence. Instructor Don Brauhn."

After attending their Operation Catapult summer session for high school seniors, Ruffin decided he would attend Rose-Hulman Institute of Technology in Indiana. He had made a good choice for himself. The school was small, about 2000 students, all studying various forms of engineering. Prospective students were assured that if admitted they would be expected to break things, even expensive equipment, and that each would be supported toward graduation with a strong writing laboratory and organized dorm-based homework sessions to boost them all over the most difficult sophomore year — when most other engineering colleges weeded their weaker admissions out.

Here is the remainder of Ruffin's first resume dictated to his *Dragon*, supporting his application for his first paid off-campus internship on a project for Cummins Engines, as a college freshman at Rose-Hulman.

Education:

Currently pursuing an EE major and a robotics certificate

Long-range goals:

To become an electrical engineer and pursue a career in electrical engineering and mechanical robotic development, alternative and sustainable energy or computer design and development.

I wish to acquire specialized skills to design and engineer equipment applicable to the fields above, while maintaining a growing and useful knowledge in scientific fields I may not encounter as frequently. I remain open to any opportunities for exposure to professional engineering experience to further broaden my horizons.

I am highly motivated by interest and curiosity; often I will drive into new subject material and not rest until I have acquired knowledge to the very limits of current understanding.

I have considerable experience working on projects in teams, and I'm particularly adept at working on teams whose members are thoroughly excited or interested in the problem or subject matter.

Extracurricular activities and/or hobbies:

Remote control car-racing and aerial enthusiast

Skilled potter at the wheel, interested in the chemistry of glazes and firing

Foreign language: Chinese (3 years)

Other Summer Activities:

Oregon Museum of Science and Industry, Summer 2004: Redwoods Ecology Adventure and John Day River Raft Adventure

Other extracurricular and community activities:

Summer 2007 — volunteered 62.25 hours at my old parochial school checking information technology wiring in 2 buildings, worked on website construction and opening and setting up a computer lab of new Apple computers.

Horsemanship: Certified Horsemanship Association Levels I and II

I have learned what I know about Computer Science on my own or in computer club and in gifted and talented programs. I am familiar with C/C++ (Robotics), have explored Java (in computer club, founding member), but not the other computer platforms yet.

Ruffin earned his undergraduate degree in electrical engineering from Rose-Hulman, and his master's in computer science from Georgia Tech. He spent a summer at Carnegie-Mellon flying drones to map the undersides of bridges in Pittsburgh, and another couple of summers working as a paid intern on the Dallas campus of Texas Instruments.

While completing his PhD, Ruffin was awarded a Google-Lime-Connect scholarship to spend several days on the Google campus networking with other accomplished students with physical or learning disabilities. He interned in Silicon Valley with a nonprofit organization to improve repeatability and reproducibility in robotic research and security using open-source robotic software. His doctoral research at the University of California San Diego focused on cyber security for robots.

For his graduation, Ruffin's lab mates at San Diego saddled him with the nickname "Dr. Hammock," as a bow to his penchant for researching and writing outdoors during the pandemic in one he strung up at his favorite spot overlooking the Torrey Pines Golf Course and the glider port.

During his time in San Diego, Evelyn and one of her daughters visited him there for a tour of his lab. Chris Foster and her son Noah snagged a tour, too. Afterwards, Ruffin, Chris, and I delivered pots of orchids to Dr. Rimland's Autism Research Institute, to honor his memory.

As his own man, Ruffin has become peripatetic, travelling to Hamburg, Tokyo, Kyoto, Seoul, Vancouver, Cancun, Copenhagen, and Singapore, while publishing to numerous scientific conferences, journals, and textbooks. Today, in his early thirties, he is as loose in the universe as anyone, a post-doctoral fellow in Venice, Italy, taking the vaporetto into his university research office, working there to found an international tech startup with his four academic business partners so they can offer the fruits of their research for wider industry adoption.

Seamus continues reading the paper by my fireplace.

I am, as I was, before Ruffin was born, writing.

APPENDIX OF ADDITIONAL DETAILED TESTING RESULTS

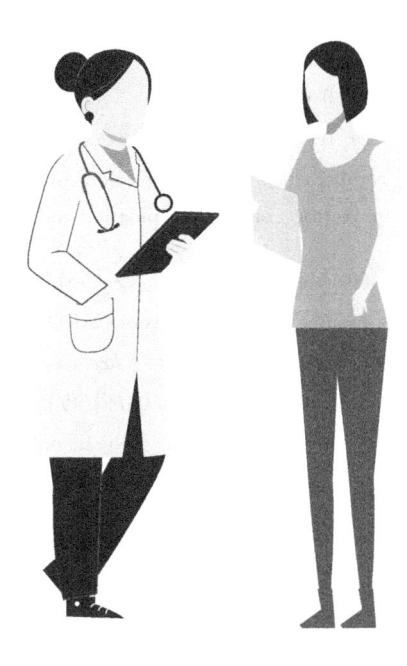

January 25, 1995: UIHC Ms. Wilding, M.S., CCC-SLP:

Ruffin age 3 years, 8 months; after 3 months of CARD training:

Peabody Picture Vocabulary Test (R) Form L

Age Equivalency:	3 years, 0 months
Percentile Rank:	18
Standard Score:	86
Stanine:	3

"This test was an evaluation of the child's ability to point to 1 picture out of 4 which best describes a single word spoken by the clinician. Standard Score Mean is 100 + or − 15.

"Ruffin's performance on the *PPVT-R* indicated a low average score for the identification of 1 picture out of 4. Ruffin again enjoyed this task and looked at all the pictures before making his choice."

Sequenced Inventory of Communication Development (SICD)

Age-months	% passed-receptive	% passed-expressive
28	100%	88%
32	100%	79%
36	80%	67%
40	64%	20%
44	33%	38%
48	0%	25%
48+	0%	20%

"This test assessed comprehension and production through a variety of language tasks, including imitation, pictures, object manipulation and answers to questions."

August 29, 1995: UIHC Ms. Wilding, M.S., CCC-SLP

Ruffin age 4 years, 4 months; after 9 months of CARD training:

Expressive One-Word Picture Vocabulary Test — Revised

Raw Score:	39 (up from 25 on 04/12/95 by Kim)
Age Equivalency:	5.0 years (up from 3.7 years on 04/12/95 by Kim)
Percentile Rank:	73 (up from 34 on 04/12/95 by Kim)
Standard Score:	109 (up from 94 on 04/12/95 by Kim)
Stanine:	6 (up from 4 on 04/12/95 by Kim)

Peabody Picture Vocabulary Test (R) Form L

Raw Score:	42
Age Equivalency:	4.0 years/months
Percentile Rank:	32
Standard Score:	93
Stanine:	4

Sequenced Inventory of Communication Development (SICD)

Age-months	% passed-receptive	% passed-expressive
32	100%	100%
36	80%	100%
40	93%	87%
44	67%	88%
48	50%	75%
48+	43%	40%

Clinical Evaluation of Language Fundamentals — Preschool (CELF-Preschool)

Receptive Subtests	Raw Score	Standard Score	Percentile Rank
Linguistic Concepts	8	6	9
Basic Concepts	16	12	75
Sentence Structure	14	7	16
Expressive Subtests			
Recalling Sentences in Context	27	9	37
Formulating Labels	22	9	37
Word Structure	11	9	37
Receptive Language Score:	93	32	
Expressive Language Score:	94	34	
Total Language Score:	93	32	

Age Equivalent: 3 years, 9 months (7-month delay)

CURRENT COMMUNICATIONS STATUS:

Speech: Developmental articulation errors. Mild high pitch.

Language: Language levels vary from approximately 3 ½ through 5 years. Single word naming and vocabulary skills are his strength with more difficulty at the more abstract levels of language and formulation skills.

RECOMMENDATIONS: We have in the body of this report indicated various concepts that are difficult for Ruffin and his mother has indicated that those will be written into his treatment program.

His mother outlined Ruffin's educational settings for the next year, and he has good opportunities for interacting with preschool children. He will have some excellent language modeling by those children in his play group and with some of the other children with whom he will be involved. He did have some good modeling with a cousin who has been here recently. His mother indicated that he did have good language growth by interacting with that child. We think it is important that he continues to have social communication opportunities.

Ruffin is a child who can take information that is presented to him and then use that in another situation. That will make it easy then to program for him certain routine kinds of language which he can use to get his social interactions going.

Ruffin also had a social group this summer which added to his confidence in language and his interaction style. He also has a variety of interests which makes him a good play partner and a good communication partner. Through practice, he will increase the number of styles he has for interaction and the issues about which he can communicate.

We talked about the vocabulary skills that we see that he needs. It seems appropriate to think about the vocabulary he will need each day in school and put that to him in a functional sense so that he has an opportunity to practice that vocabulary. It also seems appropriate to practice his various communication interaction styles and his questioning styles using the vocabulary of his classrooms. He then will have an opportunity to practice some of that language with the other children with whom he will be interacting right in the classroom settings.

Ruffin's performance on the *PPVT-R* involved his looking at 4 pictures, listening to a stimulus and then pointing to the correct picture. Here, he also showed an improvement in skills, with an approximate 1-year gain on this measure.

It is not appropriate to look in terms of year gains, but to look more at the percentile or standard score gains. We see those remain variable across the various measures. The important thing to realize is that Ruffin has made gains and they are more than the amount of time that has passed. On this measure, at this time, he is scoring at the low end of the average range for skills in a single word vocabulary recognition.

It is significant to note that during the last administration of the *PPVT-R*, Ruffin was touching each of the pictures three or four times as opposed to touching them only once. Today he had a very nice point and was addressing himself very nicely to the task, the way the task should be approached and completed. He was very skilled at looking at all the pictures before making a choice. We did not feel that he was using an impulsive style during his time with the *PPVT-R*.

Sequenced Inventory of Communication Development (SICD). This test assesses comprehension and production through a variety of language tasks, including imitation, pictures, object manipulation, and answers to questions. Ruffin scored a receptive communication age of 3 years, 4 months (a 1-year delay) and an expressive communication age of 3 years, 8 months (an 8-month delay).

It seems more appropriate to simply indicate the tasks that he was not successful on since most of the tasks that he was successful on have been recorded in the report from January. We see today that he had a little bit of difficulty with identification of "rough" and "smooth" and with identification of coins.

He was also successful at responding to commands involving 2 actions, and 2 objects, but not 3 actions. He seemed confused by all the information and tended to get the first 2 bits of the information correct. He understood the system and the strategies he needed to use but the information was just a little bit too long for him. This gives us some insight into the length of language that we need to provide to Ruffin for directions and instructions.

When we want him to be successful, we need to keep the directions to the 2-step level or give him some augmentation in the form of written plus graphic-type assists.

On the expressive language portion, Ruffin also had several important gains. He was successful again at repeating 4 unrelated numbers and 3 unrelated words. He did know that there were to be 3 unrelated words, but he was simply not able to come up with the last word. He looked stumped and was looking through his memory for that word, but it wasn't there. This again indicates to us the length of the information that we need to be presenting to Ruffin for him to be able to act on that information successfully.

Ruffin had good use of position words today and that was difficult for him last time. He also had a very good understanding of "if, what" type of questions such as, "If you fell down, what would you do?" His response was, "I feel hurt and then you get better." This indicates that he is doing some thinking about the information, coming to a conclusion, and then presenting all that information at one time. That is a good skill for Ruffin.

All things considered, on the *SICD,* we saw good growth in all of the areas we looked at.

Clinical Evaluation of Language Fundamentals — Preschool (CELF-Preschool) on which Ruffin earned an age equivalent of 3 years, 9 months (7-month delay). The *CELF-Preschool* explores the foundations of language form and content. This is a new measure for Ruffin, but we felt comfortable that he would be able to take on this new task this time with the increased amount of language he has available to him. We were successful in presenting this. This gives a good look at specific concepts which he is having difficulty with and will lead to some important programming ideas.

In looking at Ruffin's performance overall we see that he is performing at the average level for his receptive and expressive skills. In looking at the individual subtest on the receptive language portion we see that his performance on the linguistic concept subtest is just a pinch below an average performance. The linguistic concepts subtest involves a student listening to directions and then pointing to various animals that are the stimulus. Ruffin had good success when the directions were fairly concrete. As there were degrees of abstractness built into these directions, he had more difficulty. For example, specific concepts that caused him difficulty will be listed here. Those include "either," "but not the," or "point to the _____ and then _____," "next to," "after," "before," and "except."

On the recalling sentences in context subtest which involves the student simply repeating what I was modeling, Ruffin did a wonderful job here until the sentences became a bit longer. Then he tended to maintain the meaning of the sentence but not the structure. He was having some difficulty with formulating these sentences as they became longer and then we saw some false starts into the sentences as he attempted to imitate my structure. This then again is an issue of length which needs to be addressed in offering directions to him.

On one occasion Ruffin did tell me that he did not like something because it was too loud. He will need to have an explanation of what kinds of noises he might expect to hear in the classrooms, in the lunchroom, at special convocations or programs, and so on. Preparing him for these kinds of noises may assist him in being able to deal with those noises without upset. Today he did not get upset, however he did want those noises to be quieted down. Identification of what those noises are and why they are being made will assist him in being able to handle those sounds.

It seems appropriate that a buddy type system could be established where he could begin to use his communication skills to ask for information from other students in the classroom. This may work then into a system in the kindergarten and other grades where he identifies a student with whom he can check to be sure that he understands things that he is to be doing or instructions that he might not have heard correctly. This also validates his interpretation of some issues since he may have a more concrete outlook than the remainder of his classmates.

It seems appropriate to continue to work in the areas of empathy and feelings. New ideas show that those are the most valued characteristics in a communication partner. Working then on some of those seems important to peer interactions. Dealing in the area of empathy and feeling then allows young children to appreciate the fact that they may not be feeling the same way as their classmates are feeling.

Again, getting a peer buddy from the classroom would allow validation of how one should be feeling about something or being able to interpret how classmates are reacting to something and why they are reacting to that issue.

October 4, 1995: Independent Medical Evaluation at the Gundersen Clinic

Ruffin age 4 years, 6 months; after 11 months of CARD training:

ASSESSMENT RESULTS by Debbie J. Olufs, M.A. of Ruffin on the *Detroit Tests of Learning Aptitude — Primary*, an aptitude test for children ages 3-9 which measures important cognitive areas, including language, attention, and motor abilities, and is especially useful for low-functioning school-age children.

Subtests include conceptual matching, design reproduction, digit sequences, draw-a-person, letter sequences, motor directions, object sequences, oral directions, picture fragments, picture identification, sentence imitation, symbolic relations, visual discrimination, word opposites, and word sequences. It is individually administered, for 15 to 45 minutes, depending on the child's age.

Detroit Tests of Learning Aptitude — Primary

Subtest	Raw Score	Standard Score	Percentile	Age Equivalent
General Mental Ability	34	94	35%ile	4 years 1 month
Verbal	14	89	23%ile	3 years 7 months
Nonverbal	20	98	45%ile	4 years 6 months
AE	10	83	13%ile	3 years 5 months
AR	24	102	55%ile	4 years 9 months
ME	17	98	45%ile	4 years 5 months
MR	17	90	25%ile	3 years 10 months

Psychoeducational Profile-Revised, authored by Eric Schopler

Subtest	Raw Score	Age Equivalent
Imitation	15	54 months 4 years 6 months
Perception	13	63 months 5 years 3 months
Fine Motor	16	72 months 6 years 0 months
Gross Motor	18	62 months 5 years 2 months
Eye-Hand Integration	12	56 months 4 years 8 months
Cognitive Performance	23	54 months 4 years 6 months
Cognitive Verbal	18	49 months 4 years 1 month
Developmental Score	115	55-56 months 4 years 7-8 months

Woodcock-Johnson Tests of Achievement

Subtest	Grade Equivalent	Percentile	Standard Score
Science:	K.1	53%ile	101
Social Studies:	K.0-36	48%ile	99
Humanities:	K.0-20	28%ile	91

Dr. Kondrick's report also detailed Ruffin's subtest scores on the WPPSI-R IQ test she administered.

WPPSI-R

Subtest	Score	Percentile
Information	9	37%ile
Comprehension	10	50%ile
Arithmetic	9	37%ile

Object Assembly	13	84%ile
Geometric Design	14	91%ile
Block Design	16	98%ile
Vocabulary	8	25%ile
Similarities	8	25%ile
Mazes		not administered
Picture Completion	15	95%ile

Subtest scores have a mean of 10 and a standard deviation of 3. IQ and index scores have a mean of 100 and a standard deviation of 15.

Two handouts Ms. Sokolov provided were *Understanding the Language Learning Style of Children with Pervasive Developmental Disorders,* presented at the Tenth Annual Conference on the Language Disordered Child, October 24th, 1994, by Phillis Kupperman from Elmhurst, Illinois, and a little handout on memory exercises from K. Butler, "Language Processing: Halfway up the Down Staircase," from *Language Learning Disabilities in School-Age Children* (EDS 1984). As I read them, it was clear that Ruffin's current CARD drills were designed to develop his gestalt mode of language acquisition into more typically analytic modes and that they contained plenty of memory exercises.

March 21-May 2, 1996: Kim Pope, SLP

Ruffin age 5 years, 1 month; after 18 months of CARD training:

DIAGNOSTIC/EDUCATIONAL STAFFING REPORT: This is a report of the most recent speech-language testing completed with Ruffin at ACSD, completed March 21st through May 2nd, 1996.

Test of Language Development-Primary 2nd Edition (TOLD-P2)

Subtests	Standard Scores	Composites	Quotients
Picture Vocabulary	14*	Spoken Language	116
Oral Vocabulary	12	Listening	126*
Grammatic Understanding	16*	Speaking	107
Sentence Imitation	8	Semantics	118*
Grammatic Completion	12	Syntax	113
Word Discrimination	12	Phonology	112
Word Articulation	12		

*denotes scores in above average range (all other scores within average range)

Test of Auditory Comprehension of Language-Revised (TACL-R)

Subtests	Raw Scores	% Rank	Standard Score
Word Classes & Relations	38	98	131*
Grammatical Morphemes	35	93	122*
Elaborated Sentences	25	77	111
Total Score	98	92	121*

*denotes scores in above average range (other score within average range)

Ruffin has met all his speech-language objectives to criterion except for the 3-part verbal directive with each part having 2 critical elements. As of the end of April 1996, Ruffin had shown success with 3-part directives at approximately 40% accuracy. If the first 10 trials were used instead of all 15 trials, his accuracy would have been 60%. Ruffin has shown that he is able to do a 3-part directive but not up to the 85% criterion. This, however, would not be considered a critical skill for kindergarten success as teachers would not be giving 3 complex directions at 1 time to their students. If they do give 3, they would be simple directives consisting of only 1 critical element in each part (i.e., stand, go to the door, line up or sit, heads down, listen). Ruffin would not have a problem processing those directions. Attention and compliance might be another issue for him.

Ruffin's EYSE program in Lovaas will be dealing with giving Ruffin practice in this area of following directives. He will undoubtedly also get opportunities at direction following throughout his group activities this summer. Ruffin was also given some paper-crayon or pencil activities dealing with following directions to work on this summer.

After considering test results, classroom and outside classroom observations, and observations in the therapy situation both in individual and small group, Ruffin's speech-language skills are now considered to be adequate for oral communication purposes. They would also be considered adequate for classroom communications and academic progress.

January and February 1997: Lisa Shelton, MA, SLP

Ruffin age 5 years, 9-10 months; after 27-28 months of CARD training:

FORMAL LANGUAGE TESTING:

Ruffin's age at the time of testing was approximately 5 years 9 months.

The Test of Language Development-P:2 was administered in January 1997. Results were as follows: (average standard score: 8-12)

Subtest	Raw Score	Standard Score	Percentile
Picture vocabulary	19	13	84

Oral vocabulary	18	14	91
Grammatical understanding	21	13	84
Sentence imitation	9	9	37
Grammatical completion	21	12	75
Word discrimination	20	15	95
Word articulation	20	13	84

These scores equate to a spoken language quotient (SLQ) of 118. The average SLQ is between 90-110.

Boehm Test of Basic Concepts-R (Form C, Booklet 1 & 2) was administered on January 30th, 1997, and February 6th, 1997. Results were as follows:

Raw Score = 47 (possible 50)

Percentile ranking compared to a child at beginning of kindergarten year = 95%ile

Percentile ranking compared to a child at end of kindergarten year = 75%ile

Expressive One-Word Picture Vocabulary Test was administered on January 9th, 1997, with results as follows: (average standard score: 85-115)

Raw Score = 67

Language standard score = 110

Percentile = 75%ile

Language age = 6 years 11 months

Peabody Picture Vocabulary Test-R was administered on January 7th, 1997, with results as follows: (average standard score: 85-115)

Raw Score = 82

Standard Score = 115

Percentile rank = 84%ile

Age equivalent = 7 years 1 month

COMMENTS:

The results of the formal language testing indicate average or above average scores in language skills. Ruffin has achieved all his IEP goals for speech and language including drills as defined by CARD and following 3-part directives.

APPENDIX OF THEORY OF MIND DRILL LIST

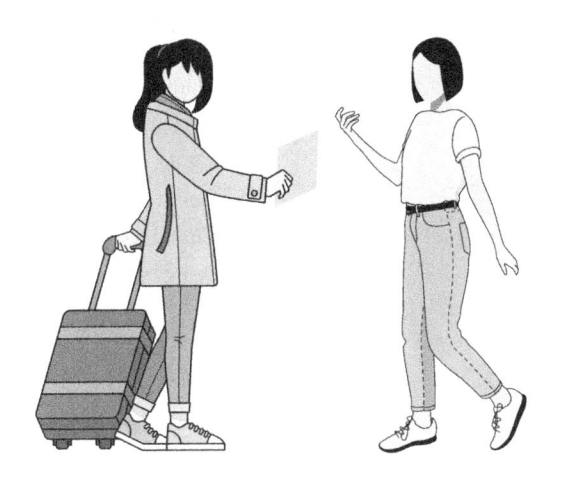

1. Theory of Mind'
2. Negations
3. Emotional Prosody
4. Finish the Story
5. If . . . what
6. Making up questions
7. Observational learning
8. What can you do with . . .?
9. What if . . .
10. Why do you like . . . Actions?
11. How do you know . . .?
12. What would you do . . .?
13. What is the difference between . . .?
14. What goes with . . .?
15. Time Concepts
16. What would you take?
17. See Something Incredible
18. What do you say?
19. Reciprocal Conversations
20. Listen to a Story
21. 'Wh' Questions
22. Thinking
23. If . . . then (Social Cues)
24. First and Last
25. Before and After
26. Same but Different
27. Impossible Tasks
28. Silly Nonsense Questions
29. Money
30. Grammatical Closure
31. Social Play
32. Social and Safety Awareness
33. Tell Me A Story
34. Staying on Topic
35. Initiating Conversation
36. Ending a Conversation
37. Social Speech
38. Senses

39. What's Missing?
40. Operational Skill Sequencing
41. Adjective Descriptions
42. Analogies
43. Definitions
44. Can you find . . .?
45. Comparisons
46. How can you tell . . .?
47. Language Promotion
48. Barrier Games
49. Rhymes
50. What is . . . made of?

Theory of Mind Drills

a) Blindfold
b) Who can see and hear?
c) Knowing
d) Sally Ann Tasks
e) Planning a Party
f) Pretending
g) Joking
h) Lies
i) White Lies
j) Figures of Speech

ACKNOWLEDGMENTS

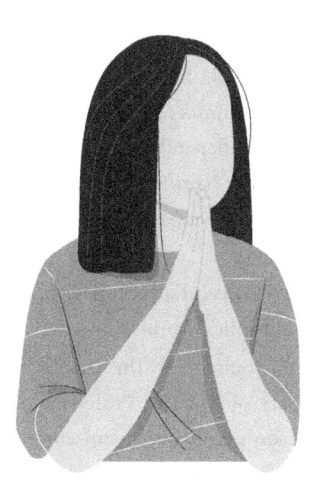

It takes a village, of course, to raise any child anywhere at any time. To raise a child through autism and to further accommodate that child to dyslexia takes the building out of a virtual village across a nation — where some will be your friends, and some will not.

Of those who were our friends, whose lives changed ours for the better, we continue to celebrate these in bright memory: Dr. O. Ivar Lovaas of UCLA's Early Autism Project, Dr. Tristram Smith, his then-recent graduate student in 1994 just beginning his own teaching career in Iowa, and Dr. Bernard Rimland of the Autism Research Institute in San Diego.

Also, some bright stars closer to our own horizon: The late Sue Baker, Iowa's longtime state autism specialist at University of Iowa's Hospital School, who although constrained in her powers, offered good advice under the table; the late "Julie" and her husband "Erik" of our town, who accepted Ruffin as a toddler into their home daycare whenever I was summoned into court; and the late Rose Ward, who lifted the burdens of housework and cooking until Ruffin was nearly 7.

Also a fallen star lost to us, my baby sister, Susan McDonald White, a fine artist, sculptor, and art conservator who sent us many useful gifts to help teach Ruffin the critical skill of pretending.

Of those who remain our friends, to whom we can continue to express gratitude these deserve their accolades:

"Dr. James Caldwell," pediatric neurologist of The Gundersen Clinic, LaCrosse, Wisconsin, who made his diagnosis early enough to allow for success in Ruffin's treatment. "Dr. Caldwell" eventually wrote the pivotal prescription for Ruffin's CARD treatment.

Other members of Gundersen's autism clinic, "Dr. Carol Reed," Kevin Josephson, M.S., Dr. Patricia A. Kondrick, "Mila Sokolov," SLP, CCCC, "Dr. Irwin Ladd," and Dr. David E. Palm also agreed to support ABA instruction as "appropriate," well into its second year, as did an earlier independent autism clinic team of evaluators at the University of Iowa, led by "Dr. Guy Norman," including Dr. Betty Simon, "Ms. Clara Wilding," SLP, CCCC, Dr. Joseph Piven, Dr. Sharon Koele, Beth Vanzee, MSW, and Deb Scott-Miller.

Dr. Glen Sallows of the Wisconsin Early Autism Project offered an early complete case review and written second medical opinion in February of 1995.

Dr. Doreen Granpeesheh, founder of The Center for Autism and Related Disorders (CARD), Autism Society of America Professional of the Year. As a practicing clinical psychologist and extraordinarily successful entrepreneurial founder of CARD in 1990, by 1994 she was an active researcher and practiced translator of academic research into the field, when with her travelling senior therapist, Evelyn Kung (also trained at UCLA) she designed the individual, early, intensive 28-month long program of applied behavior analysis (ABA) as prescribed by "Dr. Caldwell" for Ruffin.

Donna Schmidt — still a dear friend, and as nearly Ruffin's second mother as anyone — and Lisa Murphy. Together, Donna and Lisa carried out Dr. Granpeesheh and Evelyn Kung's plans rigorously and faithfully in all weathers.

Teacher RoJene Beard and special education teacher Pine Wilson implemented Dr. Granpeesheh's plan to integrate Ruffin with typically developing playmates over the summer of 1995.

Our local school district's special education teachers, "Meg Holub" and "Amy," and teacher's aide "Ella Meyer," who together with our local regional special education consultant, "Inge Nielson" from Decorah were all constrained in their powers, but offered their best special education efforts day-by-day, close to the ground, to Ruffin and me under all the administrative radar and noise of mediation and litigation.

Also, Mrs. Wonderlich's junior high school classes of volunteers who came to my home-office during Ruffin's early years to learn filing and copying, where they found much work to do, and brought flowers and much laughter.

Lois Fergus, an assistive technology specialist at the YMCA in Cedar Rapids, Iowa, who suggested when Ruffin was 3 that I buy him a Macintosh computer to run special education software programs to support his language learning.

St. Patrick's Catholic School Board and principal Peter Smith offered us a welcome respite from sharp and recurring early conflict with our local public schools and regional special education authorities by sheltering the private nursery school class taught by "Elaine Mills," and by offering K-8 small-size classes of 10-13 students, promoted as a single group along with their teachers, Mrs. Byrnes, Mrs. Thomas, Mrs. Daley, and Mrs. Fahey each over a succession of two-year periods — a small, stable and kind educational environment with after-school care that let Ruffin grow and thrive.

Dr. Kenneth Olson, our family doctor, Dr. Michael Funk, DDS, our special needs dentist at Gundersen, "Pastor David Hansen" of First Presbyterian Church, an exceptional parent himself, as well as Ruth Lembke and Diane Rissman of our local autism support group in northeast Iowa, who organized auditory integration training (AIT) to be provided by practitioner Lisa Toalson to four of our children with autism in the summer of 1995.

Robin Ouren came to watch and write about auditory integration training for the newspaper and stayed to become my legal assistant.

Andrea Shelton replaced Robin later from the unfailingly kind members of the Shelton family at our local commercial copy center who ran many free copies to be mailed: Corey Shelton, the late Don and Judy Shelton, and their daughter-in-law, Lisa Shelton, MA, SLP, who expertly finished off Ruffin's Lovaas program during latchkey aftercare at St. Patrick's Catholic school.

Jan Newmann, Ruffin's advocate in county case management, smart, empathetic and one who smoothed the way for many of us.

As I ran into a brick wall of public school resistance, Attorney Curt Sytsma and his paralegals Joan Hannum and Connie Fanslow of Iowa Protection & Advocacy Services, Inc. of Des Moines accepted Ruffin's case, and drove it unerringly as their vehicle to establishing higher legal standards — resulting in more frequent provision of year-round special education for all students with disabilities in Iowa — bringing in a 1996 decision rendered by Dr. Susan Etscheidt, our state administrative law judge.

Attorneys Scott Peters of Council Bluffs and Jane Zanglien of Texas assured that Prudential Insurance would reimburse their fair share of the costs of Ruffin's treatment.

"Attorney Caron Angelos" of Waterloo, "The Good" to my mind, eventually counseled our local school district to reimburse their fair share of Ruffin's early treatment in mediation, and after losing the 1996 due process case our district pressed her to defend before Dr. Etscheidt, gracefully and effectively advised her clients to reconsider any further opposition and agree to advance their fair share of the costs of Ruffin's continuing private school education through middle school and high school.

Attorneys Mark S. Soldat and Don Thompson, my trial partners who took up the slack when I needed to be home, and judge Stephen P. Carroll who ordered I might continue to work from home during Ruffin's early treatment.

Exceptional parents: Dave and Betty Palmer, Rick and Diane Wenndt, Dr. and Mrs. Raul Espinosa, Attorney and Mrs. James Carfagno, Jr., Dr. K. G. and Mrs. Woodward, Michael and Chris Foster, Michael and Susan Smith, Samantha Johnson, Attorney Bonnie Yates, Attorney Valerie Vanaman, Allison Hanken, and countless others who offered support through our list-serve, *The Me List*.

Regional and state allies Marion McQuaid, Mark Monson, Dee Ann L. Wilson, a state mediator, Gerry Gritzmacher, another mediator, who sometimes wavered, Dr. David Bishop of Luther College, who never did, and his student Angie Robeson, who spent the summer of 1996 with Ruffin at Decorah's Sunflower Daycare Center carrying out Dr. Granpeesheh's prescribed program for preparing Ruffin for mainstream integration before he entered kindergarten.

National parent and professional allies: Dr. Ron Huff, Linda Mayhew, Attorney Katherine Dobel, Attorney Mark Williamson and Attorney Ken Chackes.

Iowa Vocational Rehabilitation as established under *Section 504 of the Rehabilitation Act* and counselors Curt Jones, Mindy Meyers and Steven Lieberherr.

Shelley Lacey-Castelot, independent educational and assistive technology consultant who expertly assessed Ruffin's dyslexia mid-way through seventh grade and recommended early voice-recognition and optical character recognition software.

Summer Science, Technology, Engineering and Math (STEM) camp teachers Gary E. Glenn (Computer Graphics/Animated Figures), Lyle Litchey (Building Radios), Don Brauhn (Everyday Physics for the 21st Century) at the University of Iowa's Belin-Blank Center, teachers Doug Richardson (Rocketry 101) and Matthew Goodman (Not Quite C) at Iowa State University's Explorations! and Operation Catapult at Rose-Hulman Institute of Technology.

I will always be deeply grateful to many autism authors and researchers: Reed Martin, J.D., Pete Wright, J.D., Dr. Michael D. Powers, Dr. Bernard Rimland, Dr. Stephen Edelson, Dr. Dorothy Beavers, Dr. "Catherine Maurice," Dr. O. Ivar Lovaas, Dr. Tristram Smith, Clara Claibourne Park, Dr. Fred R. Volkmar, Dr. Leo Kanner, Dr. Hans Asperger, Dr. B. F. Skinner, Michele Dawson, Nancy Dalrymple, M.S., Dr. Temple Grandin, Donna Williams, Dr. Guy Berard, Anabelle Stehli, Dr. Christopher Gillberg, Dr. Mary Coleman, Dr. Vijandra K. Singh, Dr. Eric Courchesne, Dr. Simon Baron-Cohen, Dr. Uta Firth, Dr. Deborah Fein, Dr. Inge-Marie Eigsti, and Dr. Marcelo L. Berthier. I am equally grateful to their publishers.

The warmest abrazo for Sandra Cisneros who believed in the importance of my telling our story since the first day it began to pour out over a table at the Bluebird Café in Iowa City. A special thank you to Dennis Mathis who struggled to teach me to write it in prose, and to Mary Lewis, Robert Felde and Edward Brooks of my Decorah writers' group who weathered their way through many early drafts of it before and after poets Pam Uschuk and William Pitt Root invited me to join their memoir workshop. I am also grateful to have had the financial support of the Les Standiford Fellowship to attend the Writers in Paradise Conference to workshop this manuscript, and for the continuing support of my sister writers whom I met there, Carmela McIntire and Eileen Vorbach Collins.

Many thanks for the patience, precision and courage of Iurii Matviienko, the book and ebook layout expert, DPT Wizard and Indesign Pro of Kyiv, Ukraine, who designed this book, its ebook versions, its brilliant cover, and who illustrated it with a real 'storyboard' from afar and under fire.

Thank you to my siblings, Michael Thomas White, a retired electrical engineer from INTEL and Cathy Lynn Graham, M.D., a surgeon and race car enthusiast for their inspiring and supporting Ruffin in his scientific career.

Most of all, I am grateful to Ruffin whose hard work has brought him his own rewards, to his father, "Seamus," James Magner, who hung in there, and to my parents, my mother, Jane Odil White, a teacher, and my late father, Thomas Boyett White, a life-long customer service engineer for IBM who provided essential financial support during Ruffin's early treatment from age 3 to 5.

A SHORT LIST OF RECOMMENDED READING:

Bernard Rimland, Ph.D., Navy psychologist, father of a son, Mark, *Infantile Autism: The Syndrome and Its Implications for a Neural Theory of Behavior*, (Century Psychology Series Award, 1962,) still in print, an award-winning classic, still readily available and updated nicely as to all the later science in a 50th anniversary edition.

Dorothy Beavers, Ph.D., chemist, mother of a son, Leo, *Autism: Nightmare Without End*, (Ashley Books 1981, 1982), long out of print, still available on Alibris.

Catherine Maurice, Ph.D. in French literature, mother of a daughter, Anne-Marie and a son, Michel, *Let Me Hear Your Voice*, (Knopf, 1993), still in print, and readily available.

O. Ivar Lovaas, "Behavioral Treatment and Normal Educational and Intellectual Functioning in Young Autistic Children," 55 Journal of Consulting and Clinical Psychology 3 (1987).

John J. McEachin, Tristram Smith, & O. Ivar Lovaas, "Long-Term Outcome for Children with Autism Who Received Early Intensive Treatment," 97 American Journal on Mental Retardation 359 (1993).

Gary Mayerson, J.D., lawyer, father of a son, *How To Compromise With Your School District Without Compromising Your Child* and *Autism's Declaration of Independence*, (DRL Books, 2004, 2020).

Shannon Penrod, mother of a son, *AUTISM, Parent to Parent: Sanity-Saving Advice for Every Parent with a Child on the Autism Spectrum*, (Future Horizons, 2022).

Doreen Granpeesheh, Ph.D., Jonathan Tarbox, Adel C. Najdowski, and Julie Kornak, *Evidence-Based Treatment for Children with Autism: The CARD Model (Practical Resources for the Mental Health Professional)* (Academic Press, 2014).

DOCUMENTARY FILMS

Lovaas's classic 1987 video *Behavioral Treatment of Autistic Children*, now available on YouTube.

Recovered: Journeys through the Autism Spectrum and Back, a forty-five-minute documentary film by Dr. Doreen Granpeesheh (Autism Society of America Professional of the Year) about Ruffin and three other children who are loose in the universe, now available at YouTube.

A one-minute trailer for a documentary film, *Recovering Ruffin*, focused solely on Ruffin available through Good Docs.

Mary Jane White is a poet and translator who practiced law at her home in Northeast Iowa. She was born and raised in North Carolina, earned degrees from The North Carolina School of the Arts, Reed College, The University of Iowa Writers' Workshop, and studied law at Duke University, graduating from the University of Iowa. Her poetry and translations received NEA Fellowships in 1979 and 1985. She taught lyric poetry and poetry workshops briefly at the University of Iowa and at Luther College in Decorah, Iowa, and served for a decade as an Iowa Poet in the Schools, before her son, Ruffin, was born in 1991. She has been awarded writing scholarships to Bread Loaf (1979), Squaw Valley Community of Writers (2006), Bread Loaf Translators' Conference (2015), Writers in Paradise Conference (2015, 2018), Prague Summer Program for Writers (2017), Summer Literary Seminars in Tbilisi, Georgia (2018). Her first book *Starry Sky to Starry Sky* (Holy Cow! Press, 1988), contains translations of Marina Tsvetaeva's long lyric cycle, "Miles," which first appeared in *The American Poetry Review* as an inserted feature. *After Russia: Poems by Marina Tsvetaeva* (Adelaide Books, New York/Lisbon 2021) is her most recent translated work. Earlier poems and other translations have appeared widely across journals and magazines, have been included in various anthologies, and featured on Iowa Public Radio.

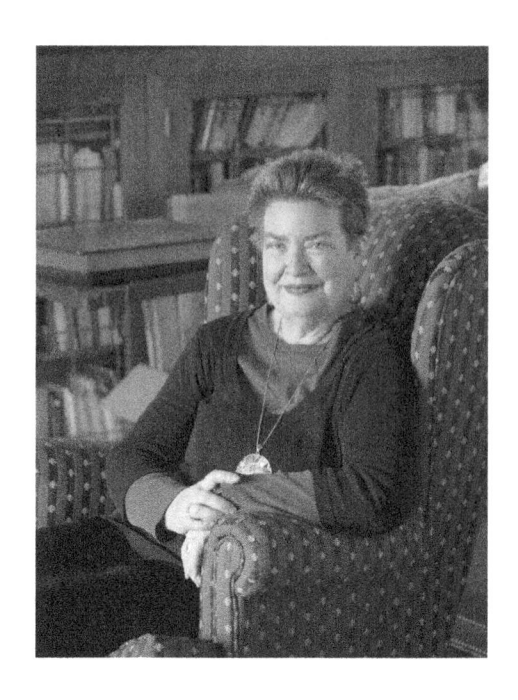

Made in the USA
Monee, IL
14 July 2024